DIETARY SUPPLEMENTS IN HEALTH PROMOTION

DIETARY SUPPLEMENTS IN HEALTH PROMOTION

Edited by
Taylor C. Wallace
George Mason University
Washington, DC, USA

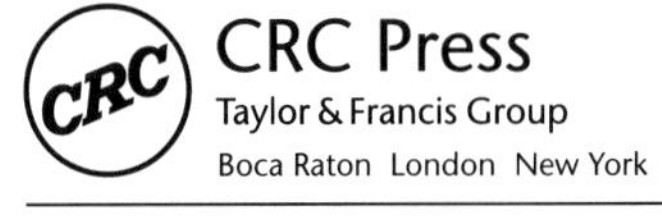

CRC Press is an imprint of the
Taylor & Francis Group, an **informa** business

CRC Press
Taylor & Francis Group
6000 Broken Sound Parkway NW, Suite 300
Boca Raton, FL 33487-2742

Printed on acid-free paper
Version Date: 20150413

International Standard Book Number-13: 978-1-4822-1034-7 (Hardback)

Visit the Taylor & Francis Web site at
http://www.taylorandfrancis.com

and the CRC Press Web site at
http://www.crcpress.com

Contents

Preface

A dietary supplement is defined in the United States as a product that is intended to supplement the diet that may contain one or more dietary ingredients, such as a vitamin or a mineral, an herb or other botanicals, an amino acid, a dietary substance for use by humans to supplement the diet by increasing the total dietary intake, or a concentrate, metabolite, constituent, extract, or combination of the preceding ingredients [1]. By definition, dietary supplements must be intended for ingestion [2]. This excludes products that may be inhaled, absorbed through the skin, etc.

The efficacy and health-promoting properties of dietary supplements vary from product to product, and to date many gaps in knowledge exist; some categories of products have extensive research portfolios illustrating their safety, efficacy, and pronounced health-promoting effects, while some categories lack even small human studies. Regardless of the amount of available scientific evidence present, consumers utilize and have faith in an array of products; this is exemplified by the rapid expansion of the dietary supplement market over the last 20 years. In 1994, there were an estimated 4000 dietary supplement products on the market in the United States. This number has now grown to over 75,000 products present day [3].

As a general guidance, I offer the following two important points for those giving clinical guidance regarding dietary supplements

1. Dietary supplements, particularly those with established Dietary Reference Intakes (DRI) [4] set by the US Institute of Medicine, Food and Nutrition Board should be used to "fill the gap" when nutrient recommended intakes are not being met through dietary intake. Heather Eicher-Miller does a superb job of identifying nutrient gaps among subpopulations of consumers in Chapter 2. This is not to suggest that higher levels of supplementation in certain situations are not beneficial, because in some instances (as you will see in many chapters within this textbook) it most certainly can be. As a general rule of thumb, I personally believe that achieving nutrient sufficiency is beneficial to overall human health and wellbeing. While dietary intake of nutrients through food is more ideal, in many instances this is neither practical nor feasible. Supplementation presents a less preferred, but practical "secondary option" to a growing population with increasingly more difficult access to and/or less preference for healthy whole food products such as fresh fruits, vegetables, nuts, whole grains, and low/non-fat dairy. The USDA National Agriculture Library has an extremely useful DRI calculator to assist healthcare professionals in calculating personalized daily nutrient recommendations for their patients [5].
2. More is not always better; consumers often get excited and think the opposite, especially when new findings showing benefit of a particular dietary supplement are widely publicized. I am a firm believer in the S-shape (sigmoid) curve, which is typical for most biochemical reactions. Such

reactions have three response zones which are likely specific to each individual nutrient or bioactive compound versus each individual health state/condition: A no-response region at the left, a relatively steep rise up to some maximum response, and finally a dose range in which further increases in intake produce no further response. The US IOM establishes tolerable upper intake limits (UL) for many nutrients [4]; likewise, several nutrients and other dietary bioactive compounds have rigorous studies indicating their safety using a lowest observed adverse effect level (LOAEL) or no observed adverse effect level (NOAEL).

The mainstream use and availability of dietary supplements create an enormous need for a balanced and credible scientific resource from top experts in the field, summarizing the various health-promoting properties connected with at least the more popular products currently in the market. This textbook seeks to offer research scientists and healthcare providers evidence-based information.

Sincerely

Taylor C. Wallace

Taylor C. Wallace, PhD, CFS, FACN
National Osteoporosis Foundation
National Bone Health Alliance
George Mason University
drtaylorwallace.com

REFERENCES

1. 108 Stat. 4325, 1994.
2. 21 CFR Parts 201(ff)(2)(A) and 411(c)(1)(B).
3. U.S. Government Accountability Office, GAO-09-250, Dietary Supplements: FDA Should Take Further Action to Improve Oversight and Consumer Understanding, 2009.
4. USDA National Agriculture Library. Dietary reference intakes. Available at: http://fnic.nal.usda.gov/dietary-guidance/dietary-reference-intakes. Accessed August 1, 2014.
5. USDA National Agriculture Library. Interactive DRI for healthcare professionals. Available at: http://fnic.nal.usda.gov/fnic/interactiveDRI/. Accessed August 1, 2014.

Editor

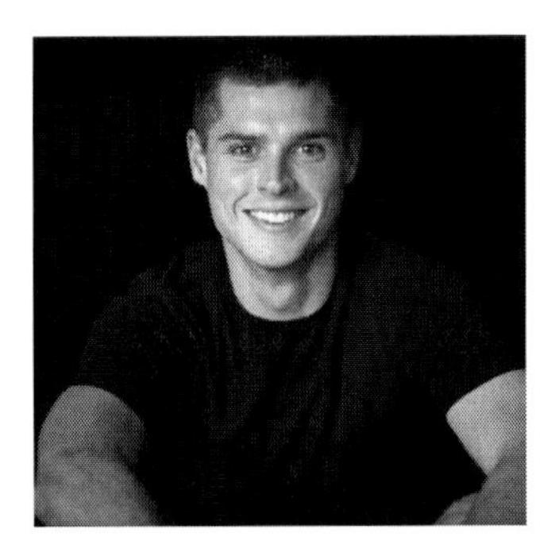

Taylor C. Wallace, PhD, CFS, FACN, is the senior director, Science Policy and Government Relations at the National Osteoporosis Foundation (NOF) and the senior director, Scientific and Clinical Programs at the National Bone Health Alliance (NBHA), a public–private partnership, managed and operated by the NOF. Dr. Wallace is responsible for ensuring that NOF's scientific, legislative, and policy programs are broad-based, comprehensive, and evidence-based, aimed at strengthening bone health, decreasing the prevalence for osteoporosis by working with various key government agencies and scientific societies toward improving tests and therapies associated with the prevention, diagnosis, and treatment of osteoporosis. In addition, Dr. Wallace provides scientific leadership, content expertise, and project management leadership in support of NBHA projects and activities such as bone turnover marker standardization and rare bone diseases.

Prior to joining NOF and NBHA, Dr. Wallace served as the senior director of Scientific and Regulatory Affairs at the Council for Responsible Nutrition (CRN), where he was responsible for providing scientific and regulatory expertise for evaluating scientific research, ensuring that legislative and policy positions were based on credible science rationale, while developing new scientific reviews and original research for the peer-reviewed literature. Dr. Wallace is also an affiliate professor in the Department of Nutrition and Food Studies at George Mason University.

His academic background includes a PhD and an MS in Food Science and Nutrition from the Ohio State University and a BS in Food Science and Technology from the University of Kentucky. In his free time, Dr. Wallace manages and operates a large food and nutrition blog, drtaylorwallace.com, where he provides science-based nutrition, food safety, and food technology information to the general public and consumer media. Dr. Wallace currently serves as a trustee and the acting treasurer of Feeding Tomorrow, the Foundation of the Institute of Food Technologists and was recently elected a fellow of the American College of Nutrition. He serves as an associate editor of the *Journal of the American College of Nutrition*. He is the editor or co-editor of three academic textbooks and more than 20 peer-reviewed publications.

Contributors

Regan Bailey
U.S. National Institutes of Health
Bethesda, Maryland

Emily R. Bovier
The University of Georgia
Athens, Georgia

Jose M. Brum
Procter & Gamble
Mason, Ohio

Weston Bussler
Plants for Human Health Institute
Kannapolis, North Carolina

Christopher M. Butt
DSM Nutritional Products
HNH-Biological Models
Boulder, Colorado

Heather A. Eicher-Miller
Department of Nutrition Science
Purdue University
West Lafayette, Indiana

George C. Fahey, Jr.
Department of Animal Sciences
University of Illinois
Urbana, Illinois

Janet E. Frick
Department of Psychology
The University of Georgia
Athens, Georgia

J. Michael Gaziano
Department of Medicine
Brigham and Women's Hospital
Harvard Medical School
and
VA Boston Healthcare System
Boston, Massachusetts

Francisco Guarner
University Hospital Vall d'Hebron
Barcelona, Spain

Billy R. Hammond, Jr.
The University of Georgia
Athen, Georgia

Gabriel Keith Harris
Food, Bioprocessing and Nutrition Sciences
NC State University
Raleigh, North Carolina

Claudia Herrera
University Hospital Vall d'Hebron
Barcelona, Spain

Joseph Hildebrand
Food, Bioprocessing and Nutrition Sciences
North Carolina State University
Raleigh, North Carolina

Bruce W. Hollis
Medical University of South Carolina
Charleston, South Carolina

Slavko Komarnytsky
Plants for Human Health Institute
Kannapolis, North Carolina

Swetha L. Kommareddy
Boston University School of Medicine
Boston, Massachusetts

Tristan E. Lipkie
Department of Nutrition Science
Purdue University
West Lafayette, Indiana

Michael I. McBurney
Friedman School of Nutrition Science and Policy
Tufts University
Boston, Massachusetts

Johnson W. McRorie, Jr.
Procter & Gamble
Mason, Ohio

and

Mississippi State University
Starkville, Mississippi

Catherine Mixon
Food, Bioprocessing and Nutrition Sciences
North Carolina State University
Raleigh, North Carolina

Clara Park
Kyungpook National University School of Medicine
Daegu, Republic of Korea

Elizabeth N. Pearce
Boston University School of Medicine
Boston, Massachusetts

Alyssa K. Phillips
Department of Nutrition Science
Purdue University
West Lafayette, Indiana

Ananda S. Prasad
Wayne State University School of Medicine
Detroit, Michigan

Susanne Rautiainen
Institute of Environmental Medicine
Karolinska Institutet
Stockholm, Sweden

Virginia Robles-Alonso
University Hospital Vall d'Hebron
Barcelona, Spain

Sarah E. Saint
Department of Psychology
The University of Georgia
Athens, Georgia

Norman Salem, Jr.
DSM Nutritional Products
HNH-Nutritional Lipids
Columbia, Maryland

Howard D. Sesso
Department of Epidemiology
Harvard School of Public Health
Boston, Massachusetts

Margaret Slavin
Department of Nutrition and Food Studies
George Mason University
Fairfax, Virginia

Sarah N. Taylor
Medical University of South Carolina
Charleston, South Carolina

Carol L. Wagner
Medical University of South Carolina
Charleston, South Carolina

Ty Wagoner
Food, Bioprocessing and Nutrition Sciences
North Carolina State University
Raleigh, North Carolina

Taylor C. Wallace
National Osteoporosis Foundation
George Mason University
Fairfax, Virginia

Connie M. Weaver
Department of Nutrition Science
Women's Global Health Institute
Purdue University
West Lafayette, Indiana

1 Trends in Health Care and Non-Communicable Diseases

Clinical Trials and Tribulations with Vitamins, Minerals, and Supplements

Jose M. Brum

CONTENTS

1.1 SUMMARY

Social, technological, and economical global factors drive three trends: (1) increase in prevalence of expensive and life-long non-communicable diseases (NCDs); (2) the high economic burden of NCDs demanding higher individual responsibility and active individual participation in disease prevention and self-care; and (3) a consequential increase in utilization of self-medication (over-the-counter medication, herbals, and supplements) with higher quality, greater safety and regulated substantiation of any health benefit claim. The convergence of these trends brings a new paradigm in the way natural remedies and OTC products will now be utilized together with lifestyle changes to decrease the prevalence of NCDs globally. As most common NCDs have modifiable risk factors, health care systems are now emphasizing on preventive measures of low costs, easy access, and high therapeutic convenience. Globally, the utilization of traditional/natural medicine and supplements is growing significantly. However, only products with proven safety and efficacy demonstrated in randomized controlled clinical trials will be able to contribute to this new preventive aspect of the health care environment.

1.2 NEW GLOBAL TREND AND SOCIOECONOMIC BURDEN OF NON-COMMUNICABLE DISEASES

The scenario of health-related conditions and the prevalence of diseases globally, have changed considerably in recent years with alarming growing trends of NCDs. Social, technological, and economical globalization factors are the transforming forces behind these trends. Higher exposure to risk factors, due to quick industrialization and inappropriate urbanization, significant lifestyle changes as well as population aging, and improvements in the ability to diagnose, have created a perfect storm scenario for an expansion of NCDs globally [1]. An aggravating factor is that NCDs are mostly incurable and require treatment over decades of a person's life span [1].

Nowadays, the leading causes of mortality in low income countries, with few exceptions in Africa, are no longer infectious diseases but heart disease, stroke, cancer, chronic respiratory diseases, diabetes, obesity, and other NCDs [1]. An age-dependent prevalence of cancer, psychiatric and neuro-degenerative diseases, and musculoskeletal diseases has also grown in high-income countries [1,2]. However, an aggravating problem for the urban poor population is that communicable diseases such as HIV/AIDS, hepatitis, tuberculosis, and even malaria are now detected together with hypertension, chronic pulmonary disease, diabetes, and obesity [1,3–5]. Rapid urbanization without appropriate infrastructure is one of the main reasons favoring the growth of NCDs in low-income communities as it has a multiplier effect on many risk factors that predispose the manifestation of diseases early in life [6].

Due to their natural life-long progression, NCDs lead to an early high mortality and a heavy societal economic burden wherever they occur. NCDs are the cause of approximately 60% of all global deaths nowadays [1]. Not surprisingly, close to 80% of the deaths caused by NCDs occur in low-income countries, generally, in a much younger population than those in high-income countries [1,7,8]. Over the coming years, the WHO predicts that NCD deaths will increase by approximately 17% globally with the greatest regional impact coming from the African and the Eastern Mediterranean countries. However, due to the size of the population the greatest absolute mortality will occur in a few Asian countries [1]. Total deaths from NCDs may reach up to 52 million people globally in 2030 [1,7,9]. Although in high-income countries such as the USA, cardiovascular diseases (CVDs) have declined in the past 20 years, this category of NCD is the most prevalent and a formidable societal burden [10]. It is expected that the projected cost of all CVD will be over 1.2 trillion dollar by 2030 [11]. The humanitarian and socioeconomic consequences of these NCDs, therefore, demand an urgent global intervention on such a trend.

1.3 MODIFIABLE RISK FACTORS

Fortunately, all these leading causes of morbidity and mortality have significant risk factors that if well controlled the onset and severity of these diseases can be delayed [12]. Some risk factors for NCDs can be controlled and modified at the community level and others at the individual level. Well-planned and controlled urbanization and health education programs have demonstrated to be effective at the community level [12]. However, it is at the individual level that the most common failures to control modifiable risk factors such as smoking, alcohol and drug abuse, and inadequate nutrition and lack of physical activity do indeed occur. In the USA, the most recent statistics showed that poor cardiovascular health behaviors are responsible for considerable fractions of CVD mortality [11]. Approximately 48% of all CVD mortality was attributable to modifiable factors such as smoking (13.7%), poor diet (13.2%), insufficient physical activity (11.9%), and abnormal fasting blood glucose levels (8.8%) [11].

From 2009 to 2010, less than 1% of Americans met at least 4 out of 5 healthy dietary goals established by the American Heart Association. Among adults (those older than 20 years), only 12.3% met the recommended AHA dietary goals for consumption of fruits and vegetables, and only 18.3% met goals for fish. These proportions were even lower in children [10,11].

The estimated prevalence of overweight and obesity in US adults is 154.7 million, which according to the statistics represented 68.2% of the adult population in 2010. Nearly 35% of US adults have body mass index (BMI) larger than 30 kg/m^2, and are by definition diseased with obesity. Among children from 2 to 19 years of age, 31.8% are overweight and obese (23.9 million) and 16.9% are obese (12.7 million) [10,11].

Based on data from 2007 to 2010, 33.0% of the US adults (78 million) have hypertension, but only 53% of those with documented hypertension have their condition controlled appropriately. In 2010, an estimated 19.7 million Americans had diagnosed diabetes mellitus, representing 8.3% of the adult population. An additional 8.2 million had undiagnosed diabetes mellitus, and 38.2% had pre-diabetes (abnormal fasting glucose levels) [10,11].

1.4 PREVENTIVE MEASURES AND POLICIES

These numbers obviously call for further implementation of serious preventive measures and higher accountability at the individual level. In fact, societal efforts in that direction are already occurring through policies and taxation efforts, demanding higher individual participation in self-care to prevent NCDs [12,13]. Measures that incentivize healthy life style, proper nutrition, and adoption of convenient and low-cost self-care preventive therapies help in decreasing the consequences of NCDs [12,13]. Recently, proposals for primary prevention of CVDs on a global scale have gained significant acceptance with health estate departments or ministries. The WHO meeting on NCDs in 2011 by the World Health Assembly sets a global target to reduce premature NCD mortality by 25% by the year 2025 [1]. In addition, the Global Cardiovascular Disease Taskforce (that includes representatives of the World Heart Federation, the American Heart Association, the American College of

Cardiology, the European Heart Network, and the European Society of Cardiology) has proposed a set of aggressive measures to be implemented at the collective level to help achieve the proposed goal by 2015. These organizations are urging governments and health care providers to adopt their global targets [13] in reducing risk factors and the prevalence of NCDs. In addition, these organizations proposed to make main drugs highly available and accessible to the public (OTC) to prevent myocardial infarction and stroke [1,13].

The European Association for Cardiovascular Prevention and Rehabilitation (a branch of the European Society of Cardiology) has aggressively recommended a paradigm shift in CVD prevention focusing on a population basis [13]. Healthy dietary habits are proposed to be supported by changes in agricultural policies and taxation. Completely smoke-free environments and second-hand smoking are proposed to be even more regulated by taxation, restrictions in sale and use, banning advertising, plain packaging, and warning labels. Physical activities are proposed to be implemented as an integral part of daily life, and controlled by taxation and subsidies. Alcohol intake, according to the proposition, is to be reduced by taxation, low availability, regulation of advertising, and low social and legal tolerance for consequences of abuse such as drunk driving [13].

1.5 POLYPILL: A SELF-CARE PROPOSAL TO BE AVAILABLE TO ALL BASED ON AGE ALONE

Proposals of using a mixture of well-established cardiovascular drugs in a single polypill format to prevent manifestation of CVDs have been tested clinically with positive results. In a recent double blind placebo controlled study, a polypill containing blood pressure (BP) medications and statin were given to people solely on the basis of age (≥50 years) for primary prevention of CVDs [14]. On an average, participants in the 12-week study experienced a 12% reduction in BP and 39% fall in LDL-cholesterol. The health implications of the results suggest that if people took a polypill for a long term starting at the age of 50, an estimated 28% of the subjects would have avoided or delayed a heart attack or stroke during their lifetime. Although, all the used medications have nontrivial side effects, the authors suggested that such option of prevention should be readily available to the public and not necessarily under prescription [14]. Several studies on the use of polypill components for primary prevention of CVD and stroke have been done and are being continued [15]. One clinical trial in patients at low risk for CVD and stroke found that a modest reduction in diastolic BP and a LDL-cholesterol correlated with a substantial 44% reduction in the relative risks of CVD. Furthermore, in high risk patients with more meaningful reductions in systolic BP and in LDL-cholesterol, a 62% relative reduction in risks of CVD was attributed to the polypill [15].

It is clear, therefore, that polypills for primary prevention, for those at risk but with no apparent disease, are being designed for easy access, convenience, and self-care [over-the-counter (OTC)] for those with 55 years of age or above [15,16]. These clinical studies proposed that early intervention on risk factors in a population basis can be cost effective for the prevention of CVD. In addition, the studies showed that several agents used in polypills have been already available for self-medication such as folic acid and aspirin (and even statins as in the UK) [16].

1.6 UTILIZATION OF SELF-CARE MEDICATION AND DIETARY SUPPLEMENTS TO DELAY ONSET OF NCDs

Medications for weight control, smoke cessation, anti-platelets (aspirin), cholesterol-lowering products, antioxidants, biotics, and herbal supplements are the available OTC options for self-care and for potential control of NCDs. However, utilization of OTC medications and dietary supplements as a venue for convenient, efficacious, and low cost therapy to delay the onset of NCDs, in a manner similar to that of polypill, has not yet been systematically explored.

In high-income countries, the utilization of traditional and herbal medications for treatment and prevention of NCDs is presently growing (USA 42%, France 49%, Canada 70%, and Germany 80%) [17]. In the Netherlands, where centralized information on medications utilization exists and the population growth has not changed much over the years, the OTC category has shown an increase from approximately 10% in 1980 to 40% in 2010 for all age brackets, whereas the prescription category has remained mostly unchanged [18].

If no prevention measures are taken, the annual tobacco-related NCD deaths globally are projected to increase from about 6 million today to 8 million in 2030 (10% of all deaths in that year) and 80% of those deaths will come from low- and middle-income countries [1]. This is certainly a situation that requires worldwide expansion of education efforts and easier access to self-medication and treatment options for smoke secession. It is estimated that, in the USA, the nicotine replacement therapy (NRT) leading to quitting attempts would avoid 40,000 premature deaths by lung cancer and CVD [not counting chronic obstructive pulmonary disease (COPD) and other tobacco-associated diseases] over a 20-year period [19]. In Australia, a review of the impact of nonprescription NRT concluded that an estimate of 68,750 successful quitters and premature deaths were prevented within 10 years, an equivalent 6875 per year, after NRT was switched to OTC in Australia [20].

Likewise, the consequences of long-term NCDs and the economic burden associated with treatment of these conditions in general, demands that a higher number of relatively safe prescription medicines be switched to OTC due to their favorable benefit to risk ratio, convenience, and lower costs [12,13]. In the USA, the FDA since the mid 1970s has allowed the switch of over 80 ingredients dosages, or indications from prescription to nonprescription with most of them occurring in the last 20 years [20].

1.7 REGULATORY ENVIRONMENT AND POLICIES

On the other hand, the growing trend in self-medication has globally triggered new regulatory efforts as well as professional safety surveillance of herbals and supplements in a similar way to the OTC medication category [20,21]. The number of participant countries of the WHO that are now imposing regulations for traditional and natural medicine has increased significantly. Before 1986, there were less than 15 countries with laws and regulations governing herbals commercialization and utilization. After 2007, more than 110 of the 193 WHO Member States had a policy in place regarding regulation and registration of traditional medicines [17,20]. The creation of international standards improved quality of products and positively affected the utilization of supplements, and favored the growth of commercialization in the countries that adopted them. The WHO indicates that the global market for traditional medicine and herbal products has expanded significantly over the last decade with growth in all regions of the world [17,20,21].

Changes in the global health care scenario are, therefore, leading to higher utilization of self-care measures in the prevention of NCDs. With the increase in reliance on self-care, self-medication, and personal responsibility for health, there is a higher need for utilization of accessible medications—OTC and supplements. The National Health and Nutrition Examination Survey (NHANES) collected data from 2003 to 2006 on all types of dietary supplements indicating that 53% of American adults took at least one dietary supplement, most commonly multivitamin/mineral supplements (taken by 39% of all adults) [22].

A high utilization of self-care therapies and products for primary or secondary prevention of NCDs are only justified if proof of efficacy, safety, and a favorable benefit to risk ratio are substantiated and documented. Consequently, high quality supplements will be in demand. Supplements produced under good manufacturing practices (GMP) with tested shelf-lives and proven consistency and standardization of constituents will also be required to demonstrate the validation of physicochemical properties of "actives" by proven analytical methods [17]. Therefore, the safety of supplements used for these purposes will be assessed by pharmaceutical standards (with toxicology studies of potential actives and clinical data). The labeling of supplements will be used more often to qualify health efficacy claims and safety; and claims will need substantiation from clinical studies. The WHO has proposed that herbal supplements and medicine biological activities should follow the International Drug Monitoring Program, which classifies and gives assessment of safety and efficacy of drugs [17]. All these trends and events that precede and follow the increase in NCDs globally and their consequences are illustrated in Figure 1.1.

Pharmacovigilance of herbal products with medicinal properties or claims will expand from passive surveillance and spontaneous reporting to active surveillance (with sentinel sites, herbal/drug event monitoring, registries, and studies registry). Determination of individual susceptibility to adverse herbal reactions or herbal–drug interactions is presently in high-income countries following models used for conventional drug development. More countries will, therefore, be forced to develop specific legislation regarding the use of herbs (as it is done in Canada and Germany) following traditional herbal references and modernized monographs [17].

In the USA, most of the supplements, herbals, vitamins, and minerals broadly utilized by the public for maintaining health, which is nothing more than delaying the onset of NCDs or aging, are regulated as food under the Dietary Supplement Health and Education Act (DSHEA) of 1994. DSHEA is outside of the requirements established by the FDA for efficacy and safety of drugs, even those available OTC. The sequences of regulatory processes or steps necessary for approval of drugs and those regulated as food under DSHEA are well established [23,24].

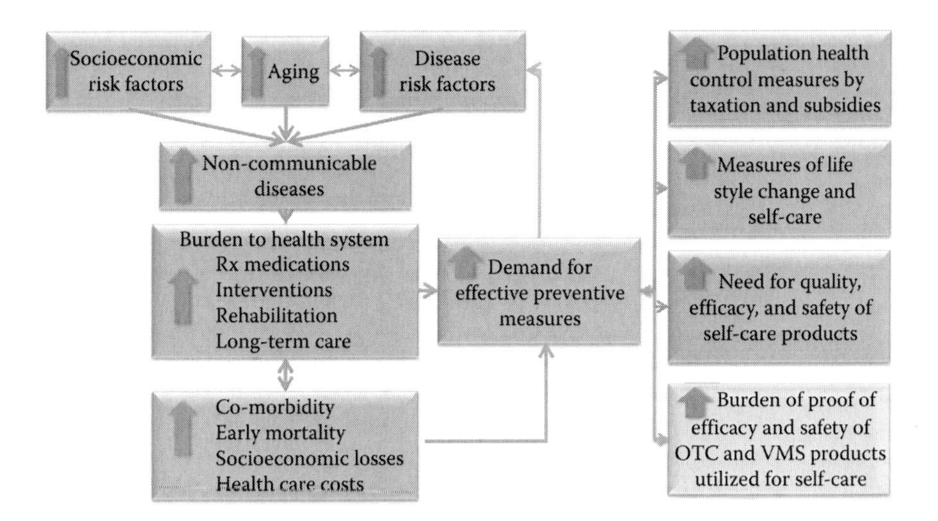

FIGURE 1.1 This figure represents the influence of the new trends regarding NCDs leading to increases in the economic burden of health care that triggers demands for self care and utilization of the OTC and supplement category in a more regulated environment to delay onset of NCDs.

In such a process, it is obvious that depending on the classification of a potential health product, a different category for proof of efficacy and safety will be demanded. These categories have quite different associated costs and time of development before approval and commercialization. These different pathways also indicated that the burden of proof of the efficacy of a supplement should be obtained in non-disease estates because a well-characterized disease treatment benefit could redefine the supplement being investigated as a drug. Under DSHEA regulation, a product can have the statements of nutritional support in the label or package regarding classical nutrient deficiency diseases as long as the prevalence of the disease in the USA is disclosed [24]. Otherwise, only the effects on structure (anatomy) or function (physiology) of the body and the potential well being achieved by consumption of a supplement are allowed by DSHEA. The statements of benefit made in the label of a supplement must also have a disclaimer that it has not been evaluated by the FDA, and that the product is not intended to diagnose, treat, cure, or prevent disease. In addition, the labeled claims must have substantiation that they are truthful and not misleading [25]. However, DSHEA does not define the requirements for substantiation of claims.

The FDA has exclusive jurisdiction over the safety of dietary supplements and primary jurisdiction over the labeling [24,25]. The FTC has primary jurisdiction over advertisement for dietary supplements and interacts with FDA regarding veracity and requirements for substantiation of claims that are advertised. In determining whether the substantiation meets the criteria or standards, these regulatory bodies will consider the meaning of the claim being made, the relationship of the evidence to the claim, the quality of the claim, and the totality of the evidence [25]. Regarding the meaning of a claim, it is equally important to substantiate an individual claim as it is the overall message. For good evidence of relationship with claim, the studies with a supplement should include design features that provide demonstration of similarities with labeling of the final product such as the formulation, serving size (dose), route of administration, and exposure to treatment [25]. The gold standard for quality of evidence, still, is the double blind placebo controlled clinical trial. However, randomized controlled clinical studies with supplements may not always be appropriate or practical.

1.8 ACCEPTABLE CRITERIA OF EFFICACY AND DIETARY SUPPLEMENT STUDIES

There are undoubtedly inherent difficulties in attempting to make dietary supplements to behave like pharmaceutical drugs in clinical trial settings. Drugs are tested for clinical efficacy only after a well-characterized profile of pharmacokinetics and pharmacodynamics variables is determined [23]. Such a process allows appropriate choices of dose and regimen that are optimized for safety and efficacy. Nevertheless, there is no clear justification for efficacy or safety aspects of supplements with medicinal claims to be tested under a less strict scientific rigor than pharmacological agents. A supplement with potential medicinal benefits should be tested under similar clinical trial rigor of drugs, but under different clinical design features to allow, appropriately, for observation of responses of low magnitude and unnecessary complex safety monitoring. Supplements should, generally like food, not be expected to cause physiological responses of such a magnitude that would be capable of jeopardizing the safety parameters. Usually, very efficacious mechanisms of action are also responsible for important side effects. Nevertheless, clinical studies with supplements should take into consideration the adequacy of sample size, the proper statistical power, the randomization and blinding procedures, the characteristics and demographics of the population, the adequacy of the primary endpoint, the duration of the intervention and follow-up, and the compliance with treatment. All these determinants of appropriateness of study should be in concordance with design features that do not diverge from the way the supplement is going to be practically used. For example, to expect significant changes in a biological parameter with a single dose is a more realistic scenario with drugs than with a single serving of a supplement.

Reproducibility of findings is another important aspect that defines the quality and totality of clinical evidence to support a claim of benefit [25]. There is no specific rule on how many studies or combinations of types of evidence are sufficient to support a health claim with a supplement. However, inconsistencies are abundant in the health-related literature and usually not easily explained by differences in methodologies, study population, and other factors. Therefore, it is expected that substantiation of a supplement claim should have at least two well-designed randomized clinical trials to fulfill the requirement for reproducibility of findings.

As claims regarding prevention or treatment of diseases are not allowed under the DSHEA regulation, the industry has attempted to extrapolate the efficacy or potential benefits from animal or in vitro studies, from traditional medicine use, or from clinical trials in patients [25]. None of these options by themselves seem to be proper to substantiate supplementation for primary prevention or health maintenance. Certainly, there is a good reason for regulatory requests that claims be substantiated in the target population. Efficacies and benefits observed in the young cannot be extrapolated to the elderly or to the pediatric populations. Therapeutic successes with secondary prevention clinical trials under disease state are difficult to demonstrate even with drugs in primary prevention with healthy subjects. One of the most efficacious drug classes to decrease total- and LDL-cholesterol is the HMG CoA reductase inhibitor class, the statins. Although the effects of the treatment with statins were clearly demonstrated to decrease the total- and LDL-cholesterol and the number of cardiovascular events in people with CVDs, it lacked demonstrable efficacy in primary prevention for a long time [26–28]. Only recently, after more than 10 years of debatable data, a meta-analysis of 19 studies is able to show that utilization of statins in primary prevention is indeed beneficial [29].

1.9 CLINICAL TRIALS AND TRIBULATIONS WITH DIETARY SUPPLEMENTS

Most people taking supplements do so to improve present health conditions or to decrease risk of manifestation of the impending NCDs such as osteoporosis, diabetes, and CVD in addition to obtaining good nutrition. Studies demonstrating efficacy of supplements in treatment of NCD are numerous. However, a recently published meta-analysis about vitamin and mineral supplements in the primary prevention of CVD and cancer showed no efficacy. Only a small trend that was close to statistical significance and directionally favoring the supplements in all-cause mortality [relative risk of 0.95 (95% CI 0.89–1.01)], and for cancer [relative risk of 0.94 (95% CI 0.89–1.00)] was observed [30]. A recent study with high-dose multivitamins and minerals for secondary prevention in patients after myocardial infarction showed no statistical benefit although all components of the composite endpoints of death, myocardial infarction, stroke, coronary revascularization, and hospitalization for angina directionally favored multivitamin use (HR 0.89, 95% CI 0.75–1.07). It is worthwhile to highlight that the trends observed in these studies were found despite the fact that the studies were done in a well-nourished population. As CVDs are multi-factorial and the subjects received proper prescription medicine treatment during the duration of the trial, it would have been more clarifying if the authors had investigated subgroups with low blood levels or deficiencies of vitamins. Unfortunately, the number of participants who dropped out of this study was extremely high (64%) making these results difficult to interpret [31]. On the other hand, another publication confirmed the benefits of primary prevention with vitamins and antioxidants on people at risk for macular degeneration. The AREDS study on Age-Related Macular Degeneration (AMD) showed that supplementation with a vitamin/zinc/antioxidant complex reduced the risk of developing advanced AMD by about 25% compared to placebo. The study was led by NIH's National Eye Institute (NEI) [32]. The American Academy of Ophthalmology now recommends the use of the AREDS formulation to reduce the risk of advanced AMD. The NEI launched a second study, AREDS 2, in 2006, to test whether the original formulation could be more efficacious and safer by adding omega-3 fatty acids;

lutein and zeaxanthin and removing beta-carotene; or reducing zinc [33]. There was no overall additional benefit from adding omega-3 fatty acids or a 5-to-1 mixture of lutein and zeaxanthin to the initial formulation. However, the study demonstrated a benefit when they analyzed two subgroups of participants. The subjects who took an AREDS formulation with lutein and zeaxanthin but no beta-carotene, had the risk of developing advanced AMD over the 5 years of the study duration reduced by approximately 18% compared with subjects who took an AREDS formulation without lutein or zeaxanthin but with beta-carotene. Removing beta carotene and adding lutein and zeaxanthin is therefore the author's advice to allow for safer formulation for smokers as a higher risk of lung cancer in smokers has been associated with beta-carotene supplementation [33]. Interestingly, a more recent update of AREDs original formulation confirmed the benefits of vitamins and antioxidants supplementation in the prevention of AMD [34].

The numerous contradictory findings and apparent low-efficacy results seen in the medical literature with supplements illustrate the need to address the complexities of a proper clinical trial with supplements. It would not be feasible and even unethical to attempt to withhold medication from those at risk for CVD to be able to discern better the magnitude of the effect of these supplements as was the case for these recent trials showing mild efficacy trends. Furthermore, earlier intervention studies allowing years of CVD outcome assessment would be more appropriate for determining the efficacy of multivitamins and supplements. However, in a condition with no other treatment alternatives to interfere with potential outcome, the true efficacy of these supplements might be more clearly manifested. This seems to be the case for subjects with signs of dry AMD who do not have available drug treatment for their condition. One would expect a far more compliant patient population and certainly a very low dropout rate from such a clinical study.

Studies with folic acid, vitamins B12 and B6 to reduce homocysteine levels are good examples of difficulties in interpreting results from clinical trials with supplements in diseased population. High levels of circulating homocysteine correlate well with thromboembolic risk and cardiovascular events [35]. Supplementations with B vitamins, indeed, decrease plasma levels of circulating homocysteine [36]. Therefore, one would expect that by decreasing the risk associated with high homocysteine levels, a decrease in cardiovascular events would be the consequence of vitamin B supplementation for patients with coronary heart disease or stroke [37]. However, the data from meta-analyses of clinical studies in patients with cardiovascular risks being treated with B vitamins have so far shown no conclusive benefit, except for the patients at risk for stroke [38]. One meta-analysis showed a mild but positive effect of vitamin B therapy against stroke [39]. A much revealing assessment of confounding factors in studies with supplements was an investigation of a subpopulation in VITATOPs, one of the largest studies on vitamin B prevention of cardiovascular events showed no benefit of vitamin B supplementation. A subgroup study analysis indicated that antiplatelet therapy, abundant in the population studied, had a masking effect on the efficacy/benefit of vitamin B [40,41]. Thus, it is plausible that patients treated for prevention of CVD with aspirin and well nourished might not have been the proper population to demonstrate a benefit of vitamin B therapy in CVDs.

1.10 DETECTING TREATMENT EFFECT IN CLINICAL TRIALS WITH DIETARY SUPPLEMENTS

It is extremely important, for those designing and preparing a study to test the efficacy of supplements, to be cognoscente of the limitations and complexities inherent to benefit and risk of supplementation. First, supplements with potential benefits are prepared to be available to all desiring self-care and therefore need to be safe enough to not add more risk to any present health condition of people taking it. In particular, safety becomes a real issue in patients being treated with prescription or even OTC medication as there is a potential for drug to active or drug to herb interactions. Benefits demonstrated with supplements in clinical studies of diseased populations can be real, and the literature has plenty of good examples. However, findings from population with a diagnosed condition need to be interpreted under professional advice regarding extrapolation of findings to a population without disease. Furthermore, benefits demonstrated in the context of disease cannot be claimed under DSHEA regulation.

The new trend of increased utilization of supplements to prevent manifestation of NCDs has increased the demand, not only by regulators but also by the consumers, for high quality and safe products with irrefutable proof of efficacy only obtainable through well-controlled clinical trials. In this complex scenario, one is left with the difficult task of attempting to demonstrate a benefit of a supplement on the structure and function of healthy bodies, which seems like an oxymoron. Not to despair, there are instances where the preventive benefits of dietary supplementation are more likely to succeed. Well-designed clinical trials in high risk but non-diseased population free of confounding factors and powerful prescription drugs might provide a better environment to demonstrate benefits of supplementation. In absence of well-defined effective dose and pharmacokinetics, it is wise to attempt first to demonstrate, with vitamins, supplements, and minerals, the ability to affect biomarkers or risk factors of disease.

The potential pathways one could then utilize to increase the probability of detecting effect or even efficacy of supplements and avoiding limitations and complications of studying NCDs are shown in Figures 1.2 and 1.3. The figure hypothesizes, in a simplistic way, that there are two types of conditions or disorders outside a disease (diagnostic) estate where supplements could appropriately demonstrate efficacy. The first type (type A, Figure 1.2) represents conditions or disorders with well-defined risk factors or biomarkers indicating imminence or natural progression of disease. Triglyceride and LDL-cholesterol, Hemoglobin $A1_c$, BP, and fasting blood glucose would be good examples of such type of conditions indicating high risk or pre-disease states. In a study with individuals under this category, an intervention with supplements, vitamins, or minerals may have a better chance to demonstrate efficacy at the higher risk end before diagnosis is well established. For example, treatments of pre-diabetes suggest that the onset of type 2 diabetes can be delayed by drug therapy or supplements [42–44]. Therefore, supplements that increase insulin sensitivity or interfere with glucose metabolism should be tested in individuals at the highest risk of diabetes, but otherwise healthy and not medicated. Similar scenario would apply for clinical studies of supplements with BP lowering effects; they should be tested in

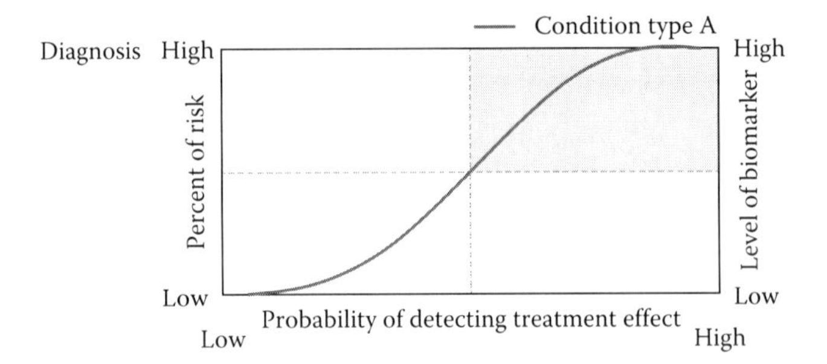

FIGURE 1.2 This is a hypothetical graph of certain (type A) health conditions and the likelihood of finding an efficacy response with vitamins, minerals, and supplements in contributing with health maintenance. Individuals at high risk of manifestation of a type A disease state (i.e., hypertension, diabetes, and obesity) would have a higher likelihood of responding (decreasing risk) in a clinical study to life style changes, diet, non-drug, and supplements.

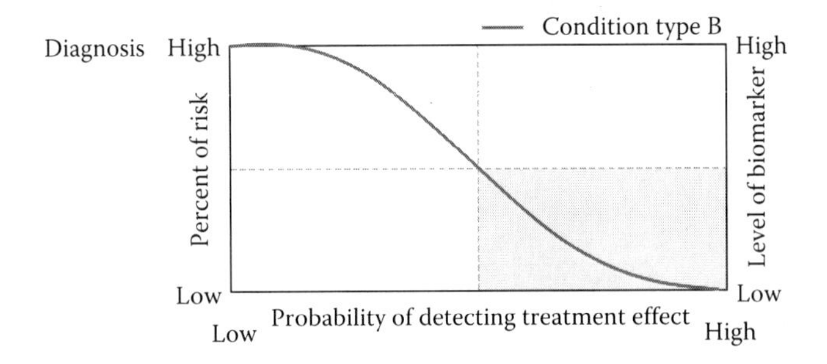

FIGURE 1.3 The figure represents a hypothetical graph of certain conditions type B (i.e., coronary artery disease and neoplasias) that would potentially respond better to non-drug treatments in clinical trials under early interventions when there is still low risk of manifestation of disease.

the higher end pre-hypertensive population. However, there are conditions and disorders that suggest the opposite; the closer one is to a complete diagnosis, the more difficult it is to intervene and consequently more difficult to show a benefit with supplements. The efficacy of supplements in these conditions (type B, Figure 1.3) should be tested first at a lower risk level when there is very little evidence of disease. This is the case for studies of primary prevention of conditions of risk leading to major CVD outcomes (stroke or myocardial infarction) or cancer outcomes. Under these conditions, it is more likely that one could observe an effect when supplementation is introduced earlier before the risk factors and underlying conditions lead to a major outcome. More benign conditions such insomnia could also be in that category. Primary insomnia is very difficult to treat and requires sleep hygiene, psychological support, and very effective sedatives [45]. Therefore, when testing the efficacy of a supplement for treatment of sleep difficulties, one needs to exclude subjects who previously failed sleep aid therapy, or who may have a diagnosis of insomnia.

Qualifying a condition in one of these two categories may facilitate premises for clinical trial design, choice of proper population, and duration of treatment. Condition of type B may require a large number of subjects and clinical trials of long duration while conditions in type A may provide a positive treatment effect in shorter term with a smaller size population sample. Nevertheless, determining if a condition to be studied should follow a type A or B designation approach requires clear understanding of physiopathology and the mechanisms of action of supplements, which are usually not available all together. Therefore, the choice is sometimes more of an art than science. In addition, there will be those disorders or conditions with population that do not fit these two designations. By default, for those conditions the choice should be tested in a population not too far from disease state but also not close to it. Figures 1.2 and 1.3 demonstrate these concepts and approaches to help in selecting population and enriching the design of clinical trials with supplements.

In conclusion, the new trend of growth regarding NCDs demands that more interventions and options for treatment of preventive nature be available globally. Furthermore, the socio-economical burden of NCDs requires an active participation and accountability of the individual to prevent these conditions that have modifiable risk factors. Self-care and self-medication will play, in the near future, a more important role in this crucial process to decrease and control the prevalence of NCDs. However, only regulated, high quality medicinal supplements with evidence-based clinical efficacy and safety will contribute significantly to this goal.

REFERENCES

1. United Nations General Assembly. Resolution adopted by the General Assembly: 66/2: Political Declaration of the High-level Meeting of the General Assembly on the Prevention and Control of Non-communicable Diseases. Adopted September 19, 2011; published January 24, 2012. Available at: http://www.who.int/nmh/events/un_ncd_summit2011/political_declaration_en.pdf.
2. Whiteford H et al. Global burden of disease attributable to mental and substance use disorders: Findings from the Global Burden of Disease Study 2010. *Lancet* 2013; 382:1575–86.
3. Koehlmoos TP et al. Global health: Chronic diseases and other emergent issues in global health. *Infect Dis Clin N Am* 2011;25:623–38.
4. Campbell T, Campbell A. Emerging disease burdens and the poor in cities of the developing world. *J Urban Health* 2007;84(1):i54–63.
5. Godfrey R, Julien M. Urbanization and health. *Clin Med* 2005;5(2):137–41.
6. WHO. Urbanization and health. *B World Health Organ* 2010;88:245–6.
7. World health statistics. 2013. World Health Organization. ISBN 978 92 4 156458 8. Available on the WHO web site at: http://www.who.int/gho/publications/world_ health_ statistics/2013/en/.
8. Fisher-Hoch S et al. Obesity, diabetes and pneumonia: The menacing interface of non-communicable and infectious diseases. *Trop Med Int Health* 2013;18:1510–9.
9. Rahim HFA et al. Health in the Arab world: A view from within 2 non-communicable diseases in the Arab world. *Lancet* 2014;383:356–67.
10. US Burden of Disease Collaborators. The State of US Health, 1990–2010 burden of diseases, injuries, and risk factors. *JAMA* 2013;310(6):591–608.
11. Go A et al. Executive summary: Heart disease and stroke statistics—2014 update: A report from the American Heart Association. *Circulation* 2014;129:399–410.

12. Interventions on diet and physical activity: What works: Summary report 2009. World Health Organization. ISBN 978 92 4 159824 8. Available at: http://www.who.int/dietphysicalactivity/whatworks/en/.
13. Smith SC et al. Our time: A call to save preventable death from cardiovascular disease (heart disease and stroke). *Global Heart* 2012;7:1–9.
14. Wald DS et al. Randomized polypill crossover trial in people aged 50 and over. PLoS ONE 2012;7(7): e41297.
15. Jørgensen T et al. Population-level changes to promote cardiovascular health. *Eur J Pre Cardiol.* Available at: http://cpr.sagepub.com/content/early/2012/05/09/2047487312441726. Published online 18 April 2012.
16. Wald NJ, Law MR. A strategy to reduce cardiovascular disease by more than 80%. *BMJ* 2003;326:1419–23.
17. WHO Traditional Medicine Strategy. 2014–2023. ISBN 978 92 4 150609 0. Available at: http://www.who.int/medicines/publications/traditional/trm_strategy14_23/en/.
18. Wong A et al. Medical innovation and age-specific trends in health care utilization: Findings and implications. *Social Sci Med* 2012;74:263–72.
19. Apelberg B et al. Estimating the risks and benefits of nicotine replacement therapy for smoking cessation in the United States. *Am J Public Health* 2010;100:341–8.
20. The Story of Self Care and Self Medication. 40 years of progress, 1970–2010. World Self Medication Industry, 2011. pp. 1–29. Available at: http://www.wsmi.org/publications.htm.
21. Robinson MM, Zhang X. The world medicines situation 2011. Traditional medications: Global situation, issues and challenges. World Health Organization, Geneva 2011.
22. Gahche J et al. Dietary supplement use among US adults has increased since NHANES III (1988–1994). *NCHS Data Brief* 2011 Apr;61:1–8.
23. Engel L, Straus S, Development of therapeutics: Opportunities within complementary and alternative medicine. *Nat Rev Drug Dis* 2002;1:229–37.
24. Public Law 103-417–Oct. 25, 1994. Dietary Supplement Health Education Act of 1994. Available at: http://ods.od.nih.gov/About/DSHEA_Wording.aspx.
25. Guidance for Industry. Substantiation for Dietary Supplement Claims Made Under Section 403 (r0 960 of Federal Food, Drug and Cosmetic Act. 74 Fed. Reg. 304 (Jan. 5, 2009). Available at: http://www.cfsan.fda.gov/~dms/dsclmgu2.html.
26. Pignone M et al. Use of lipid lowering drugs for primary prevention of coronary heart disease: Metaanalysis of randomised trials. *BMJ* 2000;321:1–5.
27. Thavendiranathan P et al. Primary prevention of cardiovascular diseases with statin therapy. A meta-analysis of randomized controlled trials. *Arch Intern Med* 2006;166:2307–13.
28. Ray K et al. Statins and all-cause mortalityin high-risk primary prevention. A meta-analysis of 11 randomized controlled trials involving 65229 participants. *Arch Intern Med* 2010;170(12):1024–31.
29. Taylor F et al. Statins for the primary prevention of cardiovascular disease. *Cochrane Data Syst Rev* 2013, Issue 1. Art. No.: CD004816. DOI: 10.1002/14651858.CD004816.pub5.
30. Lamas G et al. Oral high-dose multivitamins and minerals after myocardial infarction: A randomized trial. *Ann Intern Med* 2013;159(12):797–805.
31. Fortmann SP et al. Vitamin and mineral supplements in the primary prevention of cardiovascular disease and cancer: An updated systematic evidence review for the U.S. preventive services task force. *Ann Intern Med* 2013;159:824–34.
32. Age-related eye disease study research group, a randomized, placebo-controlled, clinical trial of high-dose supplementation with vitamins C and E, beta carotene, and zinc for age-related macular degeneration and vision loss: AREDS Report No. 8. *Arch Ophthalmol* 119 (10);2001:1417–36.

33. Chew E et al. Lutein_zeaxanthin and omega-3 fatty acids for age-related macular degeneration. The Age-Related Eye Disease Study 2 (AREDS2) randomized clinical trial. *JAMA* 2013;309(19):2005–15.
34. Chew E et al. Long-term effects of vitamins C and E, β-carotene, and zinc on age-related macular degeneration AREDS Report no. 35. *Ophthalmology* 2013;120:1604–11.
35. Malinow MR et al. Homocysteine, diet and cardiovascular diseases: A statement for healthcare professionals from the Nutrition Committee, American Heart Association. *Circulation* 1999;99:178–82.
36. Zappacosta B et al. Homocysteine lowering by folate-rich diet or pharmacological supplementations in subjects with moderate hyperhomocysteinemia. *Nutrients* 2013;5:1531–43.
37. Toole JF et al. Lowering homocysteine in patients with ischemic stroke to prevent recurrent stroke, myocardial infarction, and death. *JAMA* 2004;291:565–75.
38. Clarke R et al. Homocysteine and vascular disease: Review of published results of the homocysteine-lowering trials. *J Inherit Metab Dis* 2011;34:83–91.
39. Yang J et al. Vitamin B supplementation, homocysteine levels, and the risk of cerebrovascular disease: A meta-analysis. *Neurology* 2013;81;1298–307.
40. The VITATOPS Trial Study Group. B vitamins in patients with recent transient ischaemic attack or stroke in the VITAmins TO Prevent Stroke (VITATOPS) trial: A randomised, double-blind, parallel, placebo-controlled trial. *Lancet Neurol* 2010;9:855–65.
41. Hankey, G et al. Antiplatelet therapy and the effects of B vitamins in patients with previous stroke or transient ischaemic attack: A post-hoc subanalysis of VITATOPS, a randomised, placebo-controlled trial. *Lancet Neurol* 2012;11:512–20.
42. Lily M, Godwin M. Treating prediabetes with metformin. *Systematic review and meta-analysis. Can Fam Physician* 2009;55:363–9.
43. Pal S, Radavelli Bagatini S. Effects of psyllium on metabolic syndrome risk factors. *Obes Rev* 2012 Nov;13(11):1034–47.
44. Chutkan R et al. Viscous versus nonviscous soluble fiber supplements: Mechanisms and evidence for fiber-specific health benefits. *J Am Acad Nurse Prac* 2012;24:476–87.
45. Célyne H. Bastien. Insomnia: Neurophysiological and neuropsychological approaches. *Neuropsychol Rev* 2011;21:22–40.

2 Identifying Nutritional Gaps among Americans

Heather A. Eicher-Miller, Clara Park, and Regan Bailey

CONTENTS

2.1 INTRODUCTION

The food trends of USA have changed considerably over the past decades [1]. In addition, food is currently more affordable in the USA than in any other developed countries [2]. Processed food intake and foods consumed away from home have also increased. Despite the high availability and great variety of foods, a substantial proportion of the US population is at nutritional risk for several micronutrients.

The evidence linking diet to health is extensive and provides the foundation for determining optimum nutrient status. Scientific advancements in assessing dietary and nutrient intake have enhanced our understanding of nutrient needs across the lifespan. Nutritional assessment is comprised of measuring or monitoring data on dietary intakes, biomarkers of nutritional status, and anthropometric data. These tools can also be used to identify nutrient shortfall and excess. Given the clear role of nutrition in overall health, these measures of nutrient assessment can be used as a basis for informing and guiding individuals or groups on dietary practices.

This chapter focuses on how population-level nutrient intakes are estimated, how these estimates are compared with the dietary recommendations provided by the Dietary Reference Intakes (DRIs), and how these data are used to identify the nutrient gaps among US population groups. The four nutrient-based reference values comprising the DRIs were developed by the Food and Nutrition Board of the Institute of Medicine (IOM) and include the Estimated Average Requirement (EAR), Adequate Intake (AI), the Recommended Dietary Allowance (RDA), and the Tolerable Upper Intake Level (UL) [3]. The nutrient recommendations of interest are detailed with regard to the DRI population subgroups.

Dietary supplements are considered as a strategy for specific subpopulations to achieve nutrient recommendations that may be difficult to meet through diet alone [4]. Though supplements are not intended to substitute for foods, supplements are regarded as a simple and affordable method to achieve nutrient requirements. The efficacy of supplements to ameliorate inadequacy among the population is also discussed in this chapter.

2.2 SETTING STANDARDS FOR NUTRIENT INTAKE: THE DIETARY REFERENCE INTAKES

Essential micronutrient intake is critical for optimal growth, development, and overall health. The amount of nutrient required to support health and prevent disease may vary by several individual characteristics including: age, gender, height, weight, health and life stage (i.e., pregnancy or lactation), and genetics [3]. The exact nutrient intake to support optimum health of an individual may be very specific while the range of nutrient intakes to support optimum health for all individuals within a life stage and gender group may vary considerably. Individual nutrient needs may also be unknown, but reasonable estimates to meet the needs of healthy people are outlined by the life-stage and sex-specific DRIs [3]. DRI values are evidence based, or based on scientifically determined relationships between the dietary intake of a nutrient and biological indicators of adequacy including the prevention of acute and chronic disease in healthy populations.

Even when certain demographic characteristics are shared among the individuals comprising a group, other differences may predicate a variety of nutrient needs. Variation in the nutrient needs within a population may be represented by a distribution of requirements; the individuals comprising the population have diverse nutrient needs but these needs or the required intakes are centered around a mean. The DRIs are founded on a distribution of requirements that may be visualized as a "normal" distribution or symmetrical bell-shaped curve. The DRIs establish sentinel values in the distribution, which allow evaluation of the group's ability to meet nutrient requirements and other indicators of nutrient adequacy or excess. The values may be used as a reference, for assessment, and for planning the diets of individuals and groups. When applied, the values comprising the DRIs are designed to optimize health, prevent disease, and avoid nutrient over-consumption in healthy people [5].

The EAR is the most pertinent for determining the nutrient adequacy of a group. The EAR is defined as, "the average daily nutrient intake level that is estimated to meet the requirements of half of the healthy individuals in a particular life stage and gender group" [5]. "Average" in the EAR definition actually refers to the estimated median requirement, and as such, the EAR will be less than the true value required by half of the population, and more than the true value required by the other half of the population [5]. The AI is used when there is no sufficient knowledge to establish an EAR; and is defined as, "the recommended average daily intake level based on observed or experimentally determined approximations or estimates of nutrient intakes by a group (or groups) of apparently healthy people that are assumed to be adequate; used when an RDA cannot be determined" [5]. An interpretation of the AI may be given as the nutrient quantity that is necessary for most people of a certain gender and life stage to fulfill or exceed nutrient needs [5]. Population-level data are not recommended to be compared to the AI [6]. The establishment of a RDA is based on the EAR; and is defined as, "the average daily dietary nutrient intake level that is sufficient to meet the nutrient requirements of nearly all (97%–98%) healthy individuals in a particular life stage and gender group" [5]. Nutrient intake below the RDA may not be defined as insufficient because the RDA is beyond the requirement of almost all individuals in a specified gender and life-stage group. As a consequence, RDAs are not appropriate for use as a cut-off in the nutrient assessment of groups. RDAs are determined for those nutrients with a normal distribution of requirement and a defined EAR; an RDA is not determined for nutrients with an AI instead of an EAR. The RDA is determined by a value that is two SD above the EAR. However, special cases may exist for certain nutrients with skewed requirement distributions, as in the case of iron in menstruating women, in which the RDA is set between the 97th and 98th percentile of the requirement distribution [5].

Variations in the nutrient requirements of individual members comprising a population are inherent to a distribution. Subpopulations may exist within a larger population that share certain characteristics and which conform the group to a less diverse distribution of requirements [7]. Subpopulation requirement distributions are known to differ from the general population based on characteristics including age, sex, and life stage, just as nutrient requirements differ vastly between individuals depending on these characteristics. The DRIs include 12 sets of reference values that are specific for these characteristics, 6 of which are specific for children aged 0–18 years [5]. A set of reference values is provided for infancy that covers the first 12 months by dividing the time period into 6-month-intervals. The AIs gave an outline for all of the nutrients during the first 6 months based on an average intake of the healthy, full-term, and exclusively human milk-fed infants born to healthy mothers. One to 3 years is the age range for the toddler reference values. Toddlers experience uniquely slower growth velocity compared to infants but uniquely faster velocity compared with 4- to 5-year-olds. The studies examining this age group are few, so many of the EARs or AIs for this group have been extrapolated from the adult values. Three methods may be used to extrapolate values: adult requirements may be scaled to the 0.75 power of body mass, scaling may be based on the reference body weights, or the scaling may be based on energy intake [5]. Early childhood is the next set of reference values and includes the children aged 4–8 years. Sufficient research has been completed for many nutrients within this group of children to set EARs, RDAs, and AIs; avoiding use of the extrapolation method. Adolescence is divided into two sets of reference values, children aged from 9–13 years and 14–18 years, age groups that are based on the mean ages of the female and male growth spurts. Certain nutrient DRIs differ for males and females within an age group, such as for iron, which is needed in greater quantity for females due to the onset of menarche [5].

2.3 ASSESSING DIET TO DETERMINE USUAL NUTRIENT INTAKE

Quantification of the nutrient intake is essential for determining the prevalence of nutrient adequacy or inadequacy of the group or population; this determination involves comparing the requirement distribution with the intake distribution [7]. Dietary assessment is used to quantify the type and quantity of foods and beverages consumed. This information can then be linked with a nutrient database to facilitate calculation of the nutrient content of the individual foods or beverages that were consumed. The nutrient information of each item consumed by an individual may be added to the amount of similar nutrients contained in additionally consumed items to yield a total nutrient intake. However, this total may only represent an intake of a limited amount of time or a daily intake. A more useful measure of dietary intake for determining adequacy is the "usual" dietary intake. Usual dietary intake refers to an average intake of a nutrient over the long-term [8]. Nutrient requirements are intended to be met over time. The DRIs are derived from estimating relationships of diet to long-term outcomes such as overall health and the prevention of chronic disease; thus, usual dietary intake is a more appropriate measure for determining nutrient adequacy in the population compared with a daily intake.

Estimates of usual dietary intake may be produced by using two or more dietary assessments to quantify diet over two separate time periods or by combining the reported dietary intake information from at least two dietary assessments [8–10]. The burden of dietary assessment over an extended period of time, within and between person variation, and other forms of measurement error make usual intake very difficult to quantify [7]. A precursory determination of a mean intake for each individual will narrow the distribution towards the mean nutrient intake of the group, decreasing the chance for over-classification of deficiency [7]. Excessive variability between the individuals of the group may, however, still be present. Recent statistical modeling methods have been developed to mitigate both the variability of dietary intake for an individual over time and the variability between individuals in a group, or measurement error [8,11]. Three primary methods of dietary assessment are commonly used to determine usual dietary intake: the 24-hour dietary recall, the food record or dietary record, and food frequency questionnaires (FFQs) [12]. Each dietary assessment method has strengths and weaknesses, and each is better suited to different types of studies as described below.

2.3.1 24-Hour Dietary Recall to Quantify Nutrient Intake

The administration of a 24-hour dietary recall involves asking a participant to report everything she/he consumed in the last 24 h. Twenty-four-hour dietary recalls are considered the most precise and detailed source of dietary assessment [12]. A 24-hour dietary recall may be completed in person, by telephone, with computer assistance, or by pencil and paper and may be interview-assisted or self-administered online as in the Automated Self-Administered 24-Hour Dietary Recall (ASA-24) [13]. Usually, a model or picture of commonly consumed foods is used as a prompt for determining accurate portion sizes.

The United States Department of Agriculture (USDA) Automated Multiple Pass Method (AMPM) is a state-of-the art 24-hour dietary recall instrument currently used in the What We Eat in America (WWEIA), National Health and Nutrition Examination Survey (NHANES) that was developed to aid recollection [14]. Five passes, or series of probes are used in the AMPM to retrieve as many foods as possible consumed in the past 24 h. The AMPM takes approximately 30–45 min to complete. Diet is easily remembered in this method because foods are recalled after only 24 h and literacy is not required when the 24-hour recall is administered via interviewer. The low respondent burden makes this method useful for large studies representative of the general population.

A benefit of the 24-hour dietary recall is the limited bias resulting from systematic error. The detailed collection of information on all foods and beverages consumed does not exclude or prioritize the capture of certain dietary information [15]. A 24-hour recall is also suited to a variety of populations including those with low levels of education and children [12]. Respondent knowledge of a future 24-hour recall may increase the likelihood of alterations to diet compared with an unannounced 24-hour recall where respondents have no opportunity to modify their diets [16]. Dietary assessment by 24-hour recall is best suited to cross-sectional and surveillance studies, prospective cohort, and intervention studies. As such, the 24-hour dietary recall method of dietary assessment is included in all data collections of the nationally representative NHANES and the Continuing Survey of Food Intakes by Individuals (CSFII) [17], making this method of dietary assessment one of the most commonly used to determine nutrient gaps among Americans.

NHANES features two 24-hour recalls that were collected using the AMPM method for all of the survey years since 2002. This dietary recall was completed over the phone 3–10 days after the in-person interview at the Mobile Examination Center. In NHANES, proxy reports for children 5 years and younger and for individuals who cannot self-report. Children aged 6–11 years report with the assistance of a proxy and children older than 11 years may self-report. The dietary information collected is linked to a nutrient composition database with food descriptions, codes, and nutrient compositions. The USDA Food and Nutrient Database for Dietary Studies

(FNDDS) is the nutrient database, which allows quantification of the nutrient content of the foods reported in the dietary assessment of NHANES AMPM [18]. The nutritional content of an estimated 7000 foods are included in the FNDDS. The AMPM computerized software system allows for direct coding of the reported foods, recipe modification and development, data editing and management, and nutrient analysis of dietary data [14]. The USDA National Nutrient Database for Standard Reference is the major source of food composition data in the USA and the basis for FNDDS and other food composition databases [19]. The nutrient content of some foods contained in this database are analytically derived and other are estimated.

The dietary information collected from one 24-hour dietary recall is not a proper characterization of an individual's usual diet because of the considerable daily dietary variation exhibited by most individuals, or what may be thought of as a large within-person random error. This within-person dietary variation may be accounted for by using a second 24-hour dietary recall on a non-consecutive day of collection and by making statistical adjustments for individual variation [8,15]. An estimation of individuals meeting dietary requirements in a population or the proportion of the group meeting dietary requirements should also not be completed using the dietary data from only one 24-hour dietary recall, but rather, two or more 24-hour non-consecutive day dietary recalls. The estimate of usual dietary intake or the estimate of the intake distribution for a group may be improved with the inclusion of additional days of dietary assessment in the calculation of the estimate and statistical modifications to reduce measurement error [15].

Validation studies of the 24-hour dietary recall method have been completed by comparing energy consumption derived from recalled intakes to doubly labeled water-derived energy expenditure, or by comparisons of respondent dietary recall to trained observer food recording and weighing [12,20]. Underreporting is problematic with the 24-hour dietary recall [20,21]. Studies using energy expenditure quantified by doubly labeled water against food recalls have generally found underreporting in the range of 3%–26% for energy [20,22–28] and 11%–34% for protein against urinary nitrogen [20,27,29]. In young children, doubly labeled water studies have revealed proxy energy overreporting of approximately 7%–11% in a systematic review by Burrows et al. [30]. Subar et al. [20] compared the combined dietary data from two five-step multiple pass 24-hour recalls with doubly labeled water for energy and urinary nitrogen for protein, and found underreporting in men at 12%–14% for energy and 11%–12% for protein. In women, underreporting was slightly greater for energy at 16%–20%, while estimates for protein, at 11%–15%, were similar to the estimates for men [20]. Factors such as obesity, gender, social desirability, hunger, restrained eating, education, literacy, perceived health status, age, and race/ethnicity have been associated with underreporting [23–25,31]. Comparison of the USDA AMPM derived energy intake against doubly labeled water-derived energy expenditure has shown underreporting of energy by approximately <3% in normal weight participants. Overweight reporters exhibited both a greater prevalence of underreporting and greater percentage for which energy was underreported [32]. Compared with plausible reporters, underreporters generally provide information on fewer foods, smaller portion sizes, greater intake of low-fat and diet foods, and less mention of fat added to foods [33].

2.3.2 Using a Food Record to Quantify Nutrient Intake

Food records are methods of dietary assessment in which dietary intake is recorded after food is consumed, theoretically at the time of the eating occasion. The respondent is usually given detailed instructions on how to complete the food record, quantify the foods consumed, and provide a certain level of detail for enhanced accuracy [12]. The independent respondent recording of food requires no investigator interview, but considerable time is necessary for training respondents, reviewing, and entering data from the food records [16]. Food records are usually completed for one to not more than three or four consecutive days, a time period after which respondent fatigue becomes problematic [34]. Dietary assessment with a food record is best suited to prospective cohort studies. Similar to a single 24-hour recall, a food record must be linked with a nutrient database to determine nutrient intake. In addition, a single food record is not appropriate to estimate an individual's usual diet, or to assess the fulfillment of dietary requirements. Also similar to the 24-hour recall, at least two non-consecutive food records are necessary for a proper estimation of individual intake or achievement of dietary requirements due to the possibility of correlated intakes when food records include adjacent days [16].

The knowledge and process of recording food may also influence underreporting food by the respondent. The process of recording the food consumed has actually been shown to be a successful approach to reduce food intake [22,35]. Thus, the two disadvantages of the food record: selection of the sample and the measure of diet may be biased [12]. The immediate recording of food limits the need to remember details of the food consumed. This inherent strength of the food record is also the reason food records are sometimes considered a reference standard for other methods of dietary assessment [16,36].

Food records are not suited to all populations, such as low-literacy groups, children, low-socioeconomic status groups, and others due to the high level of detail, attention to quantity, and writing skills necessary [12]. The accuracy of the food record may vary with the sample and other characteristics of the study. Energy and protein intakes compared with energy expenditure quantified with doubly-labeled water and urinary nitrogen, respectively have shown underestimation in the range of 8%–37% [24,37–40]. Characteristics associated with underreporting using food records are education, employment grade, socio-economic status, body image, and dietary restraint [41,42]. Lower intakes of certain foods such as desserts, sweet baked goods, butter, and alcoholic beverages are declared by under-reporters compared to plausible reporters [43].

2.3.3 Using a Food Frequency Questionnaire (FFQ) to Quantify Nutrient Intake

An FFQ is a list of foods from which a respondent is asked to estimate their usual intake during a certain period of time. The time period of dietary assessment referenced by the FFQ may be modified depending on the research purposes, an advantage of the FFQ [16]. FFQs are flexible and may be used in a variety of studies including cross-sectional and surveillance, case-control, cohort, and intervention studies [12].

Because of the FFQs inquiry into previous consumption, eating behavior of the past is not influenced by knowledge of the reporting task. Most FFQs require 30–60 min to complete, but despite the ease of completion an FFQ requires complex cognitive skills that may be challenging for individuals with little education, low cognitive abilities, and low literacy skills [12,16]. FFQs are best suited to ranking individuals by nutrient, specific food, and food group intakes with regard to a certain list of foods [12,44]. The specific list of foods limits the FFQ to the population for which it was designed [16,45]. Certain cultural groups may rely heavily on certain foods that other groups do not consume; the exclusion of these foods may greatly affect the accuracy of the instrument.

The self-administered multiple choice questionnaire format of the FFQ may be scanned for data entry and has the benefit of causing a little burden to the respondent or the investigator [16]. As in other methods of dietary assessment, the FFQ must be associated with a database and dietary analysis software to approximate the nutrient or food intake. FFQs may be designed for estimating total dietary intake, food group intake, or specific nutrient intakes [12]. The FFQ may be qualitative, semi-quantitative, and quantitative. A qualitative FFQ estimates nutrient intake by querying the frequency of consumption of foods [16]. Qualitative FFQs were used more often in the 1980s [46]. Using a semi-quantitative FFQ, a reference portion size is provided when participants are asked about the frequency at which foods are consumed. The "Willett" or "Harvard" FFQ are examples of a semi-qualitative FFQs [47]. Quantitative FFQs such as the "Block" FFQ request information on the frequency of food consumed and the portion size [47].

Even a very complete and detailed FFQ is still constrained to being a list of foods and not a representation of all foods consumed. A respondent may be inhibited from remembering or listing other foods that they have consumed. The resulting dietary estimates from an FFQ generally have a high reproducibility with little within person random error compared with the 24-hour recall and dietary records. Yet, systematic error that may bias the resulting estimates is present, such as when additional foods are consumed but not quantified because they are not present in the list of foods comprising the FFQ [48]. In addition, the calculations that are completed to estimate the amount and frequency of the food lead to inherent errors. Due to this limitation, the FFQ should be used in combination with a second form of dietary assessment to estimate the mean and variance of usual dietary intake or to assess dietary adequacy and inadequacy of a group or individual [8,12,49–51].

In general, underestimation is even more problematic for energy using an FFQ compared with a 24-hour recall [12,20] when the estimates are evaluated for accuracy by comparing to the total energy expenditure derived using the doubly-labeled water method. Similarly, reported protein intakes estimated using an FFQ are not as accurate as 24-hour recall protein estimates when compared with calculations of protein intake estimated using urinary nitrogen. Research by Subar et al. [20] found highly educated men and women to underreport energy by 31%–36% and 34%–38%, respectively; and protein at 30%–34% among men and 27%–32% among women [20]. Evaluation of an FFQ is often completed by comparing the FFQ to a food record or 24-hour recall. Correlation of nutrient estimates from two instruments may be high but may be an erroneous indication of true nutrient intake due to correlated measurement error [52]. Underreporting among women using an FFQ was associated with fear of negative evaluation, weight-loss history, and percentage of energy from fat. Among men, body mass index, comparison of activity level with that of others of the same sex and age, and eating frequency were the best predictors of FFQ underreporting as reported by Tooze et al. [31].

2.4 SUMMARY

Dietary assessment is necessary for the estimation of usual nutrient intake and the evaluation of nutrient adequacy for a group or the US population. The various errors and underreporting inherent to all types of dietary assessment are important to realize when considering the accuracy, error, and limitations of estimates of usual intake. Researchers and clinicians must be careful to recognize that even the best estimates are likely to include error, and interpretation and application of the estimates should be careful not to extend the limitations of the meaning of the results or present the information as "exact". As such, dietary assessment may produce "best estimates" for which the probability of adequacy can be determined using the DRIs.

2.5 ASSESSING SUPPLEMENT INTAKE TO DETERMINE TOTAL NUTRIENT INTAKE

Assessment of total nutrient intake must entail all nutrients consumed including those consumed in the form of supplements along with those consumed from foods or reported dietary intake. Not all individuals use dietary supplements, but an analysis to determine total nutrient intake of a group or of the population should include assessment of nutrient intake from supplements. Similarly, the efficacy of supplement use to improve the nutrient intake of the population may only be investigated when nutrient intake from supplements is assessed. Similar to dietary assessment, supplement intake can be assessed using various methods. Supplement use is usually assessed using the previous month as a reference period, but may also be reflective of a daily or 12-month time period. Most assessments request information on the type (multivitamin/multimineral, single nutrient, etc.), brand name, frequency, and the dosage of supplement intake, but some also request reporting on the form in which the supplement was consumed (liquid, tablet, pill, etc.). The motivation for supplement use may also be queried. The NHANES supplement intake data are used widely to estimate nutrient intake from supplements for the general and various US subpopulations. NHANES I (1971–1975) [53] included supplement intake assessment in the 24-hour dietary recall; NHANES II (1976–1980) [54] and III (1988–1994) [55] included a 30-day dietary supplement intake assessment, replacing the 24-hour recall reference period for supplement use. A 30-day reference period for supplement intake was used in the continuous NHANES (1999–2000) and continuous NHANES (2001–present) assessment [56] during the in-house interview. Participants reporting dietary supplements are then asked to show the interviewer the bottle of the supplement, report how often he/she took each supplement during the previous month, and how much of each supplement was taken at each intake occasion. The information is recorded by the interviewer and matched to the supplement database created by the National Center for Health Statistics (NCHS). The NCHS regularly communicates with major manufacturing companies to update the NHANES nutrient database to reflect supplement reformulation [56,57]. As NHANES 2007–2008 [58], two 24-hour supplement intake recalls are completed in addition to the 30-day recall. One 24-hour recall is completed in an in-person interview with the participant in the MEC, and the other is completed over the phone, 3–10 days later. A proxy reports the supplement use for children 6 months to 16 years of age.

Pitfalls are inherent to supplement intake assessment, similar to those encountered in dietary intake assessment. For instance, lack of information in some child and adolescent groups and lack of information on dosage, frequency, and duration can result in the inconsistencies that are often present among studies. Some information gaps are due to the inability of participants to recall the various details of the supplements they use. Participants have difficulty in remembering the exact brand, type, and components of the particular supplement; and even when these are accurately recorded, it is impossible for participants to recall the various kinds and amounts of vitamins and nutrients comprising a multivitamin [59]. Participants may also not provide the current label, or may forget certain supplements, especially, if they are taking more than one. Even when bottles or labels can be recorded or photographed, discrepancy in the label and the actual content of the supplement may still exist. Another opportunity for error is present in the 5-month lag time between the market entry of the new product and updates to the NCHS database. In addition to this lag time, it is often difficult to determine whether the product consumed by the participant is the previous formula or a new formulation of the product. Participants may also inaccurately recall the time frame of intake, the amount taken for a specific period of time, the dosage, the intake routine, and if the reported brand was consistently used during the specified time period [59]. Finally, analysis of nutrient intake from diet and dietary supplements may present challenges to the normal distribution of intake due to the relatively large and discrete doses that are comprised in dietary supplements.

2.6 ASSESSING THE NUTRIENT ADEQUACY OF THE POPULATION

Self-reported diet and supplement intake assessment may be used to determine usual dietary intake or the estimate of long-term intake [9], as described above. The distribution of nutrient requirements in the population must be known in addition to the distribution of usual dietary intakes to properly assess the prevalence of inadequacy in the population or the proportion of the population with inadequate intakes. The assessment of adequacy for a population should consider the distribution of variation in the usual intake of the members of the group and account for the requirements of each life-stage and gender group. Nutrient assessment within a group of children aged 4–8 years, for example, will yield a distribution of intakes that is dramatically different from the distribution of intake within a group of pregnant women.

The EAR may be used as a cut-off for assessing the prevalence of nutrient inadequacy. Using this method, the proportion of the group with reported dietary intakes below the EAR may be considered similar to the proportion of individuals that do not meet the nutrient requirements. However, several assumptions about the group and the nutrient included in the assessment must be authenticated for this method to be appropriate: The distribution of requirements must be symmetrical, the nutrient intake distribution must be more variable compared with the nutrient requirement distribution, and there may be no correlation between intakes and requirements. The nutrient intake distributions from most groups of free-living individuals are generally consistent with these assumptions [7,60].

The EAR cut-off method (as described above) is valid for estimating the prevalence of nutrient inadequacy in a group for several reasons. When usual dietary intakes are below the EAR, the probability of inadequacy is greater than 50%. Yet, not everyone with dietary intakes below the EAR is actually consuming less nutrient than is necessary for them due to the variation in individual need. Some individuals have lower than average requirements and adequate intakes that are less than the EAR. Similarly, some individuals of the group with usual dietary intakes that exceed the EAR have greater than average individual requirements that are not met, despite their high reported dietary intake. When the assumptions for the requirement distributions described earlier for a group and a particular nutrient are valid, the proportion of individuals with lower than average requirements and higher than average requirements will be similar. In this situation, the EAR cut-off method for calculating prevalence of inadequacy is an appropriate method for approximation [7,60]. One caveat to the general adherence of most nutrients to the assumptions is manifested in the unsymmetrical distribution of iron intake for menstruating women. A statistical method, termed the "probability approach" [7,60] should be used as an alternative to the EAR cut-off in this case. Using this method, the risk of inadequacy is determined using the individual's usual dietary intake. Next, a group average of these probabilities is quantified. This average may be used as an estimate of the prevalence of inadequacy in the group. The assumptions that must be upheld for this method to be valid are that intakes and requirements are not correlated and that the distributions for the specific nutrient requirements are known [7].

Some life-stage and gender groups have an AI rather than an EAR. In this situation, caution must be used in assessing the nutrient intakes of groups. Interpretation of the AI and EAR must be distinctly different [7,60]. The lack of information on appropriate intakes limits the usefulness of the AI for determining inadequacy. The prevalence of inadequacy may not be quantified because the requirement distribution is unknown and the determination of where the AI falls in relationship to the distribution cannot be established. Limited inferences may be made about the prevalence of inadequacy in the group, but adequacy may be estimated when the mean or median intakes are at or above the AI. Comparisons may be made for where the median or mean group intake falls in relation to the AI [60].

2.7 NUTRIENT GAPS AMONG US POPULATION

The 2010 Report of the Dietary Guidelines Advisory Committee on the Dietary Guidelines for Americans [4] documents an extensive review of the published research and emerging science to determine the nutrient shortfalls of Americans. The Dietary Guidelines are published every 5 years by the US Department of Health and Human Services in conjunction with US Department of Agriculture. A systematic, evidence-based review methodology was used to select studies to inform the creation of the Dietary Guidelines for Americans 2010, to determine the nutrients that most Americans should increase and the nutrients that most Americans should decrease compared with current intake. The classification of foods and nutrients to increase and decrease were made on the basis of health promotion and reduction of the risk of chronic disease [4]. Classifications were also made based on the generalizability of study findings to the population, consistency of the findings, quality of the studies, and the impact or importance of the studied outcomes. The results of this thorough, evidence-based review indicated the nutrients to increase in the population for both adults and children included potassium, calcium, vitamin D, and fiber [4]. These nutrients can be considered shortfall nutrients or nutrient gaps for the American population. Recommendations were made for specific subpopulations: women who are capable of becoming pregnant or ones who are pregnant or nursing should increase intake of iron and folic acid while adults 50 years and older should increase their intake of vitamin B12. In addition to these nutrient gaps, significant proportions of many subpopulations do not meet the EAR for vitamins A, E, C, and magnesium. Subpopulation inadequacy may be present for vitamin B6 in older women, zinc in older adults and teenage females, and phosphorous for preteen and teenage females [4]. Vitamin K may also not be consumed in sufficient amount by certain population subgroups but the AI provided for this nutrient makes adequacy difficult to determine.

The following sections of this chapter will review the current research documenting the distribution of usual nutrient intake from food, beverages, and supplements for the "shortfall nutrients" identified above for US infants, children, adolescents, adults, and pregnant women. There may perhaps be additional shortfall of nutrients for other subpopulations, but due to lack of studies, limited representativeness, and the scope of this review, the chapter will be limited to those nutrients described above. The evaluation of nutrient intake from diet alone or from the *total* reported dietary intake, that is intake from diet along with the intake from dietary supplements will be described along with discussion regarding the usefulness of supplements to improve population-level shortfalls. The classification of children, adolescents, and adults will adhere to the study-defined age ranges and the ranges outlined in the DRIs: infancy, birth to 12 months, toddlers 1–3 years, childhood 4–8 years, puberty/adolescence 9–18 years, adulthood 19–50 years, and older adults aged 51 years and older [3].

2.8 ESTABLISHING DRIs FOR SHORTFALL NUTRIENTS IN INFANTS AND CHILDREN

The DRIs for infants were based on the nutrient needs of healthy, full-term infants born to healthy mothers who rely exclusively on human milk for the first 6 months of their life. Very few studies exist for infants to provide strong evidence for the development of DRI values, but an EAR and RDA are provided for iron and zinc that are known to be in greater demand during this stage and for which stronger evidence has been established [3].

AIs are provided for other nutrients among infants aged 0–6 months, and are based on the nutrient content from human milk consumed in increasing volume to support growth. The AIs for the subsequent 6 months of their life reflect the sum of the average amount of nutrient provided by human milk at 0.6 L/day and complementary weaning foods that are expected to be consumed at this age to support continued growth. The AI for vitamin D is an exception due to the naturally very low occurrence of vitamin D in human milk. Vitamin D is important to support bone health, calcium absorption, to prevent rickets in children [61], and to prevent osteoporosis in later adulthood. Recommended vitamin D intakes (AI) for infants aged 0–6 months and 7–12 months are set to maintain desirable serum 25-hydroxyvitamin D (25(OH)D) concentrations as human milk is not a meaningful source of vitamin D. The vitamin D recommendation for older children has been developed for intakes that preserve serum 25(OH)D concentrations while promoting normal, healthy bone accretion [61].

Calcium is another nutrient that is critical for bone growth and bone health in children that supports strong, healthy bones in adulthood. In addition, calcium is necessary for proper vascular, neuromuscular, and glandular functioning. An AI for calcium is set for infants aged 0–6 months and is assumed to be met by the intake of human milk in the absence of functional criteria for calcium status that corresponds to calcium intake in infants. The AI for older infants 7–12 months of age appertain to the intake of human milk along with the mean intake from complementary foods. A factorial approach was applied to estimate the EARs for older children from 1–18 years using data from studies of positive calcium balance and bone accretion [61].

Magnesium is necessary to maintain intracellular levels of potassium and calcium, and plays a role in the development and maintenance of bone and the health of other calcified tissues. Magnesium is a participant in over 300 enzymatic body processes [62]. The requirements for infants are based on human milk content of magnesium. Requirements for older infants 7–12 months of age are extrapolated values from younger infants with the addition of the average magnesium intake from solid foods. The requirements for children aged 1–18 years are estimated from balance studies in children and extrapolated values from these balance studies [62].

Phosphorus also supports bone and dental health and growth. In addition, phosphorus is necessary for maintaining normal body pH balance and is involved in several metabolic processes [62]. Intake requirements for phosphorus are higher in 9- to 18-year-old children compared to younger children because of the high tissue demand for phosphorus, changing rates of absorption efficiency and growth rate, and fluctuation of inorganic phosphorus in the extracellular fluid during this time of intense growth. To set an AI in the absence of functional criteria for phosphorous, the recommended intake for infants aged 0–6 months is based on mean intakes from human milk. Intake among 7–12 month infants is set with regard to the intake from human milk and solid foods. Recommendations for children 1–18 years of age are dependent on the phosphorus necessary for body accretion to support tissue composition and growth rates including corrections for absorption efficiency and urinary losses using a factorial approach [62].

The estimated vitamin K requirements for children aged 1–18 years can be attributed to the intake of vitamin K in apparently healthy populations. Uncertainty remains regarding the physiological significance of vitamin K indicators that are sensitive to diet and the extreme rarity of clinically significant vitamin K deficiency in the population. In infants, the AI for vitamin K is based on the average intake from human milk; values for 7–12 month infants are extrapolated on this basis [63].

The requirements for vitamin A are set to preserve adequate liver vitamin A stores. Vitamin A is important for a number of processes and functions including: normal vision, gene expression, reproduction, embryonic development, growth, proper function of the immune system, and to prevent vitamin A deficiency [63]. The AI for vitamin A intake in infants is relevant to the vitamin A content of human milk, and similar to other nutrients the AI in older infants (7–12 months) is extrapolated from the infant AI. In children aged 1–18 years, the AI is extrapolated from the adult data [63].

Vitamin C requirements are based on the estimated vitamin C body pool or tissue levels that are necessary to prevent antioxidant damage with minimal urinary loss. Vitamin C is necessary to prevent vitamin C deficiency or scurvy, and to provide antioxidant protection as derived from the correlation of antioxidant protection with neutrophil ascorbate concentrations and minimal urinary losses [64]. The requirements for infants 0–6 months of age were made in context to the content of human milk while older infant requirements pertain to the content of human milk and solid foods. Child recommendations are made by extrapolating the requirement set for adults.

Vitamin E is necessary for avoiding vitamin E deficiency and hydrogen peroxide-induced hemolysis. Requirements for infants 0–6 months are related to the vitamin E content of human milk and are extrapolated to older infants 7–12 months while requirements for children are extrapolated from adult values [64].

Adequate potassium for child age groups is necessary to counter excess sodium in the diet, to support healthy blood pressure, and to prevent potassium deficiency (i.e., elevated blood pressure, bone demineralization, and kidney stones) that may develop over time [65]. Potassium requirements for infants 0–6 months are set on the basis of the mean intake of potassium from human milk and intakes for infants 7–12 months reflect the mean intake from human milk plus the intake from complementary foods. The AI for children 1–18 years old is extrapolated from the adult AI on the basis of energy intake [65].

The IOM recommendations for fiber are based on total fiber intake, and do not separate the intake of "dietary fiber" and "functional fiber" [66]. "Dietary fibers" are non-digestible carbohydrates and lignin that are intrinsic and intact in plants. "Functional fiber" consists of isolated, non-digestible carbohydrates that have beneficial physiological effects in humans'. Neither an AI nor an EAR has been set for fiber in infants 0–1 years old. Requirements are related to the composition of human milk, which contains no fiber, and the lack of a theoretical justification for an AI among infants [66]. Achievement of the AI for fiber in children is helpful for relieving constipation and diverticular disease, preventing diet-related cancer, providing fuel for colonic cells, reducing levels of blood lipids and blood glucose, improving satiety while contributing little energy to the diet and helping to prevent obesity and the risk of adult-onset diabetes [66]. The fiber AI for children was extrapolated from adult values.

2.9 ESTABLISHING DRIs FOR SHORTFALL NUTRIENTS IN ADULTS

The DRI for vitamin D in younger adults (19–50 years) is set to maintain bone for the prevention of skeletal disorders later in life [61]. For older adults, the DRI is based on bone maintenance, minimized bone loss (51–70 years), and fracture prevention (>70 years). Vitamin D status of 50 nmol/L, assessed by serum 25-hydroxyvitamin D levels, is targeted to support bone health [61]. Cutaneous synthesis of vitamin D is difficult to assess as it is affected by season, latitude, time of day, sunscreen use, clothing, skin melatonin content, and other factors. Therefore, the IOM recommendations for vitamin D intake are based on the assumption of minimum sun exposure [61]. Recommendations for both younger and older adults are based on randomized control trials completed among women, as the data for men are limited [61]. Recommendations for pregnant and lactating women are consistent with the recommendations for non-pregnant/non-lactating women, due to the evidence presented by a randomized control trial and several observational studies indicating that maternal serum vitamin D status above the 50 nmol/L does not benefit maternal or infant bone mineral density [61].

Calcium is necessary for adults to maintain bone and neutral calcium balance in younger adults and older men, and to benefit bone mineral density, prevent osteoporosis, and prevent osteoporotic fractures in older adults. The recommendations for younger adults and older women are based on numerous intervention studies [61]. Recommendations for pregnant and lactating women are similar to those of non-pregnant/non-lactating women; maternal physiological changes provide the required calcium to the fetus and infant. Evidence does not support higher intake to protect maternal bone [61].

The recommendations for magnesium intake among adults are based on several balance studies that were completed to determine to the intake, necessary to maintain magnesium equilibrium and prevent negative magnesium balance. Various clinical studies have been performed in pregnant and lactating women but the results are inconsistent. The current magnesium recommendations for pregnant women include the increased requirement due to weight gain during pregnancy but the recommendations for lactating women are identical to non-lactating women [62].

Vitamin K deficiencies are rare and evidence to set an EAR and RDA are lacking [63]. The current vitamin K AI for adults is based on the median intakes surveyed from NHANES III. Vitamin K intakes were reported to be slightly lower in women compared with men, which is reflected in the lower AI for women (90 μg/day) compared to men (120 μg/day) [63]. Data from pregnant women supporting an effect of vitamin K intake on the fetus is lacking. One clinical study suggests that the dietary vitamin K intake of the lactating mother has minimal effect on the vitamin K concentration of milk [67]. In addition, the reported vitamin K intake of pregnant or lactating women is similar to or slightly lower than non-pregnant women [63]. Thus, the AIs for pregnant and lactating women are consistent with the recommendations for non-pregnant/non-lactating women.

Recommendations for vitamin A in adults assure "vitamin A reserves to cover increased needs during periods of stress and low vitamin A intake" [63]. This recommendation is calculated using the following values: percent of body vitamin A stores lost per day, minimum acceptable liver vitamin A reserves, liver weight to body weight ratio, reference weight for a specific age group and gender, ratio of total body to liver vitamin A reserves, and efficiency of storage of ingested vitamin A. The recommendations also incorporate consideration for the contributions of both carotenoids (at various levels of activity) and retinol to the total vitamin A intake. The accumulation of vitamin A in the fetal liver, the ratio of fetal liver to whole body vitamin A stores, and maternal absorption rate is additionally considered for pregnant women. Human milk (vitamin A) content is added to the recommendations of non-pregnant/non-lactating women to establish recommendations for lactating women [63].

Vitamin C requirements for adults aim to provide antioxidant protection, which is based on near-maximal neutrophil concentrations with minimal urinary loss [64]. Due to the lack of data in women, adult women's recommendations are extrapolated from values in men and based on body weight differences. Aging does not seem to affect absorption and metabolism of vitamin C, and thus the recommendations are consistent among all adult age groups. For pregnant women, the estimated vitamin C necessary for fetal transport was added to the recommendations of non-pregnant women to determine a final recommended intake. Recommendations for lactating women sum the average vitamin C produced in milk during the first 6 months of lactation with the recommendations for non-lactating women [64].

Vitamin E recommendations for adults are based on α-tocopherol intakes to prevent hydrogen peroxide-induced hemolysis [64]. Though γ-tocopherol is the most common form of vitamin E in fortified foods, biological activity has only been reported of in α-tocopherol. The vitamin E recommendations (as α-tocopherol) are based on clinical trials in men. Due to the lack of evidence for varying requirements in women and the greater fat mass of women despite smaller body weight compared to men, the requirements for vitamin E are equal for men and women. As with vitamin C, no data is available to suggest impaired absorption or utilization due to aging, and thus the requirements for younger adults and older adults are identical [64]. Pregnant women have the same requirements as non-pregnant women, but lactating women have requirements for the increased vitamin E to compensate for the amount secreted in breast milk [64].

The recommendations for potassium are set as an AI at 4700 mg/day for both men and women to lower blood pressure, blunt the adverse effects of sodium chloride on blood pressure, minimize the risk of kidney stones, and possibly reduce bone loss [65]. Potassium has received relatively less attention regarding functional and intake requirements compared with some other nutrients. Due to this lack of available research to establish an EAR, only an AI has been established for potassium. Potassium accretion during pregnancy is small and data providing a basis for a recommendation that varies from the recommendation for non-pregnant women is lacking. The AI for lactating women is set higher than the AI for adult women to compensate for milk potassium content (average 0.4 g/day), based on the assumption that the conversion of dietary potassium to milk potassium is 100% [65].

Fiber has many physiological health benefits, despite being nondigestible, which vary by the type of fiber, such as laxation, delay of gastric emptying, satiety, blood lipid normalization, attenuation of blood glucose, and prevention of coronary heart disease [66]. The AIs for total fiber are set at a level that protects against coronary heart disease and that supports a reduced risk of diabetes. The AI for fiber is equivalent for pregnant, lactating, and non-pregnant/non-lactating women [66].

Iron deficiency in pregnant women can result in fatigue, anemia, preterm birth, low-birth weight among infants, and possible cognitive impairments at birth. Iron recommendations for pregnant women are based on factorial modeling of the third trimester to build iron stores during the first trimester and meet the needs of the third trimester [63]. Iron requirements for lactating mothers were simulated by the sum of iron secreted in human milk and iron losses in non-pregnant/non-lactating women [63].

Adequate folate is essential for cell division and prevention of megaloblastic anemia during pregnancy. Folate requirements are based on intervention trials and controlled metabolic balance studies to maintain erythrocyte folate concentrations. The risk of neural tube defects (NTDs) is not covered in the recommendations for pregnant women, as NTDs form before most women know they are pregnant [68]. The DRI recommends that all women capable of becoming pregnant consume 400 μg dietary folate equivalents (DFEs) in addition to a varied diet to ensure adequacy and aid in the prevention of NTDs. Folate recommendations for pregnant women are higher compared with the recommendations for non-pregnant women for the purposes of maintaining serum folate status during pregnancy. The EAR for lactating women takes into account the folate excreted in milk and folate bioavailability in addition to accounting for the recommendations for non-lactating women [67].

2.10 NUTRIENT GAPS AMONG US CHILDREN AND ADOLESCENTS

Younger US children as a group met the EAR for more nutrients compared with adolescents and adults. However, shortfalls of many nutrients were still present for a part of the population of children and adolescents and are perhaps more concerning compared with the presence of shortfalls among adults due to the growth and development that children experience. Proper nutrient intake at specific times and in specific amounts during childhood may be necessary for children to achieve their full genetic potential in physical and mental growth and development. Thus, inadequate intake of nutrients during this critical life stage may have life-long effects.

2.10.1 Infancy

Infancy includes the first 12 months of life. The infancy stage is divided into two subgroups, age 0–6 months and age 7–12 months, based on differing growth rates during these life stages. Growth in the first 6 months is rapid compared with the 7–12 months stage. Very few studies quantifying nutrient intake for infants in the first three years of life are available. Two studies using data from the Feeding Infants and Toddlers Study (FITS) provide estimates of usual intake that were quantified from 2 to 3 separate 24-hour recalls, each collected via telephone interview. The studies included 862 infants 4–6 months old in 2002 [69], and 382 infants 0–5 months in 2008 [70]. Both studies were adjusted to be a representative of the US infants. Usual intake was estimated using the methods developed by Carriquiry et al. [9] and Nusser et al. [71], respectively. The mean usual *total* intake among US infants 0–5 months and 4–6 months exceeded the AI for the nutrients: vitamins C, B-6, B-12,

A, and K; thiamin; riboflavin; niacin; folate; calcium; phosphorus; magnesium; iron; zinc; sodium; and potassium. However, the mean usual *total* intake of vitamin D at 6.5 μg/day in 2008 and 6.4 μg/day in 2002 exceeded the previous AI of 5 μg/day but not the newly set AI of 10 μg/day [61]. In addition, the usual *total* intake of neither the 10th nor the 25th percentile met or exceed the AI for vitamin E, thiamin, niacin, folate, magnesium, iron, and zinc in 2008 [70].

The usual *total* nutrient intake for infants aged 6–11 months [70] and 7–11 months [69] was included in these studies and was similarly high in comparison with the DRIs. Mean *total* intakes in both studies for the 6–11 month and 7–11 month infants exceeded the AI for vitamins C, E, B6, B-12, A, K, thiamin, riboflavin, niacin, folate calcium, phosphorus, magnesium, sodium, and potassium [69,70]. The mean *total* vitamin D intake, again, exceeded the previous AI but neither the group mean intake nor the 75th percentile intakes exceeded the current AI of 10 μg/day [69,70]. The usual *total* intakes of neither the 10th nor the 25th percentiles met or exceeded the AI for vitamin E, magnesium, and sodium using the 2008 data [70]. An EAR is established for iron at 6.9 mg/day and for zinc at 2.5 mg/day in this 7–12 months age group. Approximately, 12% and 6% of US infants aged 6–11 months were estimated to have *total* intakes less than the EAR for iron and zinc respectively in 2008 [70].

The previous studies considered *total* nutrient intake, a study focused exclusively on the micronutrient intake among infants aged 0–5 months and 6–11 months from diet alone was not found. Dietary supplement use is very low among infants <1 year at only 11.9% as estimated by Picciano et al. using 1999–2002 NHANES data [72]. A more recent estimate using data from 2007–2010, included children <2 years old and reported an estimated 17% of children using dietary supplements. The prevalence of supplement use varies among childhood age groups, but seems to increase from infancy to approximately 45% among children 2–5 years old, the highest prevalence of supplement use among child age groups <20 years [73]. Micronutrient intake among supplement users and nonusers was contrasted in a study that included infants aged 6–11 months by Briefel et al. using FITS data from 2002 [74]. Significantly higher intakes were noted for supplement users regarding the mean usual intake of vitamin A, vitamin C, vitamin D, vitamin E, folate, vitamin B12, iron, and zinc. Among both, supplement users and nonusers, usual mean intakes, the lower 25th percentile, and even the lowest 10th percentile intakes either met or exceeded the AI for vitamin A, vitamin C, vitamin E, folate, vitamin B12, phosphorous, calcium, and potassium. The lowest 10th to 25th percentile of supplement users did not exceed the previous or current AI for vitamin D while dietary supplement nonusers mean usual intakes did exceed the previous but not the current AI for vitamin D. The EAR for iron was not met by approximately 10%–25% of supplement users and nonusers and the EAR for zinc was not met by less than 10% of all 7–11 month infants. Intakes of sodium among this life stage exceeded the AI by approximately 50%–75% of both supplement users and nonusers [74].

2.10.2 Toddlers

Toddlers aged 1–3 years are in a stage of rapid growth in height compared with older children, and thus, they are considered to be in a biologically different life stage for which unique DRIs are prescribed. In some cases, studies including toddlers have provided the necessary basis for setting an EAR. In others, an AI for the toddler lifestage was extrapolated from a child or adult EAR or AI [3].

The usual intake from diet alone for most US toddlers met the EAR for most nutrients for 2001–2002 using NHANES data. Toddlers comprise the age group whom, similar to infants, had few nutrient shortfalls, or for whom, a high proportion of the group achieved either the EAR or exceeded the AI for most nutrients compared with all other age groups. Estimates of usual intake [using the The National Cancer Institute (NCI) method] [75] from reported dietary intake alone were made using 2001–2002 data [76] in toddlers 1–3 years. Only less than 3% of all US toddlers did not meet the EAR for vitamin A, thiamin, riboflavin, niacin, vitamin B6, folate, vitamin B12, vitamin C, phosphorus, magnesium, iron, zinc, copper, and selenium, in 2001–2002 [76]. Approximately, 97% of the group exceeded the AI for sodium while 94% of US toddlers had a mean usual intake that exceeded the 500 mg AI for calcium using 2001–2002 data [76]. A similar estimate of 94% and 96% of US male and female toddlers with usual intakes that exceeded the calcium AI of 500 mg/day was calculated using 2003–2006 NHANES data [77]. A recent update of the DRIs has replaced the former AI with an EAR of 500 mg/day for calcium [61]. Despite US toddlers exceeding adequacy or requirements as a group for many nutrients, the usual intake for a few nutrients was not ideal. The usual vitamin E intake of 80% of US toddlers from diet alone did not meet the EAR in 2001–2002 and nutrients for which a vulnerable subset of the US toddler population did not surpass the AI in 2001–2002 were vitamin K at only 47% exceeding the AI, potassium at only 6% exceeding the AI, and fiber at less than 3% exceeding the AI [76]. The usual intake of vitamin D was estimated to exceed the 5 μg/day AI by 72% of male and 70% of female US infants [78], but the mean usual intake of 7.2 μg/day for males and 6.9 μg/day for females using 2005–2006 NHANES data would not exceed the recent vitamin D EAR of 10 μg/day [61,78]. The results of Briefel et al. [74] similarly identified vitamin E, potassium, vitamin D, and fiber as nutrients where a high proportion of the population did not exceed the AI or meet the EAR [74].

Approximately, 21% of US children less than 2 years reportedly used dietary supplements in 2003–2006 [77], and an estimated 39% of US children aged 1–3 years used supplements in 2003–2006 [79]. The inclusion of supplements improved the proportion of US toddlers reaching the EAR or exceeding the AI for certain nutrients when the estimates of nutrient intake from diet alone are compared with the estimates of *total* intake from diet and supplements. Estimates for *total* nutrient intake were available using data from the FITS 2008 study and represents US toddlers aged 1–3 years. The proportion of this group with vitamin E intakes that did not reach the EAR was 63%. The mean *total* usual vitamin K intake exceeded the AI for toddlers but the intake of the 25th percentile did not [70]. Neither the 50th nor the 90th percentile's mean *total* usual potassium intake (1736 mg/day and 2355 mg/day, respectively) reached the AI of 3000 mg/day. Similarly, neither the mean nor the 90th percentile usual *total* dietary fiber intake (8.7 g/day) met the AI of 19 g/day. The 10 μg/day EAR for vitamin D was not met by 10%–25% of the group [70]. Despite some methodology differences and a more recent time frame compared with the 2001–2002 estimates, the FITS 2008 estimates provide an indicator of the difference supplements make to the group attainment of nutrient intake. The estimated proportion of the population with usual *total* nutrient intake from diet and supplements that exceeded the AI or was less than the EAR was improved compared with the estimates from the diet alone but still quite high (≥10%) for vitamin E, vitamin K, potassium, fiber, and vitamin D. Out of these nutrients, only the mean nutrient intakes of vitamins E and D were significantly different between supplement users and nonusers using the 2002 FITS data [74].

2.10.3 Early Childhood

Evidence to establish DRIs for early childhood, the life stage including children aged 4–8 years, is readily available compared with the infant and toddler life stages. Various criteria were used to establish nutrient adequacy; but for nutrients where data was lacking, DRIs were developed by extrapolating data from infant or adult studies. The age range from 4 to 8 years is considered as a distinct life stage on the basis of growth velocity and endocrine status [3].

The shortfall of nutrients in young US children was similar to the shortfall of nutrients in infants and toddlers using the 2001–2002 data when diet alone was considered. Young children as a group did, however, achieve the required or adequate intake for more nutrients compared with older children and adults. Only 4% of the young children failed to meet the EAR for vitamin A, while only 3% did not meet the EAR for thiamin, riboflavin, niacin, vitamin B6, folate, vitamin B12, vitamin C, phosphorus, magnesium, iron, zinc, copper, and selenium. Approximately, 69% of the young children had a mean usual intake that exceeded the AI of 800 mg for calcium (mg/day) and >97% exceeded the AI for sodium in 2001–2002 [76]. The mean usual calcium intake using 2003–2006 data was estimated to exceed the previous AI and the current EAR of 800 mg at 1058 mg/day for males and 951 mg/day for females [78]. The usual intake of most young children (80%) did not meet the EAR for vitamin E, and approximately 14% of the young children did not exceed the AI for vitamin K. Only 3% of the young children exceeded the AI for potassium and less than 3% had intakes that were greater than the AI for fiber [76]. Mean vitamin D intake was estimated at 6.4 μg/day in males and 5.5 μg/day in females using 2005–2006 NHANES data. This mean did exceed the previous AI of 5 μg/day [78], but does not exceed the current EAR of 10 μg/day [61].

The usual nutrient intake from diet alone and *total* nutrient intake was quantified and included 1264 child participants aged 2–8 years in the NHANES 2003–2006 study [77]. Dietary supplements were reportedly used by 42% of young US children. Non-Hispanic white children had a higher prevalence of use (50%) compared with non-Hispanic black (27%) and Mexican American (29%) children. The mean nutrient intakes of US children from diet alone were not different between supplement users and nonusers. But, the proportion of non-supplement users with usual nutrient intakes that did not meet the EAR was greater than the proportion of supplement users that did not meet the EAR when reported dietary intake alone was considered among children aged 2–18 years for calcium, magnesium, phosphorus, vitamin A, and vitamin C. The *total* mean nutrient intake among males and females was higher among supplement users aged 2–8 years compared with the intakes of non-supplement users for iron, magnesium, zinc, copper, folate, vitamin B6, vitamin B12, vitamin A, vitamin C, vitamin D, and vitamin E and for calcium and selenium among females [77]. Young children who did not use supplements also had a significantly higher prevalence of inadequacy compared with young children who did use supplements with respect to their usual intake of calcium (23% for nonusers and 13% for users), vitamin A (5% for nonusers and <1% for users), vitamin C (2% for nonusers and <1% for users), vitamin D (81% for nonusers and 27% for users), and vitamin E (64% for nonusers and 3.7% for users) when intake from diet and supplements was considered [77]. Regarding these findings, the proportion of young children attaining nutrient adequacy among supplement users compared with nonusers was especially improved for calcium, vitamin D, and vitamin E. Inadequacy, however, was still prevalent for over 10% of supplement users when the *total* intakes of calcium and vitamin D were considered.

2.10.4 Puberty/Adolescence

The adolescent life stage is divided into two groups. DRIs for these life stages vary based on gender. The female and male growth spurts span across ages of 9–13 years and 14–18 years, respectively, and are accompanied by sexual development and diverse hormonal changes for which nutrient needs correspond [3].

Young adolescents aged 9–13 years as a group generally met the requirement or attained adequate intakes from diet alone for more nutrients than did adolescents aged 14–18 years and adults during 2001–2002 [76]. However, these younger adolescents as a group also did not meet the required or adequate intake for as many nutrients compared with younger children. In addition, females of both younger and older adolescents as a group met the nutrient requirements or attained adequate intakes for fewer nutrients compared with males when intake from diet alone was considered. The EAR for thiamin, riboflavin, niacin, vitamin B6, folate (DFE), vitamin B12, iron, copper, and selenium was not met by only 3% of female and male adolescents aged 9–13 years. Approximately, 9% of the females and 8% of the males aged 9–13 years had usual intakes less than the EAR for vitamin C, an estimated 10% of females and less than 3% of males did not meet the EAR for zinc, and an estimated 34% of females and 13% of males did not reach the EAR for vitamin A [76]. The magnesium and phosphorus EARs were not attained by approximately 44% and 42% of females, respectively. The proportion of males who did not meet the magnesium and phosphorous EARs was lower at only 14% and 9%, respectively. But, the proportion of both females and males who did not meet the EAR for vitamin E was high and 95% and 97%, respectively. Less than 3% of the adolescent males and females had a usual intake that exceeded the AI for potassium and fiber. The percentage of young adolescents aged 9–13 years with intakes greater than that of calcium was similarly low for females at only 6% and males at 28% based on the 2001–2002 NHANES data [76]. More recently, estimates indicate female usual calcium intake at 968 mg/day and male usual intake at 1074 mg/day using 2003–2006 NHANES data [78]. None of these estimates met the newly updated EAR of 1100 mg/day for young adolescents aged 9–13 years [61]. The AI of vitamin K was only exceeded by 9% of females and 27% of males. Adolescent usual intake exceeded the AI for sodium at approximately

97% for both males and females [76]. Vitamin D usual intake was 5.6 μg/day for males and 5.2 μg/day for females using 2005–2006 NHANES data; estimates that did not exceed the new EAR for vitamin D at 10 μg/day [61].

Supplement use among 9- to 13-year-old children was estimated at 29% and was lower compared with younger children aged 2- to 8-years-old. Mean nutrient intake from diet alone was not different for consumers of dietary supplements and non-consumers of dietary supplements, similar to the relationship between supplement and non-supplement users of young children aged 2–8 years [77]. When *total* intake was considered, male dietary supplement users had significantly higher mean intakes of calcium, iron, zinc, and copper compared with nonusers while female users had higher intakes of calcium, iron, magnesium, zinc, phosphorus, and copper compared with nonusers. Both male and female supplement users had higher mean intakes of folate, vitamins B6, B12, A, C, D, and E compared with nonusers. Differences among users and nonusers were not noted, however, for vitamin K. Estimates of the prevalence of inadequacy varied among supplement users and nonusers. Supplement users had a lower prevalence of inadequacy regarding usual intakes of calcium (66% of nonusers and 46% of users), iron (0.4% of nonusers and 0% of users), magnesium (33% of nonusers and 18% of users), zinc (7.3% of nonusers and <1% of users), folate (2.4% of nonusers and <1% of users), vitamin B6 (2.6% of nonusers and <1% of users), vitamin A (30% of nonusers and 1.5% of users), vitamin C (20% of nonusers and 1.7% of users), vitamin D (89% of nonusers and 32% of users), and vitamin E (89% of nonusers and 12% of users) when *total* intake was considered [77]. Similar to children aged 2–8 years, the use of supplements improved nutrient intakes among users for all shortfall nutrients, but the proportion of the group gaining adequacy was differentially improved among certain of the shortfall nutrients identified, these were: calcium, magnesium, vitamin A, vitamin C, vitamin D, and vitamin E. However, even among supplement users inadequate intake of calcium, magnesium, vitamin D, and vitamin E remained high at over 10% [77].

The usual nutrient intake from diet alone among older adolescents aged 14–18 years varied more between males and females compared with the 9–14 years age group. Similar nutrients may be classified as shortfalls for younger adolescent males compared with older adolescent males with the exception of magnesium, a shortfall nutrient for older adolescent males. Only 3% or fewer older adolescent males aged 14–18 years did not meet the EAR for thiamin, riboflavin, niacin, vitamin B6, vitamin B12, iron, copper, and selenium while approximately 4% did not meet the EAR for zinc and folate (DFE) [76]. The usual intake of phosphorus was not achieved by an estimated 9% of older adolescent males in 2001–2002 and 26% did not achieve the EAR for vitamin C. Nutrients where a majority of the life stage did not attain the EAR included vitamin A for 55%, vitamin E for less than 97%, and as previously mentioned, magnesium for whom 78% did not fulfill the average requirement [76]. The calcium mean usual intake of 1266 mg/day for males using 2005–2006 NHANES data [78] exceeded the EAR of 1100 mg/day but a proportion of the group may have intakes that do not fulfill the average requirement. A small proportion of 14- to 18-year-old adolescent male usual intakes exceeded the AI for vitamin K at 18%, potassium at less than 3%, and fiber at less than 3% [76]. Vitamin D was a shortfall nutrient for both males and females. The mean usual intake of females aged

14–18 years from diet alone using NHANES 2003–2006 data was approximately 3.8 μg/day while the male intake was estimated at 6.1 μg/day [78]. Neither of these estimates reached the EAR of 10 μg/day [61]. Sodium intake, unsurprisingly, was greater than the AI for over 97% of male and female adolescents aged 14–18 years using 2001–2002 data [76]. Nutrients for which only a small proportion of older female adolescents did not meet the average requirement include thiamin for which 12% did not meet the EAR, riboflavin and niacin at 6%, vitamin B6 at 16%, folate (DFE) at 19%, vitamin B12 at 8%, iron at 16%, zinc at 26%, copper at 16%, and selenium at 3% of the life stage who did not attain the average requirement. Nutrient gaps among older adolescent females were present for several nutrients including vitamin A (54% did not meet the EAR), vitamin E (97% did not meet the EAR), vitamin C (42% did not meet the EAR), phosphorus (49% did not meet the EAR), and magnesium (91% did not meet the EAR). A small proportion of older adolescent females exceeded the AI for other nutrients, including: potassium and fiber at less than 3% and vitamin K at only 13% in 2001–2002 [76]. In addition, calcium is a nutrient of concern; mean usual intakes were estimated at 876 mg/day from diet alone, falling short of the 1100 mg/day EAR [78].

The prevalence of dietary supplement use among older adolescents aged 14–18 years was estimated at 26%, and 29% for younger adolescents aged 9–13 years using 2003–2006 NHANES data [77]. As with the younger life-stage age groups, differences in the mean usual nutrient intake from diet alone were not significantly different among supplement users and non-supplement users. However, when *total* mean usual dietary intake was compared among supplement users and nonusers, mean usual intakes for supplement users were significantly higher for folate, vitamin B6, vitamin B12, vitamin A, vitamin C, vitamin D, and vitamin E. Differences in the mean usual intake of vitamin K among supplement users compared with nonusers was higher for males but not for females. The prevalence of inadequacy was higher in those who did not use supplements compared with supplement users for calcium (67% of nonusers and 38% of users), magnesium (84% of nonusers and 52% of users), zinc (12.7% of users and 1.7% of nonusers), copper (8.5% of nonusers and 2.1% of users), folate (10.9% of nonusers and 1.1% of users), vitamin B6 (10% of nonusers and <1% of users), vitamin B12 (3.1% of users and <1% of users), vitamin A (59% of nonusers and 5.9% of users), vitamin C (42% of nonusers and 7.3% of users), vitamin D (93% of nonusers and 36% of users), and vitamin E (97% of nonusers and 21% of users). Differences in the prevalence of *total* intake for supplement users and nonusers were not noted for iron, phosphorous, or selenium [77]. The proportion of older adolescents achieving adequacy for calcium, magnesium, zinc, folate, vitamin B6, vitamin A, vitamin C, vitamin D, and vitamin E was improved by at least an estimated 10% of supplement users compared with nonusers. However, as noted among younger age groups, despite supplement use the prevalence of inadequacy remained high at over 10% and even over 20% of supplement users for calcium, magnesium, vitamin D, and vitamin E.

2.10.5 Summary

Nutrient gaps exist for every age-stage group. A proportion of all of the age groups had difficulty meeting the EAR or AI for vitamins D and E. Other nutrients that were common shortfalls among the age groups, regardless of the inclusion of intake from dietary supplements, included potassium, fiber, and vitamin K. Other shortfall nutrients were only identified for certain ages or for a certain gender such as for calcium, magnesium, zinc, phosphorus, vitamin A, and vitamin C. Shortfall of nutrients generally increases in number along with age, in other words, as children age as a group, a higher proportion meet less nutrient DRIs for their age group compared with younger children. In addition, adolescent females, as a group, meet the DRIs for fewer nutrients than do their male counterparts. The consequences of these nutrient gaps may have relevance to the growth, development, and health of children and health in later adulthood.

The increases in prevalence of nutrient shortfalls are not matched by the prevalence of supplement use among child age groups that generally increase from infancy to a high at approximately 42% usage among children 2- to 8-years-old. The use of supplements did decrease the prevalence of nutrient gaps for certain nutrients among certain age groups, but even among supplement users the intakes of vitamin D and calcium were still shortfalls for many (10%) children among almost all childhood age groups.

Magnesium and phosphorus are nutrient shortfalls for older adolescent males and females aged 14–18 years, a critical life stage for bone accumulation. Similarly, the mean usual intake of neither females nor males aged 9–13 years, encompassing the period of maximum bone accumulation for females, met the EAR for calcium [78]. Mean usual vitamin D intakes for both 9–13 and 14- to 18-year-olds also did not attain the average requirement. The alignment of inadequacy for magnesium, phosphorus, vitamin D, and calcium among adolescents and especially adolescent females may have lifelong effects to bone development and the attainment of peak bone mass, increasing the risk of osteoporosis in later adulthood [61]. The manifestation of other nutrient shortfalls such as vitamins A and C during adolescence and the additional inadequate intakes of vitamin E, potassium, and fiber during the adolescent years may be particularly consequential during this time of heightened growth velocity and sexual development [80].

2.11 NUTRIENT GAPS AMONG US ADULTS

The DRI guidelines divided the age groups for adults as 19–30 years, 31–50 years, 51–70 years, and over 70 years of age [61,63–66,68]. Divisions for the age groups 19–30 years and 31–50 years are made based on the possibility of nutrient intake affecting peak bone mass during early adulthood (19–30 years) and the decrease in energy expenditure. The age group of 51–70 years is a time of active work for most adults whereas adults over 70 exhibit increasing variability between individuals in energy expenditure and other physical and physiological functions. Depending on the nutrient, recommendations may be the same or different for different age groups among adulthood [3].

Assessment of usual intake from foods in US adults aged 19–31 years using NHANES revealed that as a population, men and women had inadequate intakes of similar nutrients such as vitamin A, vitamin E, magnesium, vitamin K, vitamin D, potassium, and fiber [76,78]. Ninety-seven percent or more of US men met the EAR for thiamin, riboflavin, niacin, vitamin B6, vitamin B12, phosphorus, iron, copper, and selenium in 2001–2002 [76]. More than 90% of men met the EAR for folate and zinc [76]. Mean calcium intake of men exceeds the EAR when diet alone was considered, with 63% consuming more than the AI (1000 mg/day) in 2003–2006, which was the recommendation at the time of analysis but is lower than the current EAR (800 mg/day) [78]. Thus, a higher proportion of men in this age group would meet the current EAR by diet alone. On the other hand, 37% of men did not meet the EAR for vitamin C [76]. Mean vitamin D intake for men was 5.1 μg/day, similar to the previous AI (5 μg/day), but lower than the current EAR of 10 μg/day [78]. Only 39% of men exceeded the AI for vitamin D in 2003–2006. A high proportion of the population did not meet the EAR for vitamin A (58%), vitamin E (89%), or magnesium (55%) [76]. Less than 3% exceeded the AI for vitamin K and fiber, and only 5% exceeded the AI for potassium. However, over 97% of men exceeded the AI of sodium. On the other hand, among women in this age group, the majority of the population met the EAR for thiamin (92%), riboflavin (95%), niacin (95%), vitamin B6 (77%), folate (86%), vitamin B12 (91%), vitamin C (60%), phosphorus (96%), iron (85%), zinc (87%), copper (89%), and selenium (96%) [76]. The prevalent attainment of the EAR for the B-vitamins (thiamin, riboflavin, niacin, folate, and vitamin B12) may be influenced by the fortification of many foods in the US food supply. The mean intake of calcium from diet was 838 mg/day, which also exceeds the current EAR (800 mg/day) but was below the AI (1000 mg/day) at the time of data collection. As for vitamin D intake, 21% of women consumed more than the previous AI of 5 μg/day, but no data is available with the current EAR recommendations [78]. The EAR was not met by more than 97% for vitamin E, 58% for vitamin A, and 64% for magnesium. Only 22% of the women exceeded the EAR for vitamin K; but similar to men, less than 3% consumed more than the AI for potassium and fiber. The sodium AI was also exceeded by more than 97% of the women [76].

The rate of supplement use in 2003–2006 using NHANES data from adults aged 19–30 years was 39% [79]. Supplement intakes ranged from 34% to 39% for calcium [78], 22% to 25% for vitamins A, B, C, D (2005–2006), and E, zinc, and magnesium, and 15%–17% for selenium, chromium, and vitamin K [78,81]. Supplement users were more likely to meet the EAR compared to nonusers in this population. Among the above deficient nutrients, the percentage of women with adequate intakes was higher among users compared with nonusers for vitamin A (96% users vs. 27% nonusers), vitamin D (41% users vs. 1% nonusers), and vitamin E (87% users vs. 1% nonusers) [82]. Men showed a similar trend. The percentage of men with adequate intakes among supplement users was higher than nonusers for vitamin A (96% users vs. 35% nonusers), vitamin C (95% users vs. 51% nonusers), vitamin D (64% users vs. 6% nonusers), and vitamin E (95% users vs. 6% nonusers) [77]. In addition, the mean usual intake of vitamin A from foods was higher in supplement users compared to nonusers in women.

The nutrient adequacy of usual intake from foods in adults 31–50 years of age was similar to that of adults 19–30 years in 2001–2002. Men and women had similar patterns of inadequacy in this group. Men met the EAR for thiamin (>97%), riboflavin (>97%), niacin (>97%), vitamin B6 (>97%), folate (>97%), vitamin B12 (>97%), vitamin C (60%), phosphorus (>97%), calcium (56%), iron (>97%), zinc (96%), copper (>97%), and selenium (>97%) [76]. Inadequate nutrients include vitamin A (55% below EAR), vitamin E (90% below EAR), magnesium (61% below EAR), and may also include vitamin K (15% above AI), potassium (5% above AI), and fiber (<3% above AI) [76]. In addition, only 39% consumed more than the previous AI (5 μg/day) for vitamin D, which is half the current EAR [78]. Women, as a population in 2003–2006, had adequate intakes of thiamin (94%), riboflavin (>97%), niacin (96%), vitamin B6 (79%), folate (84%), vitamin B12 (93%), vitamin C (59%), phosphorus (>97%), iron (83%), zinc (89%), copper (92%), and selenium (>97%) [76]. The previous AI for calcium (1000 mg/day) was met by 30% of the population through food intake in 2003–2006 [78]. Though there is no published data on the percentage of the population that met the current calcium EAR (800 mg/day), one could expect that the prevalence of adequate intake should be greater, especially as the mean calcium intake from food exceeds 800 mg/day [76]. The proportion of women whose dietary intake exceeded the vitamin K AI was higher than men but still relatively low (39%) in 2001–2002. Potassium and fiber AIs were exceeded by <3 and 5% of women, respectively. Sodium intake exceeded the AI by over 97% of both men and women [76].

Forty-nine percent of adults aged 31–50 years consumed any kind of supplement during 2003–2006 [79]. During this period, use of supplement by nutrient was 45%–52% for calcium (2005–2006 [78]), 26%–30% for vitamins A, B, C, and E, zinc, and magnesium, 21%–22% for selenium, iron, chromium, and 19% for vitamin K [78,81]. Supplemental vitamin D intake prevalence was 34% with a mean supplemental dose between 6 and 7.5 μg/day (2005–2006) [78], Non-supplement users had significantly higher frequency of inadequacy compared to supplement users for folate (21% nonusers vs. 1% users), vitamin C (48% nonusers vs. 4% users), vitamin B6 (19% nonusers vs. 0.33% users), vitamin B12 (6.8% nonusers vs. 0.1% users), vitamin A (55% nonusers vs. 2.3% users), vitamin D (98% nonusers vs. 31% users), and vitamin E (98% nonusers vs. 8.6% users) [82].

The assessment of usual intake from diet alone points to similar nutrient gaps in adults aged 51–70 years compared with adults aged 31–50 years using 2001–2002 NHANES data, and lower percentages reaching sufficiency compared to younger adults [76]. In men, the EAR was reached by over 97% for riboflavin, niacin, phosphorus, iron, copper, and selenium [76]. The EAR for thiamin was met by 94%, vitamin B6 by 84%, folate by 93%, vitamin C by 61%, and zinc by 80% among men aged 51–70 years. Intakes did not meet the EAR for vitamin A (55%), vitamin E (90%), vitamin D (93%), and magnesium (70%) among men [76]. Only 22% of men in this age group exceeded the previous calcium AI of 1200 mg/day, with a mean intake of 951 mg/day, which is below the current EAR for this group (1000 mg/day) [78]. Sodium intake exceeded the AI in over 97% of the men in this age group [76]. Interestingly, 57% of women met the EAR for vitamin A. In addition, over 50% of women met the EAR for thiamin (88%), riboflavin (96%), niacin (96%), vitamin B6 (67%), folate (86%), vitamin C (71%), phosphorus (96%), iron (>97%), zinc (82%), copper (90%), and selenium (>97%). Inadequate nutrient intakes for women included vitamin E, magnesium, vitamin K, potassium, and fiber. The percentage of people not meeting the EAR for vitamin B12 was not specified in the NHANES/WWEIA 2001–2002 analyses [76]. This was due to the recommendation to consume vitamin B12 fortified foods or supplements as 10%–30% of the older population are not capable of absorbing food-bound vitamin B12. However, the report did indicate that over 95% of men and over 90% of women consumed amounts exceeding the EAR as food-bound vitamin B12. Similar to men, over 97% of women exceeded the AI for sodium [76].

Supplement intakes of men and women, aged 51–70 years, were 58% and 72%, respectively, in 2003–2006 [79]. Prevalence of supplemental intake of vitamin D was 40% with a mean supplemental dose of approximately 10 μg/day [78]. Vitamins A, B6, B12, C, and E, zinc, and magnesium supplement use ranged from 34% to 37% [79]. The prevalence of the use of vitamin K supplement was approximately 27%, selenium and chromium 29%–30%, and iron 16% [81]. Calcium supplement use differed greatly between men and women, 51% of men and 67% of women consumed calcium supplements [78]. In the years 1994–1996, inadequacy of vitamin A, vitamin C, and magnesium decreased with supplementation in men [83]. During the same time frame, vitamin B6, folate, vitamin C, and magnesium supplementation decreased the inadequacy of these nutrients in women [83]. Data from 2003–2006 indicated a lower prevalence of inadequacy in supplement users compared to nonusers for folate, vitamin C, vitamin A, vitamin B6, vitamin D, and vitamin E in both men and women and additionally for vitamin B12 in women [82].

The prevalence of vitamin A inadequacy from foods was lower among adults 71 years and older compared with younger adults, but greater proportions of adults did not meet the EAR for vitamin B6, vitamin C, magnesium, or zinc compared to younger adults [76]. Three percent or fewer men did not meet the EAR for riboflavin, niacin, phosphorus, iron, or selenium, or copper. The EAR was not met by 7% for thiamin, 23% for vitamin B6, 11% for folate, and 30% for zinc. Forty-two percent of men did not meet the vitamin C EAR, and 51% did not meet the EAR for vitamin A. Finally, 94% did not meet the EAR for vitamin E. Less than 3% of men exceeded the AI for potassium, and 3% for fiber. The prevalence of vitamin K intakes exceeding the AI was 33% [76] and only 15% of men exceeded the previous AI for calcium (1200 mg/day) through diet [78]. The mean calcium intake for this population was 871 mg/day, which is still below the current EAR (1000 mg/day). Mean vitamin D intake was 5.6 μg/day in 2005–2006, approximately 50% of the current EAR [78]. For women, 3% or less did not meet the EAR for riboflavin, selenium, and iron [76]. The prevalence of intakes under the EAR for thiamin was 12%, niacin 13%, folate 21%, phosphorus 5%, and copper 14%; the prevalence of inadequacy of vitamin A (38%), zinc (36%), vitamin C (40%), and vitamin B6 (49%) varied from the estimates among other adult age groups. Magnesium was still the most widely deficient nutrient with 82% not reaching the EAR. Furthermore, 48% of women had an intake of vitamin K that was higher than the AI guideline, but the percentage of women reaching the AI for potassium and fiber were still low at <3 to 8%, respectively [76]. Mean calcium intake was 748 mg/day and mean vitamin D intake was 4.5 μg/day in 2005–2006 in women [78]. Over 97% of the population exceeded the AI for sodium [76].

The prevalence of supplement use is higher in men 71 years and older compared to those 51–70 years, and reaches a similar prevalence of supplement use compared with that of women in 2003–2006 [79]. The proportion of the population that use vitamin B6, vitamin B12, vitamin C, vitamin K, iron, calcium, zinc, magnesium, selenium, and/or chromium containing supplements was similar to the proportion using these supplements among adults aged 51–70 years. Supplemental vitamin A usage was 33%, vitamin D was 49%, and vitamin E was 35% [79]. Sebastian et al. [83] reported those taking supplements had higher mean food intake of magnesium (men and women) and vitamin B6, folate, and vitamin E (women) in 1994–1996. In addition, a smaller proportion of supplement users had intakes below the EAR for vitamins A, B6, B12, C, and E, folate, magnesium, and zinc compared to that of non-users [83]. This is consistent with the more recent report that analyzed 2003–2006 intakes [82]. In addition, vitamin D supplement users compared to nonusers had a higher percentage of the group that met the previous AI (85% vs. 4%) [77].

2.11.1 Summary

Nutrient gaps in adults include calcium, potassium, vitamin D, magnesium, and fiber regardless of the adult age group. Vitamin E may also be a gap. In contrast to children and adolescents, the number or type of shortfall of nutrients changes minimally among different adult age groups. However, the proportion of the population meeting the vitamin B6, vitamin C, magnesium, and zinc EARs tends to decrease with age in both sexes. Surprisingly, in women, the prevalence of vitamin A deficiency decreases with age despite the unchanged recommendations. Supplement usage increases with age among adults, especially for calcium and vitamin D. In addition, supplement users are more likely to meet the recommendations by diet alone than nonusers.

2.12 NUTRIENT GAPS AMONG PREGNANT WOMEN

Surprisingly little information is available regarding the current nutrient intake of pregnant women at the national level, despite the higher nutrient needs present during pregnancy. According to the limited existing data, pregnant women meet their nutrient needs better than or at a comparable prevalence compared to non-pregnant women when recommendations are the same. According to a 2005–2006 report, 73% had usual intakes from food and water above the recommendations (AI) for calcium (vs. 28%–33% in non-pregnant women) and 46% had usual intakes from food and water below the EAR for magnesium (vs. 48%–65% in non-pregnant women) [84]. Here, we will focus on iron and folate on the grounds that for these two nutrients, adequate intake is critical during pregnancy. Recommendations for iron and folate increase beyond the amount proportionate to increased energy expenditure during pregnancy, and current intake data exists.

A frequently deficient nutrient in pregnant women is iron. To date, no studies to our knowledge have been published on the iron intake of pregnant women using the NHANES data. Unpublished analyses by Park and Eicher-Miller [85] using NHANES 1999–2010, found pregnant US women to consume 15 mg/day of iron from food and beverages. This is much below the EAR for pregnant women (23 mg/day for 14- to 19-years-old, 22 mg/day for those aged 20 and older) [63]. Similarly, Rifas-Shiman et al. [86] observed mean iron intakes in a Massachusetts cohort of pregnant women in their first trimester to be 16.7 mg/day and Siega-Riz et al. [87] reported on a North Carolina cohort with mean intakes of 20 mg iron/day during the second trimester.

The use of supplements during pregnancy in the United States is high. According to NHANES data collected in 1999–2006, about 72.5% of pregnant women take supplements containing iron with a mean supplemental iron intake of 47.7 mg/day [88]. The prevalence of supplement use among pregnant women increases as pregnancy progresses. The use of dietary supplements containing iron is approximately 56% in the first trimester, and increases to 90% by the third trimester [88]. Iron needs also dramatically increase as pregnancy progresses. This situation results in a higher prevalence of iron deficiency assessed by total body iron during the third trimester and despite a higher prevalence of iron supplementation [89].

To date, folate intake in pregnant women has not been assessed using NHANES data. Women from Massachusetts, in a study by Rifas-Shiman et al. [86] in 1999–2002, reported a mean intake of 365 μg folate/day from diet during the first trimester and women in the North Carolina report a mean 668 μg DFE/day intake during the second trimester during 1995–1998 [87]. In the latter report, the 50th percentile intake surpassed the recommended intake for pregnant women. However, NHANES (1999–2006) data reveal that similar to iron supplement intake, mean prevalence of supplements containing folic acid is 74%, increasing from 60% to 89% from the first trimester to the third trimester [88]. Mean supplemental folic acid intake is 817 μg/day in pregnant women [88].

2.12.1 Summary

Nationally representative data of nutrient intake in pregnant and lactating women are limited. Among existing studies, mean intake of iron and folate from reported dietary intake in pregnant women is below the EAR. Supplemental iron and folate usage is prevalent and mean supplemental doses are above the EARs for pregnant women ensuring adequate nutrition. More research using nationally representative data is needed to understand the nutrient gaps of this population.

2.12.2 Supplement Use among US Children and Adults

The intake of supplements among US adults has been increasing over the past 30 years in most age groups. Data from NHANES 1987, 1992, and 2000 show that the percentage of adults using vitamins and mineral supplements is on the rise (in adults ≥ age 25 years) with estimates of 23.2% (1987), 23.7% (1992), and 33.9% (2000) [90]. More recently, 49% of the US adults were estimated to be using a dietary supplement using the NHANES data from 2007–2010 [91]. This trend was consistent for both men and women and across Non-Hispanic White, Non-Hispanic Black, Hispanic, and other race/ethnicities [79,90].

Supplementation has been described as an effective way for subgroups of the population to meet requirements or to attain adequate intakes of some nutrients. Yet, the efficacy of supplementation to improve the prevalence of inadequate intakes is tempered by the negative impact that supplements impart on a proportion of the population that exceeds the UL when supplements are used, an issue of primary concern among pediatric populations. A thorough examination of the distribution of usual intake of a population must be considered, before supplements are recommended. Public health officials, practitioners, and policy makers must consider the risk of a proportion of the population exceeding the UL and balance this with the proportion of the population at risk of inadequacy when recommendations for the entire population or subpopulation are made [3].

Characteristics associated with greater vitamin and mineral supplement usage found by Millen et al. were female, non-Hispanic white, and older than 65 years ($p < 0.001$) [90]. Radimer et al. [92] also found female gender, older age, more education, non-Hispanic white, physical activity, normal or underweight, more frequent wine or spirit consumption, former smoking, and excellent or very good self-reported health to be associated with greater use of any supplement, multivitamin, or multi-mineral use in bivariate analysis [92]. The finding of positive health risk behaviors associated with supplement use was corroborated by results of a study by Balluz et al. [93] using the Behavioral Risk Factor Surveillance System (BRFSS) in 13 states in 2001. Vitamin and supplement use was found to be 1.46 times greater in participants that demonstrated "positive health risk behaviors" compared with those who did not demonstrate these behaviors ($p < 0.0001$). "Positive health risk behavior" was classified as nonsmoking, physically active, not a binge drinker or heavy drinker, not overweight or obese, and no more than one negative health behavior [93]. Similarly, Foote et al. [94] found supplement use to increase with positive health behaviors and other characteristics in gender-specific ethnic groups such as age, education, physical activity, fruit intake, and dietary fiber; and to decrease with obesity, smoking, and dietary fat intake [94]. Using NHANES 2007–2010 data, most adult and children reported using dietary supplements because of a perceived role in overall health [91].

The parents of children using supplements were found to more prevalently exhibit certain characteristics including higher levels of education [95], non-Hispanic white race/ethnicity, older, married, insured, higher household incomes, and consumers of supplements during pregnancy (for mothers) compared with parents of children not consuming supplements [96]. Supplement use among infants <1 year was low compared with other age groups at only (11.9%) with a dramatic increase for toddlers aged 1–3 years at 38.4% [72], and a continued increase for children aged 4–8 years at 42% [77]. The prevalence declined for adolescents at 29% for 9- to 13-year-olds and 26% for 14- to 18-year-olds [77]. Child supplement users compared with nonusers were also prevalently non-Hispanic white, of higher annual family incomes, and in households without smokers [72]. Adolescent supplement users were more likely to be white [97,98] female, nonsmokers, physically active, of normal weight, involved in team sports, and less frequent TV watchers when compared with nonusers [97]. Lower media/computer use, greater physical activity, lower body mass index, health insurance coverage, better access to health care, and better self-reported health were also associated with greater use of dietary supplements among US children 2–17 years of age [99]. Children who use supplements appear to have healthier lifestyles and healthier diet practices compared with nonusers, similar to the characteristics for adults. Supplement users as a group, while benefiting from supplement use, are not the individuals at greatest risk of inadequacy who tend to be members of minority groups, of low socioeconomic status, and with less healthy diets and lifestyles.

2.13 CHAPTER SUMMARY

Nutrient intake of the population must be compared against the nutrient needs in order to identify the nutrient gaps of a population. The DRIs are evidence-based recommendations, set for specific age, sex, and reproductive stage population groups according to their physiological needs with the goal to maximize health outcomes of the population. The first step in determining usual intakes of a population is dietary assessment of individuals. The most common dietary intake assessment tools are 24-hour recalls, food records, and FFQs, which are frequently connected to a database containing the nutrient content of various foods the population may consume. Reported dietary intake and reported intake from supplements are considered and compared against the recommended intakes (AI or EAR). By calculating the percentage of the population that is deficient (or that exceeds the recommendations), population nutrition gaps can be identified.

This chapter has identified several nutrient gaps in US children and adults. High percentages of children did not meet the recommendations for vitamin D and vitamin E by diet alone. In general, the proportion of children that do not meet the DRIs increase with age and female adolescents meet the DRI for fewer nutrients compared to males. A high proportion of adults did not meet recommended intakes for vitamin D, calcium, magnesium, vitamin A, vitamin E, potassium, and fiber by diet, but prevalence of deficiency for vitamin A from diet alone decreased with age among adults. Little data is available for the nutrient intakes of pregnant and lactating women. More attention to nutrient intake is necessary for women in this critical period of life to ensure the health of both the mother and child. Identifying the nutrients that are inadequately consumed in the US population is a preliminary step to determining and promoting a healthy diet for the population.

The use of supplements clearly reduces the prevalence of nutrient gaps for some nutrients in children, and is especially effective in adults. Supplement use increases from infancy to a high prevalence among children aged 2–5 years and decreases during adolescence (9–18 years), and then continues to increase throughout adulthood. As would be expected, the proportion of supplement users that do not meet the recommended intakes is lower than nonusers. For pregnant women, supplemental iron and folate intake increases with the progression of pregnancy. In addition, some characteristics, such as age, sex, race, education status, income status, and health-related behaviors, differ between supplement users and nonusers and between the parents of children consuming supplements and nonconsumers. Higher intake of certain nutrients can be encouraged not only for individuals with insufficient intake but also for specific population subgroups that have a high prevalence of inadequate intakes.

This chapter has focused on nutrient gaps; however, one should also realize that other nutrients are consumed in excess by a large proportion of the US population. Those nutrients consumed in excess by most age and gender groups in the population are outlined in the dietary guidelines as nutrients to reduce. These nutrients include: saturated fat, added sugars, cholesterol, and sodium. Continuing education and support to decrease the intake of these nutrients are needed. In addition, all of the data considered in this chapter are from dietary and supplemental intakes; biomarkers of nutritional status were not examined. Without considering biomarker data, certain nutrients might present as more problematic gaps for the population than are actually regarded (folate and vitamin D) [100].

REFERENCES

1. Wells, H.F. and J.C. Buzby, Dietary assessment of major trends in the U.S. food consumption, 1970–2005, in Economic Information Bulletin No. (EIB-33) 2008, United States Department of Agriculture Economic Research Service. p. 27.
2. United States Environmental Protection Agency, *Economic overview*. 2014 12/30/2013 [cited 2014 January 11]; Available from: http://www.epa.gov/oecaagct/ag101/economics.html
3. Otten, J.J., J.P. Hellwig, and L.D. Meyers, *DRI, dietary reference intakes: the essential guide to nutrient requirements*. 2006, Washington, DC: National Academies Press. xiii, 543 pp.
4. Dietary Guidelines Advisory Committee, Report of the dietary guidelines advisory committee on the dietary guidelines for Americans, 2010, to the Secretary of Agriculture and the Secretary of Health and Human Services. 2010, United States Department of Agriculture, Agricultural Research Service: Washington, DC.
5. Otten, J.J., J.P. Hellwig, and L.D. Meyers, *Introduction to the dietary reference intakes*, in *DRI, dietary reference intakes: The essential guide to nutrient requirements*. 2006, National Academies Press: Washington, DC, p. 5–17.
6. Murphy, S.P., S.I. Barr, and M.I. Poos, Using the new dietary reference intakes to assess diets: A map to the maze. *Nutr Rev*, 2002. **60**(9): p. 267–75.
7. Otten, J.J., J.P. Hellwig, and L.D. Meyers, *Applying the dietary reference intakes, in DRI, dietary reference intakes: The essential guide to nutrient requirements*. 2006, National Academies Press: Washington, DC, p. 19–68.
8. Dodd, K.W. et al. Statistical methods for estimating usual intake of nutrients and foods: A review of the theory. *J Am Diet Assoc*, 2006. **106**(10): p. 1640–50.
9. Carriquiry, A.L., Estimation of usual intake distributions of nutrients and foods. *J Nutr*, 2003. **133**(2): p. 601S–8S.
10. Guenther, P.M., P.S. Kott, and A.L. Carriquiry, Development of an approach for estimating usual nutrient intake distributions at the population level. *J Nutr*, 1997. **127**(6): p. 1106–12.
11. National Research Council, *Nutrient adequacy*. 1986: Washington, DC.
12. Thompson, F.E. and A. Subar, *Dietary assessment methodology*, in *Nutrition in the prevention and treatment of disease*, A.M. Coulston and C. Boushey, Editors. 2008, Academic Press: London, UK. p. 3–39.
13. Subar, A.F. et al. The Automated Self-Administered 24-hour dietary recall (ASA24): A resource for researchers, clinicians, and educators from the National Cancer Institute. *J Acad Nutr Diet*. **112**(8): p. 1134–7.
14. United States Department of Agriculture, Agricultural Research Service, USDA automated multiple-pass method. 2013 10/23/2013 [cited 2/6/2014]; Available from: http://www.ars.usda.gov/Services/docs.htm?docid=7710.
15. National Cancer Institute, Measurement Error Webinar Series. 2013 9/3/2013 [cited 2/6/2014]; Available from: http://appliedresearch.cancer.gov/measurementerror/.

16. Boushey, C.J., *Nutritional epidemiology dietary assessment methods*, in *Calcium in human health*, C. Weaver and R.P. Heaney, Editors. 2006, Humana Press: Totowa, NJ, p. 39–63.
17. United States Department of Agriculture, Agricultural Research Service, What we eat in America, NHANES 2003–2004, 2005–2006, and 2007–2008. 2013 11/13/2013 [cited 2/6/2014]; Available from: http://www.ars.usda.gov/Services/docs.htm?docid=13793.
18. Raper, N. et al. An overview of USDA's Dietary Intake Data System. *J Food Comp Anal*, 2004. 17: p. 545–555.
19. United States Department of Agriculture, Agricultural Research Service, and National Agricultural Library *USDA* National Nutrient Database for Standard Reference release *22*. 2011 12/7/2011[cited 2/6/2014]; Available from: http://www.ars.usda.gov/Services/docs.htm?docid=8964.
20. Subar, A.F. et al. Using intake biomarkers to evaluate the extent of dietary misreporting in a large sample of adults: The OPEN study. *Am J Epidemiol*, 2003. **158**(1): p. 1–13.
21. Klesges, R.C., L.H. Eck, and J.W. Ray, Who underreports dietary intake in a dietary recall? Evidence from the Second National Health and Nutrition Examination Survey. *J Consult Clin Psychol*, 1995. **63**(3): p. 438–44.
22. Trabulsi, J. and D.A. Schoeller, Evaluation of dietary assessment instruments against doubly labeled water, a biomarker of habitual energy intake. *Am J Physiol Endocrinol Metab*, 2001. **281**(5): p. E891–9.
23. Sawaya, A.L. et al. Evaluation of four methods for determining energy intake in young and older women: Comparison with doubly labeled water measurements of total energy expenditure. *Am J Clin Nutr*, 1996. **63**(4): p. 491–9.
24. Bathalon, G.P. et al. Psychological measures of eating behavior and the accuracy of 3 common dietary assessment methods in healthy postmenopausal women. *Am J Clin Nutr*, 2000. **71**(3): p. 739–45.
25. Johnson, R.K., R.P. Soultanakis, and D.E. Matthews, Literacy and body fatness are associated with underreporting of energy intake in US low-income women using the multiple-pass 24-hour recall: A doubly labeled water study. *J Am Diet Assoc*, 1998. **98**(10): p. 1136–40.
26. Tran, K.M. et al. In-person vs telephone-administered multiple-pass 24-hour recalls in women: Validation with doubly labeled water. *J Am Diet Assoc*, 2000. **100**(7): p. 777–83.
27. Kroke, A. et al. Validation of a self-administered food-frequency questionnaire administered in the European Prospective Investigation into Cancer and Nutrition (EPIC) Study: Comparison of energy, protein, and macronutrient intakes estimated with the doubly labeled water, urinary nitrogen, and repeated 24-h dietary recall methods. *Am J Clin Nutr*, 1999. **70**(4): p. 439–47.
28. Hebert, J.R. et al. Systematic errors in middle-aged women's estimates of energy intake: Comparing three self-report measures to total energy expenditure from doubly labeled water. *Ann Epidemiol*, 2002. **12**(8): p. 577–86.
29. Slimani, N. et al. Group level validation of protein intakes estimated by 24-hour diet recall and dietary questionnaires against 24-hour urinary nitrogen in the European Prospective Investigation into Cancer and Nutrition (EPIC) calibration study. *Cancer Epidemiol Biomarkers Prev*, 2003. **12**(8): p. 784–95.
30. Burrows, T.L., R.J. Martin, and C.E. Collins, A systematic review of the validity of dietary assessment methods in children when compared with the method of doubly labeled water. *J Am Diet Assoc*. **110**(10): p. 1501–10.
31. Tooze, J.A. et al. Psychosocial predictors of energy underreporting in a large doubly labeled water study. *Am J Clin Nutr*, 2004. **79**(5): p. 795–804.

32. Moshfegh, A.J. et al. The US Department of Agriculture Automated Multiple-Pass Method reduces bias in the collection of energy intakes. *Am J Clin Nutr*, 2008. **88**(2): p. 324–32.
33. Krebs-Smith, S.M. et al. Low energy reporters vs others: A comparison of reported food intakes. *Eur J Clin Nutr*, 2000. **54**(4): p. 281–7.
34. Gersovitz, M., J.P. Madden, and H. Smiciklas-Wright, Validity of the 24-hr dietary recall and seven-day record for group comparisons. *J Am Diet Assoc*, 1978. **73**(1): p. 48–55.
35. Rebro, S.M. et al. The effect of keeping food records on eating patterns. *J Am Diet Assoc*, 1998. **98**(10): p. 1163–5.
36. Thompson, F.E. and T. Byers, Dietary assessment resource manual. *J Nutr*, 1994. **124**(11 Suppl): p. 2245S–2317S.
37. Hill, R.J. and P.S. Davies, The validity of self-reported energy intake as determined using the doubly labelled water technique. *Br J Nutr*, 2001. **85**(4): p. 415–30.
38. Black, A.E. et al. Measurements of total energy expenditure provide insights into the validity of dietary measurements of energy intake. *J Am Diet Assoc*, 1993. **93**(5): p. 572–9.
39. Seale, J.L. and W.V. Rumpler, Comparison of energy expenditure measurements by diet records, energy intake balance, doubly labeled water and room calorimetry. *Eur J Clin Nutr*, 1997. **51**(12): p. 856–63.
40. Mahabir, S. et al. Calorie intake misreporting by diet record and food frequency questionnaire compared to doubly labeled water among postmenopausal women. *Eur J Clin Nutr*, 2006. **60**(4): p. 561–5.
41. Lafay, L. et al. Determinants and nature of dietary underreporting in a free-living population: The Fleurbaix Laventie Ville Sante (FLVS) Study. *Int J Obes Relat Metab Disord*, 1997. **21**(7): p. 567–73.
42. Stallone, D.D. et al. Dietary assessment in Whitehall II: The influence of reporting bias on apparent socioeconomic variation in nutrient intakes. *Eur J Clin Nutr*, 1997. **51**(12): p. 815–25.
43. Lafay, L. et al. Does energy intake underreporting involve all kinds of food or only specific food items? Results from the Fleurbaix Laventie Ville Sante (FLVS) study. *Int J Obes Relat Metab Disord*, 2000. **24**(11): p. 1500–6.
44. Subar, A.F., Developing dietary assessment tools. *J Am Diet Assoc*, 2004. **104**(5): p. 769–70.
45. Block, G. et al. A data-based approach to diet questionnaire design and testing. *Am J Epidemiol*, 1986. **124**(3): p. 453–69.
46. Chu, S.Y. et al. A comparison of frequency and quantitative dietary methods for epidemiologic studies of diet and disease. *Am J Epidemiol*, 1984. **119**(3): p. 323–34.
47. Subar, A.F. et al. Comparative validation of the Block, Willett, and National Cancer Institute food frequency questionnaires: The Eating at America's Table Study. *Am J Epidemiol*, 2001. **154**(12): p. 1089–99.
48. Schatzkin, A. et al. A comparison of a food frequency questionnaire with a 24-hour recall for use in an epidemiological cohort study: Results from the biomarker-based Observing Protein and Energy Nutrition (OPEN) study. *Int J Epidemiol*, 2003. **32**(6): p. 1054–62.
49. Jensen, J.K. et al. Development of a food frequency questionnaire to estimate calcium intake of Asian, Hispanic, and white youth. *J Am Diet Assoc*, 2004. **104**(5): p. 762–9.
50. Briefel, R.R. et al. Assessing the nation's diet: Limitations of the food frequency questionnaire. *J Am Diet Assoc*, 1992. **92**(8): p. 959–62.
51. Block, G. and A.F. Subar, Estimates of nutrient intake from a food frequency questionnaire: The 1987 National Health Interview Survey. *J Am Diet Assoc*, 1992. **92**(8): p. 969–77.
52. Kipnis, V. et al. Structure of dietary measurement error: Results of the OPEN biomarker study. *Am J Epidemiol*, 2003. **158**(1): p. 14–21; discussion 22–6.

53. Centers for Disease Control and Prevention, National Center for Health Statistics, First National Health and Nutrition Examination Survey (NHANES I), 1971–1975. 2012 9/30/2012 [cited 2/6/2014]; Available from: http://www.cdc.gov/nchs/nhanes/nhanesi.htm.
54. Centers for Disease Control and Prevention, National Center for Health Statistics, Second National Health and Nutrition Examination Survey, (NHANES II), 1976–1980. 2012 9/30/2012 [cited 2/6/2014]; Available from: http://www.cdc.gov/nchs/nhanes/nhanesii.htm.
55. Centers for Disease Control and Prevention, National Center for Health Statistics, Third National Health and Nutrition Examination Survey, (NHANES III). 1988–1994. 2013 4/25/2013 [cited 2/6/2014]; Available from: http://www.cdc.gov/nchs/nhanes/nh3data.htm.
56. Centers for Disease Control and Prevention, National Center for Health Statistics, National Health and Nutrition Examination Protocol. 1999–2000; 2012 4/6/2012 [cited 2/6/2014]; Available from: http://www.cdc.gov/nchs/nhanes/nhanes1999–2000/DSQFILE1.htm.
57. Dwyer, J., M.F. Picciano, and D.J. Raiten, Food and dietary supplement databases for What We Eat in America–NHANES. *J Nutr*, 2003. **133**(2): p. 624S–34S.
58. Centers for Disease Control and Prevention, National Center for Health Statistics. National Health and Nutrition Examination Protocol. 2007–2008; 2012 4/6/2012 [cited 2/6/2014]; Available from: http://wwwn.cdc.gov/nchs/nhanes/search/datapage.aspx?Component=Dietary&CycleBeginYear=2007.
59. Park, S.Y. et al. Allowing for variations in multivitamin supplement composition improves nutrient intake estimates for epidemiologic studies. *J Nutr*, 2006. **136**(5): p. 1359–64.
60. Barr, S.I., S.P. Murphy, and M.I. Poos, Interpreting and using the dietary references intakes in dietary assessment of individuals and groups. *J Am Diet Assoc*, 2002. **102**(6): p. 780–8.
61. National Research Council, *Dietary Reference Intakes for Calcium and Vitamin D*, ed. Ross, A.C., Taylor, C.L., Yaktine, A.L., Del Valle, H.B., 2011, Washington, DC: The National Academies Press. 482.
62. National Research Council, *Dietary reference intakes: For calcium, phosphorus, magnesium, vitamin D, and fluoride*. 1997, Washington, DC: National Academy Press. xv, 432 pp.
63. National Research Council, *Dietary Reference Intakes for Vitamin A, Vitamin K, Arsenic, Boron, Chromium, Copper, Iodine, Iron, Manganese, Molybdenum, Nickel, Silicon, Vanadium, and Zinc*. National Academy Press, 2001: Washington, DC.
64. National Research Council, *Dietary Reference Intakes: Dietary reference intakes for vitamin C, vitamin E, selenium, and carotenoids: A report*. 2000, Washington, DC: National Academy Press. xx, 506 pp., [1] folded leaf.
65. National Research Council, *Dietary Reference Intakes: Dietary reference intakes for water, potassium, sodium, chloride, and sulfate*. 2005, Washington, DC: National Academies Press. xviii, 617 pp.
66. National Research Council, *Dietary reference intakes for energy, carbohydrate, fiber, fat, fatty acids, cholesterol, protein and amino acids (macronutrients)*. 2005, Washington, DC: The National Academies Press.
67. Greer, F.R. et al. *Vitamin K status of lactating mothers, human milk, and breast-feeding infants*. Pediatrics, 1991. **88**(4): p. 751–6.
68. National Research Council, *Dietary Reference Intakes for Thiamin, Riboflavin, Niacin, Vitamin B6, Folate, Vitamin B12, Pantothenic Acid, Biotin, and Choline*. 1998, Washington, DC: The National Academies Press.
69. Devaney, B. et al. Nutrient intakes of infants and toddlers. *J Am Diet Assoc*, 2004. **104**(1 Suppl): p. s14–21.

70. Butte, N.F. et al. Nutrient intakes of US infants, toddlers, and preschoolers meet or exceed dietary reference intakes. *J Am Diet Assoc*, 2010. **110**(12 Suppl): p. S27–37.
71. Nusser, S.M. et al. A semiparametric transformation approach to estimating usual daily intake distributions. *J Am Stat Assoc*, 1996. **91**: p. 1440–9.
72. Picciano, M.F. et al. Dietary supplement use among infants, children, and adolescents in the United States, 1999–2002. *Arch Pediatr Adolesc Med*, 2007. **161**(10): p. 978–85.
73. Bailey, R.L. et al. Why US children use dietary supplements. *Pediatr Res*, 2013. **74**(6): p. 737–41.
74. Briefel, R. et al. Feeding Infants and Toddlers Study: Do vitamin and mineral supplements contribute to nutrient adequacy or excess among US infants and toddlers? *J Am Diet Assoc*, 2006. **106**(1 Suppl): p. S52–65.
75. Tooze, J.A. et al. A new statistical method for estimating the usual intake of episodically consumed foods with application to their distribution. *J Am Diet Assoc*, 2006. **106**(10): p. 1575–87.
76. Moshfegh, A., Goldman, J., Cleveland, L., What We Eat in America, NHANES 2001–2002: Usual Nutrient Intakes from Food Compared to Dietary Reference Intakes. 2005.
77. Bailey, R.L. et al. Do dietary supplements improve micronutrient sufficiency in children and adolescents? *J Pediatr*, 2012. **161**(5): p. 837–42.
78. Bailey, R.L. et al. Estimation of total usual calcium and vitamin D intakes in the United States. *J Nutr*, 2010. **140**(4): p. 817–22.
79. Bailey, R.L. et al. Dietary supplement use in the United States, 2003–2006. *J Nutr*. **141**(2): p. 261–6.
80. Dietary Guidelines Advisory Committee, Report of the Dietary Guidelines Advisroy Committee on the Dietary Guidelines for Americans, 2010 (Advisory Report), Resource 1: Children's dietary intake. 2011, United States Department of Agriculture, Agricultural Research Service: Washington, DC.
81. Bailey, R.L. et al. Dietary supplement use in the United States, 2003–2006. *J Nutr*, 2011. **141**(2): p. 261–6.
82. Bailey, R.L. et al. Examination of vitamin intakes among US adults by dietary supplement use. *J Acad Nutr Diet*, 2012. **112**(5): p. 657–663 e4.
83. Sebastian, R.S. et al. Older adults who use vitamin/mineral supplements differ from nonusers in nutrient intake adequacy and dietary attitudes. *J Am Diet Assoc*, 2007. **107**(8): p. 1322–32.
84. Moshfegh, A.J. et al. What We Eat in America, NHANES 2005–2006: Usual Nutrient Intakes from Food and Water Compared to 1997 Dietary Reference Intakes for Vitamin D, Calcium, Phosphorus, and Magnesium, United States Department of Agriculture, Agricultural Research Service, 2009.
85. Park, C.Y. and H.A. Eicher-Miller, Iron deficiency is associated with food insecurity in pregnant females in the United States: NHANES 1999–2010. (under review).
86. Rifas-Shiman, S.L. et al. Dietary quality during pregnancy varies by maternal characteristics in Project Viva: A US cohort. *J Am Diet Assoc*, 2009. **109**(6): p. 1004–11.
87. Siega-Riz, A.M., L.M. Bodnar, and D.A. Savitz, What are pregnant women eating? Nutrient and food group differences by race. *Am J Obstet Gynecol*, 2002. **186**(3): p. 480–6.
88. Branum, A.M., R. Bailey, and B.J. Singer, Dietary supplement use and folate status during pregnancy in the United States. *J Nutr*, 2013. **143**(4): p. 486–92.
89. Mei, Z. et al. Assessment of iron status in US pregnant women from the National Health and Nutrition Examination Survey (NHANES), 1999–2006. *Am J Clin Nutr*, 2011. **93**(6): p. 1312–20.
90. Millen, A.E., K.W. Dodd, and A.F. Subar, Use of vitamin, mineral, nonvitamin, and nonmineral supplements in the United States: The 1987, 1992, and 2000 National Health Interview Survey results. *J Am Diet Assoc*, 2004. **104**(6): p. 942–50.

91. Bailey, R.L. et al. Why US adults use dietary supplements. *JAMA Intern Med.* **173**(5): p. 355–61.
92. Radimer, K. et al. Dietary supplement use by US adults: Data from the National Health and Nutrition Examination Survey, 1999–2000. *Am J Epidemiol*, 2004. **160**(4): p. 339–49.
93. Balluz, L.S. et al. Vitamin or supplement use among adults, behavioral risk factor surveillance system, 13 states, 2001. Public Health Report, 2005. **120**(2): p. 117–23.
94. Foote, J.A. et al. Factors associated with dietary supplement use among healthy adults of five ethnicities: The Multiethnic Cohort Study. *Am J Epidemiol*, 2003. **157**(10): p. 888–97.
95. Eichenberger Gilmore, J.M. et al. Longitudinal patterns of vitamin and mineral supplement use in young white children. *J Am Diet Assoc*, 2005. **105**(5): p. 763–72; quiz 773–4.
96. Yu, S.M., M.D. Kogan, and P. Gergen, Vitamin-mineral supplement use among preschool children in the United States. *Pediatrics*, 1997. **100**(5): p. E4.
97. Reaves, L. et al. Vitamin supplement intake is related to dietary intake and physical activity: The Child and Adolescent Trial for Cardiovascular Health (CATCH). *J Am Diet Assoc*, 2006. **106**(12): p. 2018–23.
98. Dwyer, J.T. et al. Do adolescent vitamin-mineral supplement users have better nutrient intakes than nonusers? Observations from the CATCH tracking study. *J Am Diet Assoc*, 2001. **101**(11): p. 1340–6.
99. Shaikh, U., R.S. Byrd, and P. Auinger, Vitamin and mineral supplement use by children and adolescents in the 1999–2004 National Health and Nutrition Examination Survey: Relationship with nutrition, food security, physical activity, and health care access. *Arch Pediatr Adolesc Med*, 2009. **163**(2): p. 150–7.
100. Pfeiffer, C.M. et al. Assessing vitamin status in large population surveys by measuring biomarkers and dietary intake—two case studies: Folate and vitamin D. *Food Nutr Res.*, 2012. **56**. doi:10.3402/fnr.v56i0.5944.

3 Assessing the Potential Long-Term Effects of Multivitamin Supplements

Susanne Rautiainen, J. Michael Gaziano, and Howard D. Sesso

CONTENTS

3.1 INTRODUCTION

The recent systematic review [1] and 2014 recommendations [2] from the US Preventive Services Task Force (USPSTF) on vitamin, mineral, and multivitamin supplements have generated important dialog and scientific [3,4] and media debate regarding the role of regular, daily multivitamin use in the prevention of major chronic disease endpoints. The USPSTF concluded that "the current evidence is insufficient to assess the balance of benefits and harms of multivitamins for the prevention of cardiovascular disease (CVD) and cancer" [2]. This conclusion was not surprising given the lack of definitive, long-term, placebo-controlled, randomized clinical trials testing multivitamin supplements for their health effects. As a result, there remains a pressing need for additional data on the long-term health effects of multivitamins. Earlier guidelines on multivitamins echoed these sentiments [5,6]. At least one-third of US adults continue to take a daily multivitamin [7,8] despite pleas that "enough is enough" [4] and of a "hung jury" [3].

Many people take a daily multivitamin throughout their lifetime; unlike most other dietary supplements, multivitamin use often begins during childhood with chewables and gummies, and extends into adulthood. As a result, many people assume that taking multivitamins must confer benefits and lack risk. Yet there are major public health implications regarding persistent multivitamin use in terms of perceived benefits and financial burden, as annual vitamin supplement sales remain in billions of US dollars [9,10].

3.2 WHAT ARE MULTIVITAMIN SUPPLEMENTS, AND HOW ARE THEY USED?

3.2.1 Definition and Variability of Content

Multivitamin/mineral supplements include a wide range of lower-dose vitamins and minerals corresponding to recommended dietary allowances and/or usual dietary intakes. The primary goal of a multivitamin is typically to provide low-doses of essential vitamins and minerals to prevent deficiency. In reality, the vast majority of individuals taking multivitamins, particularly in developed countries, are less likely to suffer from vitamin and minerals deficiencies. On the other hand, individuals in developing countries where malnutrition is more prevalent would stand to benefit to a greater extent. Another consideration is age; the ability to absorb some vitamins and minerals wanes as individuals age, and accelerates particularly among those aged ≥60 years.

One major challenge when studying multivitamin use and different health outcomes across all types of research studies is the lack of a standard definition with regard to included vitamins and minerals, along with their doses [11]. Multivitamin manufacturers decide the number, dose, type, and source of the included vitamin and minerals. They also decide the brand name of their product and there are dietary supplements that are identical to multivitamins in their composition but are named differently. By definition, a "multi"-vitamin or "multi"-mineral contains >2 nutrients. Some multivitamins contain all essential vitamins and minerals; even then there are differences in the amounts provided. Other multivitamins contain many, but not all, essential vitamins and minerals, again at varying doses. Yet many of these multivitamins are still labeled as "complete."

Major multivitamin brands also tend to make subtle changes to their formulations every few years as nutritional science evolves. For example, with the increasing attention focused on the potential benefits of vitamin D on numerous health outcomes, multivitamin formulations have steadily increased their vitamin D content over the past decade. Moreover, many multivitamins have formulations targeted towards particular subgroups of individuals (e.g., men, women, children, older age) or organs (e.g., heart, eye), adding to the enormous variations in their content. Multivitamins also come in many different forms, affecting the selection, dose, and absorption of included vitamins and minerals. For example, gummy supplements typically have a more limited selection of included vitamins and minerals for their formulations, and the individual often must take at least two pills daily.

As a result, a consumer has a massive stretch of storage shelves with dozens of different multivitamin formulations to choose from, and lacks knowledge of whether particular multivitamins are more beneficial than others. Table 3.1 presents a selection of some common multivitamin formulations in the US market and the variability in content. This unfortunately complicates the interpretation and implementation of study results from the perspective of scientists, plus gives rise to confusion among the general public. Ideally, a standard definition of multivitamins would provide a big advantage with regard to interpretations of study findings and overall conclusions and how they should be communicated to the general public. Such standard definitions may begin by listing essential vitamins and minerals that should be included, along with a range of appropriate, safe doses.

3.2.2 Prevalence of Multivitamin Supplement Use

The prevalence of multivitamin use has steadily increased during the past decade in the USA [12]. In the National Health and Nutrition Examination Survey (NHANES) study, more than one-third of adults reported that they are currently taking a daily multivitamin [7]. In the Nurse's Health Study and the Health Professional Follow-up Study cohorts, multivitamins were the most commonly used supplement and the prevalence has increased from 43.1% to 73.9% and 42.7% to 71.1%, respectively [13]. Also, in the Iowa Women's Health Study of 18,346 women aged 55–69 years, the prevalence of multivitamin has increased over time (31.7% in 1986 to 62.5% in 2004) [14]. Finally, in the Physicians' Health Study (PHS) cohort, consisting of male US physicians aged ≥50 years, more than one-third of participants reported current multivitamin use based upon responses provided from 1997 to 2001 [15]. Thus, the physicians who interact with patients and provide advice on their health, including supplement choices and use, are using multivitamins themselves.

Other countries report the same trends of an increase of the prevalence in multivitamin use. In a national Swedish survey, a 70% increase in dietary supplement use occurred among adult men and women during the 1990s compared with 1980–1981 [16]. The same trend was observed in all age groups and in all socio-economic groups, except farmers. Women were more likely to take dietary supplements than men of the same age. No significant changes occurred in the use of dietary supplements during the 1980s, and the observed increase occurred mainly during the 1990s. These data are consistent with what has been observed in studies from the USA. Unfortunately, in this Swedish study it was not possible to report statistics for specific dietary supplements, but based on sales data it has been assumed that multivitamins are the most common dietary supplement used in Sweden as well.

TABLE 3.1
Comparison of Representative Vitamins and Minerals Contained in Selected Multivitamin Formulations in the United States, 2014

Vitamin or Mineral	Centrum® Silver® Adults 50+	Nature Made® Multi Complete with Iron	One A Day® Men's 50+ Healthy Advantage	One A Day® Women's 50+ Healthy Advantage
Vitamin A (IU)	2500 (40% as β-carotene)	2500 (60% as β-carotene)	3500 (20% as β-carotene)	3500 (20% as β-carotene)
Vitamin C (mg)	60	180	120	120
Vitamin D (IU)	500	1000	700	1000
Vitamin E (IU)	50	50	25.5	30
Vitamin K (μg)	30	80	20	20
Thiamin (mg)	1.5	1.5	4.5	4.5
Riboflavin (mg)	1.7	1.7	3.4	3.4
Niacin (mg)	20	20	20	20
Vitamin B6 (mg)	3	2	6	6
Folic acid (μg)	400	400	400	400
Vitamin B12 (μg)	25	6	25	25
Biotin (μg)	30	30	30	30
Pantothenic acid (mg)	10	10	15	15
Calcium (mg)	220	162	120	500
Iron (mg)	0	18	0	0
Phosphorus (mg)	20	0	0	0
Iodine (μg)	150	150	150	150
Magnesium (mg)	50	100	110	50
Zinc (mg)	11	15	24	24
Selenium (μg)	55	70	117	27
Copper (mg)	0.5	2	2.2	2.2
Manganese (mg)	2.3	4	4.2	4.2
Chromium (μg)	45	120	180	180
Molybdenum (μg)	45	75	90	90
Chloride (mg)	72	0	0	0
Potassium (mg)	80	0	0	0
Boron (μg)	150	0	0	0
Nickel (μg)	5	0	0	0
Vanadium (μg)	10	0	0	0
Silicon (mg)	2	0	0	0
Lutein (μg)	250	0	0	0
Lycopene (μg)	300	0	370	0

Taken together, multivitamins are very common in developed countries and the use continues to increase. In fact, a daily multivitamin is often recommended by physicians and other health professionals for adults and children—regardless of whether nutritional requirements are met or not. Optimally, a thorough nutritional assessment would be done to determine whether gaps in vitamin or mineral intake may be present, manifested as nutritional insufficiency or outright deficiency. It is, therefore, of great importance both from a clinical and a public health perspective to understand the actual role of multivitamins in health promotion and disease prevention.

The role of multivitamins in non-developed countries, where malnutrition is more common, is more paramount. Given the low cost of multivitamins, they represent a promising tool by which to prevent nutritional deficiencies.

3.2.3 Who Uses Multivitamins?

Many people take multivitamins in the belief that they will improve or maintain their health. Advertising plays a big role, along with recommendations from doctors, nutritionists, and other health professionals.

In many studies, multivitamin users tend to be characterized by a healthy set of lifestyle and dietary patterns [15,17–21] as part of recommendations to maintain, or improve health. This complicates the interpretation of observational studies of multivitamin use. Although these studies attempt to control for major health-related lifestyle factors in their analyses, despite the best intentions of investigators, the completeness of adjustment can never be assured. Residual confounding by additional lifestyle, dietary, and other behavioral variables in observational analyses of multivitamins cannot be completely ruled out.

For example, in the PHS cohort, it was observed that self-reported multivitamin use was positively associated with healthy lifestyle and dietary factors. At the same time, multivitamin use was associated with the likelihood of having a history of cancer, hypercholesterolemia, and hypertension [15]. In the NHANES, a multivitamin user was more likely to be older, female, Caucasian, better-educated, leaner, and more physically active [17]. Another study of 1056 women and men observed similar associations as in the NHANES [18]. Lee et al. observed that the prevalence of multivitamin use was higher among participants who were older, female, better-educated, of higher income, and had less abdominal obesity [19]. Robson et al. also observed that multivitamin use was higher among men who were older, more physically active, and leaner, and consuming more whole grains [20]. These associations stress the challenges of interpreting results from observational studies of multivitamin use and chronic disease, since any observed associations may reflect uncontrolled and residual confounding, rather than causal effects. Randomized clinical trials can overcome these limitations of observational studies, but remain confined to a specific intervention and defined study population. Thus, RCTs and observational studies must complement each other to ensure that a clear answer can emerge regarding the potential benefits or risks of daily multivitamin use in adults.

3.3 MULTIVITAMINS AND CANCER

3.3.1 Observational Studies

Vitamins and minerals included in multivitamins may prevent cancer through several plausible mechanisms. Regulation of redox homeostasis has been suggested to be fundamental for normal cells to function and survive [22,23]. Cancer cells are characterized by high levels of reactive oxygen species (ROS) [22] and the antioxidant micronutrients have been shown to protect against oxidative damage to cellular components [22]. Vitamin E is a lipid-soluble chain-breaking antioxidant exerting both anti-inflammatory and anti-carcinogenic effects [24,25]. Vitamin E also has other non-antioxidant functions including cell-signaling and anti-proliferation [24,25]. Vitamin C also has antioxidant effects and plays an important role in collagen stabilizing epithelial cells in a highly differentiated state, resulting in suppressing tumor growth [26]. Folate, vitamin B_6, and vitamin B_{12} are essential vitamins in one-carbon methylation of DNA [27,28].

Limited observational studies have investigated the association between multivitamin supplement use and total cancer incidence. In a large US prospective study of 1 million US men and women aged ≥30 years beginning in 1982, multivitamin use was associated with a 9% increased risk of total cancer mortality [29]. A large US prospective study of women and men starting in 1993–1996 observed no association between multivitamin use and total cancer mortality, in both men and women [30]. Interestingly, when using stricter criteria to assess long-term multivitamin defined as reporting usage at baseline for ≥5 years and at the follow-up questionnaire 5 years later a non-significant inverse association was observed among women but not among men. Moreover, no association was observed for CVD mortality in another prospective study of American women followed for an average of 19.0 years [31]. However, overly strong conclusions should not be drawn from this study due to the long follow-up without taking into account the duration of use and updated measurements of multivitamin use for time-varying models.

3.3.1.1 Breast Cancer

The majority of prospective observational studies examining multivitamin use in relation to the risk of breast cancer have reported no association [32,33]; however, two studies observed slightly increased risks [34,35]. The Women's Health Initiative Study included a large number of participants and assessed multivitamin use very thoroughly through interviewers and classified multivitamin according to different doses of the included ingredients. In this study, there was no association observed between multivitamins including 20–30 vitamins and minerals and nutrient levels of ≤100% Recommended Daily Allowances and invasive breast cancer [32]. In the Women's Health Study cohort, multivitamin use was not associated with the overall risk of breast cancer; however, there were some suggestions on reduced risk among women consuming alcohol or for estrogen receptor (ER)/progesterone receptor (PR) tumors [33]. However, a Swedish [34] cohort study of 35,329 women observed a 19% increased risk of total breast cancer. The association was stronger among women taking >3 multivitamin tablets per week or reporting a duration of >10 years at baseline. Moreover, consistent with the Swedish study, an American study of postmenopausal elderly women [35] observed a non-significant 18% increased risk of breast cancer. The pooled estimates from a meta-analysis summarizing cohort (RR: 0.99; 95% CI: 0.60–1.63) and case-control studies (RR: 1.00; 95% CI: 0.50–1.97) found no association between multivitamin use and breast cancer risk [36].

In summary, there is very little evidence supporting multivitamin use in the prevention of breast cancer. However, today we can only rely on the results from observational studies, and cannot therefore exclude the possibility that measurement error and confounding may have driven the results. Due to the general lack of support from observation studies, it is unclear what a newly initiated trial of multivitamins and breast cancer will yield. Given the high prevalence of multivitamin use, however, it remains important to generate such data to evaluate the totality of evidence for risks and/or benefits.

3.3.1.2 Prostate Cancer

Despite the fact that prostate cancer is the most common cancer form among men and that the use of multivitamins is wide-spread, there are very few studies investigating the association with multivitamin use and the evidence does not support taking a multivitamin to prevent prostate cancer. The majority of them have reported no association for the overall prostate cancer risk [37–40]. In the Cancer Prevention Study II including 475,726 men, multivitamin use was associated with small increased prostate cancer mortality [37]. The association was stronger for regular use for ≥15 years. However, to explore a potential impact from misclassification of multivitamin use due to the long follow-up, the authors investigated different lengths of follow-up times and observed the strongest association during the first 4 years. Thus, this could be an indication that men who died during the early years may have started taking multivitamins because they were having symptoms of advanced but undiagnosed prostate cancer [37]. In the National Institutes of Health (NIH)-AARP Diet and Health Study, multivitamin use was not associated with total cancer among 295,344 men followed for 5 years. But when investigating the frequency of multivitamin use there was some suggestion on increased risks of advanced and fatal prostate cancer on taking multivitamins more than 7 times/week [40]. However, as mentioned above, because of the short follow-up period, there is a concern that men might have started taking multivitamins due to symptoms of advanced prostate cancer. One US case-control study observed a 30% lower risk for 1–4 years of use, but no association was observed for longer durations [39].

3.3.1.3 Colorectal Cancer

Colorectal cancer is one of cancer sub-types where the evidence is most supportive for potential protective role in prevention. Multivitamin use has been inversely associated with colorectal cancer risk in several prospective cohort studies [41–43] whereas two other studies, one on colorectal cancer mortality and the other on colorectal cancer incidence, have observed no association [29,32]. In a pooled analysis of 13 cohort studies including 676,141 women and men, a 12% (95% CI: 4–19%) lower risk of colon cancer was reported [41]. However, one can argue that these results are confounded by incomplete adjustment for healthy behavior-related factors. In the Cancer Prevention Study II Nutrition Cohort of women and men, regular multivitamin use for 10 years at baseline was associated with a 29% lower mortality from colorectal cancer [42]. In the Nurses' Health Study, women who used multivitamins had 17% non-significant lower risk of colon cancer after 5–9, a 20% significant lower risk after 10–14 and 75% lower risk after 15 years of use [43]. The Women's Health Initiative Study observed that multivitamin use was not associated with the risk of colon cancer [32]. Another American study observed no association between multivitamin use and colon cancer mortality among women with no history of cancer at baseline, whereas a 46% increased risk was observed among men having previous cancer diagnosis, but this could be a result of reverse causality [29].

3.3.2 Randomized Controlled Trials

Randomized clinical trials are considered as the gold standard of study design since they can overcome the limitations of observational studies through the elimination of perceived confounding by lifestyle, dietary, and clinical factors, plus the use of placebo control and double-blinding, to provide definitive evidence on the potential causal relationship between multivitamin use and cancer and other endpoints to be discussed in this review. The design of a randomized clinical trial—small or large, short or long, choice of study population—is often underestimated and factors greatly into the interpretation of its results. No single trial has universal generalizability, but it is important for each trial to build upon the existing body of animal, clinical, and observational evidence to move the science of multivitamin supplements forward. For multivitamins, this is particularly relevant given the diversity of products available to consumers across the entire lifespan. Yet the clinical trial evidence for the long-term health effects of a common multivitamin is, remarkably, limited to US male physicians aged ≥50 years.

The PHS II is the only large-scale, long-term, placebo-controlled, double-blind randomized clinical trial that has investigated the effect of a common multivitamin on cancer [44]. In this trial, 14,641 middle-aged and older men initially aged ≥50 years (mean age, 64.3 years) were followed-up for 11.2 years. During multivitamin treatment, we confirmed that 2669 men had cancer, including 1373 cases of prostate cancer and 210 cases of colorectal cancer, with some men experiencing multiple events. A total of 2757 (18.8%) men died during follow-up, including 859 (5.9%) due to cancer.

Men taking multivitamin had a modest, significant reduction in total cancer incidence (HR, 0.92; 95% CI, 0.86–0.998; $P = 0.044$) (Figure 3.1). Nearly half of the cancers were prostate cancer, which were largely early-stage and benign due to the risk of prostate-specific antigen (PSA) testing. As a result, a multivitamin had no effect on prostate cancer (HR, 0.98; 95% CI, 0.88–1.09). The effect of a multivitamin was, therefore, stronger in significantly reducing total cancer excluding prostate cancer by 12%. A multivitamin had non-significant reductions in most other individual site-specific cancers such as colorectal (HR, 0.89), lung (HR, 0.84), and bladder (HR, 0.72) cancer, with more limited power due to smaller numbers of events. For cancer mortality, men taking a daily multivitamin had a 12% reduction that did not reach statistical significance (HR, 0.88; 95% CI, 0.77–1.01; $P = 0.07$).

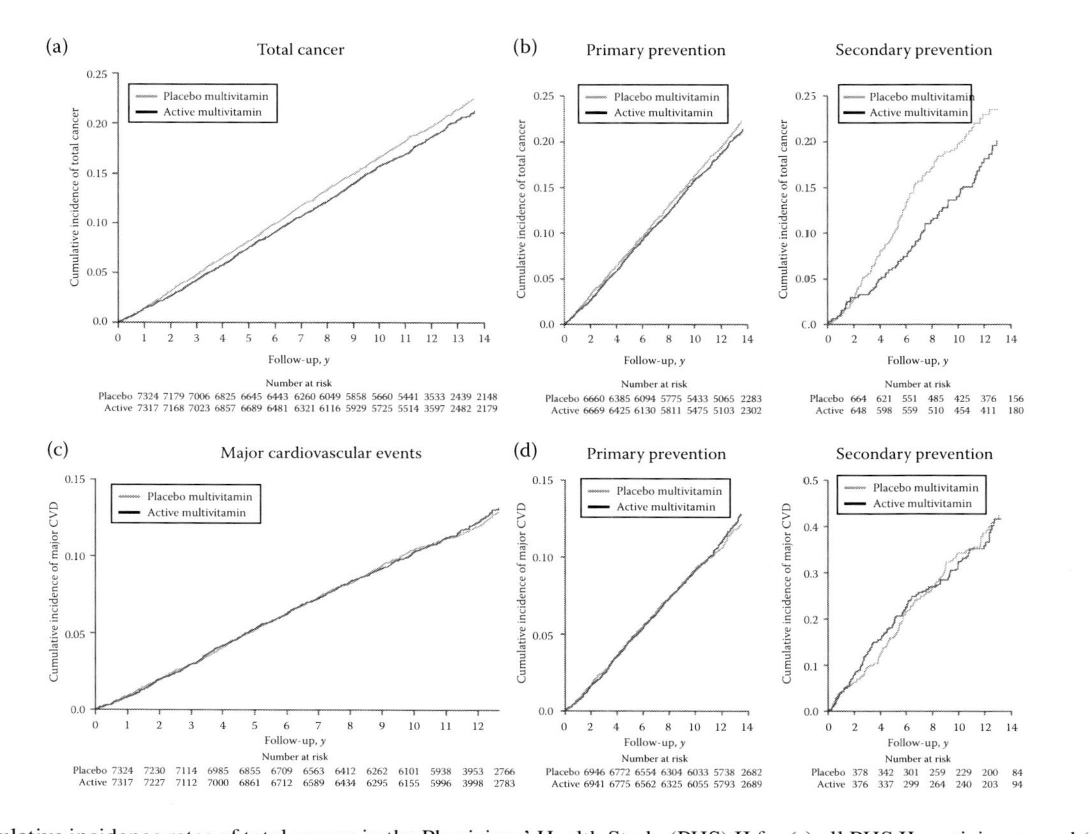

FIGURE 3.1 Cumulative incidence rates of total cancer in the Physicians' Health Study (PHS) II for (a) all PHS II participants and (b) the primary (no baseline history) or secondary (baseline history of cancer) prevention; and rates of major cardiovascular events in (c) all PHS II participants and (d) the primary (no baseline history) or secondary (baseline history of cardiovascular disease) prevention.

When taking into account the potential modifying role of key baseline clinical, lifestyle, familial, and dietary factors on the effect of a daily multivitamin on total cancer, a few interesting findings emerged regarding the age and parental history of cancer. For age, men aged ≥70 years had a stronger reduction in total cancer, with a HR of 0.82 (95% CI, 0.72–0.93), though the test for interaction was not significant (*P*, interaction = 0.06). In addition, men with no parental history of cancer had a significant beneficial effect of a daily multivitamin on total cancer (HR, 0.86, 95% CI, 0.76–0.98) (*P*, interaction = 0.012). Of note, 1312 (9.0%) men had a baseline history of cancer, in whom we found that daily multivitamin use strongly and significantly reduced total cancer by 27%, though this reduction did not significantly differ from a non-significant 6% reduction among the other 13,329 men initially free of cancer (*P*, interaction = 0.07)(Figure 3.1). This reduction in total cancer among men with a baseline history of cancer emerged within the first few years of the multivitamin intervention.

There are two other large-scale, long-term, randomized clinical trials that have tested combinations of more than three vitamins and minerals, but falling short of testing a common, low-dose daily multivitamin that includes all essential vitamins and minerals as done in PHS II. The Supplémentation en Vitamines et Minéraux Antioxydants (SU.VI.MAX) study was primary prevention randomized, placebo-controlled trial conducted among middle-aged French adults [45]. This trial tested the effect of a low-dose supplement mixture of five antioxidants (including 120 mg ascorbic acid, 30 mg vitamin E, 6 mg beta carotene, 100 μg selenium, and 20 mg zinc) and reported significant protective effect on total cancer incidence among men, but not among women. Interestingly, in this study, the effect of supplementation was stronger in men with low baseline serum vitamin C and beta-carotene levels, suggesting that people with poor nutritional status may benefit more from a low-dose vitamin/mineral supplement than those with already adequate nutrition. Moreover, the Linxian Chinese Cancer Prevention Trial, conducted among adults with low baseline nutrient status, tested a daily antioxidant supplement with low doses of ß-carotene, vitamin E, and selenium to approximate recommended dietary intakes and also found significant reductions in total, cancer, and gastric cancer mortality [46].

Overall, the limited results from randomized clinical trials to date suggest that the combination of low doses of essential vitamins and minerals included in multivitamin supplements may be promising in cancer prevention. Moreover, the results from the SU.VI.MAX and Linxian trials suggest that multivitamins may even be more effective among people with nutrient deficiencies; however, it is important to emphasize that these two trials did not test a multivitamin as done for PHS II, but was limited to middle-aged and older male physicians of high socioeconomic status. Baseline nutritional status is an important aspect of multivitamin use which previous studies have yet to comprehensively investigate in understanding the impact of multivitamin supplementation for cancer prevention.

There is also a need for research focusing on major site-specific cancers including breast, prostate, colorectal, and lung cancer. Those site-specific cancers for which diet plays a strong role, such as gastric cancer, colorectal cancer, and others, may be more apt to be related to daily multivitamin use. Further, there are less common cancers for which little is known regarding the role of multivitamins, with an opportunity to provide a low-cost, low-risk approach for cancer prevention.

3.4 MULTIVITAMINS AND CARDIOVASCULAR DISEASE

3.4.1 Observational Studies

Nutritional deficiencies are suggested to be a central component in CVD development and therefore taking a daily multivitamin could inhibit this process. Many of the included vitamins and minerals may act through several hypothesized mechanisms. Low-density lipoproteins transport antioxidants such as alpha-tocopherol and beta-carotene which may inhibit oxidative damage of these particles [47]. In vitro studies have shown that vitamin C may also protect low-density lipoproteins from oxidation by interacting with alpha-tocopherol and beta-carotene [48]. Folate, vitamin B_6, and vitamin B_{12} are important components in the homocysteine metabolism and deficiencies of these vitamins may therefore contribute to atherosclerotic and thrombotic events [49]. Vitamin D has been suggested to act through several mechanisms including actions on cardiomyocytes and by indirect effects on circulating hormone and calcium concentrations [50]. Magnesium is a cofactor included in antioxidant enzymes and therefore of importance in preventing oxidative stress but also other mechanisms involving endothelial and vascular smooth cells [51]. Endothelial selenoproteins regulates vascular tone, cell adhesion, and apoptosis, and may also be involved in inflammatory processes and atherogenesis [52].

Although multivitamins are widely used and there are several mechanistic pathways through which multivitamins could act, there is limited epidemiological evidence on how multivitamins are associated with the risk of CVD. The majority of observational studies focusing on CVD mortality suggest no association [30,31,53]. Only one US prospective cohort study, defining multivitamin use as a supplement containing at least 10 vitamins and/or minerals, observed a 16% lower risk of CVD mortality in women and men [54].

Besides CVD mortality, observational studies have mostly focused on how multivitamins are associated with coronary heart disease (CHD) [29,32,53,55–58]. One prospective cohort study of Swedish women observed that multivitamin supplement use was associated with 27% lower risk on incident myocardial infarction (MI) [55] In one Swedish case-control study, use of multivitamin supplements was associated with a statistically significant 34% lower risk of incident MI in women and a 21% lower risk in men [58]. The Nurse's Health Study reported that regular multivitamin use was associated with a 24% lower risk of incident CHD among women [56]. In the Health Professionals Follow-up Study, multivitamin use for ≥10 years was associated with 25% lower risk of CHD incidence [57]. A prospective study of women and men in the USA found that the combined use of multivitamins and vitamin A, C, or E supplements was associated with a 25% lower risk of CHD mortality, and the effect was somewhat stronger for a duration of ≥5 years [58]. In another cohort of >90,000 American women, there was an inverse association between multivitamin use and incident MI, but only among those using multivitamins containing vitamins and minerals >200% of recommended daily allowances [32]. In the PHS cohort, there was no association found between regular multivitamin use and CHD mortality [53]. To the best of our knowledge, only two prospective cohort studies have examined the association between multivitamin supplement use and the risk of stroke [29,32].

Both studies, including both women and men, reported no association between multivitamin use and stroke risk.

In summary, there is more evidence from observational epidemiologic studies supporting a role for taking multivitamins in the prevention of CHD, but not stroke. CHD and ischemic stroke share risk factors as part of the process of atherosclerosis, but may still differ in their etiology. This may explain the lack of associations for CVD mortality, which may be attributable to a higher incidence of stroke.

3.4.2 Randomized Controlled Trials

As with cancer, the PHS II is the only large-scale, long-term, randomized controlled trial that has investigated the effect of a daily multivitamin use on the risk of major cardiovascular events in 14,641 male US physicians aged ≥50 years [59].

During 11.2 years of treatment and follow-up, 1732 men had major cardiovascular events, including 652 cases of MI, 643 cases of stroke (including 527 and 94 cases of ischemic and hemorrhagic stroke, respectively), and 829 of cardiovascular death. Men taking a daily multivitamin had no effect on major cardiovascular events (HR, 1.01; 95% CI, 0.91–1.10) (Figure 3.1), as well as total MI (HR, 0.93), total stroke (HR, 1.06), ischemic stroke (HR, 1.10), and hemorrhagic stroke (HR, 1.08) compared with men taking a placebo. Only fatal MI had a significant, beneficial effect with daily multivitamin use, with a 39% reduction (HR, 0.61; 95% CI, 0.38–1.00; $P = 0.048$). However, with only 70 cases of fatal MI, lower statistical power and multiple testing for this unspecified trial limits its interpretation. Among stroke subtypes, a daily multivitamin had no significant effect on either ischemic stroke (HR, 1.10) or hemorrhagic stroke (HR, 1.08). A daily multivitamin was also not significantly associated with cardiovascular mortality (HR, 0.95). In subgroup analyses, we examined whether baseline clinical, lifestyle, and familial risk factors for CVD modified the effect of a daily multivitamin on major cardiovascular events. As seen for cancer, there was a suggestion of a differential effect by age (P, interaction = 0.041), with men aged 50–59 and ≥70 years having a non-significant 27% increase and 9% decrease on major cardiovascular events. No other risk factors modified the effect of a daily multivitamin on major cardiovascular events. There were also 754 (5.1%) men in PHS II with a baseline history of CVD, in whom we found no differences in the primary (HR, 1.02) or secondary (HR, 0.96) prevention of major cardiovascular events (Figure 3.1).

The Linxian Chinese Cancer Prevention Trial investigated the association between a wide-spectrum low-dose multivitamin supplement on the risk of stroke mortality among Chinese men and women with esophageal dysplasia, thus may have a poor micronutrient diet. In this study, multivitamin supplement use was associated with a significant 58% lower risk of stroke mortality [60]. The SU.VI.MAX trial has also tested the effect of a low-dose supplement mixture of five antioxidants (including 120 mg ascorbic acid, 30 mg vitamin E, 6 mg beta carotene, 100 μg selenium, and 20 mg zinc), but found no association with incident ischemic CVD [45]. It is important to note that neither intervention tested in the Linxian nor SU.VI.MAX trials were comparable to usual multivitamin supplements taken by consumers, or the multivitamin tested in PHS II.

The Trial to Assess Chelation Therapy (TACT) is a randomized double-blind, placebo-controlled trial in 1708 men and women with a prior MI [61]. In this study, a 28-component high-dose multivitamin supplement during almost 5 years had no effect on cardiovascular events. The doses of vitamins and minerals were at higher concentrations than usually found in commercial multivitamins. Also in the PHS II trial no effect was observed for recurrent CVD [59]. However, in this study, a multivitamin including doses of nutrients corresponding to RDA was given. These results suggest that multivitamin supplementation may not have any impact in secondary prevention of CVD. This could be explained by that atherosclerosis is a progression of many processes including dyslipidemia, endothelial dysfunction, oxidation, inflammation, and others. If multivitamins play a role in this development, the role may not be equally important for all the different processes or across all the different stages of the disease from fatty streak development to manifestation of CHD. Moreover, patients with CVD may already be well-managed medically—medicines such as statins have, besides the lipid-lowering effect, antioxidant properties as well as other beneficial effects on endothelial function—hence further benefits of multivitamin use may not be seen. The results from multivitamin use in secondary prevention may, however, not be generalized to primary prevention of CVD. To fully understand the relationship between multivitamin supplements and CVD there is a need for being more specific with regard to doses, content, and whether it is primary or secondary prevention that is studied. In this way we may avoid confusion arising in both the scientific community and general public.

3.5 MULTIVITAMINS AND EYE DISEASE

Cataract and age-related macular degeneration (AMD) are two leading causes of visual impairment in older Americans [62]. However, it may be problematic to study this outcome because cataract and AMD show a slow progression which continue for several years. Preferably studying these outcomes in an observational setting would be to have standardized eye examination performed by an ophthalmologist. However, this is usually not possible in large epidemiological studies as it is a laborious, high-cost activity. Therefore, large studies usually rely on self-reports or registries, which may contribute to misclassification of outcome. This can be very problematic in the interpretation of findings if a healthy behavior or lifestyle is driven by the study participants that use multivitamin supplements and are diagnosed with cataract or AMD since they are more likely to be screened for eye disease, and seek medical help. Thus, this may drive observed findings toward no association or even a false finding of increased risk. Observational data generally support an inverse relation between dietary and blood levels of a range of nutrients, particularly those with antioxidant capabilities, and risks of cataract and AMD [63–65]. In two prospective population-based cohorts of 24,593 Swedish women aged 49–83 years (followed-up for an average of 8.2 years) and 31,120 Swedish men aged 45–79 years (followed-up for an average of 8.4 years), multivitamin use was not associated with age-related cataract extraction [66,67]. On the other hand, in a study where standardized eye examinations were performed among 478 women from the Nurse's Health Study and the prevalence of lens opacities was less among women who had been taking a multivitamin supplement for >10 years compared to never users [68]. Moreover, a recent systematic review and meta-analysis of 12 prospective cohort studies concluded that multivitamin supplements were associated with 34% lower risk of age-related cataract, and similar reductions were reported for nuclear and cortical cataracts [69].

Results of nutritional supplementation trials have been inconsistent, and few have examined the benefits and risks of a daily multivitamin [70]. In the Age-Related Eye Disease Study (AREDS), a common daily multivitamin was tested that contained a wide range of essential vitamin and minerals, finding a reduction in any lens opacity progression. In PHS II, the effect of a daily multivitamin on the secondary endpoints of cataract and AMD [71] was found to be consistent with the AREDS trial, reporting a significant 9% reduction in cataract after a mean follow-up if 11.2 years. When investigating cataract subtypes, the association was stronger for nuclear cataracts. Moreover, in the PHS II trial, there were some suggestions that the association was stronger among older men; however, the statistical test for interaction was not significant. The PHS II is also the first randomized trial testing the effect of a multivitamin supplement on AMD, finding no effect even though more cases of AMD were seen in the multivitamin versus placebo groups [71]. Two other trials have also reported an inverse association between multivitamin use and cataract [72,73].

3.6 MULTIVITAMINS AND COGNITIVE FUNCTION

In developed countries, the aging population is growing and it is therefore of great importance to find preventive strategies for cognitive decline, which is an intermediate step towards dementia. Randomized trials investigating either the short- or long-term effect from multivitamin supplements on cognitive function have reported mixed results. A daily multivitamin given to 14,641 male physicians aged ≥50 years for an average of 8.5 years did not provide any cognitive benefit compared to the placebo group [74]. However, in an 8-week randomized trial of 51 women and men aged 50–74 years, a daily multivitamin, mineral, and herbal supplement improved cognitive function [75]. Also, a French trial, designed to primarily investigate the effect from a low-dose daily supplement including five antioxidant vitamins and minerals on ischemic CVD and cancer, a better verbal memory was reported in the active group compared to the placebo group [76]. In the Mineral and Vitamin Intervention Study (MAVIS), 910 women and men aged <65 years were randomized to either receive a daily low-dose multivitamin or placebo for 12 months [77]. There were beneficial effects on cognitive function from the multivitamin treatment. In another 6-month randomized trial of 220 women, the cognitive performance increased both in the group receiving a daily multivitamin or placebo [78].

3.7 MULTIVITAMINS AND OTHER OUTCOMES

Despite the widespread use of multivitamin supplements, basic science studies and short-term clinical trials are needed to evaluate the potential mechanisms through which multivitamins may reduce the risk of cancer and other promising endpoints. There are limited data on how the introduction of daily multivitamin use, with its low levels of essential vitamins and minerals, even affect changes in core nutritional biomarkers. Equally important is to understand how any changes in nutritional biomarkers may be affected by baseline nutritional status to potentially identify key population subgroups for intervention. Studies investigating how multivitamins affect changes in biomarkers and mechanistic pathways associated with major chronic diseases would provide a much needed perspective to which individual or combination of vitamins and minerals contained in common multivitamins may be responsible for its beneficial effects. Very little is known with regard to changes in coronary biomarkers including lipids, glucose, insulin, C-reactive protein, and others. For other chronic disease outcomes such as cancer, for which multivitamins have shown greater promise for prevention to date, established biomarkers of risk are more elusive but an important opportunity for research moving forward.

Moreover, multivitamins have not been studied well with respect to their association with intermediate endpoints for CVD such as hypertension, hypercholesterolemia, and diabetes. In cross-sectional data from PHS, the likelihood of multivitamin use was significantly higher among men with a history of hypertension [15]. Today only one randomized trial has been conducted among 128 obese Chinese women aged 18–55 years to examine changes in blood pressure. In this trial, participants were randomized to take a high-dose multivitamin, low-dose multivitamin, calcium, or placebo for 26 weeks. Women taking a high-dose multivitamin non-significantly reduced systolic blood pressure and diastolic blood pressure by 5 and 5 mmHg from baseline. Additionally, there were also significant improvements in other coronary risk factors [79,80]. It is very important to understand how multivitamin use is associated with coronary biomarkers and intermediate endpoints to better understand the biological pathway of how these supplements may act. Today, there is a big research gap within this area.

Finally, little is known on the association between multivitamin use and inflammatory disease (e.g., rheumatoid arthritis, inflammatory bowel diseases) and neurological disorders (e.g., multiple sclerosis (MS), Alzheimer's disease, Parkinson's disease). These diseases are characterized by high levels of inflammatory biomarkers and oxidative stress, and therefore multivitamins may have a preventive role because many of the nutrients included are thought to inhibit inflammatory and oxidative processes. In the Nurses' Health Study, no prospective association was observed between multivitamin use and MS; however, this study was limited by the inclusion of a small number of incident cases. Otherwise, the epidemiological and clinical studies are sparse, reflecting the fact that inflammatory and neurological disease may be hard to study because of difficulties in relying on self-reports and the availability of national registries.

3.8 CONCLUSIONS

The use of multivitamin supplements remains high in the general public, which underscores their importance and timeliness in the prevention of chronic diseases. The USPSTF concluded that there was insufficient evidence to recommend multivitamin supplements for the primary prevention of cancer and CVD. However, this recommendation was based on the results from two clinical trials, of which one (PHS II) tested a commonly used multivitamin, while the other (SU.VI.MAX) tested a limited combination of selected vitamins and minerals not found commercially. As a result, there is still a great need for complimentary evidence from basic science studies, observational studies, and clinical trials to understand whether multivitamin supplements can prevent not only total and site-specific cancers, but also CVD and its key risk factors. There is also a need to understand how the timing of multivitamin use during childhood, adolescence, and various stages of adulthood impacts its effect on cancer and other endpoints. Further, more studies are needed to distinguish the role of multivitamins in the primary versus secondary prevention of cancer, for which there were suggestive findings from PHS II. Moreover, there are almost no data for the effect of a multivitamin on inflammatory and neurological diseases.

Future studies on multivitamin use should also focus on the importance of baseline nutritional status and whether particular subgroups of individuals may be better targeted to take multivitamin supplements—or not—to prevent cancer, CVD, and other chronic diseases. The USPSTF recommendation against the use of several single high-dose vitamin or mineral supplements should not be expanded to multivitamin use given the need for more studies focusing on the role of the combination of low-dose essential vitamins and minerals contained in multivitamins in health.

REFERENCES

1. Fortmann SP, Burda BU, Senger CA, Lin JS, Whitlock EP. Vitamin and mineral supplements in the primary prevention of cardiovascular disease and cancer: An updated systematic evidence review for the U.S. Preventive Services Task Force. *Annals of Internal Medicine.* Dec 17, 2013; 159(12):824–834.
2. Moyer VA. Vitamin, mineral, and multivitamin supplements for the primary prevention of cardiovascular disease and cancer: U.S. Preventive services Task Force recommendation statement. *Annals of Internal Medicine.* Apr 15, 2014; 160(8):558–564.
3. Wassertheil-Smoller S, McGinn AP. Multivitamin and mineral supplements: Hung jury. *Womens Health (Lond Engl).* Mar 2014; 10(2):111–113.
4. Guallar E, Stranges S, Mulrow C, Appel LJ, Miller ER, 3rd. Enough is enough: Stop wasting money on vitamin and mineral supplements. *Annals of Internal Medicine.* 2013; 159:850–851.
5. *US Department of Agriculture and US Department of Health and Human Services. Report of the Dietary Guidelines Advisory Committee on the Dietary Guidelines for Americans, 2010. June 15, 2010. Available at:* http://www.cnpp.usda.gov/DGAs2010-DGACReport.htm.
6. National Institutes of Health State-of-the-science conference statement: Multivitamin/mineral supplements and chronic disease prevention. *Annals of Internal Medicine.* Sep 5, 2006; 145(5):364–371.
7. Bailey RL, Gahche JJ, Lentino CV et al. Dietary supplement use in the United States, 2003–2006. *Journal of Nutrition.* Feb 2011; 141(2):261–266.
8. Gahche J, Bailey R, Burt V et al. Dietary supplement use among U.S. adults has increased since NHANES III (1988–1994). *NCHS Data Brief.* Apr 2011(61):1–8.
9. Muth MK, Anderson DW, Domanico JL, Smith JB, Wendling B. *Economic characterization of the dietary supplement industry.* Washington, DC: Center for Food Safety and Administration, Food and Drug Administration; 1999.
10. Nutrition Business Journal. *NBJ's Supplement Business Report: An Analysis of Markers, Trends, Competition and Strategy in the U.S. Dietary Supplement Industry.* New York 2011.
11. Yetley EA. Multivitamin and multimineral dietary supplements: Definitions, characterization, bioavailability, and drug interactions. *The American Journal of Clinical Nutrition.* Jan 2007; 85(1):269S–276S.

12. Millen AE, Dodd KW, Subar AF. Use of vitamin, mineral, nonvitamin, and nonmineral supplements in the United States: The 1987, 1992, and 2000 National Health Interview Survey results. *Journal of the American Dietetic Association.* Jun 2004; 104(6):942–950.
13. Kim HJ, Giovannucci E, Rosner B, Willett WC, Cho E. Longitudinal and secular trends in dietary supplement use: Nurses' Health Study and Health Professionals Follow-Up Study, 1986–2006. *Journal of the Academy of Nutrition and Dietetics.* Mar 2014; 114(3):436–443.
14. Park K, Harnack L, Jacobs DR, Jr. Trends in dietary supplement use in a cohort of postmenopausal women from Iowa. *American Journal of Epidemiology.* Apr 1 2009; 169(7):887–892.
15. Rautiainen S, Wang L, Gaziano JM, Sesso HD. Who uses multivitamins? A cross-sectional study in the Physicians' Health Study. *European Journal of Nutrition.* Jun 2014; 53(4):1065–1072.
16. Messerer M, Johansson SE, Wolk A. Use of dietary supplements and natural remedies increased dramatically during the 1990s. *Journal of Internal Medicine.* Aug 2001; 250(2):160–166.
17. Radimer K, Bindewald B, Hughes J, Ervin B, Swanson C, Picciano MF. Dietary supplement use by US adults: Data from the National Health and Nutrition Examination Survey, 1999–2000. *American Journal of Epidemiology.* Aug 15, 2004; 160(4):339–349.
18. Block G, Jensen CD, Norkus EP et al. Usage patterns, health, and nutritional status of long-term multiple dietary supplement users: A cross-sectional study. *Nutrition Journal.* 2007; 6:30.
19. Lee JS, Kim J. Factors affecting the use of dietary supplements by Korean adults: Data from the Korean National Health and Nutrition Examination Survey III. *Journal of the American Dietetic Association.* Sep 2009; 109(9):1599–1605.
20. Robson PJ, Siou GL, Ullman R, Bryant HE. Sociodemographic, health and lifestyle characteristics reported by discrete groups of adult dietary supplement users in Alberta, Canada: Findings from The Tomorrow Project. *Public Health Nutrition.* Dec 2008; 11(12):1238–1247.
21. Reedy J, Haines PS, Campbell MK. Differences in fruit and vegetable intake among categories of dietary supplement users. *Journal of the American Dietetic Association.* Nov 2005; 105(11):1749–1756.
22. Gorrini C, Harris IS, Mak TW. Modulation of oxidative stress as an anticancer strategy. *Nature Reviews. Drug Discovery.* Dec 2013; 12(12):931–947.
23. Montero AJ, Jassem J. Cellular redox pathways as a therapeutic target in the treatment of cancer. *Drugs.* Jul 30, 2011; 71(11):1385–1396.
24. Ju J, Picinich SC, Yang Z et al. Cancer-preventive activities of tocopherols and tocotrienols. *Carcinogenesis.* Apr 2010; 31(4):533–542.
25. Cardenas E, Ghosh R. Vitamin E: A dark horse at the crossroad of cancer management. *Biochemical Pharmacology.* Oct 1, 2013; 86(7):845–852.
26. Du J, Cullen JJ, Buettner GR. Ascorbic acid: Chemistry, biology and the treatment of cancer. *Biochimica et Biophysica Acta.* Dec 2012; 1826(2):443–457.
27. Crider KS, Yang TP, Berry RJ, Bailey LB. Folate and DNA methylation: A review of molecular mechanisms and the evidence for folate's role. *Advances in Nutrition.* Jan 2012; 3(1):21–38.
28. Ulrich CM, Reed MC, Nijhout HF. Modeling folate, one-carbon metabolism, and DNA methylation. *Nutrition Reviews.* Aug 2008; 66 Suppl 1:S27–S30.
29. Watkins ML, Erickson JD, Thun MJ, Mulinare J, Heath CW, Jr. Multivitamin use and mortality in a large prospective study. *American Journal of Epidemiology.* Jul 15, 2000; 152(2):149–162.
30. Park SY, Murphy SP, Wilkens LR, Henderson BE, Kolonel LN. Multivitamin use and the risk of mortality and cancer incidence: The multiethnic cohort study. *American Journal of Epidemiology.* Apr 15, 2011; 173(8):906–914.

31. Mursu J, Robien K, Harnack LJ, Park K, Jacobs DR, Jr. Dietary supplements and mortality rate in older women: The Iowa Women's Health Study. *Archives of Internal Medicine.* Oct 10, 2011; 171(18):1625–1633.
32. Neuhouser ML, Wassertheil-Smoller S, Thomson C et al. Multivitamin use and risk of cancer and cardiovascular disease in the Women's Health Initiative cohorts. *Archives of Internal Medicine.* Feb 9, 2009; 169(3):294–304.
33. Ishitani K, Lin J, Manson JE, Buring JE, Zhang SM. A prospective study of multivitamin supplement use and risk of breast cancer. *American Journal of Epidemiology.* May 15, 2008; 167(10):1197–1206.
34. Larsson SC, Akesson A, Bergkvist L, Wolk A. Multivitamin use and breast cancer incidence in a prospective cohort of Swedish women. *The American Journal of Clinical Nutrition.* May 2010; 91(5):1268–1272.
35. Stolzenberg-Solomon RZ, Chang SC, Leitzmann MF et al. Folate intake, alcohol use, and postmenopausal breast cancer risk in the Prostate, Lung, Colorectal, and Ovarian Cancer Screening Trial. *The American Journal of Clinical Nutrition.* Apr 2006; 83(4):895–904.
36. Chan AL, Leung HW, Wang SF. Multivitamin supplement use and risk of breast cancer: A meta-analysis. *The Annals of Pharmacotherapy.* Apr 2011; 45(4):476–484.
37. Stevens VL, McCullough ML, Diver WR et al. Use of multivitamins and prostate cancer mortality in a large cohort of US men. *Cancer Causes & Control.* Aug 2005; 16(6):643–650.
38. Giovannucci E, Ascherio A, Rimm EB, Colditz GA, Stampfer MJ, Willett WC. A prospective cohort study of vasectomy and prostate cancer in US men. *JAMA: The Journal of the American Medical Association.* Feb 1993; 269(7):873–877.
39. Zhang Y, Coogan P, Palmer JR, Strom BL, Rosenberg L. Vitamin and mineral use and risk of prostate cancer: The case-control surveillance study. *Cancer Causes & Control.* Jul 2009; 20(5):691–698.
40. Lawson KA, Wright ME, Subar A et al. Multivitamin use and risk of prostate cancer in the National Institutes of Health-AARP Diet and Health Study. *Journal of the National Cancer Institute.* May 16, 2007; 99(10):754–764.
41. Park Y, Spiegelman D, Hunter DJ et al. Intakes of vitamins A, C, and E and use of multiple vitamin supplements and risk of colon cancer: A pooled analysis of prospective cohort studies. *Cancer Causes & Control.* Nov 2010; 21(11):1745–1757.
42. Jacobs EJ, Connell CJ, Patel AV et al. Multivitamin use and colon cancer mortality in the Cancer Prevention Study II cohort (United States). *Cancer Causes & Control.* Dec 2001; 12(10):927–934.
43. Giovannucci E, Stampfer MJ, Colditz GA et al. Multivitamin use, folate, and colon cancer in women in the Nurses' Health Study. *Annals of Internal Medicine.* Oct 1, 1998; 129(7):517–524.
44. Gaziano JM, Sesso HD, Christen WG et al. Multivitamins in the prevention of cancer in men: The Physicians' Health Study II randomized controlled trial. *JAMA: The Journal of the American Medical Association.* Nov 14, 2012; 308(18):1871–1880.
45. Hercberg S, Galan P, Preziosi P et al. The SU.VI.MAX Study: A randomized, placebo-controlled trial of the health effects of antioxidant vitamins and minerals. *Archives of Internal Medicine.* Nov 22, 2004; 164(21):2335–2342.
46. Blot WJ, Li JY, Taylor PR et al. Nutrition intervention trials in Linxian, China: Supplementation with specific vitamin/mineral combinations, cancer incidence, and disease- specific mortality in the general population. *Journal of the National Cancer Institute.* 1993; 85(18):1483–1492.
47. Esterbauer H, Gebicki J, Puhl H, Jurgens G. The role of lipid peroxidation and antioxidants in oxidative modification of LDL. *Free Radical Biology and Medicine.* 1992; 13(4):341–390.

48. Levine M, Rumsey SC, Daruwala R, Park JB, Wang Y. Criteria and recommendations for vitamin C intake. *JAMA: The Journal of theAmerican Medical Association.* Apr 21, 1999; 281(15):1415–1423.
49. Kaul S, Zadeh AA, Shah PK. Homocysteine hypothesis for atherothrombotic cardiovascular disease: Not validated. *Journal of the American College of Cardiology.* Sep 5, 2006;48(5):914–923.
50. McGreevy C, Williams D. New insights about vitamin D and cardiovascular disease: A narrative review. *Annals of Internal Medicine.* Dec 20, 2011; 155(12):820–826.
51. Bo S, Pisu E. Role of dietary magnesium in cardiovascular disease prevention, insulin sensitivity and diabetes. *Current Opinion in Lipidology.* Feb 2008; 19(1):50–56.
52. Brigelius-Flohe R, Banning A, Schnurr K. Selenium-dependent enzymes in endothelial cell function. *Antioxidants & Redox Signaling.* Apr 2003; 5(2):205–215.
53. Muntwyler J, Hennekens CH, Manson JE, Buring JE, Gaziano JM. Vitamin supplement use in a low-risk population of US male physicians and subsequent cardiovascular mortality. *Archives of Internal Medicine.* Jul 8, 2002; 162(13):1472–1476.
54. Pocobelli G, Peters U, Kristal AR, White E. Use of supplements of multivitamins, vitamin C, and vitamin E in relation to mortality. *American Journal of Epidemiology.* Aug 15, 2009; 170(4):472–483.
55. Rautiainen S, Akesson A, Levitan EB, Morgenstern R, Mittleman MA, Wolk A. Multivitamin use and the risk of myocardial infarction: A population-based cohort of Swedish women. *The American Journal of Clinical Nutrition.* Nov 2010; 92(5):1251–1256.
56. Rimm EB, Willett WC, Hu FB et al. Folate and vitamin B6 from diet and supplements in relation to risk of coronary heart disease among women. *JAMA: The Journal of the American Medical Association.* 1998; 279(5):359–364.
57. Rimm EB, Stampfer MJ, Ascherio A, Giovannucci E, Colditz GA, Willett WC. Vitamin E consumption and the risk of coronary heart disease in men. *The New England Journal of Medicine* 1993; 328:1450–1456.
58. Holmquist C, Larsson S, Wolk A, de Faire U. Multivitamin supplements are inversely associated with risk of myocardial infarction in men and women—Stockholm Heart Epidemiology Program (SHEEP). *Journal of Nutrition.* Aug 2003; 133(8):2650–2654.
59. Sesso HD, Christen WG, Bubes V et al. Multivitamins in the prevention of cardiovascular disease in men: The Physicians' Health Study II randomized controlled trial. *JAMA: The Journal of theAmerican Medical Association.* Nov 7, 2012; 308(17):1751–1760.
60. Mark SD, Wang W, Fraumeni JF, Jr. et al. Lowered risks of hypertension and cerebrovascular disease after vitamin/mineral supplementation: The Linxian Nutrition Intervention Trial. *American Journal of Epidemiology.* Apr 1, 1996; 143(7):658–664.
61. Lamas GA, Boineau R, Goertz C et al. Oral high-dose multivitamins and minerals after myocardial infarction: A randomized trial. *Annals of Internal Medicine.* Dec 17, 2013; 159(12):797–805.
62. Congdon NG, West KP, Jr. Nutrition and the eye. *Current Opinion in Ophthalmology.* Dec 1999; 10(6):464–473.
63. Chiu CJ, Taylor A. Nutritional antioxidants and age-related cataract and maculopathy. *Exp Eye Res.* Feb 2007; 84(2):229–245.
64. Seddon JM. Multivitamin-multimineral supplements and eye disease: Age-related macular degeneration and cataract. *The American Journal of Clinical Nutrition.* Jan 2007; 85(1):304S–307S.
65. Fletcher AE. Free radicals, antioxidants and eye diseases: Evidence from epidemiological studies on cataract and age-related macular degeneration. *Ophthalmic Research.* 2010; 44(3):191–198.

66. Rautiainen S, Lindblad BE, Morgenstern R, Wolk A. Vitamin C supplements and the risk of age-related cataract: A population-based prospective cohort study in women. *The American Journal of Clinical Nutrition.* Feb 2010; 91(2):487–493.
67. Zheng Selin J, Rautiainen S, Lindblad BE, Morgenstern R, Wolk A. High-dose supplements of vitamins C and E, low-dose multivitamins, and the risk of age-related cataract: A population-based prospective cohort study of men. *American Journal of Epidemiology.* Mar 15, 2013; 177(6):548–555.
68. Jacques PF, Chylack LT, Jr., Hankinson SE et al. Long-term nutrient intake and early age-related nuclear lens opacities. *Archives of Ophthalmology.* Jul 2001; 119(7):1009–1019.
69. Zhao LQ, Li LM, Zhu H. The Epidemiological Evidence-Based Eye Disease Study Research Group EY. The effect of multivitamin/mineral supplements on age-related cataracts: A systematic review and meta-analysis. *Nutrients.* 2014; 6(3):931–949.
70. Chew EY. Nutrition effects on ocular diseases in the aging eye. *Investigative Ophthalmology & Visual Science.* Dec 2013; 54(14):ORSF42– ORSF47.
71. Christen WG, Glynn RJ, Manson JE et al. Effects of multivitamin supplement on cataract and age-related macular degeneration in a randomized trial of male physicians. *Ophthalmology.* Feb 2014; 121(2):525–534.
72. Sperduto RD, Hu TS, Milton RC et al. The Linxian cataract studies. Two nutrition intervention trials. *Archives of Ophthalmology.* 1993; 111(9):1246–1253.
73. Maraini G, Williams SL, Sperduto RD et al. A randomized, double-masked, placebo-controlled clinical trial of multivitamin supplementation for age-related lens opacities. Clinical trial of nutritional supplements and age-related cataract report no. 3. *Ophthalmology.* Apr 2008; 115(4):599–607 e591.
74. Grodstein F, O'Brien J, Kang JH et al. Long-term multivitamin supplementation and cognitive function in men: A randomized trial. *Annals of Internal Medicine.* Dec 17, 2013; 159(12):806–814.
75. Harris E, Macpherson H, Vitetta L, Kirk J, Sali A, Pipingas A. Effects of a multivitamin, mineral and herbal supplement on cognition and blood biomarkers in older men: A randomised, placebo-controlled trial. *Human Psychopharmacology.* Jul 2012; 27(4):370–377.
76. Kesse-Guyot E, Fezeu L, Jeandel C et al. French adults' cognitive performance after daily supplementation with antioxidant vitamins and minerals at nutritional doses: A post hoc analysis of the Supplementation in Vitamins and Mineral Antioxidants (SU.VI.MAX) trial. *The American Journal of Clinical Nutrition.* Sep 2011; 94(3):892–899.
77. McNeill G, Avenell A, Campbell MK et al. Effect of multivitamin and multimineral supplementation on cognitive function in men and women aged 65 years and over: A randomised controlled trial. *Nutrition Journal.* 2007; 6:10.
78. Wolters M, Hickstein M, Flintermann A, Tewes U, Hahn A. Cognitive performance in relation to vitamin status in healthy elderly German women-the effect of 6-month multivitamin supplementation. *Preventive Medicine.* Jul 2005; 41(1):253–259.
79. Wang C, Li Y, Zhu K, Dong YM, Sun CH. Effects of supplementation with multivitamin and mineral on blood pressure and C-reactive protein in obese Chinese women with increased cardiovascular disease risk. *Asia Pacific Journal of Clinical Nutrition.* 2009; 18(1):121–130.
80. Li Y, Wang C, Zhu K, Feng RN, Sun CH. Effects of multivitamin and mineral supplementation on adiposity, energy expenditure and lipid profiles in obese Chinese women. *International Journal of Obesity (Lond).* Jun 2010; 34(6):1070–1077.

4 Prenatal Supplementation and Its Effects on Early Childhood Cognitive Outcome

Sarah E. Saint and Janet E. Frick

CONTENTS

4.1 INTRODUCTION

The most rapid developmental changes of the human lifespan occur before birth. The fetus' body is literally built from the nutrients provided by its mother, expanding the adage "you are what you eat" into "the fetus is what the mother eats." In addition, pregnancy has several sensitive periods during which nutrition can promote or impede species-typical development. Because of expanded awareness of these issues, researchers have been increasingly interested in learning how mothers' nutritional status and dietary intake of certain nutrients affect fetal development, as well as a child's propensity for disease and disability throughout their lifespan (e.g., the fetal origins hypothesis; Barker, 1995). The purpose of this chapter is to review the current literature on prenatal nutritional supplementation, with a specific emphasis on nutrients that have been shown to impact later brain and cognitive development in the growing child.

Supplementation during pregnancy has many potential health impacts to both fetus and mother, including altering the micronutrient status of the infant offspring, correcting deficiencies in the mother, and enhancing the early development of structures such as the visual and central nervous systems. Many nutrients have been studied in the quest to prevent negative birth outcomes and to optimize fetal development, and once an important nutrient is discovered, widespread supplementation and/or fortification initiatives often follow (e.g., WHO, UNICEF, and ICCIDD, 1996; Surai and Sparks, 2001; Mills and Signore, 2004). For example, the United States Centers for Disease Control and Prevention (CDC, 1992) recommends that all women of childbearing age consume 400 μg of folic acid (the synthetic form of the B vitamin folate) each day because of the substantial literature linking folic acid supplementation with significant reductions in the prevalence of neural tube defects such as spina bifida and anencephaly (see Czeizel et al., 2013 for a recent review). Neural tube defects arise during the first 3–4 weeks after conception, a period of time when most women are not yet aware that they are pregnant, which is the reasoning behind folic acid being fortified into cereal products in many countries to ensure that women of childbearing age maintain adequate blood levels of the nutrient to support typical development should they become pregnant. The United States, for example, has implemented widespread fortification of folic acid into cereals and grains since 1998 and has subsequently seen a significant drop in the number of babies born with neural tube defects (Mills and Signore, 2004).

Nevertheless, nutrients are not inherently "good" or "bad"; most nutrients have minimums that are needed to support normal bodily functioning and tolerable upper limits that can result in toxicity if exceeded. In the case of folic acid, and many other good micronutrients, research concerning the effects of high intake has been lacking. Balance is vital for optimal health as nutrients work synergistically within the body, affecting one another and the overall health of the human being they are supporting. Therefore, one complicating factor in the use of widespread fortified foods to prevent deficiency is the higher potential for exceeding the recommended dietary allowances (RDAs) or even tolerable upper limits of some micronutrients. In the United States, in particular, the consumption of large amounts of processed, micronutrient-fortified foods and the use of nutritional supplements are common (Lin and Yen, 2007; Gahche et al., 2011), making them potentially easy for Americans to unknowingly reach and exceed the RDA and even tolerable upper limits of certain micronutrients.

For example, a single serving (3/4 cup) of General Mills' "Total" cereal provides 100% of the daily value of iron, folic acid, calcium, and up to nine other vitamins and minerals, making it somewhat of a multivitamin in food form (General Mills, 2014).

Another complicating factor for understanding the impact of supplementation is that an individual's ability to absorb some nutrients can depend on stores of that nutrient in the body. Women with low iron stores are able to absorb a higher percentage of the elemental iron from a supplement (the body's way of counteracting deficiency) than are iron-replete women taking the same dose (Miret et al., 2003). This differential absorption also functions as a protective mechanism to avoid toxicity, although there are certainly upper limits to the body's ability to regulate absorption in this way. This is easy to overlook for the general consumer who is trying to get the RDA of a certain nutrient without regard to his/her own current stores and can result in wasted money (in the case of water-soluble vitamins, for example, which are excreted at excess levels) or, in extreme cases, toxicity (in the case of minerals and fat-soluble vitamins). In addition, one's nutrient status is dynamic; as a woman's nutrient stores are used up throughout pregnancy due to the excess demand from the fetus, supplementation and/or increased dietary intake becomes necessary to correct low levels and to ensure that the fetus is receiving all of the nutrients needed for optimal development. Altogether, the study of nutrition and supplementation is inherently complicated due to its synergistic nature, but the addition of fetal demands on maternal nutrient stores and maternal physiological changes that occur during pregnancy complicate this area of research even further.

4.2 ASSESSING THE IMPACT OF SUPPLEMENTATION

Given the importance (and challenges) of studying the impact of prenatal nutritional supplementation, one of the first questions to ask concerns the outcome measures by which the effects of supplementation will be evaluated. Although a large number of studies have assessed the impact of supplements on physical growth or global developmental measures, it has not been until recently that questions about the impact of nutrients on specific processes underlying brain or cognitive development have begun to emerge. This has been supported by the establishment of a solid empirical and methodological foundation of research tools that have been validated for the study of early cognition (see Colombo, 1993 for an overview). Thus, in order to evaluate the literature on the impact of prenatal supplementation on infant cognitive development, it is helpful to offer a brief review of the research tools that are most commonly employed to study infant cognition.

The history of infant cognitive assessment can be divided into two broad epochs. First, developmental research in the early twentieth century was characterized by an interest in normative development, documenting the ages at which infants and children typically reached particular developmental (primarily motor) milestones. Observational, longitudinal research characterized this period (e.g., Gesell and Ilg, 1943), and several developmental scales were developed during this time, most notably the Bayley Scales of Infant and Toddler Development (BSID; Bayley, 1969), which continues to be used to this day (Bayley, 2006). The focus of scales such as the BSID is on documenting the normative course of attainment of different developmental milestones, providing a score which compares an individual child's progress in relation to his or her same-age peers. Scales such as the BSID are useful as global measures of normative development and are available across a wide age range; the current version of the Bayley Scales can be administered as early as 1 month of age. These scales provide reliable information about normative development and are useful for evaluating if certain nutritional supplements are helping to alleviate global developmental problems that are associated with malnutrition. However, such developmental scales have limited utility when it comes to understanding more specific nutritional effects on cognitive development; the predictive validity of developmental scales toward later cognitive outcome is limited, particularly for developmental scale scores obtained from infants less than 2 years of age (see Colombo, 1993 for an overview). Developmental scales such as the Bayley are primarily composed of motor milestone items for infants under 18 months of age, and motor skill development is only coarsely related to later intelligence and cognitive outcome; it is only once developmental scales begin to incorporate language-related items (around 18 months of age) that they begin to show better prediction of later intelligence and academic outcome (McCall, 1979). Thus, developmental scales such as the BSID are best considered as global measures of developmental status, and their role in evaluating the cognitive effects of nutritional interventions may be limited (Colombo and Carlson, 2012).

As useful as developmental scales are for assessing normative development, the scientific study of infant cognition took a huge step forward in the 1960s and 1970s when new measures based on visual attention and information processing theory began to emerge (e.g., Horowitz et al., 1972). The advent of video technology (which allowed for more fine-grained analysis of moment-to-moment infant behavior), along with a shifting research zeitgeist toward interest in both individual differences and visual perception (e.g., Fantz, 1961; Fagan, 1970; Groves and Thompson, 1970), led to the development of a number of theory-driven measures of infant cognition (based on information processing theory). Although more thorough reviews of these measures are available elsewhere (Bornstein and Sigman, 1986; Colombo, 1993; McCall and Carriger, 1993), the most studied of these measures include visual habituation (a decline in look duration to a repeatedly presented stimulus), visual recognition memory (a behavioral preference for a novel stimulus compared with a familiar stimulus), and reaction time (the speed at which an infant is able to shift gaze to detect a novel stimulus). Although they differ somewhat in their theoretical underpinnings, these measures all have in common that they assess the ability of infants to detect novelty in their environment, to rapidly detect changes in their surroundings, and to compare a current stimulus with the one previously seen. Thus, they tap into various aspects of underlying cognition, which have theoretical as well as empirical validity. Importantly, these infant information processing-based measures do show modest but reliable predictive validity with later IQ and cognitive outcome (e.g., Rose et al., 1992). Although their use in studies of nutritional intervention is still not widespread (Colombo and Carlson, 2012), growing awareness of the usefulness of such cognitive/attention measures will hopefully lead to improvements in nutritional intervention studies, in which the outcome measures have theoretical as well as practical relevance to the study of cognition.

Early studies of nutritional supplementation during pregnancy measured general birth outcomes such as APGAR scores, birth weight and length, head circumference, and length of gestation, which serve as early indicators of the overall health of a pregnancy. Many reviews of nutrients that affect these global birth outcomes are available (Ramakrishnan et al., 1999, 2012a,b; Larqué et al., 2011; Lauritzen and Carlson, 2011); therefore, these studies will not be the focus of the current chapter. This chapter will also exclude studies in which the infant was supplemented after birth but the mother was not supplemented during pregnancy, although some interesting work has been done in this area (Colombo et al., 2013). Instead, we will focus on reviewing the major prenatal supplementation studies that have tested indices of infant and child cognitive development as outcome measures. The nutrients that we will cover are iron, the omega-3 fatty acid DHA, and iodine (see Table 4.1 for an overview of these nutrients' role in brain development and significant findings related to cognitive development).

4.3 IRON

4.3.1 Background

Hemoglobin is a protein in red blood cells (RBCs) that binds with oxygen in the lungs and transports it throughout the body. Iron is an integral part of hemoglobin; in fact, the oxygen taken in via the lungs directly binds with the iron molecules contained in hemoglobin, making iron necessary for adequate oxygen transport throughout the body. When an individual's iron levels become very low—usually due to blood loss, insufficient dietary intake, or low absorption of iron from food or supplements—iron deficiency anemia (IDA) results. Symptoms of IDA include fatigue, shortness of breath, trouble concentrating, and dizziness due to the decrease in the amount of oxygen that can bind to hemoglobin in the blood and thus be transported throughout the body. A human female's need for iron increases dramatically during pregnancy (27 vs. 18 mg/day non-pregnant) mainly due to blood volume expansion and formation and maintenance of the placenta (National Research Council, 2001). In addition, there is a critical need for an adequate iron supply for species-typical fetal neurogenesis and neuronal differentiation to take place, as well as proper myelination due to the fact that oligodendrocytes, the neuroglia responsible for producing myelin, require iron to function (Beard, 2008; Todorich et al., 2009). This dramatic increase in demand can make it difficult for pregnant women to obtain the necessary amount of iron from a healthy well-balanced diet alone, especially because an estimated 14% of women aged 12–49 years in the United States have low serum ferritin concentrations (<15 ng/L; used to evaluate iron stores in the body) even before they become pregnant, with rates as high as 19.9% in non-Hispanic African American women and 18.6% in Mexican American women (CDC, 2012). Although universal iron supplementation recommendations for pregnant women were once prevalent (e.g., CDC, 1998), they have since been modified to account for women's iron status and dietary intake before supplementation is recommended (WHO, 2011). The most bioavailable sources of iron (termed "heme" iron) come from animal sources, particularly red meat; however, non-heme iron (from plant sources) can be found in legumes, tofu, dried fruits, dark green leafy vegetables, and iron-fortified breads and cereals, and

TABLE 4.1
Overview of Nutrients Covered in this Chapter and Their Role in Brain Development, as Well as a Summary of the Significant Findings Covered in Infants and Children as a Result of Supplementation or Differences in Biological Measures

	Brain Development	Infant Cognitive Development	Child Cognitive Development
Iron	Iron is necessary for *myelination* (due to its role in oligodendrocyte health and functioning), *neurogenesis*, and *neuronal differentiation* (Beard, 2008; Todorich et al., 2009)	Anemic mothers: *Global Cognitive Development* (Bayley MDI at 12 months; Chang et al., 2013)	Anemic mothers: *Cognitive development* (UNIT IQ, Stroop, backward digit span), *motor development* (MABC), and *fine motor control and processing speed* (finger-tapping test at 7–9 years; Christian et al., 2010)
		Malnourished mothers: *Psychomotor development* (Bayley PDI at 7 months; Tofail et al., 2008)	Malnourished mothers: *Motor development and visual/spatial attention* (3.5 years; Prado et al., 2012) Well-nourished, non-anemic mothers: *Socio-behavioral development* (Zhou et al., 2006; Parsons et al., 2008)
DHA	DHA is found to preferentially accumulate in the developing *retina* (where it is involved in phototransduction; Jeffrey et al., 2001) and *brain* (specifically *synaptosomes*, *astrocytes*, and *myelin*; McNamara and Carlson, 2006)	*Development of attention* in infancy and toddlerhood (Colombo et al., 2004), *hand–eye coordination* (Dunstan et al., 2008), and *problem-solving* (Judge et al., 2007)	*Mental processing* (MPCOMP of K-ABC global developmental test; Helland et al., 2003; Campoy et al., 2011) and *problem-solving* (Helland et al., 2008)
Iodine	Necessary for production of *THs*, which impact: *cellular metabolism*, *myelination*, *tubulin production*, *neurogenesis*, *neuronal migration*, *axonal growth*, *dendritic branching*, *synaptogenesis*, and *glial cell differentiation and migration* (Dussault and Ruel, 1987; Williams, 2008)	Severe deficiency: *Severe intellectual disability* (cretinism; Cranefield, 1962), *neurological development*, *head circumference*, *BSID developmental quotient* (Cao et al., 1994) Mild/moderate deficiency: *Psychomotor development* (Bayley PDI; Velasco et al., 2009), *infant behavior* (Bayley Behavior Rating Scale; Velasco et al., 2009), and *Brunet-Lezine developmental quotient* (Berbel et al., 2009)	*Severe deficiency:* VMI test (O'Donnell, 2012) Mild/moderate deficiency: *ADHD prevalence* (Vermiglio et al., 2004)

non-heme iron's bioavailability can be increased by pairing its consumption with vitamin C.

The majority of prenatal iron supplementation studies have focussed on global measures of development such as birth weight and length and duration of gestation (e.g., Cogswell et al., 2003; Siega-Riz et al., 2006), with comparatively few randomized controlled trials having investigated its long-term effects on the offspring's cognitive development in infancy and childhood. Recent studies of iron supplementation in pregnant women have mainly been conducted in developing countries and have typically included a comparison group supplemented with multiple micronutrients (MMNs)—usually something close to the United Nations International Multiple Micronutrient Preparation (UNIMMAP; UNICEF, WHO, and UNU, 1999)—in addition to iron and/or iron + folic acid supplemented group(s). The UNIMMAP supplement is a comprehensive multivitamin and mineral formula containing iron, folic acid, zinc, copper, selenium, iodine, niacin, and vitamins A, D, E, C, B1, B2 (riboflavin), B6, and B12 and is typically given in populations in which micronutrient malnutrition is common, such as rural parts of India and China.

Part of the difficulty in interpreting the results of these studies is that there remains debate over the methods used to test for iron deficiency during pregnancy (Haram et al., 2001). Hemoglobin level is used in many of the studies discussed subsequently, but iron deficiency is only one potential cause of anemia, and thus a low hemoglobin (Hb) level is not sufficient to diagnose an individual with anemia, specifically due to iron deficiency. In addition, results on serum ferritin tests—one of the most commonly used tests to detect iron deficiency—can fluctuate daily and are affected by maternal plasma volume changes that occur throughout pregnancy, as well as inflammation (Haram et al., 2001). Results have also been mixed and somewhat difficult to interpret due to differences in maternal health status, ages of infants and children at testing, and outcome measures used. With that being said, the main grouping factor for studies investigating child cognitive development related to iron status in pregnant women appears to be maternal health status: studies involving women with anemia, women who are malnourished, and women who are non-anemic and well-nourished. The main studies conducted with these populations are reported here.

4.3.2 Supplementation in Mothers with Anemia

A large double-blind, randomized controlled trial conducted in rural China examined the overall effects of folic acid (400 μg), folic acid (400 μg) + iron (60 mg), and an MMN supplement (containing 30 mg of iron and 400 μg of folic acid, in addition to other micronutrients) during pregnancy on children's mental development index (MDI) scores on the BSID at 12 months of age (Li et al., 2009). The authors did not find any clinically significant differences in mental development based on supplement type; however, Chang et al. (2013) published another analysis of the same data that looked into maternal IDA as a possible moderator of the various supplements' effects on child mental development. The authors used hemoglobin levels <110 g/L in the third trimester as their indicator of IDA. As discussed previously, low hemoglobin levels can have many causes, including normal hemodilution that occurs throughout pregnancy, making their designation of IDA questionable. Not surprisingly, Chang et al. found that the children of non-anemic mothers in their sample outperformed children of anemic mothers on the MDI. Supplementation with 60 mg of iron + folic acid, however, appeared to prevent the negative effects of anemia on children's MDI scores, as they were not significantly different from those of children of non-anemic mothers. Conversely, MMN and folic acid supplements did not have the same protective effect; children of anemic mothers who received the MMN supplement had significantly lower MDI scores at 12, 18, and 24 months when compared with children of non-anemic mothers. The MMN may have been less effective at increasing the children's cognitive outcomes due to the lower dose of iron (30 mg iron in the MMN vs. 60 mg iron in the iron + folic acid supplement) as well as inhibited absorption of iron due to the presence of zinc in the MMN (Swanson, 2003), although the MMN also included vitamin C, vitamin A, and riboflavin, all of which have been shown to enhance iron absorption (UNICEF, WHO, and UNU, 1999).

A study of Nepalese mothers and their children by Christian et al. (2010) also found that relatively high doses of iron supplementation (60 mg) in mothers living in an area where iron deficiency and IDA are prevalent prevented negative effects on cognitive development in their offspring. In this sample, which was not stratified by iron or anemia status, Christian et al. found that prenatal iron (60 mg) + folic acid (400 μg) + vitamin A (100 μg) supplementation was linked to higher scores on cognitive (UNIT IQ test, Stroop task, and backward digit span task) and motor tasks [movement assessment battery for children (MABC) and a finger-tapping test of fine motor control and processing speed] at 7–9 years of age when compared with a control group of children whose mothers had received vitamin A (100 μg) alone. Of note, two other supplemented groups (60 mg iron + 400 μg folic acid + 100 μg vitamin A + 30 mg zinc, and an MMN-supplemented group that included the same quantities of iron, folic acid, vitamin A, and zinc, among other micronutrients) did not show significant differences from the control group on any measures, except for the MMN group showing significantly shorter times to complete the Stroop task.

Finally, in Indonesia, the Supplementation with Multiple Micronutrients Intervention Trial (SUMMIT) investigated the effects of MMN versus iron (30 mg) + folic acid (400 μg) supplementation during pregnancy on child development indicators 3.5 years later and found surprisingly different results (Prado et al., 2012). The researchers tested the preschoolers' motor, cognitive, and socio-emotional development using selected items from various standardized developmental assessments (such as the BSID and the Ages and Stages Questionnaire). The authors used hemoglobin <110 g/L at enrollment to designate anemia, but did not appear to stratify their analyses based on the trimester during which each woman was enrolled (an important consideration for determining expected Hb levels during a specific point in pregnancy), nor did they investigate the cause of each individual's anemia (iron, folate or B12 deficiency, blood loss, etc.). In general, and contrary to the previous two studies discussed, the children of women with anemia in this study did not appear to benefit from the iron + folic acid supplement, but those receiving the MMN supplement did benefit. Specifically, the children of anemic mothers who received the MMN supplement scored 0.23 SD higher (approximately 3 months developmental difference) on the visual attention/spatial ability test when compared with the children of anemic mothers who received iron + folic acid alone. The lack of a beneficial effect of the iron + folic acid supplement in this anemic population may be due to the fact that they only received a 30 mg dose of iron, whereas Chang et al. (2013) and Christian et al. (2010) saw significant buffering against the negative effects of anemia during pregnancy with much higher (60 mg) doses of iron supplementation. This does not fully explain why the MMN supplement seemed to help this group, counter to the results of the two previously reviewed studies, though it may be that the inclusion of vitamin C, vitamin A, and vitamin B2 (riboflavin) enhanced iron absorption more effectively than the inclusion of zinc negatively affected it. In addition, the sample of women in this study appears to have been stratified by anemia status and malnutrition status independently, such that women who were anemic may or may not have also been malnourished, which could also explain the MMN's beneficial effect in this case (this point will be discussed further in the next section on studies of malnourished mothers).

These studies illustrate the need for more specific testing of maternal iron levels throughout pregnancy to ensure that iron deficiency is present before causal effects can be proposed between iron supplementation during pregnancy and improvement of child cognitive outcome measures in the iron-deficient (with or without anemia) population. In addition, it is important to control for normal hemodilution that occurs throughout pregnancy and to adjust the rubric used to judge iron deficiency and anemia, depending on the mother's current stage of pregnancy. Finally, it remains unclear whether lower doses of iron (e.g., 30 mg) would effectively improve child cognitive development in the population of pregnant women with IDA while simultaneously reducing unpleasant side-effects, such as gastrointestinal upset; this is a question that deserves further investigation.

4.3.3 Supplementation in Malnourished Mothers

Studies of children of malnourished mothers report more consistent findings with regard to MMN supplementation positively predicting psychomotor development, and iron + folic acid alone having little-to-no beneficial effect in this population. For example, Tofail et al. (2008) supplemented pregnant women from an impoverished community in rural Bangladesh with iron (30 or 60 mg) + folate (400 μg) or an MMN supplement (which contained 30 mg iron and 400 μg folate in addition to other micronutrients) from week 14 of gestation through to delivery. All participants also received macronutrient food supplements, as this was already standard practice in this area. The authors found that the infants of low-body mass index (BMI < 18.5) mothers who received the MMN supplement during pregnancy scored significantly higher on the psychomotor development index (PDI) portion of the Bayley at 7 months of age when compared with infants of low-BMI mothers who received either of the two types of iron (30 or 60 mg) + folate supplements. In fact, children of low-BMI mothers who were supplemented with the MMN formula had scores on the PDI that were not significantly different from those of children born to normal-BMI (≥18.5) mothers, indicating that the MMN was successful in preventing the negative effects of overall malnutrition during gestation.

Prado et al. (2012), discussed previously with regard to their results in anemic mothers, also found a significant interaction between maternal malnutrition (determined by mid-upper arm circumference <23.5 cm) and supplement type with regard to children's motor and visual/spatial attention test scores in the SUMMIT study. Specifically, the children whose mothers were malnourished but received an iron + folic acid supplement scored 0.35SD lower on the motor development test (an estimated practical difference of roughly 4.5 months) and 0.35SD lower on the visual attention/spatial ability test (roughly 5 months difference) when compared with the children of malnourished mothers in the MMN group. Similar to the infants in Tofail et al. (2008), the children of malnourished mothers who received the MMN supplements during pregnancy showed no difference in scores from the well-nourished group. Again, it appears that the individuals included in the anemia and malnutrition analyses were not mutually exclusive, although an interaction between the two conditions and supplement type on child cognitive outcomes was not discussed.

In the case of malnourished mothers, research supports MMN supplementation in order to address the MMN deficiencies these mothers are experiencing. MMN supplementation in this population can buffer several of the negative cognitive and motor effects normally seen in children of mothers who are malnourished during pregnancy, whereas iron + folic acid supplementation alone has been shown to have little-to-no beneficial effect in this population.

4.3.4 Supplementation in Well-Nourished Mothers

In all of the studies mentioned previously, the children of well-nourished non-anemic mothers did not appear to be significantly affected by MMN or iron + folic acid supplementation in any of the outcome domains measured (cognitive, social, and motor). However, these women were from populations in which malnutrition and/or IDA is very common, which may mean that their risk of iron overload from supplementation was still quite a bit lower than that of women from areas where malnutrition and IDA are much less common (such as the United States). Zhou et al. (2006) investigated the effects of iron supplementation on non-anemic well-nourished Australian mothers and their offspring. The authors found no effect of routine prenatal iron (20 mg) supplementation (from 20 weeks through delivery) on children's IQ when compared with placebo, even though the rate of IDA in mothers at delivery was significantly lower in the iron-supplemented group (1% vs. 9%). They did find, however, significantly more parental reports of behavior problems on a behavioral screening tool (the Strengths and Difficulties Questionnaire, SDQ) in the iron-supplemented group. These results spurred members of the same research team to follow this sample further to see whether they could detect any long-term negative effects of prenatal iron supplementation later in childhood (Parsons et al., 2008). They tested the same group at 6–8 years of age using parent and teacher versions of the SDQ and found significantly more children from the iron-supplemented group had teacher reports of having peer problems than children in the placebo group (8% iron group vs. 2% placebo group). This follow-up study lends further support to the results they found at 4 years of age and indicates a need for future research to investigate iron supplementation in developed countries where iron deficiency is not pervasive.

4.3.5 Iron Summary

The studies covered in this section highlight the immense need for more controlled research to elucidate the circumstances under which iron supplementation (alone, with folic acid or another micronutrient, or in an MMN formula) during pregnancy prevents negative effects on the cognitive development of the child. The negative effects of anemia during pregnancy on child cognitive development were buffered in two of the studies with relatively high doses of iron (60 mg) + folic acid (Christian et al., 2010; Chang et al., 2013); infants of these mothers achieved test scores similar to those of children of non-anemic, also supplemented, mothers. Conversely, in populations afflicted with overall malnutrition (which likely includes some level of iron deficiency), iron + folic acid supplementation during pregnancy proved ineffective in buffering the negative effects on infants' and children's cognitive development when compared with an MMN formulation that seemingly addressed the MMN deficiencies that these malnourished women were experiencing. There do not seem to be any clinically significant benefits, however, to supplementing mothers who are not anemic or malnourished, and the potential negative effects of excess iron intake on the socio-behavioral development of the offspring remain unclear at this point. In all of the studies conducted in populations in which anemia and/or malnutrition were common (Tofail et al., 2008; Christian et al., 2010; Prado et al., 2012; Chang et al., 2013), the healthy, non-anemic groups were used for comparison and were all supplemented; therefore, it is difficult to say whether the supplements they were given during pregnancy impacted their offspring's cognitive development for better or for worse, although their standardized scores were indicative of normal development. In addition, the findings from Zhou et al. (2006) and Parsons et al. (2008) shed light on areas of development (specifically, socio-behavioral development in childhood) that may be affected by unnecessary iron supplementation, but were not tested in the studies that stratified mothers by anemia and/or malnutrition status for comparison. Tests of socio-behavioral development should be included in future studies now that we know this is an area that excess iron may affect. In addition, supplementing healthy non-anemic pregnant women seems like a counterintuitive strategy as many pregnant women find that iron supplements (on their own or in a prenatal multivitamin) cause them gastrointestinal upset, which may impact their appetite and their ability to take in as many nutrients from whole foods. However, in developing countries with little access to healthcare and very high rates of iron deficiency and anemia, the benefits of routine iron + folic acid supplementation on birth outcomes, child cognitive development, and maternal anemia appear to outweigh the potential and currently very understudied socio-behavioral cost of consuming unnecessary supplemental iron during pregnancy.

4.4 DHA

4.4.1 Background

Fats in the body serve three main functions: they serve as energy sources, as building blocks of phospholipid bilayers in cellular membranes, and are converted to other useful substances such as eicosanoids (chemical messengers) and hormones. A growing number of studies have shown that imbalances and deficiencies in certain fatty acids can lead to health problems. Omega-6 linoleic acid (LA) and omega-3 alpha-linolenic acid (ALA) cannot be synthesized de novo and are thus required in the human diet. Both these fatty acids are polyunsaturated, meaning that they have at least two carbon–carbon double bonds in their chemical structure, which makes them less structurally stiff, more fluid, and less able to pack together. These structural qualities improve the fluidity of cellular membranes and, in turn, benefit cellular health (in comparison to saturated or trans fats, for example). Arachidonic acid (AA; an omega-6 fatty acid) and eicosapentaenoic acid (EPA), and DHA (omega-3 fatty acids) are not considered essential because the human body can synthesize them from dietary LA and ALA; LA is metabolized into AA, whereas ALA is metabolized into EPA and then DHA. However, <1% of ALA is ultimately converted into DHA due to the two-step process required, making dietary consumption of preformed DHA (mainly via oily fish and other ocean products) the most efficient method of intake for humans (Goyens et al., 2006). Once these fatty acids are absorbed into the body, they can be converted into other compounds such as chemical messengers known as eicosanoids (see German, 2011 for a review of the functions of fatty acids), which can cause inflammatory/blood vessel dilation (when derived from omega-6 fatty acids) or anti-inflammatory/blood vessel constriction (when derived from omega-3 fatty acids) responses, making it very clear why having a balance of these fatty acids in the body is crucial for normal physiological and cellular functioning (Hadders-Algra, 2008).

In industrialized nations, the difficulty in maintaining an ideal balance in these omega-3 and omega-6 fatty acids does not usually come from deficiency in the omega-6 group, as oils rich in these fatty acids (i.e., palm, soybean, rapeseed, and sunflower oils) are common in the processed foods ubiquitous in the American diet (Dunstan et al., 2008). In contrast, omega-3 fatty acids are found in high amounts in only a limited number of sources. The richest source of omega-3 fatty acids is cold-water fatty fish (e.g., salmon, sardines, and mackerel; Scientific Advisory Committee on Nutrition, 2004), although seeds (e.g., flaxseed) and nuts are good plant-based alternatives (Lane et al., 2014). Dietary sources of preformed DHA, however, are even scarcer and are largely limited to cold-water fatty fish and algal oil, which is a source suitable for vegetarians (Arterburn et al., 2008; Lane et al., 2014). It can be particularly difficult for pregnant women concerned about mercury contamination in fish to consume enough omega-3 fatty acids to maintain proper balance without supplementation of purified fish oil or algal oil capsules (Strain et al., 2012). This is especially important during pregnancy because the developing fetus is unable to efficiently convert ALA into DHA, making it even more important for pregnant women to obtain preformed DHA from their diet (or supplements) to aid in efficient transfer to the fetus (Salem et al., 1996; Sun et al., 2007).

DHA has been shown to preferentially accumulate in the cells of the fetal brain (e.g., myelin, astrocytes, and synaptosomes) and retina (where it is involved in phototransduction), especially during the third trimester, and is transferred to infants after birth via breast milk to the extent that it is present in the mother's diet (Jeffrey et al., 2001; see McNamara and Carlson, 2006 for a review). Prenatal DHA supplementation has been associated with increased gestational length and birth weight (e.g., Smuts et al., 2003; Olsen et al., 2007), whereas infant formula supplemented with DHA has been shown to improve visual functioning in young infants (Birch et al., 1992; Carlson and Werkman, 1993). Following suit, researchers began investigating the effects of maternal DHA dietary content and blood levels on the child's later cognitive development (e.g., Ghys et al., 2002; Bakker et al., 2003; Gale et al., 2008; Oken et al., 2008a,b; Boucher and Burden, 2011). It was not until relatively recently, however, that researchers have attempted to manipulate prenatal DHA levels via maternal supplementation in order to explore the potential effects on cognitive outcomes in infants and longer-term development in toddlers and children.

Seven major clinical trials have examined the effects of maternal DHA supplementation (via capsules or a functional food) on subsequent infant and child cognitive development. Five of these studies have measured developmental indicators in infants and children under 3 years of age, whereas two have focussed on more long-term effects shown in school-aged children (specifically 4–7 years old). The developmental indicators used for each study vary, which has made comparison across studies difficult and has led to the overall lack of consensus regarding which developmental processes are affected by DHA and in what dosages it is most helpful prenatally. These studies are reviewed subsequently, with findings organized by the age group in which outcomes were measured.

4.4.2 Prenatal Supplementation Studies and Infant/Toddler (<3 Years) Development

Colombo et al. (2004) studied the development of attention (using measures that have been verified in other research to be predictive of childhood IQ, as explained earlier in this chapter) in infants who had been enrolled in a previous prenatal DHA supplementation trial (Smuts et al., 2003). In this previous study, Smuts et al. supplemented mothers with either high DHA eggs (containing 135 mg per egg) or normal DHA eggs (containing 35 mg per egg) from 24–28 weeks of gestation through delivery. Colombo et al. (2004) tested these infants' habituation and novelty-preference responses at 4, 6, and 8 months of age and did not find DHA/egg group membership to be a significant predictor of infants' performance on these cognitive tasks. They did, however, find that maternal RBC phospholipid DHA levels at birth (stratified into high vs. low groups at the median) were significantly and positively predictive of infant visual attention (although infant birth RBC phospholipid levels were surprisingly not predictive of infant performance). The infants whose mothers had high DHA levels at delivery showed shorter peak look durations during habituation at 4 and 6 months, which is an indication that they needed less time to process the stimuli (i.e., more mature attentional response). In addition, at 12 and 18 months of age, the infants of mothers with high DHA levels spent more time looking to orient themselves to a toy placed in front of them and exhibited sustained attention for a higher percentage of the overall time that the task took place (i.e., more mature focussed attention). When the toddlers' distractibility and attention patterns were measured during a free-play session at 12 and 18 months, more advanced attention continued to be observed in the children of mothers who had high RBC DHA levels at delivery. These toddlers took longer to turn to a distractor (video clips presented at intermittent intervals), and when they did turn to it, they looked at it for a significantly shorter amount of time before returning to focus attention on a toy in front of them. In other words, the infants of mothers who had higher DHA levels at delivery were less distractible during a focussed attention task, suggesting that maternal DHA status was related to infant cognitive response after birth. The authors note that further data will be required to elucidate why supplement group and the infants' own RBC DHA levels at birth were not significant predictors of performance.

A study of Australian mothers and their children examined moderately high doses of DHA and EPA supplementation (2200 and 1100 mg, respectively), compared with 2700 mg olive oil capsules (a monounsaturated fatty acid) in pregnant women from 20 weeks of gestation through birth (Dunstan et al., 2008). The authors followed-up on the children of these mothers at 2.5 years of age and tested their behavioral (Child Behavior Checklist), cognitive (Griffiths Mental Development Scales, GMDS), and language development (Language Development Survey and Peabody Picture Vocabulary Test). The children from the fish oil-supplemented group showed significantly higher hand–eye coordination scores on the GMDS; however, none of the other tests showed significant differences based on supplement group alone. When newborn cord blood fatty acid levels were used to predict later performance, AA (an omega-6 fatty acid) content was negatively correlated with the overall performance on the GMDS, and children whose cord blood had contained higher levels of omega-3 versus omega-6 fatty acids showed superior performance on the later hand–eye coordination subtest. These findings support those of Colombo et al. (2004) regarding blood levels of fatty acids being more predictive of developmental outcomes than supplementation status and also identify hand–eye coordination as another specific area of development that omega-3 fatty acid intake may impact, perhaps due to faster processing speed and more mature attentional development (e.g., Colombo et al., 2004; Willatts et al., 2013).

Judge et al. (2007) conducted a randomized trial using a functional food (DHA cereal bars containing 300 mg DHA in 8:1 DHA:EPA ratio or corn oil cereal bars containing 1.7 g of fat, but no DHA; average of 5 weeks consumed) from 24 weeks of gestation through delivery. The authors tested infants at 9 months of age on a problem-solving task (a combination of the commonly used support and cover tasks that are used to test infants' knowledge of object permanence and object relations; see Willatts, 1984) and the Fagan test of infant intelligence, which primarily tests recognition memory via habituation/novelty-preference tasks (Fagan and Detterman, 1992). Infants of mothers who had received the DHA cereal bars during pregnancy performed significantly better on the support and cover problem-solving task, bolstering the practice of testing more specific areas of cognitive development that DHA may impact. The infants in this study did not significantly differ on the Fagan memory task, although this may have been due to the test being conducted at 9 months of age, which may be too late in infancy to see differences in recognition memory via habituation/novelty-preference tasks. The supplemented and non-supplemented infants in Colombo et al. (2004) performed equally well at 8 months of age, yet had significant differences in their performance earlier at 4 and 6 months.

When supplementation status and standardized developmental assessments (as opposed to blood levels of DHA and more specific cognitive tests) are the main variables studied in DHA intervention studies, researchers have largely reported insignificant findings, potentially due to the lack of specificity inherent in both measures, in addition to a higher prevalence of methodological challenges. For example, Tofail et al. (2006) examined 10-month-old infants' developmental scores on the Bayley II MDI and PDI in relation to their mothers' supplementation status during pregnancy. Bangladeshi women were supplemented with an omega-3 fish oil capsule (1200 mg DHA/1800 mg EPA) or a soy oil capsule (2250 mg LA/270 mg ALA) from 25 weeks of gestation through delivery.* Regression models indicated that supplement type was not a significant predictor of Bayley MDI or PDI scores after accounting for many other significant variables (such as age, quality of stimulation at home, birth weight, gestational age, and BMI of mothers), although the number of variables in this model left very little variance available for supplement type to account for on a global test of developmental status. In addition, the researchers were able to follow-up on only 62% of the infants in the original sample, and there were significant demographic differences between the two groups; infants who were lost to follow-up were from families with lower income and were smaller in size at birth, which is unfortunate as these infants would have been most likely to show a benefit from supplementation. Finally, the authors posit that supplement type may not have significantly predicted Bayley scores due to the fact that they did not use a true placebo control and that supplementation occurred from 25 weeks through delivery, which may not have been early or long enough for significant effects to occur.

In Australia, Makrides et al. (2010) looked at the effects of supplementation early in pregnancy (sometime before 21 weeks of gestation through delivery) on Bayley III Cognitive and Language scores at 18 months of age. The supplements contained 800 mg of DHA and 100 mg of EPA, whereas the control contained 500 mg of vegetable oils in saturated:polyunsaturated:monounsaturated fat ratios typical of the diet in that area. The authors found significantly fewer scores, indicating delayed cognitive development in the fish oil group; however, there were no overall differences in mean cognitive and language scores of the children in each supplement group. This may have been due to the dosage being insufficient to fully correct for Australian women's very low dietary intake of omega-3 long-chain polyunsaturated fatty acids, according to the authors. Differences in individual absorption may also have hidden potential effects in this and the previous study by Tofail et al. suggesting that measurement of DHA status, rather than analysis based on supplementation group, may better elucidate the effects of prenatal DHA status on infant cognitive development.

In summary, studies of prenatal supplementation of DHA and its effects on early cognitive development have resulted in mixed findings. Results have been fairly consistent that biological indicators of DHA status (maternal RBC phospholipid and cord blood measures) predict performance on tests of specific domains of attention and cognitive development. However, studies using DHA supplementation status to predict performance on global assessments of developmental status have not been conducted. In addition, differences in sample characteristics (e.g., country of residence, diet, BMI, and absorption abilities) and duration and timing of supplementation (starting before the third trimester or after) may have contributed to the mixed

* The soy oil capsule was a pseudo-control, as humans can (inefficiently) transform ALA into EPA and DHA as previously mentioned, but was used because of its prevalence in the diet of the Bangladesh community (Tofail et al., 2006).

results. Overall, however, when specific, sensitive tools are used to assess cognitive processes, significant developmental differences based on DHA status have been observed (e.g., Colombo et al., 2004; Judge et al., 2007; Dunstan et al., 2008; see Colombo, 2001 for more on the topic of infant cognitive testing methods that are best-suited for DHA research).

4.4.3 Prenatal Supplementation Studies and School-Age Development (4+ Years)

Two major randomized trials of the long-term effects of prenatal omega-3 fatty acid supplementation have been conducted in the past 15 years. Helland et al. (2003) supplemented Norwegian mothers with cod liver oil (1183 mg DHA/803 mg EPA) or corn oil (4747 mg LA/92 mg ALA) from 18 weeks of gestation through 3 months postpartum and measured the children's cognitive development via the Kaufman Assessment Battery for Children (K-ABC) at 4 and 7 years of age. At the 4-year follow-up, the children from the cod liver oil-supplemented group scored significantly higher (four points) on the Mental Processing Composite (MPCOMP) of the K-ABC and showed similarly sized, though statistically insignificant, advantages in areas of sequential and simultaneous processing (measures of children's ability to problem-solve in different ways), as well as non-verbal abilities. When the children turned seven, Helland et al. (2008) found that the differences in K-ABC scores based on the supplement group were no longer seen; however, maternal plasma phospholipid DHA content (a measure comparable to the maternal RBC phospholipid DHA content) at 35 weeks of gestation and breast milk content at 3 months postpartum were still significant predictors of the 7-year-old children's sequential processing performance. The authors posit that the gains that the children experienced due to maternal supplementation during pregnancy may have helped them to perform better early on in development; however, those gains may have been overshadowed by environmental differences (e.g., dietary differences, educational resources, and socioeconomic status) that became increasingly more salient for the child's cognitive development as childhood progressed. Accordingly, the authors found that parent education was also a significant predictor of age 7 sequential processing scores.

A similar randomized controlled trial was conducted by Campoy et al. (2011) in Germany, Hungary, and Spain. The authors supplemented mothers from 20 weeks of gestation through delivery with DHA (500 mg) + EPA (150 mg), 5-methyltetrahydrofolate (400 μg, a methylated form of folic acid) alone or with DHA (500 mg) + EPA (150 mg), or a placebo and assessed the children's cognitive development at 6.5 years of age using the K-ABC. All of the mothers were encouraged to breastfeed; however, if any chose not to or needed to supplement with formula, the infant received a formula with DHA and AA if they were enrolled in the treatment group or a formula without DHA and AA if they were from the placebo group. Similar to the findings of Helland et al. (2008), the authors did not find any significant difference on the K-ABC tests based on the supplement group. This may be due to the authors' encouragement of the mothers in both groups to breast feed; mothers who chose to breastfeed would have passed DHA on to their infants after birth via their breast milk, regardless of the supplementation group. However, children of mothers who had high

RBC DHA levels at delivery were significantly more likely to have an MPCOMP score above the 50th percentile, whereas children of mothers with higher overall AA (an omega-6 fatty acid) versus DHA RBC levels at delivery were significantly more likely to have an MPCOMP score below the 50th percentile, further supporting the stratification of DHA status based on biological markers as opposed to assigned supplement group to predict developmental differences.

Many of the studies that have investigated the effects of DHA supplementation on long-term child cognitive development have focussed on infant supplementation via formula, instead of maternal DHA supplementation during pregnancy. The few studies that have supplemented mothers during pregnancy have found biological measurements of DHA status to be the most predictive, which is not surprising as biological measures are more representative of the amount of DHA that was actually absorbed by the mother's body, and therefore available to the fetus, than is supplement group. The results of these studies also support the position that a well-balanced omega-3 to omega-6 ratio during pregnancy is important for fetal development to set the stage for normal brain development later in life; however, further research in this area of long-term effects on specific areas of cognitive development is needed before any strong conclusions can be made.

4.4.4 DHA Summary

The studies reviewed here have identified several specific areas of development that DHA may influence: problem solving, hand–eye coordination, sequential processing, and attention. For example, Colombo et al. (2004) and Judge et al. (2007) found the early development of attention, which later impacts and predicts overall intelligence and executive functioning (Colombo, 1993), to be an area in which DHA appears to be significantly helpful. Conversely, it appears that global measures such as the K-ABC and Bayley may be too broad to detect the very specific cognitive differences in infants and children that DHA status during pregnancy affects; the studies that used global outcome measures (the K-ABC and Bayley II or III, for example) early in life did not show significant effects of supplementation on performance, whereas the two that used specific skill-based measures (the support and cover problem solving task and habituation/novelty preference task, for example) did find significant effects of DHA levels or supplementation on performance. Now that research has uncovered several specific areas of cognitive functioning that DHA seems to affect, future studies can utilize more focussed cognitive tests in order to gain further insight into the role that DHA plays in fetal brain development.

A second overall theme that has come from this literature emphasizes blood levels of DHA over supplementation group as the most valid predictor of infant and child cognitive development. One might think that the two would be equally reflective of DHA status; however, administration of a supplement does not guarantee that it is absorbed well or that it is being transferred to the fetus and not primarily being used to correct maternal levels. As blood levels are more reflective than supplement group of DHA absorption, future research should utilize these measures to control for individual differences in maternal absorption and transfer and simultaneously attempt to elucidate the circumstances under which maternal and infant RBCDHA levels differ in their ability to predict future cognitive development. More work is needed to investigate the effects of prenatal DHA supplementation on cognitive outcomes in childhood; a few that have been done are fairly consistent, but there are too few to make definitive claims about long-term effects at this point.

4.5 IODINE

4.5.1 Background

Iodine is needed for the synthesis of thyroid hormones (THs), which in turn regulate cellular metabolism throughout the human body. Within the thyroid, iodine released from the blood binds with the individual amino acids that make up thyroglobulin (a protein), and these iodinated amino acids are then clipped to form THs, the most abundant of which is thyroxine (T4). Because iodine is not an endogenous compound and is necessary for TH production, it is considered an essential nutrient that must be supplied via diet or supplementation. When the thyroid does not have enough iodine to synthesize the required THs, the thyroid may enlarge itself in an attempt to obtain more iodine from the blood, resulting in goiter and a diagnosis of hypothyroidism (underactive thyroid functioning). As THs play such an important role in the body's metabolism, hypothyroidism commonly leads to symptoms such as lethargy, weight gain, thermoregulation abnormalities in the extremities, difficulty concentrating, and memory problems—all of which are indicative of a slower-than-normal metabolism.

During pregnancy, maternal iodine deficiency can have serious negative effects on the fetus. The fetus relies heavily on the mother for THs until mid-gestation (18–20 weeks), when the fetal hypothalamic–pituitary–thyroid (HPT) axis is more mature and functional (Obregon et al., 2007). Even after the HPT axis is functional, however, the fetus still relies on the mother to provide the iodine necessary to synthesize its own TH. During periods of rapid brain development, such as those that occur during gestation, slowing of the cellular metabolism due to low levels of THs can significantly impede neural development. In particular, THs are involved in neurogenesis, neuronal migration, axonal growth, dendritic branching, synaptogenesis, and glial cell differentiation and migration, in addition to regulating the rate at which myelination and tubulin production occur in the developing brain (Dussault and Ruel, 1987; Williams, 2008); hypothyroidism due to iodine deficiency results in slowing of these processes. Under conditions of severe prenatal iodine deficiency, these processes can be slowed to the point that they cause serious and permanent cognitive damage and result in a condition known as cretinism, characterized by significant intellectual disability, spastic motor functioning, deaf-mutism, and squint (Cranefield, 1962). In addition, the existence of TH receptors in the fetal brain during the first trimester of pregnancy indicates that THs play a role in neural development very early on in pregnancy (Obregon et al., 2007). Iodine supplementation programs utilizing iodized salt, potassium iodide (KI) tablets, and oral or intramuscular doses of iodinated oil initiated by the WHO and UNICEF have significantly reduced the incidence of iodine deficiency disorders (including cretinism) around the world; however, it remains a public health problem in many nations with low soil and water iodine concentrations and little access to meat, dairy, iodized salt, and ocean products (WHO, UNICEF, and ICCIDD, 2007).

During pregnancy, there is an increased need for iodine for two main reasons. First, the mother needs more iodine to produce more THs to supply the fetus with all of its required TH throughout the first and into some of the second trimester. In addition, the mother provides the fetus with the iodine necessary for it to synthesize much of its own TH (to the extent that the HPT axis of the fetus is functional) in the second half of gestation. Secondly, pregnancy induces an increased rate of clearance of iodine via the kidneys due to increased estrogen levels, making higher levels of iodine intake necessary to keep the mother and fetus iodine-replete and euthyroid (having a normal functioning thyroid). In addition, pregnant women with special dietary habits, such as vegetarians and vegans, may have a higher likelihood of experiencing iodine deficiency during pregnancy (Phillips, 2005) as iodine is largely found in animal products (cheese, milk, eggs, salt water fish, and shell fish; Haldimann et al., 2005), although iodized salt, soy milk, seaweed, and iodine-fortified foods may be good non-animal sources of iodine for this population (National Research Council, 2001).

4.5.2 Severe Iodine Deficiency

Although the link between severe iodine deficiency during pregnancy and disrupted fetal neurodevelopment has been extensively researched and reviewed (e.g., Cranefield, 1962; Pharoah et al., 1971; Hetzel, 2000; Morreale de Escobar et al., 2004), further research is needed to pinpoint the specific time periods during (or even prior to) pregnancy in which supplementation is needed in order to avoid the negative cognitive effects associated with deficiency. A few reviews of the literature in this area have been completed recently (Zimmerman 2009, 2012; Melse-Boonstra and Jaiwswal, 2010; Zhou et al., 2013), and they all generally support the practice of supplementing women who live in areas where severe iodine deficiency is prevalent. Furthermore, they suggest that the earlier the supplementation is given (in order to ensure that maternal stores are sufficient to last through the entire pregnancy), the better the offspring's outcomes are. With that being said, there remains a need for studies using more sensitive attention and cognitive processing measures (as opposed to global developmental and intelligence assessments) to enable more specific functional deficits to be detected in cases in which overt cretinism is not apparent (Melse-Boonstra and Jaiswal, 2010).

One of the earliest longitudinal iodine supplementation studies was conducted in Papua New Guinea by Pharoah et al. (1971). The researchers gave a single (relatively high) intramuscular dose of 4 mL iodinated oil to women and children living in an area with a high prevalence of endemic cretinism. Women who became pregnant after the injection were part of the supplemented group, and their children were compared with children of women in the trial who had not been supplemented prior to (or during) pregnancy. A much lower rate of endemic cretinism was observed in the supplemented group (7 out of 412 children examined vs. 26 out of 406), and from this, the authors concluded that there is a critical period during the first trimester of pregnancy during which sufficient iodine stores are necessary in order for typical neural development to follow (Pharoah et al., 1971).

Another longitudinal supplementation study provides support for the hypothesis that supplementation in iodine-deficient populations is required early in (if not before) pregnancy to prevent atypical development. Cao et al. (1994) and O'Donnell et al. (2002) looked at the importance of the timing of supplementation during pregnancy on developmental outcomes in an area of severe iodine deficiency in China. Of note, the women supplemented with single doses of oral iodinated oil (400 mg) beginning in their second trimester delivered infants with significantly fewer neurological abnormalities (2% vs. 9%) and significantly larger head circumferences at 1–2 years of age when compared with infants who were treated after birth or those whose mothers were treated in the third trimester (Cao et al., 1994). In addition, infants whose mothers had been treated during the second trimester had significantly higher developmental quotients on the BSID when compared with infants who had not been treated prenatally or after birth, whereas the scores of infants who had been supplemented during the third trimester or after delivery were only marginally higher than those of infants who had never been supplemented (Cao et al., 1994).

O'Donnell et al. (2012) later examined developmental outcomes in these children using several measures of psychological development and compared 6-year-old children whose mothers were supplemented prenatally with 6-year-old children who were first supplemented at 2 years of age. The authors continued to find that, in this area of severe iodine deficiency, the earlier the supplementation occurred, the better were the children's developmental outcomes. Specifically, those treated early in pregnancy (first or second trimester) had significantly higher scores (average of 86.2—early pregnancy vs. 81.5—third trimester vs. 72.1—comparison group) on the Developmental Test of Visual Motor Integration (VMI) than children from the comparison group, although all three groups were close to or in excess of 1SD below the standardized mean for this test (mean 100, SD 15), which is perhaps a testament to the severe nature of their iodine deficiency. However, the percentage of children showing significant impairment on the VMI who were supplemented in the second trimester was significantly lower than that of those who were supplemented in the third trimester or at 2 years of age (6.3%—early pregnancy vs. 18.8%—third trimester vs. 75%—comparison group).

4.5.3 Mild/Moderate Iodine Deficiency

The study of prenatal iodine supplementation and child cognitive development in areas of mild-to-moderate iodine deficiency is still new, and trials of excessive iodine intake in humans during pregnancy are non-existent, as it would be unsafe and unethical to intentionally dose mothers above the tolerable upper limit. However, evidence of mild learning and memory deficits was recently found in rat pups whose mothers were fed excessive iodine during pregnancy (Zhang et al., 2012), reinforcing the need for observational studies in humans to elucidate the effects of excessive or high iodine intake during pregnancy on offspring development. A recent review by Trumpff et al. (2013) includes a section that covers supplementation in areas of Europe classified as having mild iodine deficiency; therefore, our discussion will be limited to a few of the key studies in this area that have resulted in consistent findings.

Both Velasco et al. (2009) and Berbel et al. (2009) found evidence of more typical development in the infants of Spanish mothers supplemented orally with potassium iodide (KI). The controlled trial by Velasco et al. (2009) supplemented pregnant women daily from their first trimester on through lactation with 300 μg of KI and evaluated infants' development in both groups using the BSID and a Behavior Rating Scale. They found significant differences in the Bayley PDI based on group membership, although breastfeeding status turned out to be a confounding variable, with infants in the supplemented group who were breastfed achieving the highest PDI values.* In addition, infants from the potassium iodide-supplemented group significantly exhibited more behaviors typical of their age group in several areas of the Bayley Behavior Rating Scale (reaction to persons, reaction to mother, cooperation, activity, arousal, and producing sounds by banging). Berbel et al. (2009) found similar results in their study of pregnant women with mild hypothyroxinemia (low levels of circulating thyroxine, T4) in an area of Spain where iodine deficiency is highly prevalent. The authors supplemented these women with 200 μg KI daily either early (4–6 weeks) or later (12–14 weeks) in pregnancy and through lactation or after delivery and through lactation. Infant outcome was tested at 18 months post-partum using the Brunet-Lezine scales (a global developmental test) and showed that children of mothers supplemented early in pregnancy had significantly higher developmental quotients when compared with the other two supplemented groups. In addition, the group of mothers supplemented early in pregnancy showed a significantly higher percentage of children with normal or advanced performance and no children with delayed performance on the test (compared with a 25% and 36.8% incidence in those supplemented late in pregnancy or after delivery, respectively).

Finally, in a very small prospective study investigating the effects of maternal iodine status on child cognitive development, Vermiglio et al. (2004) found a 68.7% prevalence (11 of 16 children) of attention deficit hyperactivity disorder (ADHD) in children of mothers from a moderately iodine-deficient area of Sicily, whereas none of the 11 children of women from an iodine-sufficient area presented with the disorder. In addition, the children from the moderately iodine-deficient area had significantly lower IQ scores (92 vs. 110; > 1SD lower) on the WISC-III, whereas the subset of children with ADHD from this area showed an even more striking difference of 22 points when compared with the children from the iodine-sufficient area. Although not a controlled supplementation trial, this study does provide further support for the investigation of attention as an area of cognitive development that may be impacted negatively by low iodine status during pregnancy.

* The infants from the supplemented group were also significantly younger at BSID testing than the control group (12.44 ± 4.96 months—control group vs. 5.47 ± 2.86 months—supplemented group), which is troublesome as the 5-month and 12-month BSID have very different emphases (the 5-month test is heavily focussed on motor development, whereas the 12-month test includes areas such as language and communication that are largely absent in the 5-month test). The authors used the Bayley's standardized indices (MDI and PDI) to compare the groups' scores, which control for the age differences at testing to a point.

4.5.4 Iodine Summary

In summary, the evidence behind severe iodine deficiency causing severe cognitive and motor deficits is clear and well established; however, there is a need for further research in iodine-replete and mild-to-moderately iodine-deficient pregnant women to determine whether routine supplementation (via prenatal vitamins, for instance) is helpful and without side effects in these populations. In addition, further elucidation of the specific weeks of early gestation during which maternal iodine sufficiency is critical would be helpful in informing public health initiatives and would also determine whether routine supplementation in iodine-deficient populations "prior to" pregnancy, as has been implemented with folic acid, would be more effective. Finally, in a recent review of the effects of iodine deficiency during critical developmental stages (prenatal, infancy, and childhood) on cognitive development, Melse-Boonstra and Jaiswal (2010) called for the use of more focussed tests of the many components of cognitive development instead of global IQ and developmental quotient tests in order to provide a more detailed picture of the effects of insufficient iodine during pregnancy on the offspring (see Murcia et al., 2011; Santiago et al., 2013), echoing the call from Colombo (2001) with regard to research on DHA and the development of attention.

4.6 OTHER NUTRIENTS WITH EMERGING LITERATURES

The nutrients covered in this chapter are only a few of the nutrients that appear to affect brain development *in utero*, and new lines of research are emerging, which show promise in identifying other important nutritional predictors of early brain and cognitive development. Certain nutrients, such as zinc and the carotenoids lutein and zeaxanthin, have been studied extensively but ultimately were excluded from this review due to the fact that their impact on neurodevelopment based on prenatal supplementation is currently unclear. For example, the most recent zinc supplementation trials have not found significant differences in cognitive development based on supplementation status (e.g., Hamadani et al., 2002; Tamura et al., 2003; Black et al., 2013), even though zinc is believed to play a role in neurogenesis, neuronal migration, and synaptogenesis (Bhatnagar and Taneja, 2001) and has been shown to affect attentional and motor development in the past (see Bhatnagar and Taneja, 2001 for a review).

Other nutrients holding great promise in the realm of prenatal supplementation are the macular carotenoids lutein and zeaxanthin (LZ), which are dietary-derived nutrients that comprise the yellow pigment in the retina known as "macular pigment" and which are also found throughout neural tissue (Frick et al., 2009; Hammond, 2012). Although many carotenoids are found in nature and have also been studied in their role in human health, L and Z can only be obtained through dietary sources (primarily plant-based sources such as green and yellow vegetables and colored fruits; see Hammond, 2012). These carotenoids have been studied extensively in adults and have been shown to play many essential roles in visual function and processing speed (e.g., Renzi et al., 2013). Importantly, a number of LZ supplementation studies in adults have found measurable improvements in visual function as well as more general cognitive processing in supplemented groups compared with placebo groups (e.g., Renzi et al., 2014). The relevance to prenatal supplementation is that for the fetus, the carotenoids

L and Z are obtained from maternal stores, which in turn are largely dependent on maternal dietary intake, as these carotenoids cannot be manufactured by the body (see Hammond, 2012). After birth, however, young infants are completely dependent on their diet (i.e., their milk source in the early months) for these carotenoids, and this is where interesting questions emerge, because L and Z are found in human breast milk (in levels corresponding to maternal dietary intake; Cena et al., 2009), but are absent in most commercial infant formulas (Frick et al., 2009). Lutein is the dominant carotenoid found in the brain throughout prenatal and postnatal development (Vishwanathan et al., 2011; Hammond, 2012), and its prevalence throughout embryonic and neural tissues suggests that it may play an important role in visual and neural function throughout the lifespan and not just later in life, as it has primarily been studied (for example, in relation to macular degeneration; Olson et al., 2011). Thus, current research is examining the relation between maternal LZ levels, infant LZ levels, and infant visual and neural function (e.g., Henriksen et al., 2013; Frick et al., 2013). Based on findings with adults, it is expected that LZ status will be related to overall cognitive function, but more data are needed to address these predictions (Hammond and Frick, 2007).

4.7 DISCUSSION

As human beings grow, the complexity of the environmental and genetic interactions that impact development increases. For example, mothers' nutritional status during pregnancy can have very long-lasting effects on development in the case of teratogens and nutritional deficiencies in key nutrients (such as folate during neural tube closure), but nutritional differences outside of these areas can have more subtle and difficult-to-detect effects due to large variation in environmental influences as life progresses. In addition, due to the fact that the human body strives to maintain homeostasis, these subtle effects can go largely unnoticed because of compensatory mechanisms that work to keep the body functioning. It is for these reasons that more hypothesis-driven testing is needed to look for specific deficits or advantages related to functioning due to nutritional differences in addition to more general assessment of global developmental status (e.g., Colombo et al., 2004; Judge et al., 2007; Christian et al., 2010). Laboratory-based tasks are well-established to test the development of specific facets of cognition, such as attention, disengagement, and distractibility, and are worthwhile measures to include in future studies of prenatal supplementation and its effects on infant and child cognitive outcomes, although global tests such as the Bayley are still useful for documenting overall developmental progress, particularly in malnourished populations who are expected to suffer deficits without supplementation. In addition, longitudinal study of participants is vital to detect differences in developmental areas that do not follow a linear trend, such as the triphasic development of look duration during visual habituation (Colombo et al., 1999).

As the iron supplementation studies have shown us, it is important to factor in women's nutrient stores/current status, as well as any other health maladies (e.g., overall malnutrition, anemia, and infection), when deciding whether to recommend supplementation. For example, close spacing between pregnancies and breastfeeding may leave mothers mildly or frankly deficient in a number of nutrients, without time to recover her stores before a new pregnancy increases the demand placed on her body again. Individual differences in parity, breastfeeding status, diet, and health status need to be critically evaluated as potential moderating variables in prenatal supplementation studies. In addition, as the impact of a supplement ultimately depends on the ability of the mother's body to absorb it, biological measures of nutrient status may be more predictive of child cognitive outcomes than supplement group alone, as individual differences in the many potential moderating variables just mentioned can vary widely within a sample. For example, when Colombo et al. (2004) used biologically measured DHA status as a predictor of infant and toddler cognitive development, they found significant effects; when they used supplement group as a predictor, they did not.

Finally, the majority of research on supplementation during pregnancy has occurred in deficient populations, which does not necessarily translate to healthy, well-nourished populations. There is an overwhelming lack of research on supplementation of micronutrients and beneficial fats in non-deficient pregnant women, which is largely due to a lack of funding availability for the study of healthy populations. In addition, ethical considerations make it difficult to study excessive intake in humans in a controlled manner, although there are animal models that explore this topic. Nevertheless, supplementation studies in impoverished, nutrient-deficient populations are sometimes used to support generalized recommendations for supplement use during pregnancy in healthy populations, which is inappropriate and risky in our opinion. Thankfully, this trend toward generalized supplementation recommendations has evolved and become more sensitive to potential individual differences in nutrient stores and health status during pregnancy (e.g., WHO, 2011).

ACKNOWLEDGMENTS

This chapter was completed while the first author was a doctoral student in the Behavioral and Brain Sciences Program in the Department of Psychology, under the direction of the second author. The authors thank the other members of the UGA Infant Visual Attention Lab for feedback on earlier versions of this manuscript, especially Quinn Tracy, Kaitlyn Barrow, Laura Beckwith, Emily Harris, Victoria Moreira, Mallory Osborne, and Mark Wendolowski. Both authors have also benefitted from many discussions with Randy Hammond, Alex Anderson, Emily Bovier, and Laura Fletcher on these topics; their contributions are gratefully acknowledged.

REFERENCES

Arterburn, L. M., Oken, H., Bailey Hall, E. Hamersley, J., Kuratko, C. N., and Hoffman, J. P. 2008. Algal-oil capsules and cooked salmon: Nutritionally equivalent sources of docosahexaenoic acid. *Journal of the American Dietetic Association*, *108*(7), 1204–1209.

Bakker, E. C., Ghys, J., Kester, D. M., Vles, J. S. H., Dubas, J. S., Blanco, C. E., and Hornstra, G. 2003. Long-chain polyunsaturated fatty acids at birth and cognitive function at 7 y of age. *European Journal of Clinical Nutrition*, *57*(1), 89–95.

Barker, D. J. 1995. Fetal origins of coronary heart disease. *British Medical Journal*, *311*, 171–174.

Bayley, N. 1969. *The Bayley Scales of Infant Development: Birth to Two Years*. New York: The Psychological Corporation.

Bayley, N. 2006. *Bayley Scales of Infant and Toddler Development: Bayley-III* (Vol. 7). Harcourt Assessment, Psych. Corporation.

Beard, J. 2008. Why iron deficiency is important in infant development. *The Journal of Nutrition, 138*(2), 2534–2536.

Berbel, P., Mestre, J., Santamaría, A. et al. 2009. Delayed neurobehavioral development in children born to pregnant women with mild hypothyroxinemia during the first month of gestation: The importance of early iodine supplementation. *Thyroid, 19*(5), 511–519.

Bhatnagar, S. and Taneja, S. 2001. Zinc and cognitive development. *British Journal of Nutrition, 85*(S2), S139–S145.

Birch, E. E., Birch, D. G., Hoffman, D. R., and Uauy, R. 1992. Dietary essential fatty acid supply and visual acuity development. *Investigative Ophthalmology and Visual Science, 33*(11), 3242–3253.

Black, M., Sazawal, S., Black, R. E., Khosla, S., Kumar, J., and Menon, V. 2013. Cognitive and motor development among small-for-gestational-age infants: Impact of zinc supplementation, birth weight, and caregiving practices. *Pediatrics, 113*(5), 1297–1305.

Bornstein, M. H. and Sigman, M. D. 1986. Continuity in mental development from infancy. *Child Development, 57*(2), 251–274.

Boucher, O. and Burden, M. 2011. Neurophysiologic and neurobehavioral evidence of beneficial effects of prenatal omega-3 fatty acid intake on memory function at school age. *The American Journal of Clinical Nutrition, 93*, 1025–1037.

Campoy, C., Escolano-Margarit, M. V., Ramos, R. et al. 2011. Effects of prenatal fish-oil and 5-methyltetrahydrofolate supplementation on cognitive development of children at 6.5 y of age. *The American Journal of Clinical Nutrition, 94*(3), 1880–1888.

Cao, X. Y., Jiang, X. M., Dou, Z. H., Rakeman, M. A., Zhang, M. L., O'Donnell, K., Ma, T., Amette, K., DeLong, N., and DeLong, G. R. 1994. Timing of vulnerability of the brain to iodine deficiency in endemic cretinism. *New England Journal of Medicine, 331*(26), 1739–1744.

Carlson, S. and Werkman, S. 1993. Visual-acuity development in healthy preterm infants: Effect of marine-oil supplementation. *The American Journal of Clinical Nutrition, 58*, 35–42.

Cena, H., Castellazzi, A. M., Pietri, A. et al. 2009. Lutein concentration in human milk during early lactation and its relationship with dietary lutein intake. *Public Health Nutrition, 12*, 1878–1884, doi:10.1017/S1368980009004807.

Centers for Disease Control and Prevention (CDC). 1992. *Recommendations for the use of folic acid to reduce the number of cases of spina bifida and other neural tube defects.* MMWR 41(no. RR-14).

Centers for Disease Control and Prevention (CDC). 1998. *Recommendations to prevent and control iron deficiency in the United States.* MMWR 47(no. RR-3), pp. 1–36.

Centers for Disease Control and Prevention (CDC). 2012. *Second National Report on biochemical indicators of diet and nutrition in the U.S. population*, pp. 1–480.

Chang, S., Zeng, L., Brouwer, I. D., Kok, F. J., and Yan, H. 2013. Effect of iron deficiency anemia in pregnancy on child mental development in rural China. *Pediatrics, 131*(3), e755–e763.

Christian, P., Murray-Kolb, L. E., Katry, S. K. et al. 2010. Prenatal micronutrient supplementation and intellectual and motor function in early school-aged children in Nepal. *The Journal of the American Medical Association, 304*(24), 2716–2723.

Cogswell, M. E., Parvanta, I., Ickes, L., Yip, R., and Brittenham, G. M. 2003. Iron supplementation during pregnancy, anemia, and birth weight: A randomized controlled trial. *The American Journal of Clinical Nutrition, 78*(4), 773–781.

Colombo, J. 1993. *Infant Cognition: Predicting Later Intellectual Functioning*. London, UK: Sage Publications.

Colombo, J. 2001. Recent advances in infant cognition: Implications for long-chain polyunsaturated fatty acid supplementation studies. *Lipids, 36*(9), 919–926.

Colombo, J. and Carlson, S. 2012. Is the measure the message: The BSID and Nutritional Interventions. *Pediatrics*, *129*, 1166.

Colombo, J., Carlson, S., Cheatham, C. L. et al. 2013. Long-term effects of LCPUFA supplementation on childhood cognitive outcomes. *The American Journal of Clinical Nutrition*, *98*(2), 403–412.

Colombo, J., Harlan, J. E., Mitchell, D. W., Richman, W. A., Maikranz, J. M., and Shaddy, D. J. 1999. *Look Duration in Infancy: Evidence for a Triphasic Developmental Course*. Albuquerque, NM: Society for Research in Child Development.

Colombo, J., Kannass, K., Shaddy, D. J. et al. 2004. DHA and the development of attention in infancy and toddlerhood. *Child Development*, *75*(4), 1254–1267.

Cranefield, P. F. 1962. The discovery of cretinism. *Bulletin of the History of Medicine*, 36, 489–511.

Czeizel, A. E., Dudás, I., Vereczkey, A., and Bánhidy, F. 2013. Folate deficiency and folic acid supplementation: The prevention of neural-tube defects and congenital heart defects. *Nutrients*, *5*(11), 4760–4775.

Dunstan, J. A., Simmer, K., Dixon, G., and Prescott, S. L. 2008. Cognitive assessment of children at age 2(1/2) years after maternal fish oil supplementation in pregnancy: Arandomised controlled trial. *Archives of Disease in Childhood: Fetal and Neonatal Edition*, *93*(1), F45–F50.

Dussault, J. H. and Ruel, J. 1987. Thyroid hormones and brain development. *Annual Review of Physiology*, *49*, 321–334.

Fagan, J. F. 1970. Memory in the infant. *Journal of Experimental Child Psychology*, *9*, 217–226.

Fagan, J. F. and Detterman, D. K. 1992. The Fagan test of infant intelligence: A technical summary. *Journal of Applied Developmental Psychology*, *13*, 173–193.

Fantz, R. L. 1961. The origin of form perception. *Scientific American*, *204*, 66–72.

Frick, J. E., Dengler, M., and Hammond, B. R. 2009. Effects of dietary intake of lutein and zeaxanthin on maturation of the human visual system. *Agro Food Industry Hi-Tech*, *20*, 18–20.

Frick, J. E., Saint, S., O'Brien, K., and Hammond, B. R. 2013. The effects of lutein on infant brain development: Assessment using a novel temporal device. *European Journal of Ophthalmology*, *23*, 608.

Gahche, J., Bailey, R., Burt, V. et al. 2011. Dietary supplement use among U.S. adults has increased since NHANES III (1988–1994). *NCHS Data Brief*, *61*, 1–8.

Gale, C. R., Robinson, S. M., Godfrey, K. M., Law, C. M., Schlotz, W., and O'Callaghan, F. J. 2008. Oily fish intake during pregnancy—Association with lower hyperactivity but not with higher full-scale IQ in offspring. *Journal of Child Psychology and Psychiatry, and Allied Disciplines*, *49*(10), 1061–1068.

General Mills. 2014. *Total: 100% Nutrition*. Retrieved from http://www.totalcereal.com/nutrition.aspx.

German, J. B. 2011. Dietary lipids from an evolutionary perspective: Sources, structures and functions. *Maternal and Child Nutrition*, *7*(Suppl 2), 2–16.

Gesell, A. and Ilg, F. E. 1943. *Infant and Child in the Culture of Today*. New York: Harper.

Ghys, A., Bakker, E., Hornstra, G., and van den Hout, M. 2002. Red blood cell and plasma phospholipid arachidonic and docosahexaenoic acid levels at birth and cognitive development at 4 years of age. *Early Human Development*, *69*, 83–90.

Goyens, P. L. L., Spilker, M. E., Zock, P. L., Katan, M. B., and Mensink, R. P. 2006. Conversion of alpha-linolenic acid in humans is influenced by the absolute amounts of alpha-linolenic acid and linoleic acid in the diet and not by their ratio. *The American Journal of Clinical Nutrition*, *84*(1), 44–53.

Groves, P. M. and Thompson, R. F. 1970. Habituation: A dual-process theory. *Psychological Review*, *77*, 419–450.

Hadders-Algra, M. 2008. Prenatal long-chain polyunsaturated fatty acid status: The importance of a balanced intake of docosahexaenoic acid and arachidonic acid. *Journal of Perinatal Medicine*, *36*(2), 101–109.
Haldimann, M., Alt, A., Blanc, A., and Blondeau, K. 2005. Iodine content of food groups. *Journal of Food Composition and Analysis*, *18*(6), 461–471.
Hamadani, J. D., Fuchs, G. J., Osendarp, S. J. M., Huda, S. N., and Grantham-McGregor, S. M. 2002. Zinc supplementation during pregnancy and effects on mental development and behaviour of infants: A follow-up study. *Lancet*, *360*(9329), 290–294.
Hammond, B. R. 2012. The dietary carotenoids lutein and zeaxanthin in pre- and post-natal development. *Functional Food Reviews*, *4*(3), 130–137.
Hammond, B. R. and Frick, J. E. 2007. Nutritional protection of the developing retina. *The Hong Kong Practitioner*, *29*, 200–207.
Haram, K., Nilsen, S. T., and Ulvik, R. J. 2001. Iron supplementation in pregnancy—Evidence and controversies. *Acta Obstetricia et Gynecologica Scandinavica*, *80*(8), 683–688.
Helland, I. B., Smith, L., Blomén, B., Saarem, K., Saugstad, O. D., and Drevon, C. A. 2008. Effect of supplementing pregnant and lactating mothers with n-3 very-long-chain fatty acids on children's IQ and body mass index at 7 years of age. *Pediatrics*, *122*(2), e472–e479.
Helland, I. B., Smith, L., Saarem, K., Saugstad, O. D., and Drevon, C. A. 2003. Maternal supplementation with very-long-chain n-3 fatty acids during pregnancy and lactation-augments children's IQ at 4 years of age. *Pediatrics*, *111*(1), e39–e44.
Henriksen, B. S., Chan, G., Hoffman, R. O., Sharifzaden, M., Ermakov, I. V., Gellerman, W., and Bernstein, P. S. 2013. Interrelationships between maternal carotenoid status and newborn infant macular pigment optical density and carotenoid status. *Investigative Ophthalmology and Visual Science*, *54*(8), 5568–5578.
Hetzel, B. S. 1971. Neurological damage to the fetus resulting from severe iodine deficiency during pregnancy. *The Lancet*, 308–310.
Hetzel, B. 2000. Iodine and neuropsychological development. *The Journal of Nutrition*, *130*, 493S–495S.
Horowitz, F. D., Paden, L. Y., Bhana, K., Aitchison, R., and Self, P. A. 1972. Developmental changes in infant visual fixation to differing complexity levels among cross-sectionally and longitudinally studied infants. *Developmental Psychology*, *7*, 88–89.
Jeffrey, B. G., Weisinger, H. S., Neuringer, M., and Mitchell, D. C. 2001. The role of docosahexaenoic acid in retinal function. *Lipids*, *36*(9), 859–871.
Judge, M. P., Harel, O., and Lammi-Keefe, C. J. 2007. Maternal consumption of a docosahexaenoic acid-containing functional food during pregnancy: Benefit for infant performance on problem-solving but not on recognition memory tasks at age 9 mo. *The American Journal of Clinical Nutrition*, *85*(6), 1572–1577.
Lane, K., Derbyshire, E., Li, W., and Brennan, C. 2014. Bioavailability and potential uses of vegetarian sources of omega-3 fatty acids: A review of the literature. *Critical Reviews in Food Science and Nutrition*, *54*(5), 572–579.
Larqué, E., Demmelmair, H., Gil-Sanchez, A. et al. 2011. Placental transfer of fatty acids and fetal implications. *The American Journal of Clinical Nutrition*, *94*, 1908–1913.
Lauritzen, L. and Carlson, S. E. 2011. Maternal fatty acid status during pregnancy and lactation and relation to newborn and infant status. *Maternal and Child Nutrition*, *7*(Suppl 2), 41–58.
Li, Q., Yan, H., Zeng, L. et al. 2009. Effects of maternal multimicronutrient supplementation on the mental development of infants in rural western China: Follow-up evaluation of a double-blind, randomized, controlled trial. *Pediatrics*, *123*(4), e685–e692.
Lin, B. and Yen, S. T. 2007. *The U.S. Grain Consumption Landscape: Who Eats Grain, in What Form, Where, and How Much?* United States Department of Agriculture: Economic Research Report Number 50.

Makrides, M., Gibson, R., and McPhee, A. 2010. Effect of DHA supplementation during pregnancy on maternal depression and neurodevelopment of young children: A randomized controlled trial. *Journal of the American Medical Association*, *304*(15), 1675–1683.

McCall, R. B. 1979. The development of intellectual functioning in infancy and the prediction of later IQ. In J. D. Osofsky (Ed.), *Handbook of Infant Development* (pp. 707–741). New York: John Wiley.

McCall, R. B. and Carriger, M. S. 1993. A meta-analysis of infant habituation and recognition memory performance as predictors of later IQ. *Child Development*, *64*(1), 57–79.

McNamara, R. K. and Carlson, S. E. 2006. Role of omega-3 fatty acids in brain development and function: Potential implications for the pathogenesis and prevention of psychopathology. *Prostaglandins, Leukotrienes and Essential Fatty Acids*, *75*(4), 329–349.

Melse-Boonstra, A. and Jaiswal, N. 2010. Iodine deficiency in pregnancy, infancy and childhood and its consequences for brain development. *Best Practice and Research. Clinical Endocrinology and Metabolism*, *24*(1), 29–38.

Mills, J. L. and Signore, C. 2004. Neural tube defect rates before and after food fortification with folic acid. *Birth Defects Research. Part A, Clinical and Molecular Teratology*, *70*, 844–845.

Miret, S., Simpson, R. J., and McKie, A. T. 2003. Physiology and molecular biology of dietary iron absorption. *Annual Review of Nutrition*, *23*, 283–301.

Morreale de Escobar, G., Obregón, M. J., and Escobar del Rey, F. 2004. Role of thyroid hormone during early brain development. *European Journal of Endocrinology*, *151*(Suppl 3), U25–U37.

Murcia, M., Rebagliato, M., Iñiguez, C. et al. 2011. Effect of iodine supplementation during pregnancy on infant neurodevelopment at 1 year of age. *American Journal of Epidemiology*, *173*(7), 804–812.

National Research Council. 2001. *Dietary Reference Intakes for Vitamin A, Vitamin K, Arsenic, Boron, Chromium, Copper, Iodine, Iron, Manganese, Molybdenum, Nickel, Silicon, Vanadium, and Zinc*. Washington, DC: The National Academies Press.

Obregon, M. J., Calvo, R. M., Escobar del Rey, F., and Morreale de Escobar, G. 2007. Ontogenesis of thyroid function and interactions with maternal function. *Endocrine Development*, *10*, 86–98.

O'Donnell, K. J., Rakeman, M. A., Zhi-Hong, D., Xue-Yi, C., Mei, Z. Y., DeLong, N., Brenner, G., Tai, M., Dong, W., and DeLong, G. R. 2002. Effects of iodine supplementation during pregnancy on child growth and development at school age. *Developmental Medicine and Child Neurology*, *44*(2), 76–81.

Oken, E., Østerdal, M. L., Gillman, M. W. et al. 2008a. Associations of maternal fish intake during pregnancy and breastfeeding duration with attainment of developmental milestones in early childhood: A study from the Danish National Birth Cohort. *The American Journal of Clinical Nutrition*, *88*(3), 789–796.

Oken, E., Radesky, J. S., Wright, R. O. et al. 2008b. Maternal fish intake during pregnancy, blood mercury levels, and child cognition at age 3 years in a US cohort. *American Journal of Epidemiology*, *167*(10), 1171–1181.

Olson, J. H., Erie, J. C., and Bakri, S. J. 2011. Nutritional supplementation and age-related macular degeneration. *Seminars in Ophthalmology*, *26*(3), 131–136.

Olsen, S. F., Østerdal, M. L., Salvig, J. D., Weber, T., Tabor, A., and Secher, N. J. 2007. Duration of pregnancy in relation to fish oil supplementation and habitual fish intake: A randomised clinical trial with fish oil. *European Journal of Clinical Nutrition*, *61*(8), 976–985.

Parsons, A. G., Zhou, S. J., Spurrier, N. J., and Makrides, M. 2008. Effect of iron supplementation during pregnancy on the behaviour of children at early school age: Long-term follow-up of a randomised controlled trial. *The British Journal of Nutrition*, *99*(5), 1133–1139.

Pharoah, P. O. D., Buttfield, I. H., Hetzel, B. S. 1971. Neurological damage to the fetus resulting from severe iodine deficiency during pregnancy. *The Lancet*, *297*(7694), 308–310.

Phillips, F. 2005. Vegetarian nutrition. *Nutrition Bulletin*, *30*(2), 132–167.

Prado, E. L., Alcock, K. J., Muadz, H., Ullman, M. T., and Shankar, A. H. 2012. Maternal multiple micronutrient supplements and child cognition: A randomized trial in Indonesia. *Pediatrics*, *130*(3), e536–e546.

Ramakrishnan, U., Grant, F. K., Goldenberg, T., Bui, V., Imdad, A., and Bhutta, Z. A. 2012a. Effect of multiple micronutrient supplementation on pregnancy and infant outcomes: A systematic review. *Paediatric and Perinatal Epidemiology*, *26*(Suppl 1), 153–167.

Ramakrishnan, U., Grant, F., Goldenberg, T., Zongrone, A., and Martorell, R. 2012b. Effect of women's nutrition before and during early pregnancy on maternal and infant outcomes: A systematic review. *Paediatric and Perinatal Epidemiology*, *26*(Suppl 1), 285–301.

Ramakrishnan, U., Manjrekar, R., Rivera, J., González-Cossío, T., and Martorell, R. 1999. Micronutrients and pregnancy outcome: Are view of the literature. *Nutrition Research*, *19*(1), 103–159.

Renzi, L., Bovier, E., and Hammond, B. R. 2013. A role for the macular carotenoids in visual motor response. *Nutritional Neuroscience*, 16, 262–268.

Renzi, L. M., Dengler, M. J., Puente, A., Miller, L. S., and Hammond, B. R. 2014. Relationships between macular pigment optical density and cognitive function in unimpaired and mildly cognitively impaired older adults. *Neurobiology of Aging*, *35*(7), 1695–1699.

Rose, S. A., Feldman, J. F., and Wallace, I. F. 1992. Infant information processing in relation to six-year cognitive outcomes. *Child Development*, *63*, 1126–1141. doi: 10.1111/j.1467-8624.1992.tb01684.

Salem, N., Wegher, B., Mena, P., and Uauy, R. 1996. Arachidonic and docosahexaenoic acids are biosynthesized from their 18-carbon precursors in human infants. *Proceedings of the National Academy of Sciences of the United States of America*, *93*(1), 49–54.

Santiago, P., Velasco, I., Muela, J. A. et al. 2013. Infant neurocognitive development is independent of the use of iodised salt or iodine supplements given during pregnancy. *The British Journal of Nutrition*, *110*(5), 831–839.

Scientific Advisory Committee on Nutrition. 2004. *Advice on Fish Consumption: Benefits & Risks*. London.

Siega-Riz, A. M., Hartzema, A. G., Turnbull, C., Thorp, J., McDonald, T., and Cogswell, M. E. 2006. The effects of prophylactic iron given in prenatal supplements on iron status and birth outcomes: A randomized controlled trial. *American Journal of Obstetrics and Gynecology*, *194*(2), 512–519.

Smuts, C. M., Huang, M., Mundy, D., Plasse, T., Major, S., and Carlson, S. E. 2003. A randomized trial of docosahexaenoic acid supplementation during the third trimester of pregnancy. *Obstetrics and Gynecology*, *101*(3), 469–479.

Strain, J. J., Davidson, P. W., Thurston, S. W. et al. 2012. Maternal PUFA status but not prenatal methylmercury exposure is associated with children's language functions at age five years in the Seychelles. *The Journal of Nutrition*, *142*, 1943–1949.

Sun, Q., Ma, J., Campos, H., Hankinson, S. E., and Hu, F. B. 2007. Comparison between plasma and erythrocyte fatty acid content as biomarkers of fatty acid intake in US women. *The American Journal of Clinical Nutrition*, *86*(1), 74–81.

Surai, P. and Sparks, N. H. 2001. Designer eggs: From improvement of egg composition to functional food. *Trends in Food Science and Technology*, *12*(1), 7–16.

Swanson, C. A. 2003. Iron intake and regulation: Implications for iron deficiency and iron overload. *Alcohol*, *30*, 99–102.

Tamura, T., Goldenberg, R. L., Ramey, S. L., Nelson, K. G., and Chapman, V. R. 2003. Effect of zinc supplementation of pregnant women on the mental and psychomotor development of their children at 5 y of age. *The American Journal of Clinical Nutrition*, *77*(6), 1512–1516.

Todorich, B., Pasquini, J. M., Garcia, C. I., Paez, P. M., and Connor, J. R. 2009. Oligodendrocytes and myelination: The role of iron. *Glia*, *57*(5), 467–478.

Tofail, F., Kabir, I., Hamadani, J. D., Chowdhury, F., Yesmin, S., Mehreen, F., and Huda, S. N. 2006. Supplementation of fish-oil and soy-oil during pregnancy and psychomotor development of infants. *Journal of Health, Population, and Nutrition*, *24*(1), 48–56.

Tofail, F., Persson, L. A., El Arifeen, S. et al. 2008. Effects of prenatal food and micronutrient supplementation on infant development: A randomized trial from the Maternal and Infant Nutrition Interventions, Matlab (MINIMat) study. *The American Journal of Clinical Nutrition*, *87*(3), 704–711.

Trumpff, C., De Schepper, J., Tafforeau, J., Van Oyen, H., Vanderfaeillie, J., and Vandevijvere, S. 2013. Mild iodine deficiency in pregnancy in Europe and its consequences for cognitive and psychomotor development of children: A review. *Journal of Trace Elements in Medicine and Biology: Organ of the Society for Minerals and Trace Elements (GMS)*, *27*(3), 174–183.

UNICEF, WHO, and UNU. 1999. *Composition of a Multi-micronutrient Supplement to be Used in Pilot Programmes Among Pregnant Women in Developing Countries*. New York: UNICEF.

Velasco, I., Carreira, M., Santiago, P. et al. 2009. Effect of iodine prophylaxis during pregnancy on neurocognitive development of children during the first two years of life. *The Journal of Clinical Endocrinology and Metabolism*, *94*(9), 3234–3241.

Vermiglio, F., Lo Presti, V. P., Moleti, M. et al. 2004. Attention deficit and hyperactivity disorders in the offspring of mothers exposed to mild–moderate iodine deficiency: A possible novel iodine deficiency disorder in developed countries. *The Journal of Clinical Endocrinology and Metabolism*, *89*(12), 6054–6060.

Vishwanathan, R., Kuchan, M., and Johnson, E. 2011. Lutein is the predominant carotenoid in infant brain. *Acta Biologica Cracoviensia Series Botanica*, *53*(Suppl. 1), 29.

WHO. 2011. *Guideline: Intermittent Iron and Folic Acid Supplementation in Menstruating Women*. Geneva: World Health Organization.

WHO, UNICEF, and ICCIDD. 1996. *Recommended Iodine Levels in Salt and Guidelines for Monitoring Their Adequacy and Effectiveness*. Geneva: World Health Organization.

WHO, UNICEF, and ICCIDD. 2007. *Assessment of Iodine Deficiency Disorders and Monitoring Their Elimination: A Guide for Programme Managers* (*3rd ed.*). Geneva: World Health Organization.

Willatts, P. 1984. Stages in the development of intentional search by young infants. *Developmental Psychology*, *20*(3), 389.

Willatts, P., Forsyth, S., Agostoni, C., Casaer, P., Riva, E., and Boehm, G. 2013. Effects of long-chain PUFA supplementation in infant formula on cognitive function in later childhood. *The American Journal of clinical nutrition*, *98*(2), 536S–542S.

Williams, G. R. 2008. Neurodevelopmental and neurophysiological actions of thyroid hormone. *Journal of Neuroendocrinology*, *20*(6), 784–794.

Zhang, L., Teng, W., Liu, Y. et al. 2012. Effect of maternal excessive iodine intake on neurodevelopment and cognitive function in rat offspring. *BMC Neuroscience*, *13*(1), 121.

Zhou, S. J., Anderson, A. J., Gibson, R. A., and Makrides, M. 2013. Effect of iodine supplementation in pregnancy on child development and other clinical outcomes: A systematic review of randomized controlled trials. *The American Journal of Clinical Nutrition*, *98*, 1241–1254.

Zhou, S. J., Gibson, R. A., Crowther, C. A., Baghurst, P., and Makrides, M. 2006. Effect of iron supplementation during pregnancy on the intelligence quotient and behavior of children at 4 y of age: Long-term follow-up of a randomized controlled trial. *The American Journal of Clinical Nutrition*, *83*(5), 1112–1117.

Zimmermann, M. B. 2009. Iodine deficiency in pregnancy and the effects of maternal iodine supplementation on the offspring: A review. *The American Journal of Clinical Nutrition*, *89*(2), 668S–672S.

Zimmermann, M. B. 2012. The effects of iodine deficiency in pregnancy and infancy. *Paediatric and Perinatal Epidemiology*, *26*(s1), 108–117.

5 Dietary Supplements in Active Individuals and Athletes

Taylor C. Wallace

CONTENTS

5.1 INCREASED MACRONUTRIENT AND MICRONUTRIENT REQUIREMENTS OF ACTIVE INDIVIDUALS

A few decades ago sports nutrition science was in its early infancy; however, today, many science-based solutions are available in the form of functional foods and dietary supplements. It is important to understand that some populations of active individuals, such as combat personnel, first responders, and athletes, may have greater nutritional requirements when compared with the general population. In the United States and Canada, dietary reference intakes (DRIs) are calculated using "reference people" of specific height, weight, sex, physical activity, and environmental conditions; however, many active individuals do not fit into these standard reference categories. For this reason, military DRIs were derived from the existing DRIs, taking into account increased physical activity and environmental stress factors faced by these individuals [1].

Whether running cross-country, lifting weights, swimming sprints, or playing tennis, active individuals expend more energy than the average individual, and therefore, their bodies need additional nutrients to recover from intense physical activity. Optimal nutrition and the appropriate selection of foods and fluids, timing of intake, and supplemental choices enhance athletic performance and recovery from exercise [2]. Energy needs, especially protein and carbohydrate intakes, must be met during times of intense activity to help to maintain body weight, replenish glycogen stores, and in the case of protein, help to build and repair tissue (e.g. muscle). Adequate energy intakes during periods of high-intensity or long-term exercise can help maximize results, while warding off common problems such as loss of muscle mass, failure to gain bone density, menstrual dysfunction, injury, and fatigue, among others. In particular, low energy consumption in female athletes and military personnel (e.g. >1800–2000 kcal/day) is a major nutritional concern as a constant state of negative energy balance can lead to weight loss, impaired menstrual function, and disruption of endocrine function [3]. When energy intakes are limited, lean tissue and fat are used to fuel the body, resulting in loss of strength, endurance, and musculoskeletal function [4]. Low energy intakes are also associated with poor micronutrient intakes and resultant metabolic dysfunctions (e.g. lowered resting metabolic rate).

Micronutrients play an essential role in energy production, maintenance of bone, protection from oxidative damage, cell function, and, most importantly, repair of muscle tissue during recovery. Routine exercise may increase the turnover and loss of these micronutrients from the body; as a result, greater intakes may be required. In a perfect world, vitamin and mineral intakes should be obtained from consuming a variety of nutrient-rich whole foods; however, similar to the diets of most non-athletes, many athletes restrict energy intakes, use severe weight-loss practices, and/or consume unbalanced diets with low micronutrient densities. These individuals may benefit from a daily multivitamin–multimineral supplement and/or other micronutrient supplements such as calcium, if, for instance, adequate dairy is not being consumed, or iron in the case of menstruating vegetarian female athletes. Adequate intake of B-vitamins helps ensure optimal energy production (i.e. thiamin, riboflavin, niacin, B_6, pantothenic acid, and biotin) and repair of muscle tissue (i.e. folate and B_{12}) [5]. Recent data suggest that exercise may increase an active individual's B-vitamin needs as much as two times the current DRI amounts [5]. Micronutrients that exhibit antioxidant properties (e.g. vitamins C and E, β-carotene, and selenium) may be increasingly beneficial to active individuals as they play an important role in protecting cells from oxidative stress; exercise has been hypothesized to increase oxygen intake by 10–15-fold, exerting increased oxidative stress on muscles and other cells [6]. Calcium and vitamin D are extremely important for bone accretion and maintenance, which are important for avoiding stress fractures. Calcium is also extremely important for regulation of muscle contraction. The 2010 US Dietary Guidelines for Americans recommend that adults consume three cups of low- or non-fat milk daily to achieve adequate calcium from the diet [7]. As calcium is a "bulky" mineral, only very small amounts are present in most daily multivitamin–multimineral supplements; therefore, additional supplementation (approximately 300 mg per absent serving of dairy) may be warranted to help achieve recommended intakes. Iron is required for formation of oxygen-carrying proteins (i.e. hemoglobin and myoglobin), and iron depletion (low iron stores) is one of the most prevalent nutrient deficiencies observed in athletes, especially among menstruating women [8]. Iron requirements for endurance athletes can be increased by up to approximately 75% [9], and athletes who are vegetarian often show a higher prevalence of iron deficiency. Magnesium plays a variety of roles in cellular metabolism, regulation of membrane stability, and neuromuscular, cardiovascular, immune, and hormonal functions [10]; deficiency impairs endurance performance by increasing oxygen requirements. Similar to calcium, magnesium is a "bulky" mineral, and only very small amounts are present in most daily multivitamin–multimineral supplements; therefore, additional supplementation may be warranted to help achieve recommended intakes. Zinc deficiencies are not widely present in the US population [11]; however, it does play a substantial role in the growth, building, and repair of muscle tissue.

5.1.1 Dietary Supplement Use among Athletes

Athletes use dietary supplements to increase energy, maintain strength, enhance performance, sustain health and immune system function, and/or prevent nutritional deficiencies [12]. Several studies estimate that dietary supplement use among athletes is common and varies between 59% and 88%. The most common supplements used by athletes include multivitamin–multimineral supplements, protein, and energy drinks; however, the type of supplement and amounts used vary between age groups, genders, and different sports [13–15]. A recent study of Norwegian athletes reported a large difference in supplement use between different sporting groups: power sport athletes frequently used supplemental creatine, protein/amino acids, vitamins, and minerals, whereas cross-country skiers had the most frequent intake of iron, vitamin C, and fish oils [16]. A recent study suggests that dietary supplement use has decreased among Olympic athletes from approximately 81% in 2002 to 73% in 2009. Athletes in speed, power, and endurance events reported use of any dietary supplement significantly more often than those competing in team events in both 2002 and 2009. The frequency of dietary supplement use also increased with athletes' age. Approximately 63% of the athletes under the age of 21 years reported use of dietary supplements, compared with 83% in 21–24-year olds and 90% in those above 24 years [17].

According to the National Council for Youth Sports, there are approximately 44 million youth athletes participating in organized sports annually in the United States as of 2008 [18]. Many youth athletes take or have considered using dietary supplements to enhance sports performance [19]. Among children less than 18 years who use dietary supplements for sports performance, 94.5% reported use of multivitamin–multimineral supplements, followed by fish oil/omega-3, creatine, and fiber. Males and Caucasians reported greater usage [20]. Parents and coaches were among the most likely individuals to recommend dietary supplements to adolescent athletes [21]. Although there is ample scientific evidence to support appropriate nutrition and hydration practices among youth athletes, supplement use in youth, particularly adolescents, should be to fill nutritional gaps (i.e. to ensure that youth athletes are obtaining adequate levels of macro- and micronutrients) when the diet is not sufficient. It is extremely important for physicians, dieticians, healthcare providers, coaches, and parents of youth athletes to monitor intakes of any kind of supplement in youth athletes.

5.1.2 Dietary Supplement Use among Military Personnel

Recent data from the US Department of Defense show that approximately 60% of the active duty military personnel report use of a dietary supplement at least once a week over the previous 12 months. Products with a combination of vitamins and minerals are among the most frequently used dietary supplements in both the general active duty population and special military subpopulations. A high percentage of these subjects reported "improvement of health" or "to supplement the diet" as reasons for their use of multivitamin–multimineral supplements (76%) or individual vitamin and mineral supplements (65%) [22]. A recent study of US military and coastguard personnel found that users of multivitamin–multimineral and protein/amino acid supplements were more likely to report positive mood states such as being awake, cheerful, friendly, clearheaded, and coordinated when compared with non-users [23]. Outside of typical macronutrient- and micronutrient-based supplements, approximately 21% and 18% of active duty personnel indicate the frequent use of body building and weight-loss supplements, respectively [24]. About 22% of military respondents, including 23% of air force personnel and 18% of army personnel, reported frequent use of 1,3-dimethylamylamine (DMAA) in 2012 [25], prior to the removing of the product from the market by Food and Drug Administration (FDA) in 2014. Male deployers have been shown to be more likely to use bodybuilding supplements, whereas female deployers use more weight-loss supplements. Active duty men and women reporting less than five or more hours of sleep per night have also reported greater use of energy supplements. Deployment experience and younger age were significantly associated with increased odds of reporting bodybuilding, energy, and/or weight-loss supplement use. Men and women reporting use of at least one type of supplement were more likely to use additional types of supplements. Individuals who were engaged in strength training were more likely to use bodybuilding, energy, and weight-loss supplements, with odds for use of bodybuilding supplements being the largest [25].

5.1.3 Banned Substances

Athletes, in particular, should be familiar with current restrictions for what is permissible by their appropriate sports' governing authority, as groups such as the National Collegiate Athletic Association, the International Olympic Committee (IOC), and other professional sports leagues have different requirements. The World Anti-Doping Agency (WADA) and the US Anti-Doping Agency are independent groups responsible for coordinating and monitoring the fight against doping in sport. WADA publishes a list of prohibited substances that may be a useful reference tool for athletes (www.wada-ama.org). Completely legal products (both OTC medicines and dietary supplements) may be banned by one or more sports' governing body, but may be legally purchased by consumers. As many substances may have multiple common and scientific names, it is important for athletes to do the research, especially if any particular substance on the label is unfamiliar.

5.1.4 Tainted Products and Third-Party Certification

In recent years, the US FDA has identified hundreds of products identified as dietary supplements or conventional foods with hidden drugs and/or chemicals. Additionally, the Medical Commission of the IOC recently found that of 634 tested non-hormonal nutritional supplements from 13 countries, 14.8% contained substances that would have led to a positive doping test but were not listed on the label [26]. Tainted products are widespread, typically marketed for bodybuilding and weight loss, but also for sexual enhancement [27]. Tainted products may not only cause an athlete to test positive for an illegal and/or banned substance, but they may also put them at an increased risk for health complications (e.g. interactions with other medications). Labeling claims such as "barely legal," "won't be available much longer," "legal alternative to [anabolic steroid]," and/or "in limited supply" are likely characteristics that indicate that a product may be tainted. Although the Internet can be a viable option for purchasing quality products, many products identified by the FDA as problematic are exclusively sold through Internet sites from "fly-by-night" companies [28].

Large nationally recognized brands have a lot at stake and consequently invest a lot of time and resources into ensuring that their products are free of unlabeled and/or illegal substances. Many use third-party certification systems that award a seal to companies passing rigorous product examination. There are five primary third-party certifiers/verifiers in the United States (Figure 5.1).

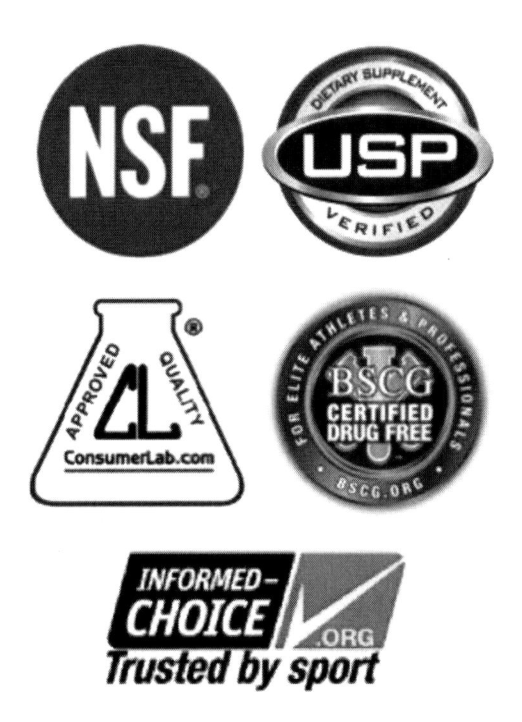

FIGURE 5.1 Common third-party certification seals used on sports nutrition products.

1. US Pharmacopeial Convention (USP)—www.usp.org
2. NSF International—www.nsf.org
3. Banned Substances Control Group—www.bscg.org
4. Informed-Choice—www.informed-choice.org
5. Consumer Lab—www.consumerlab.com

Although dietary supplements are required by law to follow current good manufacturing practices, third-party certification further ensures that sports nutrition supplements and foods are screened for hundreds of banned or prohibited substances such as narcotics, steroids, stimulants, hormones, and other related substances along with diuretics and other masking agents. Third-party certifiers monitor prohibitive lists of substances, such as WADA, NCAA, NFL, MLB, etc. on an ongoing basis. Certification means that supplement manufacturers, as well as their suppliers, have met stringent independent certification process guidelines to ensure that their products are free of any substance that is not listed on the Supplement Facts Panel. The FDA published a guidance document for third-party certifiers in 2009 [29].

5.1.5 Adverse Event Reporting for Dietary Supplements

The 2006 Dietary Supplement and Nonprescription Drug Consumer Protection Act requires manufacturers, packers, and/or distributors to submit all serious adverse events associated with the use of a dietary supplement to FDA using the standard FDA MedWatch form FDA 3500A [30]. The law defines serious adverse events as an adverse event that "results in death; a life-threatening experience; inpatient hospitalization; a persistent or significant disability or incapacity; or a congenital anomaly or birth defect; or requires, based on reasonable medical judgment, a medical or surgical intervention to prevent an outcome described" [31]. Dietary supplement labels must include the contact information (the domestic address or phone number) for the supplement's manufacturer, packer, or distributor—referred to as the "responsible person" who is charged with reporting serious adverse events to FDA [32]. The responsible person must submit a serious adverse event to FDA not later than 15 business days after the report is received; any new medical information related to a previously submitted adverse event report must be submitted to the agency within 1 year of the initial report and within 15 days of receipt [33]. The law also requires companies to maintain records related to all adverse event reports, both serious and non-serious, for a period of 6 years and authorizes FDA to inspect these records to ensure compliance with these record-keeping requirements [34]. Healthcare professionals and consumers may voluntarily report serious adverse events to FDA by calling 1800-FDA-1088 and requesting a Voluntary Reporting Form 3500. It is important to note that FDA's MedWatch system and the poison control centers do not share information; it is important for healthcare professionals to report serious adverse events to FDA via MedWatch.

5.2 POPULAR SPORTS NUTRITION PRODUCTS

Nutrition and health professionals are often asked to evaluate sports nutrition supplements and foods that active individuals such as military personnel and athletes currently use or are considering using. When evaluating sports nutrition products, three major areas of concern must be addressed.

1. Safety and efficacy of the product
2. Doping status of the product or substances contained within the product
3. Quality of the product

The most unreasonable position for a health professional giving nutrition guidance to an athlete is automatically discouraging use of any/all sports nutrition products, as this leaves the individual open to exploring other less credible alternative sources of information (e.g. websites, word-of-mouth, etc.) about products. Understanding the science behind more mainstream sports nutrition products gives the health professional ability to adequately council athletes on safe and healthy alternatives to the many poor-quality and/or tainted products on the market. To accomplish this, it is extremely important that health professionals be up-to-date on banned substances lists and third-party certification programs, as outlined previously.

This section seeks to provide a brief evidence-based summary of the safety and efficacy in relation to common sports nutrition products on the market, excluding vitamin and mineral supplements, which are discussed briefly in the sections above and throughout other chapters in this textbook.

It is always important to further review the scientific literature and to meticulously examine the quantity and quality of studies provided to support the safety and effectiveness of a product. All supportive research should be published in a peer-reviewed journal that is indexed in the National Library of Medicine database (PubMed) (www.ncbi.nlm.nih.gov/pubmed). Multiple human studies reporting similar outcomes (i.e. reproducible results) offer the best insight into the safety and efficacy of any particular product. However, one should keep in mind that there are many caveats when studying nutritional interventions that may led to null outcomes, such as the absence of a true placebo or knowledge of baseline nutritional status [35]. This is why assessing the entire body of scientific evidence is important. Guidance should not be given based solely on an individual published manuscript or a group of manuscripts published by a single individual or laboratory group. The Bradford-Hill criteria for causation [36] can act as a useful tool for assessing the association of a particular exposure in relation to any particular risk and/or benefit outcome. At minimum, consider the following components of the Bradford-Hill criteria when evaluating a collection of peer-reviewed scientific literatures.

- *Strength of association*: small associations do not mean that there is not a causal effect; however, the larger the association the more likely it is causal (smaller associations are more likely to suffer from confounding).
- *Consistency*: consistent findings among various samples/studies strengthen the likelihood of a causal effect.
- *Biological gradient or "dose response"*: greater exposure should generally lead to greater incidence of the effect.
- *Plausibility*: an established plausible biological mechanism between cause and effect gives greater confidence that the outcome is not by chance.

The Academy of Nutrition and Dietetics (AND) practice paper on dietary supplements provides additional guidelines for appraising the scientific validity of research [37].

5.2.1 Protein

Muscle growth happens as a result of combined exercise and proper nutrition. To attain peak levels of performance, active individuals clearly need to be aware of their dietary intake of protein; a large body of evidence supports that appropriate intakes of protein/amino acids can help support increased rates of protein synthesis and positive protein balance following endurance exercise [38]. Studies have consistently demonstrated the acute benefits of protein supplementation on post-exercise muscle anabolism [39]. National and international dietary guidelines consistently recommend that adults need no more than 0.8–0.9 g/kg/day of protein [40,41] to satisfy their nutritional requirement (equivalent to about 56 and 46 g/day for men and women, respectively). However, a number of recent reviews, including a position stand by the *American College of Sports Medicine* [42], scrutinize the use of current dietary recommendations for protein among active individuals such as athletes. There is general consensus that protein needs of active individuals are higher than those of sedentary persons. Intakes of 1.2–1.4 g/kg/day for endurance athletes and 1.2–1.7 g/kg/day for power athletes have been suggested as an appropriate requirement for active individuals [2,41], which is equivalent to approximately 84–119 g and 66–94 g for active men and women, respectively. Endurance athletes tend to synthesize more protein for fuel, whereas strength athletes retain more for muscle development. Although it is not difficult to obtain sufficient protein intakes from food, protein shakes and/or amino acid supplements may be advantageous in situations such as in which an athlete does not have time for a full meal post workout. Skeletal muscles reach peak mass by the third decade of life, and with each subsequent decade, muscle fibers decrease in size and number. This process speeds up in the later years of life. As protein is the building block for muscle tissue, it makes sense that adequate intakes are important for building and maintaining muscle throughout the lifespan.

Protein quality is measured using a variety of ways; however, the most accepted and understood index is the protein digestibility-corrected amino acid score (PDCAAS). Using the PDCAAS, a number of proteins are classified as "high quality," based on the amino acid requirements of humans and their ability to digest it. A PDCAAS rating of 1.0 is the highest and 0 is the lowest. Casein (milk protein), whey (milk protein), egg white (albumin), and isolated soy protein all have a 1.0 rating (Table 5.1). Most meat proteins are also considered high quality.

5.2.2 Branched-Chain Amino Acids

Branched-chain amino acids are essential nutrients that the body obtains from proteins found in food, especially meat, dairy products, and legumes. There are three branched-chain amino acids: leucine, isoleucine, and valine. "Branched-chain" refers to the chemical structure of these amino acids. They account for about 30%–40% of the dietary essential amino acids in body protein and 14%–18% of the total

TABLE 5.1
PDCAAS Quality Rankings of Commonly Consumed Food Proteins

Protein Type	PDCAAS Rating
Milk (casein)	1.0
Milk (whey)	1.0
Egg whites (albumin)	1.0
Soy	1.0
Beef	0.92
Black beans	0.75
Peanuts	0.52
Wheat (gluten)	0.25

Source: Adapted from the US Dairy Export Council, Reference Manual for US Whey Products, 2nd edition, 1999.

amino acids in muscle proteins [43,44]. They are the only amino acids oxidized for energy during exercise; this process nullifies their effects, which is why in theory supplementation can have positive outcomes. Recent studies have demonstrated that branched-chain amino acids, especially leucine, play a very important role in protein metabolism; leucine promotes protein synthesis and inhibits protein degradation [45]. Oral supplementation with branched-chain amino acids has been reported to increase intracellular and arterial branch-chain amino acid levels during exercise, resulting in the suppression of endogenous muscle protein breakdown [46]. Oral administration of branched-chain amino acids also suppresses the rise in serum creatine kinase activity for several days after exercise [47]. These findings suggest that branched-chain amino acids may reduce muscle damage induced by exercise. A study of 30 healthy young female and male adults suggests that ingestion of 5 g of branched-chain amino acids before exercise can reduce delayed-onset muscle soreness and muscle fatigue in individuals for several days after exercise [48].

5.2.3 Caffeine

Caffeine, a methylated xanthine (1,3,7-trimethylxanthine), is the most widely used mild central nervous system stimulant, naturally present in many common conventional foods, including coffee, tea, and cacao, among others. Coffee and tea remain the chief sources of caffeine in the US diet; coffee and brewed tea contain approximately 65–125 and 20–90 mg of caffeine per 8 oz. serving [49]. However, energy beverages and caffeine-containing dietary supplements have been on the rise in the general population, but more notably among athletes and tactical populations. Caffeine has recently been added to a growing number of readily available products including, but not limited to energy beverages, weight-loss supplements, chewing gum, and others for its stimulant effects. Perhaps, no substance has been the subject of more conflicting scientific reports in recent years. For healthy adults, FDA has cited 400 mg/day as an amount not generally associated with dangerous, negative effects [50]. Currently, there are more than 25 published reviews supporting the safety of caffeine; the weight of evidence does not support a positive relationship between caffeine consumption and adverse effects, including reproductive or vascular events in healthy individuals consuming at levels under 400 mg/day [51] (individuals with impaired vascular and/or cerebrovascular function should talk with a medical professional about their caffeine intake). A recent systematic review and a meta-analysis of observational studies evaluating 115,993 individuals found no association between chronic caffeine exposure and the risk of atrial fibrillation [52]. Caffeine may also act as a gastrointestinal irritant for those with gastritis, esophagitis, irritable bowel syndrome, inflammatory bowel disease, ulcerative colitis, Crohn's disease, and/or other related disorders.

Performance benefits attributed to caffeine include physical endurance, reduction of fatigue, and enhancing mental alertness and concentration [53]. Many studies confirm caffeine's ability to enhance mood and alertness [54], exercise performance [55], the speed at which information is processed, awareness, attention, and reaction time [56]. At safe levels, caffeine through its wide-ranging physiological and psychological effects increases endurance in well-trained athletes. Abstaining from caffeine at least 7 days before use will give the greatest chance of optimizing the ergogenic effect [57].

As many individuals are sensitive to caffeine, several trade associations and industry groups such as the American Beverage Association (the leading beverage trade association) and Council for Responsible Nutrition (the leading dietary supplement trade association) have developed guidelines (industry self-regulation) to address disclosure of caffeine content and set forth consumer advisories to promote the safe, responsible use of beverage products and dietary supplements [58,59]. Many national brands and companies who are members of these industry groups abide to these voluntary guidelines. Table 5.2 compares the amount of caffeine in a variety of popular beverage products.

5.2.4 Creatine Monohydrate

Creatine is a nitrogenous organic acid that occurs naturally in vertebrates and helps to supply energy to all cells in the body, primarily muscle. In humans, over 95% of the body's creatine content is stored in the skeletal muscle, where creatine or more specifically phosphocreatine plays a major role in a muscle's ability to perform and maintain short duration, high-intensity exercise [60]. In athletes and active individuals, the demand for adenosine triphospate (ATP) is elevated during exercise due to the nature of effort. Phosphocreatine is an energy substrate required for ATP regeneration [61]. In this regard, several human studies have shown that creatine supplementation increases phosphocreatine skeletal muscle content [62]. Creatine monohydrate is an increasingly popular dietary supplement that significantly increases high-intensity exercise capacity and lean body mass during athletic training. A large body of human and animal research suggests supplemental creatine to have a consistent ergogenic effect, particularly with exercises or activities requiring high-intensity, short bursts of energy. A recent meta-analysis indicates that creatine

TABLE 5.2
Caffeine (mg/8 oz.) Comparison in a Variety of Popular Beverage Products

Source of Caffeine	Caffeine (mg)[a]	Caffeine Range (mg)[a]
	Coffee	
Decaffeinated	5	3–12
Instant	93	27–173
Plain, brewed	133	102–200
Espresso	320	240–720
	Tea	
Tea, brewed	53	40–120
Green	45	30–50
Black	47	25–110
	Soft Drinks	
Coca-Cola Classic	23	NA
Pepsi-Cola	25	NA
Diet Coke	31	NA
Diet Pepsi	35	NA
Mountain Dew	37	NA
Dr. Pepper	41	NA
Sprite	0	NA
	Energy Drinks	
Amp	72	NA
Full Throttle	72	NA
Red Bull	76	NA
Monster	80	NA
Rockstar	80	NA

[a] Caffeine contents (mg) expressed per 8 oz. serving.

supplementation combined with resistance training has a positive effect on muscle mass and upper body strength when compared with resistance training alone. It also showed promise for improving bone mineral density, suggesting that the combination could be an effective intervention to improve aging musculoskeletal health (i.e. sarcopenia) [63].

Recent case reports have suggested that creatine users are at a greater risk of numerous adverse events including kidney and liver impairment and musculoskeletal injury, even though the current scientific literature is not supportive of these claims. A recent risk assessment indicated that the evidence of safety is strong at intakes of up to 5 g/day for chronic supplementation. Although much higher levels have been tested under acute conditions without adverse effects and may be safe, the data for intake above 5 g/day are not sufficient for a confident conclusion of long-term safety [64]. Contrary to popular belief, emerging scientific evidence supports the hypothesis that creatine users have a lower rate of injury compared with non-creatine users. A recent small human study evaluated the impact of creatine supplementation on injury incidence during 3 years of NCAA Division IA college football training and competition and found that the occurrence of cramping, heat illness or dehydration, muscle tightness and pulls/strains, non-contact joint injuries, contact injuries, illness, number of missed practices due to injury, and players lost for the season were "generally lower or proportional to the creatine use rate" among athletes [65]. A scientific status review conducted by the International Society of Sports Nutrition supports that "creatine monohydrate supplementation is not only safe, but possibly beneficial in regard to preventing injury" among athletes adhering established guidelines [66].

5.2.5 DMAA (1,3-Dimethylamylamine)

The pharmaceutical amphetamine-like derivative 1,3-DMAA first introduced by Eli Lilly and Company in 1948 as a nasal inhalant for rhinitis (irritation and inflammation of the mucous membrane) has been recently incorporated into approximately 200 sports supplements [67]. The most popular brands containing DMAA include Jack3d™ and OxyElite Pro™, both marketed by USP Labs and both detained by the FDA in July 2013 [68] (however, some can still be found on Amazon and other online retail stores). Dietary supplements by law in the United States must contain "dietary ingredients" that have been traditionally present in the food supply [69]. For instance, synthetic beta-carotene can be legally manufactured and sold in a dietary supplement because it is naturally present in commonly consumed foods such as carrots. Remarkably, the evidence to support the incorporation of DMAA into dietary supplement products hinges on a single study, attempting to assess the chemical constituents of geranium oil, published almost two decades ago in the now defunct *Journal of the Guizhou Institute of Technology* [70]. Over a half dozen recent peer-reviewed studies have not been able to reproduce this finding.

Dietary supplements containing DMAA have been linked to multiple serious adverse health consequences, including panic attacks, seizures, stress-induced cardiomyopathy, and death [71]. The substance has also been used as a "party drug," implicated in at least one hemorrhagic stroke in New Zealand. Several chemical and common names exist for DMAA on dietary supplement products, including but not limited to

- 1,3-DMAA
- 1,3-Dimethylamylamine
- 1,3-Dimethylpentylamine
- 2-Amino-4-methylhexane
- 2-Hexanamine, 4-methyl-(9CI)
- 4-Methyl-2-hexanamine
- 4-Methyl-2-hexylamine
- Dimethylamylamine
- Geranamine

- Methylhexanamine
- Methylhexanenamine
- InChIKey = YAHRDLICUYEDAU-UHFFFAOYSA-N

Some products will also list *Pelargonium graveolens* extract or geranium extract, which may also indicate that the product contains DMAA [72]. The FDA keeps an updated list of products that have received warning letters advising them to discontinue the sale of their products containing DMAA (available at: http://www.fda.gov/Food/DietarySupplements/QADietarySupplements/ucm346576.htm). DMAA has been banned by every sports governing authority and may cause an individual to test false positive for amphetamines. It is important to note that many other similar compounds have also been synthesized and incorporated into dietary supplement products. If a dietary supplement label contains a compound similar to those substances listed earlier, it is advisable to avoid and/or discontinue use of the product.

REFERENCES

1. Arensberg ME, Costello R, Deuster PA, Jones D, Twillman G. Summit on human performance and dietary supplements summary report. Nutr Today. 2014;49(1):7–15.
2. Academy of Nutrition and Dietetics. Position of the Academy of Nutrition and Dietetics, Dieticians of Canada, and American College of Sports Medicine: Nutrition and athletic performance. J Acad Nutr Diet. 2009;109(3):509–527.
3. Beals K, Manore M. Nutritional considerations for the female athlete. In: *Advances in Sports and Exercise Science Series*. Philadelphia, PA: Elsevier. 2007:187–206.
4. Burke LM, Loucks AB, Broad N. Energy and carbohydrate for training and recovery. J Sports Sci. 2006;24:675–685.
5. Woolf K, Manore MM. B-vitamins and exercise: Does exercise alter requirements? Int J Sport Nutr Exerc Metab. 2006;16:453–484.
6. Powers SK, DeRuisseau KC, Quindry J, Hamilton KL. Dietary antioxidants and exercise. J Sports Sci. 2004;22:81–94.
7. U.S. Department of Agriculture and U.S. Department of Health and Human Services. Dietary Guidelines for Americans, 2010. 7th Edition, Washington, DC: U.S. Government Printing Office. December 2010.
8. Haymes E. Iron. In: Driskell J, Wolinsky I, eds. *Sports Nutrition; Vitamins and Trace Elements*. New York, NY: CRC Press. 2006:203–216.
9. Whiting SJ, Barabash WA. Dietary reference intakes for the micronutrients: Considerations for physical activity. Appl Physiol Nutr Metab. 2006;31:80–85.
10. Institute of Medicine, Food and Nutrition Board. *Dietary Reference Intakes for Calcium, Phosphorus, Magnesium, Vitamin D, and Fluoride*. Washington, DC: National Academies Press, 1997.
11. Wallace TC, McBurney M, Fulgoni VL III. Multivitamin/mineral supplement contribution to micronutrient intakes in the United States, 2007–2010. J Am Coll Nutr. 2014; 33(2):94–102.
12. Dascombe BJ, Karunaratna M, Cartoon J, Fergie B, Goodman C. Nutritional supplementation habits and perceptions of elite athletes within a state-based sporting institute. J Sci Med Sport 2010;13:274–280.
13. Erdman KA, Fung TS, Doyle-Baker PK, Verhoef MJ, Reimer RA. Dietary supplementation of high-performance Canadian athletes by age and gender. Clin J Sport Med. 2007;17:458–464.

14. Duellman MC, Lukaszuk JM, Prawitz AD, Brandenburg JP. Protein supplement users among high school athletes have misconceptions about effectiveness. J Strength Cond Res. 2008;22:1124–1129.
15. Striegel H, Simon P, Wurster C, Niess AM, Ulrich R. The use of nutritional supplements among master athletes. Int J Sports Med. 2006;27:236–241.
16. Ronsen O, Sundgot-Borgen J, Maehlum S. Supplement use and nutritional habits in Norwegian elite athletes. Scand J Med Sci Sports 1999, 9:28–35.
17. Heikkinen A, Alaranta A, Helenius I, Vasankari T. Use of dietary supplements in Olympic athletes is decreasing: A follow-up study between 2002 and 2009. J Int Soc Sports Nutr. 2011;8:1.
18. National Council on Youth Sports. Report on trends and participation in organized youth sports. 2008. Retrieved 31 March 2014. Available from http://69.13.130.212/pdfs/2008/2008-ncys-market-research-report.pdf.
19. Bell A, Dorsch K, McCreary D, Hovey R. A look at nutritional supplement use in adolescents. J Adolescent Health 2004;34:508–516.
20. Evans MW, Ndetan H, Perko M, Williams R, Walker C. Dietary supplement use by children and adolescents in the United States to enhance sport performance: Results of the National Health Interview Survey. J Prim Prevent. 2012;33:3–12.
21. Dunn M, Eddy JM, Wang MQ, Nagy S, Perko MA, Bartee RT. The influence of significant others on attitudes, subjective norms, and intentions regarding dietary supplement use among adolescent athletes. Adolescence. 2001;35:583–591.
22. Marriott BM. Dietary supplement use by active duty military personnel: A world wide sample. Institute of Medicine Committee on Dietary Supplement Use by Military Personnel meeting. Washington, DC, 13 February 2007.
23. Austin KG, McGraw SM, Lieberman H. Dietary supplement use is associated with positive mood states in US Military and Coast Guard personnel. FASEB J. 2013;27:242.7.
24. Austin KG, McGraw S, Carvey C, Lieberman HR. Use of dietary supplements containing 1,3 dimethylamylamine by military personnel. FASEB J. 2012;26:Ib415.
25. Jacobson IG, Horton J, Smith B, Wells TS, Boyko EJ, Lieberman HR, Ryan MAK, Smith TC. Bodybuilding, energy, and weight-loss supplements are associated with deployment and physical activity in U.S. military personnel. Ann Epidemiol. 2012;22:318–330.
26. Geyer H, Parr MK, Mareck U, Reinhart U, Schrader Y, Schänzer W. Analysis of non-hormonal nutritional supplements for anabolic-androgenic steroids—Results of an international study. Int J Sports Med. 2004;25:124–129.
27. U.S. Food and Drug Administration. Tainted dietary supplements and foods: Responsibilities of retailers and distributors. 2010. Accessed on March 31, 2014. Available from http://www.fda.gov/downloads/Drugs/ResourcesForYou/Consumers/Buying Using MedicineSafely/MedicationHealthFraud/UCM230993.pdf.
28. Council for Responsible Nutrition. Backgrounder: one dozen tips for consumers. 2011. Accessed on March 31, 2014. Available from http://www.crnusa.org/FDAunity/tips.html.
29. U.S. Food and Drug Administration. Voluntary third-party certification programs for foods and feeds: Guidance for industry. Accessed on April 15, 2014. Available from http://www.fda.gov/regulatoryinformation/guidances/ucm125431.htm.
30. Dietary Supplement and Nonprescription Drug Consumer Protection Act, 120 Stat. 469, 2006.
31. Federal Food, Drug and Cosmetic Act, §761(a)(2).
32. Federal Food, Drug and Cosmetic Act, §761(b)(1).
33. Federal Food, Drug and Cosmetic Act, §761(c)(2).
34. Federal Food, Drug and Cosmetic Act, §761(c).
35. Heaney RP. Nutrients, endpoints, and the problem of proof. J Nutr. 2008;138:1591–1595.
36. Hill AB. The environment and disease: Association or causation? Proc R Soc Med. 1965;58:295–300.

37. Academy of Nutrition and Dietetics. Practice paper of the American Dietetic Association: Dietary supplements. *J Acad Nutr Diet*. 2005;102:460–470.
38. Burd NA, Tang JE, Moore DR. Exercise training and protein metabolism: Influences of contraction, protein intake, and sex-based differences. J Appl Physiol. 2009;106: 1692–1701.
39. Pasiakos SM, Lieberman HR, McLellan TM. Effects of protein supplements on muscle damage, soreness and recovery of muscle function and physical performance: A systematic review. Sports Med. 2014;44:655–670.
40. Institute of Medicine. *Dietary Reference Intakes for Energy, Carbohydrate, Fiber, Fat, Fatty Acids, Cholesterol, Protein and Amino Acids*. Washington, DC: National Academies Press, 2005.
41. WHO Technical Report Series 935. Protein and amino acid requirements in human nutrition: Report of a joint FAO/WHO/UNU expert consultation. Report of a Joint WHO/FAO/UNU Expert Consultation. 2011.
42. Rodriguez NR, Di Marco NM, Langley S. American College of Sports Medicine position stand. Nutrition and athletic performance. *Med Sci Sport Exer.* 2009;41: 709–731.
43. Riazi R, Wykes LJ, Ball RO, Pencharz PB. The total branched-chain amino acid requirement in young healthy adult men determined by indicator amino acid oxidation by use of L-[1-^{13}C]phenylalanine. J Nutr. 2003;133:1383–1389.
44. Layman DK, Baum JI. Dietary protein impact on glycemic control during weight loss. J Nutr. 2004;134(Suppl):S968–S973.
45. Bolster DR, Jefferson LS, Kimball SR. Regulation of protein synthesis associated with skeletal muscle hypertrophy by insulin-, amino acid- and exercise-induced signaling. Proc Nutr Soc. 2004;63:351–356.
46. MacLean DA, Graham TE, Saltin B. Branched-chain amino acids augment ammonia metabolism while attenuating protein breakdown during exercise. Am J Physiol. 1994;267:E1010–E1022.
47. Coombes JS, McNaughton LR. Effects of branced-chain amino acid supplementation on serum creatine kinase and lactate dehydrogenase after prolonged exercise. *J Sports Med Phys Fitness*. 2000;40:240–246.
48. Shimomura Y, Yamamoto Y, Bajotto G, Sato J, Murakami T, Shimomura N, Kobayashi H, Mawatari K. Nutraceutical effects of branched-chain amino acids on skeletal muscle. J Nutr. 2006;136:529S–532S.
49. International Food Information Council. Fact sheet: Caffeine and health. Accessed on August 1, 2013. Available from http://www.foodinsight.org/Resources/Detail.aspx?topic=Fact_Sheet_Caffeine_and_Health.
50. U.S. Food and Drug Administration. For consumers: FDA to investigate added caffeine. Accessed on July 30, 2013. Available from http://www.fda.gov/ForConsumers/ConsumerUpdates/ucm350570.htm.
51. Peck JD, Leviton A, Cowan LD. A review of the epidemiologic evidence concerning the reproductive health effects of caffeine consumption: A 2000–2009 update. Food Chem Toxicol. 2010;48(10):2549–2576.
52. Caldeira D, Martins C, Alves LB, Pereira H, Ferreira JJ, Costa Joao. Caffeine does not increase the risk of atrial fibrillation: A systematic review and meta-analysis of observational studies. Heart 2013;99:1383–1389.
53. Heckman MA, Weil J, De Mejia EG. Caffeine (1,3,7-trimethylxanthine) in foods: A comprehensive review on consumption, functionality, safety, and regulatory matters. J Food Sci. 2010;75(3):R77–R87.
54. Lorist M, Tops MM. Caffeine, fatigue and cognition. Brain Cogn. 2003;53:82–94.
55. Doherty M, Smith PM. Effects of caffeine ingestion on exercise testing: A meta-analysis. Int J Sport Nutr Exerc Metab. 2004;14:626–646.

56. Cysneiros RM, Farkas D, Harmatz JS, Von Moltke LL, Greenblatt DJ. Pharmacokinetic and pharmacodynamic interactions between zolpidem and caffeine. Clin Pharmacol Ther. 2007;82:54–62.
57. Ganio MS, Klau JF, Casa DJ, Armstrong LE, Maresh CM. Effect of caffeine on sport-specific endurance performance: A systematic review. J Strength Cond Res. 2009;23(1):315–324.
58. American Beverage Association. ABA guidance for the responsible labeling and marketing of energy drinks. Accessed on June 5, 2014. Available from http://www.ameribev.org/files/339_Energy%20Drink%20Guidelines%20(final).pdf.
59. Council for Responsible Nutrition. CRN recommended guidelines for caffeine-containing dietary supplements. Accessed on June 4, 2014. Available from http://www.crnusa.org/caffeine/guidelines.html.
60. Baker JS, McCormick MC, Robergs RA. Interaction among skeletal muscle metabolic energy systems during intense exercise. J Nutr Metab. 2010;2010:905612.
61. Clark JF. Creatine and phosphocreatine: A review of their use in exercise and sport. J Athl Train. 1997;32:45–51.
62. van Loon LJ, Oosterlaar AM, Hartgens F, Hesselink MK, Snow RJ, Wagenmakers AJ. Effects of creatine loading and prolonged creatine supplementation on body composition, fuel selection, sprint and endurance performance in humans. Clin Sci (Lond). 2003;104:153–162.
63. Candow DG, Chilibeck PD, Forbes SC. Creatine supplementation and aging musculoskeletal health. Endocrine 2014;45:354–361.
64. Shao A, Hathcock JN. Risk assessment for creatine monohydrate. Regul Toxicol Pharm. 2006;45(3):242–251.
65. Greenwood M, Kreider RB, Greenwood L, Byars A. Cramping and injury incidence in collegiate football players are reduced by creatine supplementation. *J Athl Train.* 2003;38:216–219.
66. Buford TW, Kreider RB, Stout JR, Greenwood M, Campbell B, Spano M, Ziegenfuss T, Lopez H, Landis J, Antonio J. International society of sports nutrition position stand: Creatine supplementation and exercise. *J Int Soc Sports Nutr.* 2007;4:6.
67. Cohen P. DMAA as a dietary supplement ingredient. JAMA Intern Med. 2012; 172(13):1038–1039.
68. Gee P, Jackson S, Easton J. Another bitter pill: A case of toxicity from DMAA party pills. NZ Med J. 2010;123(1327):124–127.
69. Federal Food, Drug and Cosmetic Act, §413(a).
70. Ping Z, Jun Q, Qing L. A study on the chemical constituents of geranium oil [in Mandarin]. J Guizhou Inst Tech. 1996;25(1):82–85.
71. Salinger L, Daniels B, Sangalli B, Bayer M. Recreational use of bodybuilding supplement resulting in severe cardiotoxicity. Clin Toxicol. 2011;49(6):573–574.
72. U.S. Food and Drug Administration. DMAA in dietary supplements. Accessed on April 24, 2014. Available from http://www.fda.gov/Food/DietarySupplements/QADietarySupplements/ucm346576.htm.
73. U.S. Dairy Export Council, Reference Manual for U.S. Whey Products, 2nd edition, 1999.

6 Calcium and Vitamin D

Nutritional Role and the Benefits and Risks of Dietary Supplements in Health Promotion

Alyssa K. Phillips, Tristan E. Lipkie, and Connie M. Weaver

CONTENTS

6.1 BIOLOGICAL FUNCTIONS

Although calcium is regarded as a nutrient of concern predominantly for bone health, it is essential to nearly all cell types in its function as a secondary messenger for signal transduction. Over 99% of calcium in the body is in teeth and bone, which acts as the reservoir in times of low dietary intake. Serum calcium concentration in humans is homeostatically maintained within a tightly controlled range of approximately 9–10 mg/dL, and when blood levels dip, bone mineral is mobilized for immediate need in cellular functions, thereby sacrificing long-term health outcomes of bone. Vitamin D is a prohormone of 1,25-dihydroxyvitamin D (calcitriol), which contributes to the homeostatic control of serum calcium through the vitamin D receptor (VDR). Although emerging evidence suggests that vitamin D may have non-skeletal health outcomes, the well-established role of vitamin D is in calcium homeostasis and bone health. For further discussion of non-skeletal effects of vitamin D, refer to the following chapter. Vitamin D is hydroxylated in the liver to 25-hydroxyvitamin D (25OHD). Serum 25OHD concentration is the clinical indicator of vitamin D status as 25OHD has a half-life of 2–3 weeks in circulation.

Calcium homeostasis is achieved through a hormone-driven balance of physiological adaptations, including alterations in intestinal absorption, bone formation, and kidney reabsorption. The principle regulators of this process include parathyroid hormone (PTH) and calcitriol, whereby calcitriol is synthesized in response to low serum calcium through the calcium–PTH–vitamin D axis. Low serum calcium stimulates release of PTH from parathyroid chief cells, which subsequently enhances synthesis of calcitriol from 25OHD in the kidney. Calcitriol then activates VDR in the intestine to enhance calcium absorption, in the kidney to enhance calcium retention, and in osteoclast cells to release calcium from the bone mineral matrix. Randomized controlled trials (RCTs) and animal models indicate that vitamin D is not required to maintain bone health if calcium intake is sufficient (Reid et al., 2013). Bone loss by VDR null mice was reversed with calcium + phosphorus supplementation (Masuyama et al., 2003), and mice with intestine-specific VDR expression (otherwise VDR null in other tissues including bone and kidney) had normal serum calcium levels and greater bone mineral density (BMD) than control mice (Xue and Fleet, 2009). These experiments, in addition to the observation that VDR is expressed by osteosclasts (absorptive bone cells) and not osteoblasts (mineralizing bone cells), suggest that the function of vitamin D is to maintain serum calcium, not to maintain bone health directly. Severe vitamin D deficiency affects bone health when serum 25OHD concentration is too low (<25 nmol/L) for adequate production of calcitriol, thereby preventing upregulation of intestinal calcium absorption (Need et al., 2008).

6.2 RECOMMENDED INTAKES

The Institute of Medicine (IOM) updated the dietary reference intakes (DRIs) for calcium and vitamin D in 2011 (Ross et al., 2011). An essential nutrient, calcium, must be obtained through exogenous sources including calcium-containing foods and supplements. The intake recommendations for calcium are set at levels demonstrated to maintain calcium retention and to prevent bone loss (Ross et al., 2011). The IOM committee concluded that the evidence was not sufficient to consider possible non-skeletal health outcomes of calcium and vitamin D in the development of the new DRIs. The current estimated average requirements (EARs) set to meet the needs of 50% of the population recommend 1100 mg/day for pre-teens and adolescents 9–18 years, 800 mg/day for adults 19–50, 800 mg/day for males 51–70, and 1000 mg/day for women 51–70 as well as for all adults over 71 years. The current recommended dietary allowance (RDA) values set to meet the requirements of 97.5% of the population also vary depending on life stage and sex and are as follows: 700 mg/day for children 1–3 years, 1000 mg/day for children 4–8 years, 1300 mg/day for pre-teens and adolescents 9–18 years, 1000 mg/day for adults 19–50, 1000 mg/day for men 51–70 years, 1200 mg/day for men 71+ years, and 1200 mg/day for women 51+ years. The upper limit of safety for calcium is between 2000 and 3000 mg/day, in which the risk for developing kidney stones may increase when consumption exceeds these levels.

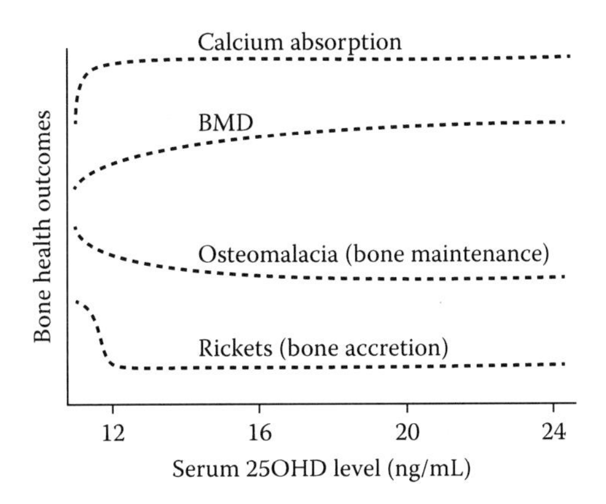

FIGURE 6.1 Skeletal outcomes of serum 25OHD status reach a plateau of effect between 40 and 50 nmol/L (16–20 ng/mL). (Adapted from Rosen, C. J. et al. 2012. *Journal of Clinical Endocrinology and Metabolism* 97(4): 1146–1152.)

The IOM committee derived DRIs for vitamin D based on optimizing calcium absorption and BMD while minimizing risk for osteomalacia (lack of bone accretion) and rickets (Figure 6.1) (Rosen et al., 2012). The EAR for vitamin D is 400 IU/day for all life-stage groups, and the RDA is 600 IU/day for ages 1–70 or 800 IU for age 71+. Corresponding serum 25OHD status for the EAR is 37.5 nmol/L (15 ng/mL) and for the RDA is 50 nmol/L (20 ng/mL). The upper limit of safety set by the IOM is 4000 IU/day, which was adjusted from the no-observed-adverse-effect level of 10,000 IU/day. Effects of vitamin D toxicity are related to hypercalcemia such as kidney damage and tissue calcification (Ross et al., 2010).

6.3 INTAKES

6.3.1 Calcium

Dietary sources of calcium include dairy products, leafy green vegetables, and whole grain products. However, the calcium in vegetables and whole grains is less bioavailable as it is tightly bound to phytate, which inhibits its intestinal absorption (Gueguen and Pointillart, 2000). As such, most countries have dietary guidelines that emphasize two to three cups of milk per day to achieve adequate dietary calcium intakes (Weaver et al., 2013). Individuals who do not consume dairy may have difficulty achieving their recommended dietary calcium intakes. As a result, calcium is widely recognized as a shortfall nutrient and calcium inadequacy is not uncommon. NHANES data collected in 2009–2010 revealed that women ≥51 years are particularly vulnerable to the dietary calcium shortfall as 72%–76% did not meet the EAR through food sources (Figure 6.2). Additionally, 69% of men over 70 years did not meet the EAR for calcium. Pre-teens and adolescent girls were also alarmingly inadequate, with 54% of girls aged 6–12 and 74% of girls aged 13–18 years not reaching the EAR for calcium through the consumption of calcium-containing foods.

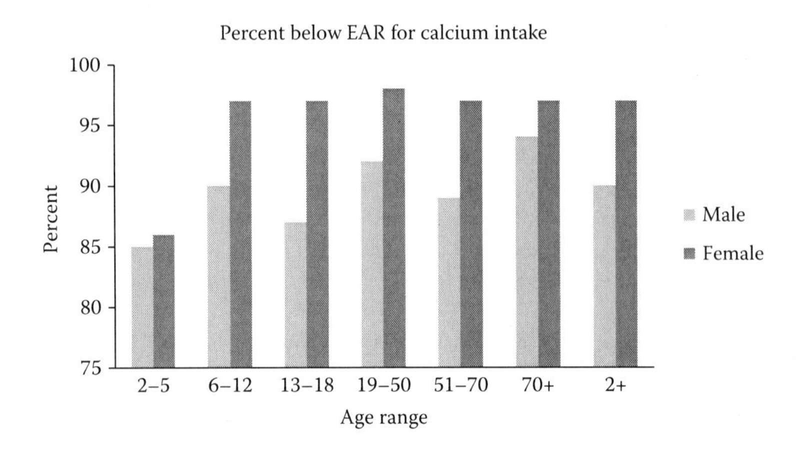

FIGURE 6.2 Percentage of Americans with calcium intake below the EAR by NCI Usual Intake Method from NHANES 2009–2010 (from foods only).

As a result of the widely recognized calcium inadequacy in the United States, calcium supplementation has been advocated and is common practice, particularly in the prevention and management of osteoporosis. About 43% of people in the United States taking supplemental calcium (Bailey et al., 2010). Among women over 50 years of age, this number jumps to approximately 66%. Although the use of supplementation remains common, recent concern over a potential link between calcium supplementation and cardiovascular risk has been blamed, at least in part, for the decrease in US consumers using calcium supplements from 22% in 2011 to 17% in 2012 (CRN, 2012). The calcium controversy will be addressed in subsequent sections of this chapter.

6.3.2 Vitamin D

Intakes of vitamin D tend to be inadequate as few foods are rich in vitamin D. Vitamin D is often reported as international units (IU), where 40 IU = 1 μg. Mean vitamin D intakes are estimated to be 150–220 IU/day mostly from milk (44%–45% of intake), fish and meat (15%–20%), and fortified ready-to-eat cereals (4%–8%) (Hill et al., 2012; O'Neil et al., 2012). Vitamin D is unique in that there is a significant nondietary source. Exposure of skin to ultraviolet B (UVB) catalyzes synthesis of vitamin D_3 from 7-dehydrocholesterol. Estimates of intake equivalents from cutaneous synthesis can be complicated as 25OHD response depends on season, latitude, time of exposure, skin pigmentation, and area of skin exposed (Chen et al., 2007). Exposure of about 0.5 erythemal dose (about half the exposure required to induce slightly pink skin) raises serum $25OHD_3$ 2–5 nmol/L (Bogh et al., 2011) and is equivalent to ingesting around 3000 IU vitamin D_3 (Hossein-nezhad and Holick, 2013).

Gaps between recommended intakes and actual intakes are significant, as are gaps for 25OHD status. Data from NHANES 2009–2010 suggest that 90% of males and over 95% of females age 2+ consume less than the EAR. Although these data may be misleading as it does not consider vitamin D from cutaneous synthesis,

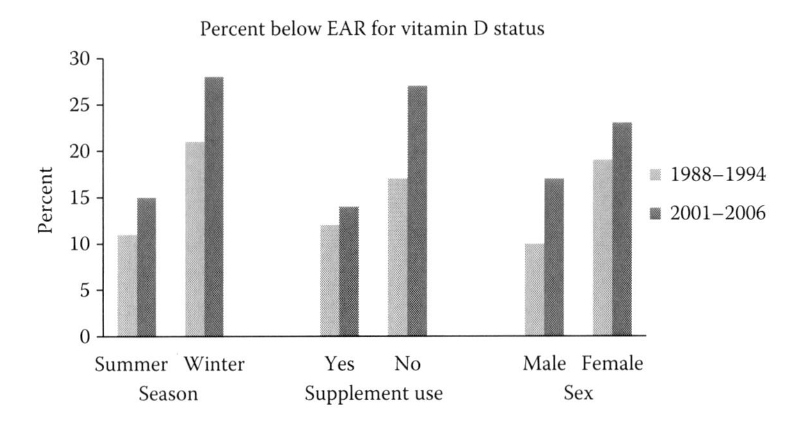

FIGURE 6.3 Percentage of Americans with 25-hydroxyvitamin D status <40 nmol/L from NHANES 1988–1994 and 2001–2006. (Adapted from Ganji, V., Zhang, X., and Tangpricha, V. 2012. *Journal of Nutrition* 142(3): 498–507.)

surveys of vitamin D status also reflect inadequacy, albeit less severe. Data from NHANES 2001–2006 suggest that 20% of the US population were deficient with serum 25OHD < 40 nmol/L (approximately EAR) and 32% were insufficient with <50 nmol/L (RDA), both increasing since the 1988–1994 survey (Figure 6.3) (Ganji et al., 2012). The gap is larger in winter than in summer due to seasonal fluctuations in sun exposure and cutaneous vitamin D synthesis (Looker et al., 2008). Certain populations have elevated risk for vitamin D deficiency, including elderly (MacLaughlin and Holick, 1985), those that live at high latitude, and lactose-intolerant and vegan individuals that do not consume milk and fish (Ho-Pham et al., 2012).

These gaps suggest a role for vitamin D supplements for Americans to fulfill the dietary requirement. Most over-the-counter supplements in the United States contain vitamin D_3 unless specifically formulated to be vegan, whereas prescriptions contain D_2 (Holick, 2007). About 37% of respondents to NHANES 2005–2006 used a supplement containing vitamin D, which increased its intake from about 200–250 IU/day from diet alone to 280–360 IU/day for adults age 18+ (Bailey et al., 2010). Vitamin D supplement use increased in the Nurses' Health Study and Health Professionals Follow-up study from 2% to 32% in women from 1986 to 2006 (Kim et al., 2013), and the CRN estimates that 20% of adults take vitamin D (CRN, 2012).

6.4 EVIDENCE FOR SUPPLEMENTATION

The ability of calcium and vitamin D supplements to improve bone health depends on the gap between dietary intake and physiological need. Calcium is excreted once intake exceeds a certain threshold. Therefore, supplemental intake above the individual's physiological need will not improve bone outcomes. Supplemental vitamin D will continue to be absorbed above the physiological need, but once sufficient vitamin D is available to maintain calcium balance and to minimize bone turnover, little additional benefit on bone health is attained from supplemental intake. Although calcium intake and vitamin D intake have been moderately associated with intermediate indicators such as BMD and serum PTH, evidence on end outcomes including fracture risk is less consistent. Much of the inconsistency in clinical and epidemiological evidence for calcium and vitamin D is due to varying baseline status of subjects between and within studies. Few RCTs have used adequate status (or intake) as exclusion criteria; therefore, null results may be due to supplementation of subjects above the threshold for benefit. Sub-group analysis of subjects with deficient status (or insufficient intake) may be the strongest evidence for supplementation due to the lack of RCTs targeting deficient populations.

The Women's Health Initiative (WHI) calcium + vitamin D trial (CaD) is the largest and longest RCT to assess fracture risk (Jackson et al., 2006). Over 36,000 women received either placebo or 1000 mg calcium + 400 IU vitamin D per day (divided into two doses to be taken with meals) for an average of 7 years. Participants were allowed to take additional calcium and/or vitamin D supplements throughout the trial, and as a result baseline intakes nearly met the EARs at baseline (1150 mg/day calcium and 365 IU/day vitamin D). Participants receiving supplements had 1.06% greater hip BMD, but no improvement in lumbar spine BMD, total BMD, hip fracture risk, spine fracture risk, or total fracture risk (Cauley, 2013). Improved hip BMD was associated with altered geometry and increased cross-sectional area of the hip at the narrow neck (Jackson et al., 2011). Limiting analysis to adherent participants revealed a benefit to hip fracture [hazard ratio (HR) 0.71, 95% confidence interval (CI) 0.52–0.97] (Cauley, 2013). As participants who were allowed to continue supplement use were likely above the threshold to receive additional benefit, subgroup analysis of non-users is more appropriate for developing supplementation recommendations. Hip fracture HR among women not taking supplements at baseline and adherent to the intervention for 5+ years was 0.24 (95% CI 0.07–0.84), i.e. calcium + vitamin D supplements reduced hip fracture by 76% (Prentice et al., 2013). Although this subgroup analysis of the WHI CaD trial may be subject to loss of complete randomization, it strongly indicates that calcium + vitamin D supplementation reduces fracture risk in women not meeting the EARs through diet alone.

Meta-analyses show similar results as most are dominated by the WHI CaD trial. One assessing people aged 50+ years found that calcium + vitamin D reduced total fracture risk by 12%, or 24% in studies with 80% or greater compliance, thereby excluding the WHI CaD trial (Tang et al., 2007). Patient-level meta-analysis of 68,500 participants from seven trials, including the WHI CaD trial, shows that calcium + vitamin D reduced hip and overall fracture risk, but supplementation with vitamin D alone was not effective (DIPART, 2010). Similarly, a systematic Cochrane review of studies on postmenopausal women found that calcium + vitamin D effectively reduced hip fracture risk, but not vitamin D alone (Avenell et al., 2009). However, NHANES III data show that vitamin D status is associated with fracture risk. Osteoporotic fracture risk increased 26%–27% with each standard deviation decrease in vitamin D status, and hip fracture risk was 2.63 times greater for subjects with 25OHD status <30 nmol/L in comparison to those with >30 nmol/L (Looker, 2013). Calcium without vitamin D also did not reduce fracture risk in meta-analysis (Bischoff-Ferrari et al., 2007). Overall, evidence suggests that calcium + vitamin D supplementation for 5+ years is required to significantly reduce fracture risk (Chung et al., 2009; Prentice et al., 2013).

The US Preventative Services Task Force recommends against ≤1000 mg calcium + ≤400 IU vitamin D supplementation in older, non-institutionalized adults who do not have osteoporosis or vitamin D deficiency (Moyer, 2013). Meta-analysis for the task force shows that calcium + vitamin D reduced fracture risk in older adults, but the effect was not significant in non-institutionalized adults (Chung et al., 2011). The National Osteoporosis Foundation responded with concern that this recommendation may lead to an increase in fractures if older adults stop taking supplements (NOF, 2013). Osteoporotic hip fracture in the elderly significantly raises mortality risk in the first year after fracture and reduces quality of life (Gonzalez-Rozas et al., 2012; Valizadeh et al., 2012). Vitamin D + calcium supplementation may at least be warranted during winter months as intervention prevents seasonal decline in 25OHD and BMD (Meier et al., 2004). Although evidence for supplementation is criticized for sub-group analysis, supplementation seems to be required for certain individuals to fill gaps of dietary intake and to maintain bone health.

6.5 BIOAVAILABILITY FROM SUPPLEMENTS AND FOOD SOURCES

6.5.1 Calcium

Intestinal absorption and subsequent availability of calcium to the body are affected by both dietary and non-dietary factors. Dietary contributions to calcium bioavailability include habitual calcium intake levels, vitamin D status, the total amount of calcium consumed at one time, and interactions of calcium with other food components that may be consumed concurrently. Non-dietary factors include age, life stage, the use of certain medications, and some conditions of the intestines. Intestinal calcium absorption has been demonstrated to decrease with advanced age (60+ years) and with post-menopausal status due to estrogen deficiency (Nordin et al., 2004), whereas calcium absorption increases during pregnancy and after weaning (Kalkwarf et al., 1996). Two commonly used forms of calcium supplements include calcium citrate and calcium carbonate. As calcium carbonate depends on gastric acid for optimal absorption, calcium carbonate is poorly absorbed on an empty stomach in individuals with achlorhydria, a condition in which stomach acid production is deficient (Recker, 1985). Calcium absorption is restored when calcium carbonate is given with a meal or if calcium citrate is administered. Calcium absorption is also significantly impacted by habitual calcium intakes. In times of low calcium consumption, active vitamin D-dependent transcellular calcium absorption in the duodenum is upregulated. However, when calcium intakes are adequate or high, this active absorption process is downregulated, and passive paracellular absorption along the small intestine prevails. Because the active transcellular intestinal absorption becomes saturated with high calcium intakes, the percentage of total calcium that is absorbed decreases. Thus, although more calcium is ultimately absorbed with increasing intakes, the efficiency of this process is decreased. However, adaptation is limited and cannot completely compensate for low dietary intake. It has been recommended that individuals consume calcium supplements in doses of ≤500 mg at one time to maximize the absorption efficiency. The bioavailability of calcium from one cup of cow's milk, a relatively well-absorbed source of calcium, is about 30%–35%

(Nickel et al., 1996). In healthy people, the bioavailability of calcium from calcium supplements has been shown to be as good as or better than that of milk and other dairy products (Talbot et al., 1999).

6.5.2 Vitamin D

Vitamin D is absorbed like other fat-soluble nutrients via the lymphatic system (Schachter et al., 1964). Bioavailability of vitamin D from supplements depends on dissolution of the supplement (Grossmann and Tangpricha, 2010) and also upon subsequent solubilization of vitamin D into mixed lipid micelles (Reboul and Borel, 2011). As with other lipids, emerging evidence suggests that epithelial vitamin D uptake is not a diffusive process. Cholesterol transports Scavenger receptor class B member 1 (SR-B1), Niemann–Pick C1-like 1 protein (NPC1L1), and Cluster Determinant 36 (CD36) are all likely involved (Reboul et al., 2011). Coingestion of lipid is regarded as an important factor in lipophilic nutrient bioavailability. However, serum vitamin D_2 response was similar for 25,000 IU doses of corn oil on toast, skim milk, and whole milk (Tangpricha et al., 2003). An early rat study suggests that fatty acids and monoglycerides enhance chylomicron synthesis and the secretion of vitamin D into the lymph rather than enhancing intestinal absorption (Thompson et al., 1969). The amount and composition of a meal coingested with supplements and vitamin D-rich foods likely affect vitamin D bioavailability, but have been little studied.

Change in 25-hydroxyvitamin D status is currently the most widely used indicator of vitamin D bioavailability from foods and supplements. A meta-analysis (Grossmann and Tangpricha, 2010) indicated that the vehicle of vitamin D supplementation may influence bioavailability (Figure 6.4). The increase in subjects' 25OHD status was about 4 nmol/L per 100 IU administered daily in studies utilizing oil vehicles, compared with 2.7 nmol/L per 100 IU from studies using powder tablets and only 0.5 nmol/L per

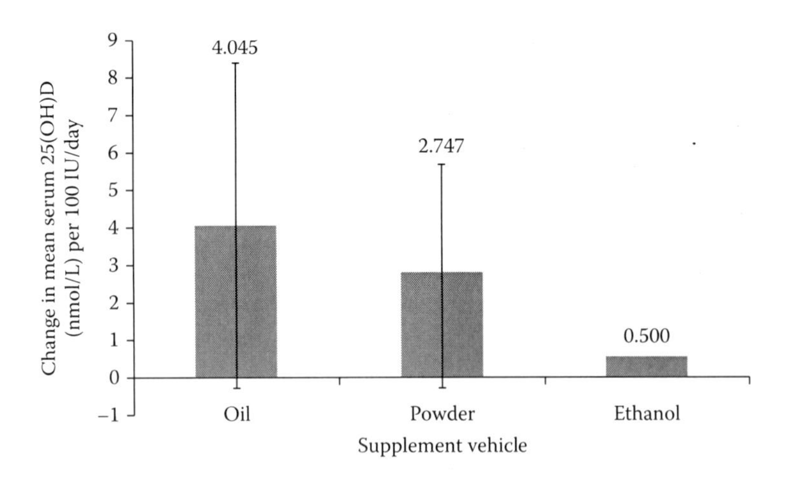

FIGURE 6.4 Change in vitamin D status from 100 IU/day supplemental vitamin D. (Adapted from Grossmann, R. E. and Tangpricha, V. 2010. *Molecular Nutrition and Food Research* 54: 1055–1061.)

100 IU from a single study using ethanol vehicle (Grossmann and Tangpricha, 2010). Meta-analysis of vitamin D fortified foods is confounded by many factors such as baseline vitamin D status, but data suggest a similar average serum 25OHD increase of 2.5 nmol/L per 100 IU ingested daily from foods (Black et al., 2012). The efficacy of vitamin D_2 versus vitamin D_3 is highly contentious. A systematic review of RCTs indicates that vitamin D_3 is more effective than vitamin D_2 in raising total 25OHD status when given as a single or minimal bolus dose, but the vitamers are equal when supplements are consumed daily (Tripkovic et al., 2012).

Serum 25OHD alone is not a sufficient indicator of vitamin D status when considering diverse populations and genetic variation. In the Healthy Aging in Neighborhoods of Diversity across the Life Span (HANDLS) study, Black Americans had significantly lower 25OHD levels than White Americans (15.6 vs. 25.8 ng/mL), despite higher BMD and serum calcium, which is consistent with other observations that Blacks are at lower risk for fracture (Powe et al., 2013). As Blacks had proportionally lower levels of vitamin D binding protein, it is hypothesized that the ratio of 25OHD to vitamin D binding protein might better reflect bioavailable 25OHD and vitamin D status; yet, this still needs to be validated across a wider range of ethnic populations.

6.6 RISKS ASSOCIATED WITH CALCIUM AND VITAMIN D SUPPLEMENTATION

Traditionally thought to have only minimal potential side effects including gastrointestinal upset and kidney stones, recent secondary analyses have called into question the safety of calcium supplements pertaining to cardiovascular health. Previously, calcium was thought to have cardioprotective effects by beneficially altering blood pressure and blood lipids (Reid et al., 2005; van Mierlo et al., 2006). More recently, a meta-analysis of RCTs demonstrated an approximate 30% increased risk of myocardial infarction in healthy adults allocated to calcium supplements compared with placebo (Bolland et al., 2010). The validity of these findings has been debated (Heaney et al., 2012; Lewis et al., 2012; Weaver, 2013) primarily due to the use of non-adjudicated endpoints, secondary analysis of trials designed to investigate bone outcomes, a lack of baseline cardiovascular data, and a lack of demonstrated physiological mechanism. Nonetheless, one proposed mechanism by which calcium supplements may be detrimental to cardiovascular health is through the acceleration of vascular calcification. To date, studies have failed to show associations between calcium intake and coronary artery calcium scores in adults (Manson et al., 2010; Kim et al., 2012; Samelson et al., 2012). Furthermore, the previously mentioned WHI CaD trial, one of the largest clinical trials of calcium and vitamin D, did not demonstrate an increased risk of myocardial infarction, coronary heart disease, total heart disease, stroke, and overall cardiovascular disease (CVD) with supplement allocation (Prentice et al., 2013). Notably, in subgroup analysis of those adherent to study pills, calcium and vitamin D were associated with an overall decreased risk for hip fracture, breast cancer, and total invasive cancer (Figure 6.5). There have not been any long-term RCTs in adults that have investigated the effect of calcium intake on cardiovascular outcomes as a primary endpoint. Thus, a definitive conclusion regarding a causal relationship between calcium intake and cardiovascular risk cannot be drawn.

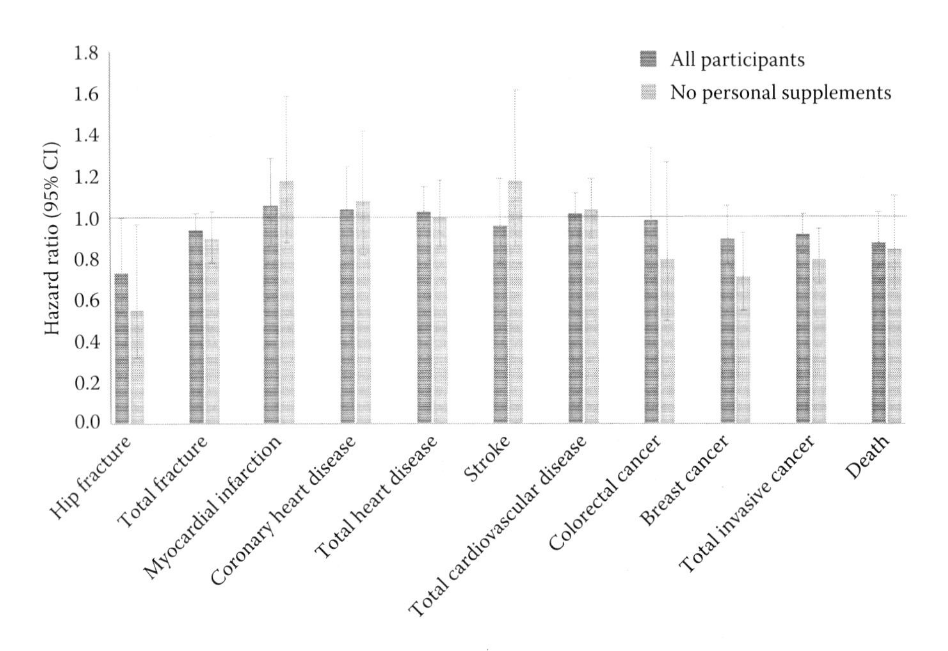

FIGURE 6.5 Overall HRs for clinical outcomes from the WHI CaD trial for subjects adherent to study pills. Results reflect data from all participants assigned to calcium and vitamin D (dark gray) and subgroup analysis of those not taking personal supplements (light gray). Data are expressed as HRs with 95% CIs.

However, the collective evidence from observational studies and trials does not warrant concern over calcium supplementation with regard to cardiovascular safety. One other concern over calcium supplements is an increase in kidney stone development. However, the USPSTF has recently concluded that this risk is minimal (Moyer, 2013).

Vitamin D supplementation is associated with reduced risks of CVD and mortality and therefore less contentious than calcium supplementation. Low vitamin D status was associated with increased risks of all-cause mortality in NHANES III data (Melamed et al., 2008). Furthermore, low 25OHD status has been associated with an increased risk of fatal cardiovascular events (Perna et al., 2013) and arterial disease (vande Luijtgaarden et al., 2012). As for supplement usage, all-cause mortality risk in older adults (median 70 h) after 3 years of intervention was reduced 7% by vitamin D + calcium, but not by vitamin D alone in a meta-analysis (Rejnmark et al., 2012). The observation that vitamin D + calcium is more effective than vitamin D alone in reducing mortality risk seems contradictory to the observation that calcium supplementation is associated with increased mortality risk (Bolland et al., 2010) and might suggest that the actions of calcium and vitamin D against mortality are complementary.

6.7 CONCLUSIONS

Bone is the primary reservoir for calcium, and negative calcium balance decreases BMD. The 2011 IOM committee sets the DRIs on evidence for skeletal outcomes as evidence for non-skeletal outcomes was insufficient. Calcium + vitamin D is effective in preventing osteoporotic bone fractures following 5+ years of supplement usage when dietary intakes do not meet recommendations. Bioavailability of these nutrients from supplements is comparable to food sources. Trends of supplement usage indicate that vitamin D supplementation is increasing, whereas calcium usage is decreasing due to a perceived increased risk for cardiovascular events. However, secondary analyses that suggest calcium supplementation increases cardiovascular risk have not been supported by mechanistic evidence or clinical interventions with cardiovascular primary outcomes. Further, calcium + vitamin D supplementation has been shown to decrease mortality. Supplements seem to safely and effectively fulfill gaps of calcium and vitamin D intake from food sources, so long as the 2011 DRIs are followed.

REFERENCES

Avenell, A., Gillespie, W. J., Gillespie, L. D., and O'Connell, D. 2009. Vitamin D and vitamin D analogues for preventing fractures associated with involutional and post-menopausal osteoporosis. *Cochrane Database of Systematic Reviews* (2): CD000227.

Bailey, R. L., Dodd, K. W., Goldman, J. A., Gahche, J. J., Dwyer, J. T., Moshfegh, A. J., Sempos, C. T., and Picciano, M. F. 2010. Estimation of total usual calcium and vitamin D intakes in the United States. *Journal of Nutrition* 140(4): 817–822.

Bischoff-Ferrari, H. A., Dawson-Hughes, B., Baron, J. A., Burckhardt, P., Li, R., Spiegelman, D., Specker, B., Orav, J. E., Wong, J. B., Staehelin, H. B. et al. 2007. Calcium intake and hip fracture risk in men and women: A meta-analysis of prospective cohort studies and randomized controlled trials. *American Journal of Clinical Nutrition* 86(6): 1780–1790.

Black, L. J., Seamans, K. M., Cashman, K. D., and Kiely, M. 2012. An updated systematic review and meta-analysis of the efficacy of vitamin D food fortification. *Journal of Nutrition* 142(6): 1102–1108.

Bogh, M. K., Schmedes, A. V., Philipsen, P. A., Thieden, E., and Wulf, H. C. 2011. Vitamin D production depends on ultraviolet-B dose but not on dose rate: A randomized controlled trial. *Experimental Dermatology* 20(1): 14–18.

Bolland, M. J., Avenell, A., Baron, J. A., Grey, A., MacLennan, G. S., Gamble, G. D., and Reid, I. R. 2010. Effect of calcium supplements on risk of myocardial infarction and cardiovascular events: Meta-analysis. *British Medical Journal (Clinical Research Ed.)* 341: c3691.

Cauley, J. A. 2013. The Women's Health Initiative: Hormone Therapy and Calcium/Vitamin D Supplementation Trials. *Current Osteoporosis Reports* 11(3): 171–178.

Chen, T. C., Chimeh, F., Lu, Z., Mathieu, J., Person, K. S., Zhang, A., Kohn, N., Martinello, S., Berkowitz, R., and Holick, M. F. 2007. Factors that influence the cutaneous synthesis and dietary sources of vitamin D. *Archives of Biochemistry and Biophysics* 460(2): 213–217.

Chung, M., Balk, E. M., Brendel, M., Ip, S., Lau, J., Lee, J., Lichtenstein, A., Patel, K., Raman, G., Tatsioni, A. et al. 2009. Vitamin D and calcium: A systematic review of health outcomes. *Evidence Report Technology Assessment (Full Rep)* (183): 1–420.

Chung, M., Lee, J., Terasawa, T., Lau, J., and Trikalinos, T. A. 2011. Vitamin D with or without calcium supplementation for prevention of cancer and fractures: An updated meta-analysis for the U.S. Preventive Services Task Force. *Annals of Internal Medicine* 155(12): 827–838.

CRN. 2012. 2012 CRN Consumer Survey on Dietary Supplements. Council for Responsible Nutrition.

DIPART. 2010. Patient level pooled analysis of 68 500 patients from seven major vitamin D fracture trials in US and Europe. *British Medical Journal (Clinical Research Ed.)* 340: b5463.

Ganji, V., Zhang, X., and Tangpricha, V. 2012. Serum 25-hydroxyvitamin D concentrations and prevalence estimates of hypovitaminosis D in the U.S. population based on assay-adjusted data. *Journal of Nutrition* 142(3): 498–507.

Gonzalez-Rozas, M., Perez-Castrillon, J. L., Gonzalez-Sagrado, M., Ruiz-Mambrilla, M., and Garcia-Alonso, M. 2012. Risk of mortality and predisposing factors after osteoporotic hip fracture: A one-year follow-up study. *Aging Clinical and Experimental Research* 24(2): 181–187.

Grossmann, R. E. and Tangpricha, V. 2010. Evaluation of vehicle substances on vitamin D bioavailability: A systematic review. *Molecular Nutrition and Food Research* 54: 1055–1061.

Gueguen, L. and Pointillart, A. 2000. The bioavailability of dietary calcium. *Journal of the American College of Nutrition* 19(2 Suppl): 119S–136S.

Heaney, R. P., Kopecky, S., Maki, K. C., Hathcock, J., Mackay, D., and Wallace, T. C. 2012. A review of calcium supplements and cardiovascular disease risk. *Advances in Nutrition* 3(6): 763–771.

Hill, K. M., Jonnalagadda, S. S., Albertson, A. M., Joshi, N. A., and Weaver, C. M. 2012. Top food sources contributing to vitamin D intake and the association of ready-to-eat cereal and breakfast consumption habits to vitamin D intake in Canadians and United States Americans. *Journal of Food Science* 77(8): H170–H175.

Holick, M. F. 2007. Vitamin D deficiency. *New England Journal of Medicine* 357(3): 266–281.

Ho-Pham, L. T., Vu, B. Q., Lai, T. Q., Nguyen, N. D., and Nguyen, T. V. 2012. Vegetarianism, bone loss, fracture and vitamin D: A longitudinal study in Asian vegans and non-vegans. *European Journal of Clinical Nutrition* 66(1): 75–82.

Hossein-nezhad, A. and Holick, M. F. 2013. Vitamin D for health: A global perspective. *Mayo Clinic Proceedings* 88(7): 720–755.

Jackson, R. D., LaCroix, A. Z., Gass, M., Wallace, R. B., Robbins, J., Lewis, C. E., Bassford, T., Beresford, S. A., Black, H. R., Blanchette, P. et al. 2006. Calcium plus vitamin D supplementation and the risk of fractures. *New England Journal of Medicine* 354(7): 669–683.

Jackson, R. D., Wright, N. C., Beck, T. J., Sherrill, D., Cauley, J. A., Lewis, C. E., LaCroix, A. Z., LeBoff, M. S., Going, S., Bassford, T. et al. 2011. Calcium plus vitamin D supplementation has limited effects on femoral geometric strength in older postmenopausal women: The Women's Health Initiative. *Calcified Tissue International* 88(3): 198–208.

Kalkwarf, H. J., Specker, B. L., Heubi, J. E., Vieira, N. E., and Yergey, A. L. 1996. Intestinal calcium absorption of women during lactation and after weaning. *American Journal of Clinical Nutrition* 63(4): 526–531.

Kim, H. J., Giovannucci, E., Rosner, B., Willett, W. C., and Cho, E. 2013. Longitudinal and secular trends in dietary supplement use: Nurses' Health Study and Health Professionals Follow-up Study, 1986–2006. *Journal of the Academy of Nutrition and Dietetics* 114(3): 436–443.

Kim, J. H., Yoon, J. W., Kim, K. W., Lee, E. J., Lee, W., Cho, S. H., and Shin, C. S. 2012. Increased dietary calcium intake is not associated with coronary artery calcification. *International Journal of Cardiology* 157(3): 429–431.

Lewis, J. R., Zhu, K., and Prince, R. L. 2012. Adverse events from calcium supplementation: Relationship to errors in myocardial infarction self-reporting in randomized controlled trials of calcium supplementation. *Journal of Bone and Mineral Research* 27(3): 719–722.

Looker, A. C. 2013. Serum 25-hydroxyvitamin D and risk of major osteoporotic fractures in older U.S. adults. *Journal of Bone and Mineral Research* 28(5): 997–1006.

Looker, A. C., Pfeiffer, C. M., Lacher, D. A., Schleicher, R. L., Picciano, M. F., and Yetley, E. A. 2008. Serum 25-hydroxyvitamin D status of the US population: 1988–1994 compared with 2000–2004. *American Journal of Clinical Nutrition* 88(6): 1519–1527.

MacLaughlin, J. and Holick, M. F. 1985. Aging decreases the capacity of human skin to produce vitamin D3. *Journal of Clinical Investigation* 76(4): 1536–1538.

Manson, J. E., Allison, M. A., Carr, J. J., Langer, R. D., Cochrane, B. B., Hendrix, S. L., Hsia, J., Hunt, J. R., Lewis, C. E., Margolis, K. L. et al. 2010. Calcium/vitamin D supplementation and coronary artery calcification in the Women's Health Initiative. *Menopause* 17(4): 683–691.

Masuyama, R., Nakaya, Y., Katsumata, S., Kajita, Y., Uehara, M., Tanaka, S., Sakai, A., Kato, S., Nakamura, T., and Suzuki, K. 2003. Dietary calcium and phosphorus ratio regulates bone mineralization and turnover in vitamin D receptor knockout mice by affecting intestinal calcium and phosphorus absorption. *Journal of Bone and Mineral Research* 18(7): 1217–1226.

Meier, C., Woitge, H. W., Witte, K., Lemmer, B., and Seibel, M. J. 2004. Supplementation with oral vitamin D3 and calcium during winter prevents seasonal bone loss: A randomized controlled open-label prospective trial. *Journal of Bone and Mineral Research* 19(8): 1221–1230.

Melamed, M. L., Michos, E. D., Post, W., and Astor, B. 2008. 25-Hydroxyvitamin D levels and the risk of mortality in the general population. *Archives of Internal Medicine* 168(15): 1629–1637.

Moyer, V. A. 2013. Vitamin D and calcium supplementation to prevent fractures in adults: U.S. Preventive Services Task Force recommendation statement. *Annals of Internal Medicine* 158(9): 691–696.

Need, A. G., O'Loughlin, P. D., Morris, H. A., Coates, P. S., Horowitz, M., and Nordin, B. E. 2008. Vitamin D metabolites and calcium absorption in severe vitamin D deficiency. *Journal of Bone and Mineral Research* 23(11): 1859–1863.

Nickel, K. P., Martin, B. R., Smith, D. L., Smith, J. B., Miller, G. D., and Weaver, C. M. 1996. Calcium bioavailability from bovine milk and dairy products in premenopausal women using intrinsic and extrinsic labeling techniques. *Journal of Nutrition* 126(5): 1406–1411.

NOF. 2013. NOF Responds to the U.S. Preventive Services Task Force Recommendations on Calcium and Vitamin D. National Osteoporosis Foundation.

Nordin, B. E., Need, A. G., Morris, H. A., O'Loughlin, P. D., and Horowitz, M. 2004. Effect of age on calcium absorption in postmenopausal women. *American Journal of Clinical Nutrition* 80(4): 998–1002.

O'Neil, C. E., Keast, D. R., Fulgoni, V. L., and Nicklas, T. A. 2012. Food sources of energy and nutrients among adults in the US: NHANES 2003–2006. *Nutrients* 4(12): 2097–2120.

Perna, L., Schottker, B., Holleczek, B., and Brenner, H. 2013. Serum 25-hydroxyvitamin D and incidence of fatal and non-fatal cardiovascular events: A prospective study with repeated measurements. *Journal of Clinical Endocrinology and Metabolism* 98(12): 4908–4915.

Powe, C. E., Evans, M. K., Wenger, J., Zonderman, A. B., Berg, A. H., Nalls, M., Tamez, H., Zhang, D., Bhan, I., Karumanchi, S. A. et al. 2013. Vitamin D-binding protein and vitamin D status of Black Americans and White Americans. *New England Journal of Medicine* 369(21): 1991–2000.

Prentice, R. L., Pettinger, M. B., Jackson, R. D., Wactawski-Wende, J., Lacroix, A. Z., Anderson, G. L., Chlebowski, R. T., Manson, J. E., Van Horn, L., Vitolins, M. Z. et al. 2013. Health risks and benefits from calcium and vitamin D supplementation: Women's Health Initiative clinical trial and cohort study. *Osteoporosis International* 24(2): 567–580.

Reboul, E. and Borel, P. 2011. Proteins involved in uptake, intracellular transport and basolateral secretion of fat-soluble vitamins and carotenoids by mammalian enterocytes. *Progress in Lipid Research* 50(4): 388–402.

Reboul, E., Goncalves, A., Comera, C., Bott, R., Nowicki, M., Landrier, J. F., Jourdheuil-Rahmani, D., Dufour, C., Collet, X., and Borel, P. 2011. Vitamin D intestinal absorption is not a simple passive diffusion: Evidences for involvement of cholesterol transporters. *Molecular Nutrition and Food Research* 55(5): 691–702.

Recker, R. R. 1985. Calcium absorption and achlorhydria. *New England Journal of Medicine* 313(2): 70–73.

Reid, I. R., Bolland, M. J., and Grey, A. 2013. Effects of vitamin D supplements on bone mineral density: A systematic review and meta-analysis. *The Lancet* 383(9912): 146–155.

Reid, I. R., Horne, A., Mason, B., Ames, R., Bava, U., and Gamble, G. D. 2005. Effects of calcium supplementation on body weight and blood pressure in normal older women: A randomized controlled trial. *Journal of Clinical Endocrinology and Metabolism* 90(7): 3824–3829.

Rejnmark, L., Avenell, A., Masud, T., Anderson, F., Meyer, H. E., Sanders, K. M., Salovaara, K., Cooper, C., Smith, H. E., Jacobs, E. T. et al. 2012. Vitamin D with calcium reduces mortality: Patient level pooled analysis of 70,528 patients from eight major vitamin D trials. *Journal of Clinical Endocrinology and Metabolism* 97(8): 2670–2681.

Rosen, C. J., Abrams, S. A., Aloia, J. F., Brannon, P. M., Clinton, S. K., Durazo-Arvizu, R. A., Gallagher, J. C., Gallo, R. L., Jones, G., Kovacs, C. S. et al. 2012. IOM committee members respond to Endocrine Society vitamin D guideline. *Journal of Clinical Endocrinology and Metabolism* 97(4): 1146–1152.

Ross, A. C., Abrams, S. A., Aloia, J. F., Brannon, P. M., Clinton, S. K., Durazo-Arvizu, R. A., Gallagher, J. C., Gallo, R. L., Jones, G., Kovacs, C. S. et al. 2010. Dietary reference intakes for calcium and vitamin D. Institue of Medicine.

Ross, A. C., Manson, J. E., Abrams, S. A., Aloia, J. F., Brannon, P. M., Clinton, S. K., Durazo-Arvizu, R. A., Gallagher, J. C., Gallo, R. L., Jones, G. et al. 2011. The 2011 report on dietary reference intakes for calcium and vitamin D from the Institute of Medicine: What clinicians need to know. *Journal of Clinical Endocrinology and Metabolism* 96(1): 53–58.

Samelson, E. J., Booth, S. L., Fox, C. S., Tucker, K. L., Wang, T. J., Hoffmann, U., Cupples, L. A., O'Donnell, C. J., and Kiel, D. P. 2012. Calcium intake is not associated with increased coronary artery calcification: The Framingham Study. *American Journal of Clinical Nutrition* 96(6): 1274–1280.

Schachter, D., Finkelstein, J. D., and Kowarski, S. 1964. Metabolism of vitamin D. I. Preparation of radioactive vitamin D and its intestinal absorption in the rat. *Journal of Clinical Investigation* 43: 787–796.

Talbot, J. R., Guardo, P., Seccia, S., Gear, L., Lubary, D. R., Saad, G., Roberts, M. L., Fradinger, E., Marino, A., and Zanchetta, J. R. 1999. Calcium bioavailability and parathyroid hormone acute changes after oral intake of dairy and nondairy products in healthy volunteers. *Osteoporosis International* 10(2): 137–142.

Tang, B. M., Eslick, G. D., Nowson, C., Smith, C., and Bensoussan, A. 2007. Use of calcium or calcium in combination with vitamin D supplementation to prevent fractures and bone loss in people aged 50 years and older: A meta-analysis. *Lancet* 370(9588): 657–666.

Tangpricha, V., Koutkia, P., Rieke, S. M., Chen, T. C., Perez, A. A., and Holick, M. F. 2003. Fortification of orange juice with vitamin D: A novel approach for enhancing vitamin D nutritional health. *American Journal of Clinical Nutrition* 77(6): 1478–1483.

Thompson, G. R., Ockner, R. K., and Isselbacher, K. J. 1969. Effect of mixed micellar lipid on the absorption of cholesterol and vitamin D3 into lymph. *Journal of Clinical Investigation* 48(1): 87–95.

Tripkovic, L., Lambert, H., Hart, K., Smith, C. P., Bucca, G., Penson, S., Chope, G., Hypponen, E., Berry, J., Vieth, R. et al. 2012. Comparison of vitamin D2 and vitamin D3 supplementation in raising serum 25-hydroxyvitamin D status: A systematic review and meta-analysis. *American Journal of Clinical Nutrition* 95(6): 1357–1364.

Valizadeh, M., Mazloomzadeh, S., Golmohammadi, S., and Larijani, B. 2012. Mortality after low trauma hip fracture: A prospective cohort study. *BMC Musculoskeletal Disorders* 13: 143.

van de Luijtgaarden, K. M., Voute, M. T., Hoeks, S. E., Bakker, E. J., Chonchol, M., Stolker, R. J., Rouwet, E. V., and Verhagen, H. J. 2012. Vitamin D deficiency may be an independent risk factor for arterial disease. *European Journal of Vascular and Endovascular Surgery* 44(3): 301–306.

van Mierlo, L. A., Arends, L. R., Streppel, M. T., Zeegers, M. P., Kok, F. J., Grobbee, D. E., and Geleijnse, J. M. 2006. Blood pressure response to calcium supplementation: A eta-analysis of randomized controlled trials. *Journal of Human Hypertension* 20(8): 571–580.

Weaver, C. 2013. Calcium is not only safe but important for health. In *Nutritional Influences on Bone Health*, 359–363 (Eds P. Burckhardt, B. Dawson-Hughes, and C. M. Weaver). London: Springer.

Weaver, C. M., Wijesinha-Bettoni, R., McMahon, D., and Spence, L. 2013. Milk and dairy products as part of the diet. In *Milk and Diary Products in Human Nutrition*, 103–183 (Eds E. Muehlhoff, A. Bennet, and D. McMahon). Rome: Food and Agriculture Organization.

Xue, Y. and Fleet, J. C. 2009. Intestinal vitamin D receptor is required for normal calcium and bone metabolism in mice. *Gastroenterology* 136(4): 1317–1327, e1311–e1312.

7 Vitamin D Requirements during Pregnancy and Lactation

Lessons Learned and Unanswered Questions

Carol L. Wagner, Sarah N. Taylor, and Bruce W. Hollis

CONTENTS

Vitamin D requirements during pregnancy and lactation were unvarying for decades: Women were thought to obtain all that they needed from their prenatal vitamin containing 400 IU vitamin D. Data have accumulated that demonstrate otherwise. In this chapter, we review the differences in vitamin D metabolism during pregnancy and lactation and the implications of these differences on vitamin D sufficiency important for both the mother and her developing fetus during pregnancy and for both the mother and her breastfeeding infant during lactation. A summary of relevant clinical trials that have been conducted to answer the question of what amount of vitamin D is necessary to optimize its metabolism during pregnancy and lactation will also be reviewed. More questions than answers remain, however, regarding the impact of vitamin D on immune function and inflammation during pregnancy and lactation and the long-term implications of vitamin D on the health of the child.

7.1 INTRODUCTION

The controversy that surrounds vitamin D and what is needed to maintain optimal health is perhaps most contended during pregnancy and lactation. With such physiological changes that define both pregnancy and lactation, it is no wonder that vitamin D metabolism should be included in the list of changes that occur. Why? Because vitamin D actions during pregnancy and lactation reflect its role as a pre-prohormone, serving as the substrate for one of the most potent hormones in the body—$1,25(OH)_2D$, whose non-traditional endocrine effects are just beginning to be understood.

Until the 1990s, the criterion for appropriate vitamin D nutrition was simply the absence of overt rickets or osteomalacia [1]. To prevent rickets and osteomalacia, an expert panel convened by the Institute of Medicine in 1997 recommended that infants and adults receive 400 and 200 IU vitamin D/day, respectively [2]. The effectiveness of 400 IU vitamin D/day given as a teaspoon of cod liver oil in children in preventing rickets was a time-honored remedy and treatment since the 1930s [3,4]. There was little evidence, however, to support the daily vitamin D dose for adults of 200 IU in achieving vitamin D sufficiency without adequate sunlight exposure. Such a dose was later shown to be inconsequential in all but the most deficient adult individuals [5,6]. Even less was known about the needs of the pregnant and lactating women and that of the developing fetuses and breastfed infants [2,7].

What little was known about vitamin D requirements during pregnancy came from supplementation studies that began in the 1980s [8–15]. Deficiency in certain groups of women, especially those who had darker pigmentation or with limited sunlight exposure due to clothing worn for cultural reasons, was noted, and doses up to 1000 IU/day were shown to do little to reverse that deficiency [8–10,16,17]. Further, reports of vitamin D-associated rickets among exclusively breastfed infants, particularly those who had darker pigmentation, began to surface [18–20] and led some to question whether or not a prenatal vitamin containing between 200 and 400 IU vitamin D taken during pregnancy and lactation was adequate with today's lifestyles [21].

Although 200 IU vitamin D/day was considered adequate for non-pregnant and non-lactating women [22], it was a commonly held belief until recently that all of the needs of the pregnant and lactating women could be met by taking a prenatal vitamin containing 400 IU vitamin D_3 [2,7]. There was some discussion in years past that a woman could be vitamin D-deficient, particularly if she moved from a more moderate climate to the one more northerly, if she had darker pigmentation and/or if she wore clothing that restricted her sunlight exposure [23,24], but such deficiency was thought to be rare. Furthermore, based on the data to prevent osteomalacia, deficiency was defined as a total circulating 25(OH)D concentration of less than 8 ng/mL (<20 nmol/L) [2]. It was not until a paper published by the Center for Disease Control (CDC) in 2002 on the prevalence of vitamin D deficiency among women in their childbearing years that any credence was given to the premise that the degree of vitamin D deficiency in a westernized country such as the United States was more widespread than had previously been thought [22]. Utilizing the Third National Health and Nutrition Examination Survey, 1988–1994 (NHANES-III) database,

Nesby-O'Dell et al. [22] measured total circulating 25(OH)D concentrations in 1546 African–American women and 1426 white women aged 15–49 years who were not pregnant. Hypovitaminosis D was defined as a serum 25(OH)D concentration ≤15 ng/mL (37.5 nmol/L). More than 40% of the African–American women in this large cohort met the criterion for vitamin D deficiency having a 25(OH)D concentration of ≤15 ng/mL, compared with 4.2% of white women [22]. In addition, among the 243 African–Americans who consumed what was considered at the time to be the adequate intake of vitamin D from supplements (200 IU/day), approximately 28% met the definition of hypovitaminosis D. Yet, despite these findings, one was left wondering what the clinical significance of such deficiency was and whether or not there were any discernible health effects, either short- or long-term.

With severe vitamin D deficiency states, fetal growth impairment was noted; it was well known that vitamin D impacted bone development and the risk of rickets, and it was the derangement of calcium metabolism and bone formation that was thought to have impacted fetal growth [8,13]. Beyond calcium and bone metabolism, little was known about vitamin D's non-endocrine roles. There were certainly data around the turn of the twentieth century by Mellanby and co-workers [25–27], which suggested that vitamin D deficiency in children and in animal models was associated with increased risks of respiratory infections, but even Mellanby (and his co-workers) had somewhat discounted the effect of vitamin D on infection risk as noted in a paper published by this group of investigators in 1931: "On experimental grounds we are inclined to believe that vitamin D has little anti-infective action... The possibility cannot be denied, however, that the results described [of their combined vitamin A (375 Carr and Price blue units/day) and vitamin D (12,500 IU/day) treatment in the last month of pregnancy] may be due in part at least, to the presence of increased vitamin D in the diet (p. 598)" [28]. It took another 60 years before the (re)discovery of vitamin D's role in immune function set the stage for an expansion of scientific inquiry into vitamin D's role in immune function in an unprecedented manner [29–35]. Elaboration of inflammatory and immune markers as a function of vitamin D status led some to consider that higher target concentrations of vitamin D were necessary to maintain optimal health, but again, little was known and remains unknown about the role of vitamin D during pregnancy and lactation on immune function and what normal really was.

Additional studies began to emerge that showed in fact there were far more deficient or marginally sufficient pregnant women than there were vitamin D-sufficient pregnant women [36–41], but was this occurring because of a different set point in defining vitamin D deficiency? Controversy arose regarding what defined deficiency, and once the scientific community agreed that the concentration of total circulating 25(OH)D was the indicator of vitamin D sufficiency (due to its longer half-life of 2–3 weeks, its relative ease of measurement, and lower cost than measuring the parent compound vitamin D whose half-life is a mere 12 h), the question then became what should 25(OH)D concentrations really be [42,43]? Should one aim for a concentration of 15 g/mL (37.5 ng/mL) as was the concentration used by the CDC in the 2002 article [22], 20 ng/mL (50 nmol/L), or 30 ng/mL (80 nmol/L), as suggested by Hollis and Wagner [21] in 2004? Does this sufficiency definition change during pregnancy? If there were issues surrounding recommendations during pregnancy, what would one then advise during lactation [44]? To answer some of these questions, we must review the unique metabolism of vitamin D during pregnancy and along that continuum—during lactation.

7.2 VITAMIN D METABOLISM DURING PREGNANCY

Vitamin D is the precursor to 25(OH)D, which is then metabolized further by the kidneys and the placenta to the active form 1,25(OH)$_2$D. It has been known for some time that circulating 25(OH)D freely crosses from maternal circulation to fetal circulation via the placenta, which possesses vitamin D receptors and the enzyme CYP27B1, essential for the conversion of 25(OH)D to 1,25(OH)$_2$D [45]. Although the kidneys are the main source of 1,25(OH)$_2$D throughout the lifespan, the placenta does contribute to the pool of vitamin D metabolites that surge through both maternal and fetal circulations.

In their recent review of vitamin D, Hollis and Wagner [46] point out, however, that the parent compound vitamin D plays a significant role in providing substrate to cells for internalization: vitamin D is vastly more accessible than 25(OH)D for internalization throughout the body with the exception of cells in the kidney and parathyroid gland, for example, that utilize the megalin–cubilin system [47] and which maintain the vitamin D endocrine system. Cells that process vitamin D through paracrine/autocrine actions are dependent on delivery of the vitamin D substrate and how tightly bound it is to the carrier protein, vitamin D-binding protein (VDBP) [46]. For example, availability of circulating 25(OH)D to cells is reduced because it is tightly bound to VDBP. In contrast, vitamin D is far more bioavailable as it is less tightly bound to VDBP, allowing entrance of vitamin D into the cell more easily than 25(OH)D. Once in the cell, vitamin D is then converted to 25(OH)D and then to its active form 1,25(OH)$_2$D. There is no evidence to suggest that this is altered during pregnancy, although the concentration of VDBP during pregnancy is increased [48]. With respect to the conversion of vitamin D to 25(OH)D, this metabolic conversion appears to be similar in pregnant and non-pregnant women and follows first- and zero-order enzyme kinetics (Figure 7.1) [49].

In any discussion about vitamin D deficiency, parathyroid hormone (PTH) is mentioned because it upregulates 1-α-hydroxylase, the enzyme responsible for 1-α-hydroxylation of 25(OH)D, converting 25(OH)D to 1,25(OH)$_2$D. In individuals who have vitamin D deficiency, the body increases the production of PTH to maintain 1,25(OH)$_2$D and calcium homeostasis. If vitamin D deficiency is sustained, secondary hyperparathyroidism will result. Yet, during pregnancy, this association is diminished due to the uncoupling of vitamin D metabolism from calcium [49]. Pregnant women attain "supraphysiological" concentrations of 1,25(OH)$_2$D in the first weeks of gestation [50], sometimes exceeding 700 pmol/L in our NICHD study [36], and yet never exhibit hypercalciuria or hypercalcemia. It is not surprising then that during pregnancy PTH as a marker of vitamin D status is a less reliable predictor than that in non-pregnant women [51] and typically will decrease as 25(OH)D increases at the lower end of values [49,51,52].

What was most interesting from our recent NICHD vitamin D pregnancy trial was the discovery that to optimize 1,25(OH)$_2$D production (which, as was just discussed,

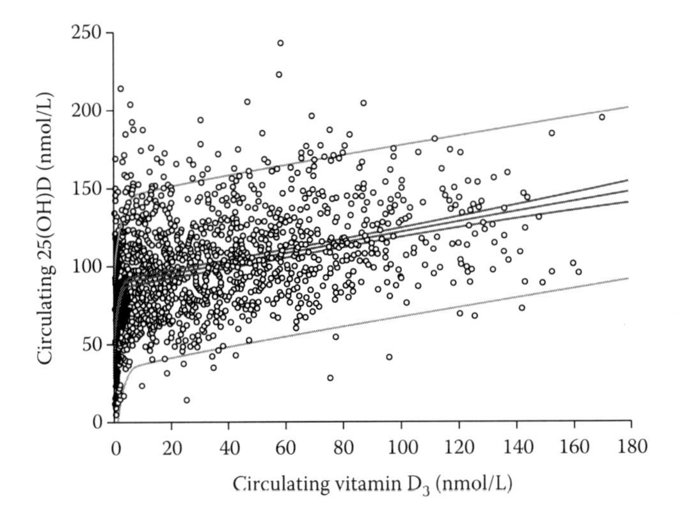

FIGURE 7.1 Demonstrates the relationship between circulating vitamin D_3 to control the production of 25(OH)D during pregnancy. (Adapted from Hollis BW. et al., *Journal of Bone and Mineral Research: The Official Journal of the American Society for Bone and Mineral Research*. 2011;26(10):2341–57.)

soars early-on in pregnancy), total circulating 25(OH)D should be at least 40 ng/mL (100 nmol/L) [49]. As shown in Figure 7.2, this relationship exhibits first- and zero-order enzyme kinetics. It is also of great interest that production of circulating $1,25(OH)_2D$ in the fetus is linked directly to circulating 25(OH)D [53]. This increase in circulating $1,25(OH)_2D$ concentration has, in particular, been attributed

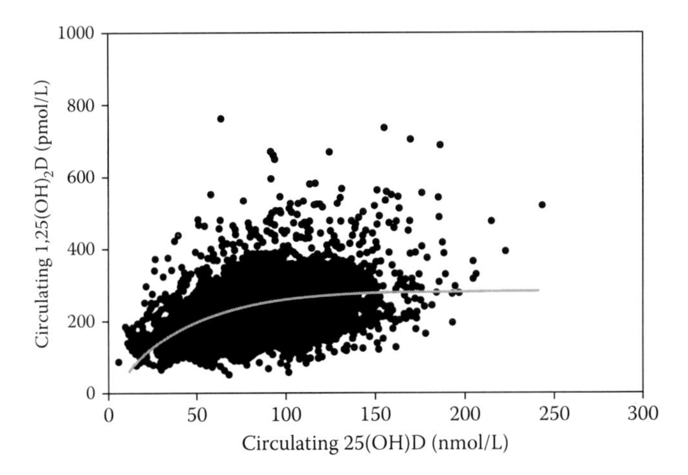

FIGURE 7.2 Demonstrates the relationship of circulating 25(OH)D to control the production of $1,25(OH)_2D$ during pregnancy. All data points for all subjects in all groups were included in this analysis. (Adapted from Hollis BW. et al., *Journal of Bone and Mineral Research: The Official Journal of the American Society for Bone and Mineral Research*. 2011;26(10):2341–57.)

to an increase in the serum VDBP, which would regulate the amount of "free" $1,25(OH)_2D$ available in the circulation [54]. Although this rise in DBP during pregnancy has been shown to be 46%–103%, depending on the assay employed [55], it cannot account for the 2–3-fold increase in circulating $1,25(OH)_2D$ [49]. In an earlier study by Bikle et al. [48], free $1,25(OH)_2D$ levels were found to be increased during pregnancy, despite the significant increase in DBP levels, and our recent data agree with this premise [49]. Why this association exists solely during pregnancy remains unclear and is the focus of active research endeavors.

As a corollary to the extraordinary change in vitamin D metabolism during pregnancy, it has been known for some time that unique during pregnancy, maternal and neonatal 25(OH)D and $1,25(OH)_2D$ are strongly associated [53]. From early in gestation, serum $1,25(OH)_2D$ concentrations rise much higher and are driven by substrate—25(OH)D—availability (Figure 7.2). It is important to again note that this substrate dependence of $1,25(OH)_2D$ production is neither observed in normal human physiology driven by classic calcium homeostasis nor seen in any other time in the lifecycle except pregnancy and in the newborn infant.

7.3 ACHIEVING SUFFICIENCY DURING PREGNANCY: RESULTS OF CLINICAL TRIALS THROUGH THE DECADES

When considering what is the "norm" for vitamin D status, Luxwolda et al. [56] studied native tribal Africans who have an average of 5–9 h of sunlight exposure per day. This group achieved a mean circulating 25(OH)D level of 46 ng/mL (115 nmol/L). In another study by this group that included 139 East African pregnant women, the mean 25(OH)D was 55.4 ng/mL (138.5 ± 31.8 nmol/L) during pregnancy and 54.4 ng/mL (135.9 ± 31.8 nmol/L) at delivery [57]. The cord blood 25(OH)D concentration was 31.6 ng/mL (79.0 ± 26.4 nmol/L), well above the mean of cord blood values found in western countries [49,58,59]. Mothers 3 days postpartum, almost all of whom were lactating, had a mean 25(OH)D value of 36.6 ng/mL (91.5 ± 26.8 nmol/L), which remained stable at 3 months postpartum. In our recent randomized clinical trial, pregnant women receiving 4000 IU vitamin D_3/day attained an average circulating 25(OH)D level of 44.4 ng/mL (111 nmol/L) [49], similar to what is achieved through sunlight alone with a certain level of sun exposure. If one wants to recapitulate what occurs in individuals living in a sun-rich environment with hours of exposure, the goal should be to achieve a circulating 25(OH)D concentration of at least 40 ng/mL (100 nmol/L); however, it is achieved, be it solar exposure and/or diet/supplementation.

Studies performed in the 1980s with up to 1000 IU vitamin D/day given or bolus doses given in the last trimester compared with placebo showed minimal effectiveness of the various therapies in meeting the needs of the pregnant women to attain sufficiency throughout pregnancy [8–10,16,60]. This led to the idea that higher daily supplementation doses would be needed to achieve sufficiency in the pregnant mother, but at what cost? There was significant fear that vitamin D at doses higher than 400 IU/day would act as a teratogen [61–69]. There had been reports of mothers supplemented with higher doses of vitamin D during pregnancy, who had children with a constellation of findings: idiopathic hypercalcemia of infancy, elfin facies and ears, and supravalvular aortic stenosis [62–69]. Later, with the advent of molecular genetics, it was found that these children had Williams syndrome with a translocation of the elastin gene on chromosome 7 [70,71], which often involves an abnormal, exaggerated response to vitamin D and altered metabolism leading to "idiopathic" hypercalcemia [71–73]. The "teratogenic" effect of vitamin D observed in the 1950s was really a genetic disorder; however, this association, despite its fallacy coupled with true vitamin D toxicity when hundreds of thousands of units are consumed, sets the stage for a concern among clinicians of vitamin D's use beyond the teaspoon-equivalent of cod liver oil or 400 IU/day.

It took another decade before data were available in non-pregnant adults about the safety and efficacy of higher doses of vitamin D in preventing deficiencies and in sustaining sufficiency that would support the use of similar doses during pregnancy. Vieth [5] published a landmark study in 1999 and another in 2001 [6] of the safety of daily vitamin D supplementation up to 4000 IU/day. Similarly, Heaney et al. [74] published pharmacokinetic data about vitamin D supplementation in male subjects living in Omaha, Nebraska in the winter months with doses up to 10,000 IU/day. It became evident that vitamin D supplementation up to 10,000 IU/day was safe and that total circulating 25(OH)D in subjects plateaued by 3 months, with sustained normocalcemia up to 5 months [5,6,74]. These important studies provided critical data that supported higher dosing of vitamin D during pregnancy to achieve sufficiency.

Following receipt of an Investigational New Drug number from the FDA (#66,346), Hollis and co-workers began to assess the vitamin D requirements of women during their first trimester of pregnancy. In their two published randomized controlled trials, Hollis et al. [49] and Wagner et al. [75] found that higher total circulating 25(OH)D was associated with improved vitamin D status throughout pregnancy. In the first trial sponsored by NICHD, women were randomized to receive 400, 2000, or 4000 IU vitamin D_3/day starting at 12 weeks of gestation [49]. Women were followed monthly to assess health status and vitamin D-related metabolic parameters. It was found that 4000 IU vitamin D/day was superior to 2000 or 400 IU/day, and 2000 IU/day was superior to 400 IU/day in achieving vitamin D sufficiency throughout pregnancy. Women taking 400 IU vitamin D/day had a minimal change in their 25(OH)D concentrations; those in the 2000 IU group were often deficient through 20–24 weeks compared with the 4000 IU group. The number of neonates who were deficient at birth defined as a total circulating concentration of 25(OH)D <20 ng/mL was greater in the lower dose groups. There was no toxicity associated with the higher vitamin D dosing: Women in the three treatment groups did not differ in terms of serum calcium, phosphorus, creatinine, and urinary calcium-to-creatinine ratios.

In another trial funded by the Thrasher Research Fund and conducted by Wagner et al. [59], women who received their health care in two community health centers were randomized to receive either 2000 or 4000 IU vitamin D_3/day starting at 12–16 weeks of gestation, following a 1-month run-in dose of 2000 IU/day. A total of 257 pregnant women were enrolled and randomized to 2000 vs. 4000 IU/day, following a 1-month run-in dose of 2000 IU/day. As in the NICHD trial described earlier, participants were monitored for hypercalciuria, hypercalcemia, and 25(OH)D status. Maternal 25(OH)D (n = 161) increased from approximately 23 ng/mL (57.5 nmol/L) at baseline to 36 ng/mL (90 nmol/L) and 38 ng/mL (95 nmol/L) in the 2000 and 4000 IU groups, respectively. Although the change in maternal 25(OH)D from baseline did not differ between the groups, the increase in monthly 25(OH)D differed between the groups with the greater change in the 4000 IU group ($p < 0.01$). No supplementation-related adverse events occurred. The mean cord blood 25(OH)D was 22 ng/mL (55 nmol/L) in 2000 IU and 27 ng/mL (67.5 nmol/L) in 4000 IU groups ($p = 0.024$).

Both the NICHD and the Thrasher Research Fund pregnancy vitamin D supplementation trials utilized common questionnaires and vitamin D tablets from the same manufacturing lot, allowing the two datasets to be combined using a common data dictionary, thus increasing the sample size and power to detect differences between the groups [75]. It was again found that 4000 IU vitamin D/day was superior to either 400 or 2000 IU/day in achieving vitamin D sufficiency throughout pregnancy.

Other trials conducted throughout the world support the effectiveness of higher vitamin D dosing regimens in improving maternal vitamin D status. In a study conducted in the United Arab of Emirates by Dawodu et al. [76], Arab women were randomized at 12–16 weeks of gestation to 400, 2000, and 4000 IU/day vitamin D through pregnancy. Of 192 enrolled, 162 (84%) continued to delivery. Mean serum 25(OH)D of 8.2 ng/mL (20.5 nmol/L) at enrollment was consistent with severe deficiency. Mean serum 25(OH)D concentrations at delivery and in cord blood were significantly higher in the 2000 and 4000 IU/day than in the 400 IU/day group ($p < 0.001$) and was highest in the 4000 IU/day group. When using the threshold 25(OH)D concentrations of 32 ng/mL (80 nmol/L) and 20 ng/mL (50 nmol/L), the percentage of mothers who achieved these thresholds was greatest in the 4000 IU/day group. Safety measurements were similar in the group, and no adverse event occurred, which was related to vitamin D supplementation. The investigators concluded that vitamin D supplementation at doses of 2000 and 4000 IU/day appeared safe, and similar to the study of Hollis et al. 4000 IU/day was most effective in optimizing serum 25(OH)D concentrations in mothers and their infants.

Roth et al. reported the results of a clinical trial conducted in Dhaka where 160 women were randomized to receive 35,000 IU/week (=5000 IU/day) or placebo until delivery. Maternal mean 25(OH)D was significantly higher at delivery after vitamin D vs. placebo (134 vs. 39 nmol/L, $p < 0.001$; $N = 133$); as expected, cord 25(OH)D was significantly higher following vitamin D vs. placebo (103 vs. 39 nmol/L, $p < 0.001$; $N = 132$). In this study, there was no evidence of maternal hypercalcemia or vitamin D-related serious adverse events, and major adverse birth and neonatal outcomes were non-significantly less common in the vitamin D-treated group.

7.4 HEALTH EFFECTS OF VITAMIN D DURING PREGNANCY

As mentioned earlier, what is unique during pregnancy is that total circulating concentrations of $1,25(OH)_2D$ are more than double/triple by 10–12 weeks of gestation compared to what they are in the non-pregnant state [49]. Despite this dramatic increase in the active hormone, serum calcium concentrations remain stable and within normal range. How could this be and more importantly, why does this occur? It is postulated that the sustained high concentration of $1,25(OH)_2D$ during pregnancy serves an important role in stabilizing the immune function in the mother to prevent rejection of the fetus [77,78]. Yet, this remains conjecture at this point because the discovery of vitamin D's role in both innate and adaptive immune functions is relatively recent [33,79]. There is, however, mounting evidence that supports this premise: women who are vitamin D-deficient are more likely to have preeclampsia [80–84], infection [59,85,86], and preterm labor and preterm birth [59,75,87], all of which have been associated with states of vitamin D deficiency.

When randomized clinical trials or comparative effectiveness trials involving vitamin D supplementation during pregnancy have been analyzed for vitamin D's putative effect on maternal and fetal health, certain trends have emerged. The first hint that vitamin D deficiency during pregnancy impacted fetal development came from studies conducted in the early 1980s. Brooke et al. [8,16], who studied British mothers of Asian descent, found a greater incidence of small-for-gestational-age (SGA) infants born to mothers who received placebo, compared with mothers who received 1000 IU vitamin D_2/day during the final trimester of pregnancy. Neonates in the placebo group also had a greater fontanelle area than did the supplemented group. It must be noted that the placebo group in this study showed profound hypovitaminosis D.

Follow-up studies by Brooke et al. [9] again were conducted in Asian mothers who were provided with either placebo or 1000 IU vitamin D_2/day during the last trimester of pregnancy. The follow-up data provided evidence that, during the first year of life, the infants of the maternal placebo group gained less weight and had a lower rate of linear growth than did those of the maternal supplemented group. Cockburn et al. [88] undertook a large vitamin D supplementation study of 1000 pregnant subjects in the United Kingdom who were supplemented with 400 IU vitamin D_2/day or received a placebo from week 12 of gestation onward. Based on pharmacokinetics of vitamin D, it is not surprising that serum concentrations of 25(OH)D in the supplemented group were only slightly higher than those in the placebo group. A defect in dental enamel formation was observed in a higher proportion of children at 3 years of age in the maternal placebo group.

Maxwell et al. [10] conducted a clinical trial involving Asian women living in London who received 1000 IU/day of vitamin D during the last trimester of pregnancy. Supplemented mothers had greater weight gain and, at term, had significantly higher plasma concentrations of retinol-binding protein and thyroid-binding prealbumin, indicators of protein-calorie nutritional status. Almost twice as many infants of the unsupplemented group weighed <2500 g at birth and had significantly lower retinol-binding protein concentrations than did infants of the supplemented mothers.

Brunvard et al. [89] followed 30 pregnant Pakistani women who were free of chronic diseases and had uncomplicated pregnancies. Nearly, all of the women had low (<15 ng/mL) circulating 25(OH)D concentrations, and 50% exhibited secondary hyperparathyroidism. The maternal circulating PTH concentration was inversely related to the neonatal crown–heel length. These authors concluded that maternal vitamin D deficiency affected fetal growth through an effect on maternal calcium homeostasis.

Similar effects of vitamin D status on fetal growth were found in a more recent study by Hashemipour et al. [90] in their randomized controlled trial of 160 healthy pregnant women, of whom 81% were vitamin D-deficient at baseline. This team of investigators based in Iran studied the effect of vitamin D administration on maternal and neonatal serum calcium and vitamin D concentrations. Women were randomized to receive a daily multivitamin containing 400 IU plus 200 mg elemental calcium (control group) vs. 50,000 IU oral vitamin D_3 every 2 weeks for a total of 8 weeks starting at 26–28 weeks of gestation as well as the daily intervention given to the control group (average daily total of 3971 IU/day). At delivery, maternal 25(OH)D was significantly higher in the intervention group. Maternal weight gain during pregnancy was greater in the intervention group and significantly correlated with serum 25(OH)D and inversely correlated with body mass index (BMI) at the time of enrollment. Growth parameters in the neonates of mothers in the intervention group were significantly greater than those in the control group; effects that persisted even after controlling for other maternal factors such as age, BMI, gravidity, and gestational age at delivery. These findings are supported by earlier as well as more recent studies: Marya et al. [14] in 1988 and Kalra et al. [91] in 2012 showed improved growth effects of vitamin D interventions as a function of timing during gestation as either a single large bolus of vitamin D given in the second trimester or two boluses during the second and third trimesters. In contrast, Mallet et al. who randomized women to receive 0, 200, or 1000 IU vitamin D/day, showed no effect on neonatal weight.

Based on the aforementioned studies, it would appear that the baseline starting 25(OH)D and the resulting 25(OH)D concentration that is achieved are the two predictors of fetal growth effect. There may be a threshold 25(OH)D concentration above which no further effect is seen in neonatal growth. In both the NICHD and Thrasher Research Fund trials, there were no differences in neonatal anthropomorphic measures as a function of maternal vitamin D treatment, but those studies in which profound deficiency was found and then corrected appeared to have the greatest effect on neonatal growth indices.

In a recent systematic review and meta-analysis by Thorne-Lyman and Fawzi [17] that assessed the association between vitamin D status during pregnancy and maternal, neonatal, and infant health outcomes, there was suggestion that vitamin D has a protective effect on low birth weight [three trials, risk ratio = 0.40 (95% confidence interval 0.23, 0.71)]. There was a trend where daily supplementation led to fewer SGA infants, but this did not reach significance. There were only two trials that met criteria for inclusion in the analysis for preterm delivery, and no effect was noted as a function of vitamin D supplementation. The conclusion was that there remains little evidence from trials to evaluate the effect of vitamin D supplementation during pregnancy on maternal, perinatal, and infant health outcomes [17]. This was the conclusion of a recent meta-analysis by the World Health Organization as well [92]. Both meta-analyses suggest that more clinical data are necessary to ascertain the true effect of vitamin D on the mother and her developing fetus.

In an attempt to uncover potential effects of vitamin D during pregnancy with a greater sample size and thus power to detect differences, the NICHD [49] and Thrasher Research Fund [59] vitamin D pregnancy trials' data were combined and then analyzed on an intent-to-treat basis [75]. The studies had used a common data dictionary, questionnaires, and vitamin D dispensed from the same lot number. In the combined cohort, there were 110 in the 400 IU group, 201 in the 2000 IU group, and 193 in the 4000 IU group. No differences were found between groups in baseline 25(OH)D; however, delivery and cord blood values were greater in the 4000 IU group ($p < 0.0001$), an effect that persisted even after controlling for race and study.

Although maternal supplementation with vitamin D at 2000 and 4000 IU/day during pregnancy improved maternal/neonatal vitamin D status, a greater percentage was vitamin D replete throughout pregnancy in the 4000 IU group ($p < 0.0001$) [59]. There was a trend in which the 4000 IU group had decreased rates of comorbidities of pregnancy. Evidence of risk reduction in infection, preterm labor, and preterm birth was suggestive, requiring additional studies powered for these endpoints.

It is important to note that more than a third of women in both the NICHD and the Thrasher Research Fund vitamin D pregnancy trials did not take their vitamin D supplement, which impacted the intent-to-treat analysis. When the combined datasets were analyzed on the basis of 25(OH)D at various time points during pregnancy, there emerged stronger health associations with vitamin D [75]. After controlling for race and study site, preterm birth and labor were inversely associated with predelivery and mean 25(OH)D, but not with baseline 25(OH)D. There was a strong association between comorbidities of pregnancy and final maternal 25(OH)D: an effect that persisted even after controlling for race and study ($p = 0.006$). Furthermore, for every 10 ng/mL increase in maternal 25(OH)D at delivery resulted in reduced odds of infection and preterm birth without preeclampsia, but these did not reach statistical significance. When the four main comorbidities of pregnancy were combined, for every 10 ng/mL increase in maternal 25(OH)D at delivery, the odds ratio was reduced to 0.84 ($p = 0.006$). Maternal delivery 25(OH)D was inversely associated with any comorbidity of pregnancy, with fewer events as 25(OH)D increased.

Soheilykhah et al. [93] studied varying doses of vitamin D during pregnancy and their effect on insulin resistance. In their initial case–control study, 54 Iranian women with diagnosed gestational diabetes mellitus (GDM) and 39 women with one abnormal oral glucose tolerance test [impaired glucose tolerance (IGT)] were compared with 111 non-GDM control women, in whom GDM was excluded by glucose challenge tests. Controls were matched for gestational age, age, and BMI with both the IGT and GDM groups. Maternal serum 25(OH)D in GDM and IGT groups at 24–28 weeks of gestation was significantly lower than that in non-GDM controls ($p = 0.001$); 83% of GDM compared with 71% of controls met the definition of vitamin D deficiency (<20 ng/mL; $p = 0.03$), and, in fact, women with GDM had a 2.7-fold increased risk of significant deficiency [defined as 25(OH)D <15 ng/mL] compared with the control group. In comparison, in an observational, cross-sectional study by Whitelaw et al. in the United Kingdom involving 1467 women, of whom 137 developed gestational diabetes, there was only a weak association between 25(OH)D and fasting plasma glucose but not with fasting insulin, post-challenge glucose. The issue is that 81% of the cohort met the definition of vitamin D deficiency [25(OH)D <20 ng/mL], making it difficult to discern those with gestational diabetes with and without vitamin D deficiency. In addition, of the 137 women, 114 women had raised post-challenge glucose only, six with raised fasting only, and 17 with both being abnormal. It is only with a prospective, interventional trial that the issue of vitamin D's effect on insulin resistance and the development of gestational diabetes can be properly addressed.

Going beyond the observational trials, Soheilykhah et al. [94] again studied the effects of different doses of vitamin D on insulin resistance during pregnancy. Women ($n = 120$) less than 12 weeks of gestation were randomized into three treatment groups: group A, 200 IU vitamin D daily (control group); group B, 50,000 IU vitamin D monthly; and group C, 50,000 IU vitamin D every 2 weeks until delivery. The serum levels of fasting blood sugar, insulin, calcium, and 25(OH)D were measured before and after intervention, and the homeostatic model assessment of insulin resistance (HOMA-IR) as a surrogate measure of insulin resistance. Serum 25(OH)D increased most dramatically in group C from 7.3 to 34.1 ng/mL and to a slightly lesser extent in group B from 7.3 to 27.2 ng/mL; group A, however, had only a slight increase from 8.3 to 17.7 ng/mL ($p < 0.001$). The mean differences of insulin and HOMA-IR before and after intervention in groups A and C were significant ($p = 0.01$ and 0.02, respectively). The results of this study suggest that supplementation of pregnant women with 50,000 IU vitamin D every 2 weeks improved insulin resistance significantly. This is one of the first reports of how vitamin D administered during pregnancy impacts outcome.

What can one ascertain from the increasing number of vitamin D studies that have been performed during pregnancy? Is it still ethical to prescribe 400 IU/day to a pregnant woman and expect her to achieve a total circulating 25(OH)D concentration of 40 ng/mL, the threshold necessary to optimize conversion of 25(OH)D to $1,25(OH)_2D$? Does complacency and fear of change set us in another direction? Do we say that generations of individuals have thrived on the regimen, so why change? Yet, we know that every major health adverse outcome in the United States has worsened in the past two decades and so clearly something is not quite right. Rates of preterm birth in the United States continue despite our best efforts to reverse this trend. The United States ranks lower on any major health indicator than most developed countries throughout the world. When data are presented that suggest a simple intervention such as vitamin D supplementation will correct deficiencies in women and has the potential to reverse serious morbidities of pregnancy without toxicity, the answer is: “More studies need to be performed.” Again, at what expense? It is the expense of the women who are pregnant and their unborn children. It is the expense of the society that continues to pay more than US $60,000 per preterm birth, with many infants whose care costs escalate into hundreds of thousands of dollars, and yet, we persist in saying that vitamin D is not the magic bullet and could potentially harm. Emerging data suggest otherwise, and while we sit debating this issue, literally, millions of women throughout the world remain vitamin D-deficient. At the very least, we must mandate that pregnant women, all pregnant women throughout the world, achieve the minimum 25(OH)D concentration that is suggested by the Institute of Medicine, 20 ng/mL (50 nmol/L). Once that goal is achieved, the next step is to achieve a total circulating 25(OH)D concentration of at least 40 ng/mL to optimize its conversion to $1,25(OH)_2D$.

What is set into motion during pregnancy continues during lactation. If a mother is vitamin D-deficient during pregnancy, then her developing fetus will be deficient and so will her newborn infant [21,44,95–97]. Neonatal total circulating 25(OH)D at delivery is 0.7–0.8 that of maternal 25(OH)D [49,59]. The problems of deficiency that manifest during pregnancy become compounded during lactation: As the mother who is providing breast milk to her newborn infant remains deficient, her breast milk is deficient and her infant can only receive a certain amount of vitamin D that is far below what is necessary to achieve sufficiency. The stage is set for profound vitamin D deficiency in the infant. In the next section, we discuss these and other issues regarding vitamin D sufficiency during lactation for both the mother and her breastfeeding infant.

7.5 VITAMIN D REQUIREMENTS DURING LACTATION

For the past three decades, it has been maintained that human milk is "marginally sufficient" in vitamin D necessitating supplementation of breastfed infants [2,42,98–100]. Initial work on the vitamin D content of human milk first measured only the 25(OH)D moiety and thus showed it to be woefully inadequate in vitamin D [101]. At that time, the parent vitamin D could not be measured due to inadequate methodology [102,103]. The main moiety transferred into breast milk is not 25(OH)D, but rather vitamin D itself. The basic problem, though, has been that when studying breast milk, typically, there has been little circulating vitamin D in the mothers because they had poor oral intake and limited UV exposure [21], impacting on what was measured in the breast milk: when mother herself is vitamin D-deficient, there is little vitamin D for transfer into the mother's milk [21,44,94,104]. This led to an incorrect premise about human milk as being marginally sufficient [102], which was corrected only when experiments demonstrating that both UV exposure and increased maternal vitamin D supplementation could produce profound increases in both circulating and milk concentrations of vitamin D but minimal changes in concentrations of 25(OH)D [105,106].

Additional insight into the transfer of vitamin D into breast milk came from the work of Greer and Hollis [106]. They studied a hypoparathyroid patient taking 100,000 IU vitamin D_2/day who went through two normal pregnancies and deliveries and breastfed her infants. Her milk contained nearly 8000 IU/L of antirachitic activity (concentrations of vitamin D and its metabolites), mostly as vitamin D_2 with relatively little 25(OH)D_2 content [106]. This mother's milk contained vitamin D_2 at 28% of the circulating concentration when compared with 25(OH)D_2, which was found at only 1.3% of the circulating concentration [106], an observation confirmed in lactating women with "normal" vitamin D status [107]. Thus, it was clear that the parent compound is transferred from maternal circulation into her breast milk much more efficiently than 25(OH)D. The following relationship has been observed: For every 1000 IU vitamin D_3/day provided to a lactating woman, about 80 IU/L will appear in her breast milk [46]. Thus, to provide 400–500 IU/day for their infants, nursing mothers require 6000 IU vitamin D_3/day. It was only recently that this premise was tested [95,96,108]. Prior to the NICHD vitamin D lactation trial, recommended intakes for nursing mothers were 400 IU/day, and intakes above 2000 IU/day were considered harmful [2]. For this reason, for more than a decade, vitamin D supplementation of the breastfeeding infant has been recommended [98,109].

Infant supplementation with 400 IU vitamin D_3/day will achieve sufficiency in the vast majority of infants if mother is adherent to supplementation. Maternal supplementation varies by country and by community. In a large study of infant feeding practices by Perrine et al. [110] in the United States, adherence to the American Academy of Pediatrics' recommendation (that all infants receiving <1 L of formula per day should receive 400 IU vitamin D/day) fell far below even 20%. In comparison, adherence among mothers in British Columbia, Canada showed that of the 90% of infants who were receiving breast milk at 2 months of age, 80% were also receiving vitamin D supplementation [111]. This approach addresses the needs of the breastfeeding infant without taking into account the needs of the lactating mother, nor does it address why maternal milk is marginally sufficient or even deficient in vitamin D.

To address the issue of vitamin D sufficiency in both mother and her breastfeeding infant, two vitamin D trials involving lactating women and their infants overseen by Hollis and Wagner [44,95] provided pilot data and paved the way for a larger two-site NICHD vitamin D supplementation during lactation trial [95,108]. The first pilot study was designed to establish vitamin D transfer from the mother to her milk and then to her recipient, fully breastfeeding infant. Women were randomized to receive either 1600 or 3600 IU vitamin D_2 and continue to take their prenatal vitamin containing 400 IU vitamin D_3 for a total of either 2000 or 4000 IU vitamin D/day. Both mother and infant were followed for 3 months. It was found that women taking the 4000 IU/day regimen had better vitamin D status, had higher milk antirachitic activity, and their recipient infants had higher 25(OH)D_2 concentrations than those in the 2000 IU group. The study confirmed that the vitamin D moiety that passes most freely into breast milk is not 25(OH)D but rather vitamin D itself. In addition, it was learned that 4000 IU vitamin D/day was not sufficient to achieve adequate vitamin D concentrations in the milk. This led to the second pilot study by our group.

In the second pilot study by Wagner et al. [95], women ($n = 19$) were randomized to either 400 or 6400 IU vitamin D_3/day. Infants whose mothers were in the 400 IU group received 300 IU vitamin D/day, whereas infants whose mothers were in the 6400 IU group received placebo. The findings were as predicted: Women in the 6400 IU group achieved higher total circulating 25(OH)D concentrations than those in the 400 IU group. Specifically, 6400 IU vitamin D_3/day safely and significantly increased maternal circulating 25(OH)D and vitamin D from baseline, compared with controls ($p < 0.0028$ and 0.0043, respectively). Mean milk antirachitic activity of mothers receiving 400 IU vitamin D/day decreased to a nadir of 46 IU/L at visit 4 and varied little during the study period (46–79 IU/L), whereas the mean activity in the 6400 IU/day group increased from 82 to 873 IU/L ($p < 0.0003$). Another important finding was that during the fall and winter months with limited sun exposure, an intake of 400 IU vitamin D_3/day did not sustain circulating maternal 25(OH)D and thus supplied only extremely limited amounts of vitamin D to the nursing infant via breast milk. The infants did not differ in their vitamin D status: Both the vitamin D-supplemented infants and those whose sole source of vitamin D was their mothers' breast milk (the maternal 6400 IU group) achieved similar 25(OH)D concentrations at 4 and 7 months of age. There was no toxicity associated with the higher vitamin D dosing; however, the sample size was small. To ascertain both safety and effectiveness, a two-site comparative effectiveness trial sponsored by NICHD was conducted in 2006–2012.

Some studies challenge the concept that maternal vitamin D supplementation should be daily rather than sporadic as a bolus. The main issue with maternal daily dosing is adherence. In some areas of the world, maternal adherence to daily supplements is less than 40% [112] and in other areas, it is greater than 90% [111]. Bolus dosing has the advantage of being given in a clinic in which one can assure 100% adherence. Saadi et al. [113] first evaluated the effectiveness of daily vitamin D (2000 IU/day) vs. monthly (60,000 IU) in a group of healthy breastfeeding mothers ($n = 90$) and a group of nulliparous women ($n = 88$). The mothers and nulliparous women who received daily vs. monthly vitamin D had comparable 25(OH)D by the end of a 3-month study period; however, on both dosing schedules, there was persistent, significant vitamin D deficiency noted [113]. In a follow-up study by the same group [114], healthy breastfeeding mothers ($n = 90$) again were randomized to receive either 2000 IU vitamin D_2/day or monthly boluses of 60,000 IU vitamin D_2. All of their infants ($n = 92$) received 400 IU daily of vitamin D_2 for the 3-month study period. Most infants had baseline 25(OH)D <15 ng/mL (<37.5 nmol/L); however, at the end of the 3-month study period, serum 25(OH)D concentrations had increased significantly from baseline in both groups. Milk antirachitic activity increased from undetectable (<20 IU/L) to a median of 50.9 IU/L. The authors concluded that combined maternal (either daily or monthly dosing schedules) and infant daily supplementation was associated with a 3-fold increase in infant serum 25(OH)D concentrations and with a 64% reduction in the prevalence of vitamin D deficiency without causing hypervitaminosis D in either group.

A recent study by Oberhelman et al. [104] compared a single monthly supplement to a daily maternal supplement in increasing breast milk vitamin D to achieve the endpoint of its sufficiency in their infants. Exclusively breastfeeding mothers ($n = 40$) were randomized to receive 5000 IU/day of vitamin D_3 for 28 days or 150,000 IU once and were followed prospectively for 28 days. In mothers given daily cholecalciferol (oral vitamin D), concentrations of serum and breast milk cholecalciferol attained steady concentrations of 18 and 8 ng/mL, respectively, from day 3 through 28. In mothers given the single dose, serum and breast milk cholecalciferol (vitamin D) peaked at 160 and 40 ng/mL, respectively, at day 1 before rapidly declining. Maternal milk and serum cholecalciferol concentrations were related ($r = 0.87$). The infant mean serum 25(OH)D concentration increased from 16.9 to 39.2 ng/mL in the single-dose group and from 16.3 to 38.7 ng/mL in the daily dose group ($p = 0.88$). All infants achieved serum 25(OH)D concentrations of more than 20 ng/mL. The conclusion of this team of investigators was that either single-dose or daily dose cholecalciferol supplementation of mothers provided breast milk concentrations that resulted in vitamin D sufficiency in breastfed infants. Although the sample size was small and the follow-up was through 28 days, the findings are provocative.

Preliminary results from the two-site NICHD vitamin D supplementation during lactation trial suggest that maternal vitamin D supplementation with 6400 IU/day is safe and effective in achieving vitamin D sufficiency in the exclusively breastfed infants and comparable to what is achieved when an exclusively breastfed infant is receiving 400 IU vitamin D_3/day as a supplement [96,108]. In this study, 476 mother/infant dyads were enrolled and randomized into three treatment groups: 206 in the 400 IU group, 71 in 2400 IU group, and 199 in 6400 IU group. The 2400 IU group was stopped in 2009 as the treatment failed to increase infant 25(OH)D concentrations, resulting in a higher number of infants in that treatment arm with vitamin D deficiency (<20 ng/mL): 31% in the 2400 IU group vs. 6% in the 400 IU group and 5% in the 6000 IU group. In the remaining two groups (400 vs. 6400 IU), maternal vitamin D status at baseline differed by race/ethnicity, education, socioeconomic status (SES), and by latitude, but not by treatment; baseline maternal 25(OH)D concentrations were 29 ng/mL in the 400 IU group vs. 30 ng/mL in the 6400 IU group ($p = 0.1$). Of the 177 mothers who continued to fully breastfeed through 7 months ($n = 83$, 400 IU group and $n = 94$, 6400 IU group), as early as 2 months into treatment, maternal 25(OH)D differed between the two groups that was sustained to 7 months postpartum ($p < 0.0001$). As predicted, however, there were no differences in infant 25(OH)D concentrations by treatment: 45 ng/mL in the 400 IU groups vs. 43 ng/mL in the 6400 IU group ($p = 0.4$). No differences in any of the safety measures by treatment (serum calcium, phosphorus, and urinary calcium/creatinine) were noted in the mothers and infants, except in the 25(OH)D concentration. Thus, preliminary analyses from this study support the premise that maternal vitamin D supplementation with 6400 IU/day alone safely improved maternal vitamin D status during 6 months of full breastfeeding and was equivalent to maternal/infant vitamin D supplementation of 400 IU/day in achieving infant vitamin D sufficiency. Such findings have implications for vitamin D recommendations for both the mother and her infant during lactation.

Of interest are the factors that predict maternal and infant vitamin D status during lactation. Using the NICHD vitamin D lactation study data described earlier, a series of preliminary separate analyses were undertaken to determine which factors independently predicted maternal and infant vitamin D status in women living at two diverse latitudes: Charleston, SC(32°N) and Rochester, NY(43.2°N) [115]. In multiple regression models predicting 25(OH)D and including race, insurance status, vitamin D dose at baseline, education, and acute maternal illness during the past month, the factors that were independently positively associated with baseline maternal 25(OH)D were Caucasian ($p < 0.0001$), privately insured ($p < 0.0001$), and summer season ($p = 0.0008$). When predicting baseline infant 25(OH)D, only season ($p < 0.0001$) and latitude ($p = 0.024$) were independently positively associated. At 7 months of lactation, maternal 25(OH)D was positively associated with being Caucasian ($p = 0.0051$), privately insured ($p = 0.037$), and with the higher dose of 6400 IU/day ($p < 0.0001$). At 7 months, infant 25(OH)D was independently associated with race ($p = 0.02$), but not with maternal education, treatment, race, latitude, or insurance status. The strongest predictor of vitamin D status in both mother and her breastfeeding infant during sustained lactation was maternal supplementation with 6400 IU/day.

There is compelling evidence that suggests if mother is vitamin D replete with total circulating 25(OH)D concentrations in the range of women who have ample sunlight exposure, milk antirachitic activity will be sufficient to provide adequate concentrations of vitamin D to her recipient infant, foregoing the need for infant vitamin D supplementation. The work of Hollis and Wagner, Saadi et al. and Oberhelman et al. independently supports this premise. It is essential that women who choose to breastfeed are aware of their options in achieving vitamin D sufficiency not only for their breastfeeding infants but also for themselves.

7.6 SUMMARY

Vitamin D requirements during pregnancy must take into account the needs not only of the mother but also that of her developing fetus. This relationship continues during lactation, such that the mother becomes the sole source of vitamin D for her unsupplemented breastfeeding infant. Whereas in pregnancy, there is a direct relationship between total circulating 25(OH)D and $1,25(OH)_2D$; such a relationship is not seen during lactation or any other time during the lifecycle. To optimize the conversion of 25(OH)D to $1,25(OH)_2D$, a woman should attain a 25(OH)D concentration of at least 40 ng/mL (100 nmol/L) during pregnancy.

The impact of vitamin D deficiency on the health of the pregnant woman and her developing fetus is just beginning to be understood. At the very least, a woman should attain a 25(OH)D concentration that will allow her to have optimal conversion of $1,25(OH)_2D$, the active hormone that is more than twice the concentration during pregnancy than it is during the non-pregnant state.

It is clear from work conducted during the past three decades that human milk can be and is often deficient in vitamin D. This is not because there is something inherently wrong or bad with human milk; rather, it is a reflection of maternal vitamin D status. Mother is the reservoir of vitamin D for her breastfeeding infant; if she is deficient, so will her infant. Therefore, during lactation, for a mother to have adequate transfer of vitamin D in her breast milk and thus to her recipient breastfeeding infant, mother should attain a 25(OH)D concentration of at least 45 ng/mL, a concentration consistently and safely achieved on a daily vitamin D supplement of 6000 IU.

Although much remains to be learned about vitamin D's health effects during pregnancy on mother and her developing fetus in the short as well as in the long-term, it is reasonable to recommend that no pregnant woman should be vitamin D-deficient, nor she should have suboptimal 25(OH)D substrate, the essential precursor to $1,25(OH)_2D$. Similarly, a lactating woman should receive adequate vitamin D to ensure that her milk has ample vitamin D for her breastfeeding infant. As more intensive research is conducted to understand vitamin D's effect on immune function and health, our recommendations will be expanded and refined.

REFERENCES

1. Weick MT. A history of rickets in the United States. *The American Journal of Clinical Nutrition*. 1967;20(11):1234–41. Epub 1967/11/01. PubMed PMID: 4862158.
2. Food and Nutrition Board. Standing Committee on the Scientific Evaluation of Dietary Reference Intakes. *Dietary Reference Intakes for Calcium, Phosphorus, Magnesium, Vitamin D, and Fluoride*. Washington, DC: National Academy Press; 1997.
3. Park E. The etiology of rickets. *Physiological Reviews*. 1923;3:106–19.
4. Park EA. The therapy of rickets. *JAMA: The Journal of the American Medical Association*. 1940;115(5):370–9.
5. Vieth R. Vitamin D supplementation, 25-hydroxy-vitamin D concentrations, and safety. *The American Journal of Clinical Nutrition*. 1999;69:842–56.
6. Vieth R, Chan PC, MacFarlane GD. Efficacy and safety of vitamin D3 intake exceeding the lowest observed adverse effect level. *The American Journal of Clinical Nutrition*. 2001;73(2):288–94. Epub 2001/02/07. PubMed PMID: 11157326.
7. Institute of Medicine. *Nutrition During Lactation*. Washington, DC: National Academy Press; 1991. 309 p.
8. Brooke OG, Brown IRF, Bone CDM, Carter ND, Cleeve HJW, Maxwell JD, Robinson VP, Winder SM. Vitamin D supplements in pregnant Asian women: Effects on calcium status and fetal growth. *British Medical Journal*. 1980;1:751–4.

9. Brooke O, Brown I, Cleeve H, Sood A. Observations on the vitamin D state of pregnant Asian women in London. *British Journal of Obstetrics and Gynaecology.* 1981;88:18–26.
10. Maxwell J, Ang L, Brooke O, Brown I. Vitamin D supplements enhance weight gain and nutritional status in pregnant Asians. *British Journal of Obstetrics and Gynaecology.* 1981;88:987–91.
11. Marya R, Rathee S, Lata V, Mudgil S. Effects of vitamin D supplementation in pregnancy. *Gynecologic and Obstetric Investigation.* 1981;12:155–61.
12. Markestad T, Aksnes L, Ulstein M, Aarskog D. 25-Hydroxyvitamin D and 1,25-dihydroxy vitamin D of D_2 and D_3 origin in maternal and umbilical cord serum after vitamin D_2 supplementation in human pregnancy. *The American Journal of Clinical Nutrition.* 1984;40:1057–63.
13. Mallet E, Gugi B, Brunelle P, Henocq A, Basuyau J, Lemeur H. Vitamin D supplementation in pregnancy: A controlled trial of two methods. *Obstetrics and Gynecology.* 1986;68:300–4.
14. Marya R, Rathee S, Dua V, Sangwan K. Effect of vitamin D supplementation during pregnancy on foetal growth. *Indian Journal of Medical Research.* 1988;88:488–92.
15. Brunvand L, Quigstad E, Urdal P, Haug E. Vitamin D deficiency and fetal growth. *Early Human Development.* 1996;45:27–33.
16. Brooke OG, Butters F, Wood C. Intrauterine vitamin D nutrition and postnatal growth in Asian infants. *British Medical Journal.* 1981;283:1024.
17. Thorne-Lyman A, Fawzi WW. Vitamin D during pregnancy and maternal, neonatal and nfant health outcomes: A systematic review and meta-analysis. *Paediatric and Perinatal Epidemiology.* 2012;26(Suppl 1):75–90. Epub 2012/07/07. doi: 10.1111/j.1365-3016.2012.01283.x. PubMed PMID: 22742603; PubMed Central PMCID: PMC3843348.
18. Sills I, Skuza K, Horlick M, Schwartz M, Rapaport R. Vitamin D deficiency rickets. Reports of its demise are exaggerated. *Clinical Pediatrics.* 1994;33:491–3.
19. Tomashek KM, Nesby S, Scanlon KS, Cogswell ME, Powell KE, Parashar UD, Mellinger-Birdsong A, Grummer-Strawn LM, Dietz WH. Nutritional rickets in Georgia. *Pediatrics.* 2001;107(4):E45. Epub 2001/05/23. PubMed PMID: 11335766.
20. Weisberg P, Scanlon KS, Li R, Cogswell ME. Nutritional rickets among children in the United States: Review of cases reported between 1986 and 2003. *The American Journal of Clinical Nutrition.* 2004;80(6 Suppl):1697S–705S. PubMed PMID: 15585790.
21. Hollis B, Wagner C. Assessment of dietary vitamin D requirements during pregnancy and lactation. *The American Journal of Clinical Nutrition.* 2004;79:717–26.
22. Nesby-O'Dell S, Scanlon K, Cogswell M, Gillespie C, Hollis B, Looker A, Allen C, Doughertly C, Gunter E, Bowman B. Hypovitaminosis D prevalence and determinants among African American and white women of reproductive age: Third National Health and Nutrition Examination Survey: 1988–1994. *American Journal of Clinical Nutrition.* 2002;76:187–92.
23. Moncrieff M, Fadahunsi TO. Congenital rickets due to maternal vitamin D deficiency. *Archives of Disease in Childhood.* 1974;49(10):810–1. PubMed PMID: 4429363.
24. Grover SR, Morley R. Vitamin D deficiency in veiled or dark-skinned pregnant women. *Medical Journal of Australia.* 2001;175(5):251–2. Epub 2001/10/06. PubMed PMID: 11587255.
25. Mellanby E. An experimental investigation on rickets. *Lancet.* 1919;1:407–12.
26. Mellanby E. Experimental rickets. *Medical Research (Great Britain) Special Report Series.* 1921;SRS-61:1–78.
27. Beser E, Cakmakci T. Factors affecting the morbidity of vitamin D deficiency rickets and primary protection. *East African Medical Journal.* 1994;71(6):358–62. Epub 1994/06/01. PubMed PMID: 7835254.

28. Green HN, Pindar D, Davis G, Mellanby E. Diet as a prophylactic agent against puerperal sepsis. *British Medical Journal*. 1931;2(3691):595–8. Epub 1931/10/03. PubMed PMID: 20776417; PubMed Central PMCID: PMC2315000.
29. Poulter LW, Rook GA, Steele J, Condez A. Influence of 1,25-(OH)2 vitamin D3 and gamma interferon on the phenotype of human peripheral blood monocyte-derived macrophages. *Infection and Immunity*. 1987;55(9):2017–20. Epub 1987/09/01. PubMed PMID: 3114140.
30. Rook GA. The role of vitamin D in tuberculosis. *American Review of Respiratory Disease*. 1988;138(4):768–70. Epub 1988/10/01. PubMed PMID: 2849343.
31. Lemire JM, Adams JS. 1,25-Dihydroxyvitamin D3 inhibits the passive transfer of cellular immunity by a myelin basic protein-specific T cell clone. *Journal of Bone and Mineral Research: The Official Journal of the American Society for Bone and Mineral Research*. 1992;7(2):171–7. Epub 1992/02/01. doi: 10.1002/jbmr.5650070208. PubMed PMID: 1373930.
32. Hewison M, Gacad MA, Lemire J, Adams JS. Vitamin D as a cytokine and hematopoetic factor. *Reviews in Endocrine and Metabolic Disorders*. 2001;2(2):217–27. Epub 2001/11/14. PubMed PMID: 11705327.
33. Liu PT, Stenger S, Li H, Wenzel L, Tan BH, Krutzik SR, Ochoa MT. et al. Toll-like receptor triggering of a vitamin D-mediated human antimicrobial response. *Science*. 2006;311(5768):1770–3. PubMed PMID: 16497887.
34. Cannell JJ, Vieth R, Umhau JC, Holick MF, Grant WB, Madronich S, Garland CF, Giovannucci E. Epidemic influenza and vitamin D. *Epidemiology and Infection*. 2006;134(6):1129–40. PubMed PMID: 16959053.
35. Adams JS. Vitamin D as a defensin. *Journal of Musculoskeletal and Neuronal Interactions*. 2006;6(4):344–6. Epub 2006/12/23. PubMed PMID: 17185816.
36. Johnson DD, Wagner CL, Hulsey TC, McNeil RB, Ebeling M, Hollis BW. Vitamin D deficiency and insufficiency is common during pregnancy. *American Journal of Perinatology*. 2011;28(1):7–12. Epub 2010/07/20. doi: 10.1055/s-0030-1262505. PubMed PMID: 20640974.
37. Hamilton SA, McNeil R, Hollis BW, Davis DJ, Winkler J, Cook C, Warner G, Bivens B, McShane P, Wagner CL. Profound vitamin D deficiency in a diverse group of women during pregnancy living in a sun-rich environment at latitude 32 degrees N. *International Journal of Endocrinology*. 2010;917428. Epub 2011/01/05. doi: 10.1155/2010/917428. PubMed PMID: 21197089; PubMed Central PMCID: PMC3004407.
38. Song SJ, Zhou L, Si S, Liu J, Zhou J, Feng K, Wu J, Zhang W. The high prevalence of vitamin D deficiency and its related maternal factors in pregnant women in Beijing. *PLoS One*. 2013;8(12):e85081. Epub 2014/01/05. doi: 10.1371/journal.pone.0085081. PubMed PMID: 24386450; PubMed Central PMCID: PMC3873449.
39. Song SJ, Si S, Liu J, Chen X, Zhou L, Jia G, Liu G. et al. Vitamin D status in Chinese pregnant women and their newborns in Beijing and their relationships to birth size. *Public Health Nutrition*. 2013;16(4):687–92. Epub 2012/11/24. doi: 10.1017/S1368980012003084. PubMed PMID: 23174124.
40. Dawodu A, Wagner CL. Mother–child vitamin D deficiency: An international perspective. *Archives of Disease in Childhood*. 2007;92(9):737–40. Epub 2007/08/24. doi: 92/9/737 [pii] 10.1136/adc.2007.122689. PubMed PMID: 17715433; PubMed Central PMCID: PMC2084036.
41. Dawodu A. What's new in mother–infant vitamin D deficiency: A 21st century perspective. *Medical Principles and Practice: International Journal of the Kuwait University*, Health Science Centre. 2012;21(1):2–3. Epub 2011/10/26. doi: 10.1159/000331904. PubMed PMID: 22025133.
42. Food and Nutrition Board. Standing Committee on the Scientific Evaluation of Dietary Reference Intakes. *Dietary Reference Intakes for Vitamin D and Calcium*. Washington, DC: National Academy Press; 2010.

43. Holick MF, Binkley NC, Bischoff-Ferrari HA, Gordon CM, Hanley DA, Heaney RP, Murad MH, Weaver CM. Evaluation, treatment, and prevention of vitamin D deficiency: An Endocrine Society Clinical Practice Guideline. *The Journal of Clinical Endocrinology and Metabolism*. 2011;96(12):3908. Epub 2011/06/08. doi: jc.2011-0385 [pii] 10.1210/jc.2011-0385. PubMed PMID: 21646368.
44. Hollis BW, Wagner CL. Vitamin D requirements during lactation: High-dose maternal supplementation as therapy to prevent hypovitaminosis D for both the mother and the nursing infant. *The American Journal of Clinical Nutrition*. 2004;80(6 Suppl):1752S–8S. Epub 2004/12/09. doi: 80/6/1752S [pii]. PubMed PMID: 15585800.
45. Liu NQ, Hewison M. Vitamin D, the placenta and pregnancy. *Archives of Biochemistry and Biophysics*. 2012;523(1):37–47. Epub 2011/12/14. doi: 10.1016/j.abb.2011.11.018. PubMed PMID: 22155151.
46. Hollis BW, Wagner CL. The role of the parent compound vitamin D with respect to metabolism and function: Why clinical dose intervals can affect clinical outcomes. *The Journal of Clinical Endocrinology and Metabolism*. 2013;98(12):4619–28. Epub 2013/10/10. doi: 10.1210/jc.2013-2653. PubMed PMID: 24106283; PubMed Central PMCID: PMC3849670.
47. Nykjaer A, Dragun D, Walther D, Vorum H, Jacobsen C, Herz J, Melsen F, Christensen EI, Willnow TE. An endocytic pathway essential for renal uptake and activation of the steroid 25-(OH) vitamin D3. *Cell*. 1999;96(4):507–15. Epub 1999/03/03. PubMed PMID: 10052453.
48. Bikle DD, Gee E, Halloran B, Haddad JG. Free 1,25-dihydroxyvitamin D levels in serum from normal subjects, pregnant subjects, and subjects with liver disease. *The Journal of Clinical Investigation*. 1984;74(6):1966–71. Epub 1984/12/01. doi: 10.1172/JCI111617. PubMed PMID: 6549014; PubMed Central PMCID: PMC425383.
49. Hollis BW, Johnson D, Hulsey TC, Ebeling M, Wagner CL. Vitamin D supplementation during pregnancy: Double-blind, randomized clinical trial of safety and effectiveness. *Journal of Bone and Mineral Research: The Official Journal of the American Society for Bone and Mineral Research*. 2011;26(10):2341–57. Epub 2011/06/28. doi: 10.1002/jbmr.463. PubMed PMID: 21706518; PubMed Central PMCID: PMC3183324.
50. Kumar R, Cohen WR, Silva P, Epstein FH. Elevated 1,25-dihydroxyvitamin D plasma levels in normal human pregnancy and lactation. *The Journal of Clinical Investigation*. 1979;63(2):342–4. Epub 1979/02/01. doi: 10.1172/JCI109308. PubMed PMID: 429557; PubMed Central PMCID: PMC371958.
51. Wagner CL, Hollis BW. Beyond PTH: Assessing vitamin D status during early pregnancy. *Clinical Endocrinology*. 2011;75(3):285–6. Epub 2011/07/05. doi: 10.1111/j.1365-2265.2011.04164.x. PubMed PMID: 21722152.
52. Wagner CL, Hollis BW. The relationship between PTH and 25-hydroxy vitamin D early in pregnancy. *Clinical Endocrinology*. 2011. doi: 10.1111/j.1365-2265.2011.04164.x.
53. Walker VP, Zhang X, Rastegar I, Liu PT, Hollis BW, Adams JS, Modlin RL. Cord blood vitamin D status impacts innate immune responses. *The Journal of Clinical Endocrinology and Metabolism*. 2011;96(6):1835–43. Epub 2011/04/08. doi: jc.2010-1559 [pii] 10.1210/jc.2010-1559. PubMed PMID: 21470993.
54. Bouillon R, Van Assche FA, Van Baelen H, Heyns W, DeMoor P. Influence of the vitamin D-binding protein on serum concentrations of 1,25$(OH)_2$D. *The Journal of Clinical Investigation*. 1981;67:589–96.
55. Haughton M, Mason R. Immunonephelometric assay of vitamin D-binding protein. *Clinical Chemistry*. 1992;38:1796.
56. Luxwolda MF, Kuipers RS, Kema IP, Janneke Dijck-Brouwer DA, Muskiet FA. Traditionally living populations in East Africa have a mean serum 25-hydroxyvitamin D concentration of 115 nmol/l. *The British Journal of Nutrition*. 2012;108(9):1557–61. Epub 2012/01/24. doi: 10.1017/S0007114511007161. PubMed PMID: 22264449.

57. Luxwolda MF, Kuipers RS, Kema IP, van der Veer E, Dijck-Brouwer DA, Muskiet FA. Vitamin D status indicators in indigenous populations in East Africa. *European Journal of Nutrition*. 2013;52(3):1115–25. Epub 2012/08/11. doi: 10.1007/s00394-012-0421-6. PubMed PMID: 22878781.
58. Basile LA, Taylor SN, Wagner CL, Quinones L, Hollis BW. Neonatal vitamin D status at birth at latitude 32 degrees 72′: Evidence of deficiency. *Journal of Perinatology*. 2007;27(9):568–71. Epub 2007/07/13. doi: 7211796 [pii] 10.1038/sj.jp.7211796. PubMed PMID: 17625571.
59. Wagner CL, McNeil R, Hamilton SA, Winkler J, Rodriguez Cook C, Warner G, Bivens B. et al. A randomized trial of vitamin D supplementation in 2 community health center networks in South Carolina. *American Journal of Obstetrics and Gynecology*. 2013;208(2):137. e1–13. Epub 2012/11/08. doi: 10.1016/j.ajog.2012.10.888. PubMed PMID: 23131462.
60. Delvin EE, Salle BL, Glorieux FH, Adeleine P, David LS. Vitamin D supplementation during pregnancy: Effect on neonatal calcium homeostasis. *The Journal of Pediatrics*. 1986;109(2):328–34. PubMed PMID: 3488384.
61. American Academy of Pediatrics. Committee on Nutrition. The prophylactic requirement and the toxicity of vitamin D. 1963.
62. Williams J, Barratt-Boyes B, Lowe J. Supravalvular aortic stenosis. *Circulation*. 1961; 24:1311–8.
63. Beuren A, Apitz J, Harmjanz D. Supravalvular aortic stenosis in association with mental retardation and certain facial appearance. *Circulation*. 1962;26:1235–40.
64. Garcia RE, Friedman WF, Kaback M, Rowe RD. Idiopathic hypercalcemia and supravalvular aortic stenosis: Documentation of a new syndrome. *TheNew England Journal of Medicine*. 1964;271:117–20.
65. Friedman WF, Roberts WC. Vitamin D and the supravalvular aortic stenosis syndrome. The transplacental effects of vitamin D on the aorta of the rabbit. *Circulation*. 1966;34:77–86.
66. Friedman WF. Vitamin D as a cause of the supravalvular aortic stenosis syndrome. *American Heart Journal*. 1967;73:718–20.
67. Antia AV, Wiltse HE, Rowe RD, Pitt EL, Levin S, Ottesen OE, Cooke RE. Pathogenesis of the supravalvular aortic stenosis syndrome. *Journal of Pediatrics*. 1967;71:431–41.
68. Friedman WF, Mills LS. The production of “elfin facies” and abnormal dentition by vitamin D during pregnancy: Relationship to the supravalvular aortic stenosis syndrome. *Proceedings of the Society for Pediatric Research*. 1967;37:80.
69. Friedman WF, Mills L. The relationship between vitamin D and the craniofacial and dental anomalies of the supravalvular aortic stenosis syndrome. *Pediatrics*. 1969;43:12–8.
70. Curran ME, Atkinson DL, Ewart AK, Morris CA, Leppert MF, Keating MT. The elastin gene is disrupted by a translocation associated with supravalvular aortic stenosis. *Cell*. 1993;73(1):159–68. Epub 1993/04/09. doi: 0092-8674(93)90168-P [pii]. PubMed PMID: 8096434.
71. Aravena T, Castillo S, Carrasco X, Mena I, Lopez J, Rojas JP, Rosembert C, Schroter C, Aboitiz F. Williams syndrome: Clinical, cytogenetical, neurophysiological and neuroanatomic study. *Revista médica de Chile*. 2002;130(6):631–7.
72. Ewart AK, Jin W, Atkinson D, Morris CA, Keating MT. Supravalvular aortic stenosis associated with a deletion disrupting the elastin gene. *The Journal of Clinical Investigation*. 1994;93(3):1071–7. Epub 1994/03/01. doi: 10.1172/JCI117057. PubMed PMID: 8132745; PubMed Central PMCID: PMC294040.
73. Mathias RS. Rickets in an infant with Williams syndrome. *Pediatric Nephrology*. 2000;14:489–92.
74. Heaney R, Davies K, Chen T, Holick M, Barger-Lux M. Human serum 25-hydroxycholecalciferol response to extended oral dosing with cholecalciferol. *The American Journal of Clinical Nutrition*. 2003;77:204–10.

75. Wagner CL, McNeil RB, Johnson DD, Hulsey TC, Ebeling M, Robinson C, Hamilton SA, Hollis BW. Health characteristics and outcomes of two randomized vitamin D supplementation trials during pregnancy: A combined analysis. *The Journal of Steroid Biochemistry and Molecular Biology*. 2013;136:313–20. Epub 2013/01/15. doi: 10.1016/j.jsbmb.2013.01.002. PubMed PMID: 23314242.
76. Dawodu A, Saadi HF, Bekdache G, Javed Y, Altaye M, Hollis BW. Randomized controlled trial (RCT) of vitamin D supplementation in pregnancy in a population with endemic vitamin D deficiency. *The Journal of Clinical Endocrinology and Metabolism*. 2013;98(6):2337–46. Epub 2013/04/06. doi: 10.1210/jc.2013-1154. PubMed PMID: 23559082.
77. Hollis BW, Wagner CL. Vitamin D and pregnancy: Skeletal effects, nonskeletal effects, and birth outcomes. *Calcified Tissue International*. 2013;92(2):128–39. Epub 2012/05/25. doi: 10.1007/s00223-012-9607-4. PubMed PMID: 22623177.
78. Wagner CL, Taylor SN, Dawodu A, Johnson DD, Hollis BW. Vitamin D and its role during pregnancy in attaining optimal health of mother and fetus. *Nutrients*. 2012;4(3):208–30. Epub 2012/06/06. doi: 10.3390/nu4030208. PubMed PMID: 22666547; PubMed Central PMCID: PMC3347028.
79. Christakos S, Hewison M, Gardner DG, Wagner CL, Sergeev IN, Rutten E, Pittas AG, Boland R, Ferrucci L, Bikle DD. Vitamin D: beyond bone. *Annals of the New York Academy of Sciences*. 2013;1287:45–58. Epub 2013/05/21. doi: 10.1111/nyas.12129. PubMed PMID: 23682710; PubMed Central PMCID: PMC3717170.
80. Hypponen E. Vitamin D for the prevention of preeclampsia? A hypothesis. *Nutrition Reviews*. 2005;63(7):225–32. PubMed PMID: 16121476.
81. Bodnar LM, Catov JM, Simhan HN, Holick MF, Powers RW, Roberts JM. Maternal vitamin D deficiency increases the risk of preeclampsia. *The Journal of Clinical Endocrinology and Metabolism*. 2007;92(9):3517–22. Epub 2007.
82. Robinson CJ, Alanis MC, Wagner CL, Hollis BW, Johnson DD. Plasma 25-hydroxyvitamin D levels in early-onset severe preeclampsia. *American Journal of Obstetrics and Gynecology*. 2010;203(4):366.e1–6. Epub 2010/08/10. doi: S0002-9378(10)00811-2 [pii] 10.1016/j.ajog.2010.06.036. PubMed PMID: 20692641.
83. Robinson CJ, Wagner CL, Hollis BW, Baatz JE, Johnson DD. Association of maternal vitamin D and placenta growth factor with the diagnosis of early onset severe preeclampsia. *American Journal of Perinatology*. 2013;30(3):167–72. Epub 2012/08/10. doi: 10.1055/s-0032-1322514. PubMed PMID: 22875657.
84. Bodnar LM, Simhan HN, Catov JM, Roberts JM, Platt RW, Diesel JC, Klebanoff MA. Maternal vitamin D status and the risk of mild and severe preeclampsia. *Epidemiology*. 2014;25(2):207–14. Epub 2014/01/25. doi: 10.1097/EDE.0000000000000039. PubMed PMID: 24457526.
85. Bodnar LM, Krohn MA, Simhan HN. Maternal vitamin D deficiency is associated with bacterial vaginosis in the first trimester of pregnancy. *The Journal of Nutrition*. 2009;139(6):1157–61. Epub 2009/04/10. doi: 10.3945/jn.108.103168. PubMed PMID: 19357214; PubMed Central PMCID: PMC2682987.
86. Hensel KJ, Randis TM, Gelber SE, Ratner AJ. Pregnancy-specific association of vitamin D deficiency and bacterial vaginosis. *American Journal of Obstetrics and Gynecology*. 2011;204(1):41.e1–9. Epub 2010/10/05. doi: 10.1016/j.ajog.2010.08.013. PubMed PMID: 20887971.
87. Bodnar LM, Klebanoff MA, Gernand AD, Platt RW, Parks WT, Catov JM, Simhan HN. Maternal vitamin D status and spontaneous preterm birth by placental histology in the US Collaborative Perinatal Project. *American Journal of Epidemiology*. 2014;179(2): 168–76. Epub 2013/10/15. doi: 10.1093/aje/kwt237. PubMed PMID: 24124195; PubMed Central PMCID: PMC3873106.

88. Cockburn F, Belton N, Purvis R, Giles M, Brown J, Turner T, Wilkinson E. et al. Maternal vitamin D intake and mineral metabolism in mothers and their newborn infants. *British Medical Journal*. 1980;231:1–10.
89. Brunvand L, Shah SS, Bergström S, Haug E. Vitamin D deficiency in pregnancy is not associated with obstructed labor. A study among Pakistani women in Karachi. *Acta obstetricia et gynecologica Scandinavica*. 1998 Mar;77(3):303–6.
90. Hashemipour S, Ziaee A, Javadi A, Movahed F, Elmizadeh K, Javadi EH, Lalooha F. Effect of treatment of vitamin D deficiency and insufficiency during pregnancy on fetal growth indices and maternal weight gain: A randomized clinical trial. *European Journal of Obstetrics and Gynecology and Reproductive Biology*. 2014;172:15–9. Epub 2013/11/12. doi: 10.1016/j.ejogrb.2013.10.010. PubMed PMID: 24210789.
91. Kalra P, Das V, Agarwal A, Kumar M, Ramesh V, Bhatia E, Gupta S, Singh S, Saxena P, Bhatia V. Effect of vitamin D supplementation during pregnancy on neonatal mineral homeostasis and anthropometry of the newborn and infant. *The British Journal of Nutrition*. 2012;108(6):1052–8. Epub 2012/01/04. doi: 10.1017/S0007114511006246. PubMed PMID: 22212646.
92. De-Regil LM, Palacios C, Ansary A, Kulier R, Pena-Rosas JP. Vitamin D supplementation for women during pregnancy. The Cochrane database of systematic reviews. 2012;2:CD008873. Epub 2012/02/18. doi: 10.1002/14651858.CD008873.pub2. PubMed PMID: 22336854; PubMed Central PMCID: PMC3747784.
93. Soheilykhah S, Mojibian M, Rashidi M, Rahimi-Saghand S, Jafari F. Maternal vitamin D status in gestational diabetes mellitus. *Nutrition in Clinical Practice*. 2010;25(5):524–7. Epub 2010/10/22. doi: 10.1177/0884533610379851. PubMed PMID: 20962313.
94. Soheilykhah S, Mojibian M, Moghadam MJ, Shojaoddiny-Ardekani A. The effect of different doses of vitamin D supplementation on insulin resistance during pregnancy. *Gynecological Endocrinology*. 2013;29(4):396–9. Epub 2013/01/29. doi: 10.3109/09513590.2012.752456. PubMed PMID: 23350644.
95. Wagner CL, Hulsey TC, Fanning D, Ebeling M, Hollis BW. High-dose vitamin D3 supplementation in a cohort of breastfeeding mothers and their infants: A 6-month follow-up pilot study. *Breastfeeding Medicine*. 2006;1(2):59–70. Epub 2007/07/31. doi: 10.1089/bfm.2006.1.59. PubMed PMID: 17661565.
96. Wagner C, ed. Current concepts in vitamin D requirements for mother and her breastfeeding infant. *International Society for Research in Human Milk and Lactation*, Breastfeeding Medicine, Trieste, Italy; 2013.
97. Wagner CL, Howard CR, Hulsey TC, Lawrence RA, Ebeling M, Shary J, Smith PG, Morella K, Taylor SN, Hollis BW. Maternal and infant vitamin D status during lactation: Is latitude important? *Health*. 2013;5:2004.
98. Gartner L, Greer F. American Academy of Pediatrics. Section on Breastfeeding Medicine and Committee on Nutrition. Prevention of rickets and vitamin D deficiency: New guidelines for vitamin D intake. *Pediatrics*. 2003;111(4):908–10.
99. Greer FR. Issues in establishing vitamin D recommendations for infants and children. *The American Journal of Clinical Nutrition*. 2004;80(6):1759S–62S.
100. Misra M, Pacaud D, Petryk A, Collett-Solberg PF, Kappy M; Drug and Therapeutics Committee of the Lawson Wilkins Pediatric Endocrine Society. Vitamin D deficiency in children and its management: Review of current knowledge and recommendations. *Pediatrics*. 2008;122(2):398–417. Epub 2008/08/05. doi: 10.1542/peds.2007-1894. PubMed PMID: 18676559.
101. Harris BS, Bunket JWM. Vitamin D potency of human breast milk. *American Journal of Public Health*. 1939;29:744–7.
102. Hollis B, Roos B, Lambert P. Vitamin D and its metabolites in human and bovine milk. *The Journal of Nutrition*. 1981;111:1240–8.

103. Greer FR, Ho M, Dodson D, Tsang RC. Lack of 25-hydroxyvitamin D and 1,25-dihydroxyvitamin D in human milk. *The Journal of Pediatrics*. 1981;99(2):233–5. Epub 1981/08/01. PubMed PMID: 6973018.
104. Oberhelman SS, Meekins ME, Fischer PR, Lee BR, Singh RJ, Cha SS, Gardner BM, Pettifor JM, Croghan IT, Thacher TD. Maternal vitamin D supplementation to improve the vitamin D status of breast-fed infants: A randomized controlled trial. *Mayo Clinic Proceedings*. 2013;88(12):1378–87. Epub 2013/12/03. doi: 10.1016/j.mayocp.2013.09.012. PubMed PMID: 24290111.
105. Greer FR, Hollis BW, Cripps DJ, Tsang RC. Effects of maternal ultraviolet B irradiation on vitamin D content of human milk. *Journal of Pediatrics*. 1984;105:431–3.
106. Greer FR, Hollis BW, Napoli JL. High concentrations of vitamin D_2 in human milk associated with pharmacologic doses of vitamin D_2. *Journal of Pediatrics*. 1984;105:61–4.
107. Hollis BW, Pittard WB, Reinhardt TA. Relationships among vitamin D, 25(OH)D, and vitamin D-binding protein concentrations in the plasma and milk of human subjects. *The Journal of Clinical Endocrinology and Metabolism*. 1986;62:41–4.
108. Wagner CL, Howard CR, Hulsey T, Ebeling M, Shary J, Smith P, Childs C. et al. Results of NICHD two-site maternal vitamin D supplementation randomized controlled trial during lactation [abstract; platform presentation]. Pediatric Academic Societies, Washington, DC; 2013.
109. Wagner CL, Greer FR. Prevention of rickets and vitamin D deficiency in infants, children, and adolescents. *Pediatrics*. 2008;122(5):1142–52. Epub 2008/11/04. doi: 122/5/1142 [pii] 10.1542/peds.2008-1862. PubMed PMID: 18977996.
110. Perrine CG, Sharma AJ, Jefferds ME, Serdula MK, Scanlon KS. Adherence to vitamin D recommendations among US infants. *Pediatrics*. 2010;125(4):627–32. Epub 2010/03/24. doi: 10.1542/peds.2009-2571. PubMed PMID: 20308221.
111. Crocker B, Green TJ, Barr SI, Beckingham B, Bhagat R, Dabrowska B, Douthwaite R. et al. Very high vitamin D supplementation rates among infants aged 2 months in Vancouver and Richmond, British Columbia, Canada. *BMC Public Health*. 2011;11:905. Epub 2011/12/14. doi: 10.1186/1471-2458-11-905. PubMed PMID: 22151789; PubMed Central PMCID: PMC3265491.
112. Dawodu A, Agarwal M, Patel M, Ezimokhai M. Serum 25-hydroxyvitamin D and calcium homeostasis in the United Arab Emirates mothers and neonates: A preliminary report. *Middle East Paediatrics*. 1997;2:9–12.
113. Saadi H, Dawodu A, Afandi B, Zayed R, Benedict S, Nagelkerke N. Efficacy of daily and monthly high-dose calciferol in vitamin D deficient nulliparous and lactating women. *The American Journal of Clinical Nutrition*. 2007;85(6):1565–71.
114. Saadi HF, Dawodu A, Afandi B, Zayed R, Benedict S, Nagelkerke N, Hollis BW. Effect of combined maternal and infant vitamin D supplementation on vitamin D status of exclusively breastfed infants. *Maternal and Child Nutrition*. 2009;5(1):25–32. Epub 2009/01/24. doi: 10.1111/j.1740-8709.2008.00145.x. PubMed PMID: 19161542.
115. Wagner C, Howard C, Hulsey T, Ebeling M, Taylor S, Lawrence R, Hollis B, eds. *Predicting Maternal and Infant Vitamin D Status During Lactation: Effect of Vitamin D Supplementation and Other Factors*. Pediatric Academic Societies, Washington, DC; 2013.

8 Fiber Supplements and Clinically Meaningful Health Benefits

Identifying the Physiochemical Characteristics of Fiber that Drive Specific Physiologic Effects

Johnson W. McRorie, Jr. and George C. Fahey, Jr.

CONTENTS

8.1 INTRODUCTION

While there is no globally-accepted definition of dietary fiber, the Institute of Medicine (IOM) developed the following set of working definitions for fiber in the food supply: "*Dietary fiber* consists of non-digestible carbohydrates and lignin that are intrinsic and intact in plants" [1]. *Functional fiber* consists of isolated, non-digestible carbohydrates that have beneficial physiological effects in humans. The isolated fibers found in the vast majority of dietary supplements would, therefore, be considered "functional fiber," with the prerequisite of clinical evidence supporting the latter part of the statement, "… that have beneficial physiological effects in humans." Consistent with these definitions, this chapter will focus on the health benefits of dietary fiber supplements, as evidenced by the physiologic effects observed in well-controlled clinical studies. Unlike prescription and over-the-counter medications, fiber supplements have no requirements for pre-market approval by the Food and Drug Administration (FDA), so it can be challenging to determine which fiber supplements have well-controlled clinical evidence to support specific health claims. It is, therefore, important to have a working knowledge of the physical characteristics of fiber that drive specific physiologic effects so as to accurately discern which products provide a clinically meaningful health benefit supported by published clinical data.

It is widely recognized that dietary fiber is "good for you," [2–7], and that fruits, vegetables, and whole grains can be a good source of dietary fiber [3,7,8], but it can be a challenge to consume a sufficient quantity of these dietary sources of fiber daily to meet USDA recommendations for fiber consumption. Most servings of fruits, vegetables, and whole grains contain only 1–3 g of dietary fiber [9]. A recent (2014) review of data from the National Health and Nutrition Examination Survey database showed that only 8% of adults and 3% of children (including adolescents) consumed at least 3 whole grain ounce equivalents per day (≥3 whole grain ounce equivalents per day considered high consumption) [8]. The IOM Adequate Intake guidelines recommend 14 g dietary fiber per 1000 kcal consumed, which is about 25 g/day for women and 38 g/day for men [1]. In contrast to this recommendation, the vast majority (90%) of the United States population does not consume enough dietary fiber [10]. The average American consumes only 15 g of dietary fiber per day [11] and, for those on a low carbohydrate diet, total fiber intake may be less than 10 g/day [12]. Epidemiologic studies show that dietary fiber is strongly associated with a reduced risk of heart attack, stroke, and cardiovascular disease [13,14]. Given the low success rate in achieving recommended levels of fiber intake by consumption of high fiber foods, it is reasonable to consider fiber supplements as a convenient and concentrated source of fiber, which can facilitate meeting that goal.

It is important to recognize that, when considering the health benefits of dietary fiber, there is a key distinction between "replacement" and "supplementation." If a substantial portion of a diet is *replaced* by healthier, high fiber dietary components, then both the total calories consumed and the glycemic index of the diet [15] would be reduced, leading to a conclusion in epidemiological studies that a wide variety of fiber sources (e.g., fruits, vegetables, whole grains) can provide a detectable health benefit. It remains unclear, however, how much of that benefit is directly attributable to the effects of the dietary fiber, versus the elimination of less healthy components of the diet, a reduced calorie intake, and increased consumption of healthy constituents other than fiber derived from fruits, vegetables, and whole grains. In contrast to *replacement*, which includes a variety of fiber sources, a fiber *supplement* is typically an isolated fiber source that is consumed in addition to an existing diet. It therefore becomes essential to appreciate the unique physiochemical characteristics of each fiber supplement, and how these characteristics are, or are not, associated with one or more clinically meaningful health benefits. While some fiber supplements have extensive, reproducible clinical evidence for clinically meaningful health benefits, other fiber supplements do not. The term "fiber supplement" implies a benefit to one's health when consumed on a regular (e.g., daily) basis, but not all fiber supplements have clinical data at physiologic doses to support a clinically meaningful health benefit.

There are numerous *in vitro* and pre-clinical (animal) studies in the literature that suggest a health benefit is *possible* in humans, but evidence for a clinically meaningful health benefit should only be derived from well-controlled clinical studies. Individual clinical studies will be discussed, but the term "clinically demonstrated" will be reserved for fiber supplements with two or more well-controlled clinical studies that provide reproducible evidence of a health benefit. Further, health benefits should be demonstrated at doses that can reasonably and comfortably be consumed on a daily basis to facilitate long-term compliance. A fiber supplement is intended to *supplement* the fiber in a diet, not replace the dietary fiber naturally found in fruits, vegetables, and whole grains, which have other beneficial constituents that may not be found in a fiber supplement. The "Nutrition Facts" panel on food products characterizes a product as an "excellent" source of dietary fiber if it contains 5 g of fiber per serving. If consumed 4-times per day, an excellent source of fiber would provide 20 g fiber per day, representing 71% of the recommended fiber intake for a given day (based on 28 g fiber/2000 kcal) [16]. Therefore, it is a reasonable expectation that a fiber supplement should be capable of demonstrating a clinically meaningful health benefit at a total dose of 20 g/day or less. A fiber supplement that requires a total daily dose of fiber in excess of 20 g to detect a physiologic effect will not be considered to have a clinically meaningful health benefit.

While solubility (soluble versus insoluble) is commonly used to characterize dietary fiber, clinical evidence supporting specific health benefits, such as cholesterol lowering, improved glycemic control, and improvement in constipation and diarrhea, has often been inconsistent based on this single characterization. This inconsistency in the literature may be due to an under-appreciation of the importance of additional characteristics of specific fiber types, including particle size of insoluble fiber, viscosity/gel-formation for soluble fiber, and how processing might have altered the final product versus the original raw fiber. When considering the health benefits of fiber supplements, it is important to understand the physical characteristics of the marketed product for each fiber supplement, and the resulting health benefits that each product can, or cannot, provide. Health benefits derived from fiber supplements are primarily a function of the fiber's physical effects in the small bowel (e.g., cholesterol lowering, improved glycemic control, satiety/weight loss) and in the large bowel (improved stool form and reduced symptoms in constipation, diarrhea, and irritable bowel syndrome (IBS)). There are three main characteristics of fiber supplements that drive clinical efficacy: solubility, viscosity/gel-formation, and degree/rate of fermentation. Solubility defines whether a fiber supplement will dissolve in water (soluble) or remain as discreet insoluble particles [17]. Most fibers are not exclusively soluble or insoluble, so for the purposes of this chapter, the predominant characteristic will be discussed (e.g., a fiber that is 70% soluble will be considered a soluble fiber). For soluble fibers, viscosity refers to the ability of some polysaccharides to "thicken" when hydrated, in a concentration dependent manner [17–20]. Gel-formation refers to the ability of a subset of soluble viscous fibers to form cross-links, resulting in a visco-elastic gel [17,20]. Fermentation refers to degree to which a dietary fiber, after resisting digestion in the small bowel, can be degraded by gut bacteria, producing byproducts such as short chain fatty acids and gas [5].

Based on solubility, viscosity, and fermentation, fiber supplements can be divided into four clinically meaningful categories:

1. Insoluble (e.g., wheat bran): does not dissolve in water (no water-holding capacity); is poorly fermented, and can exert a laxative effect by mechanical irritation/stimulation of gut mucosa *if* particles are sufficiently large and coarse, but does not gel to attenuate diarrhea and the mechanical irritation could make diarrhea symptoms worse; small smooth particles (e.g., wheat bran flour/bread) have no significant laxative effect; do not significantly affect chyme viscosity, so would not reduce cholesterol concentration or improve glycemic control at physiologic doses.
2. Soluble non-viscous (e.g., inulin, oligosaccharides, resistant starches, wheat dextrin): dissolves in water; does not cause a significant increase in viscosity; does not form a gel (no significant cholesterol lowering effect, no significant improvement in glycemic control at physiologic doses); is rapidly fermented [rapid gas formation, energy harvest (calorie uptake) from fermentation by-products]; no significant laxative effect at physiologic doses; does not form a gel to attenuate diarrhea.
3. Soluble viscous/gel-forming, readily fermented (e.g., β-glucan, guar gum): dissolves in water, forms a viscous gel; increased chyme viscosity may improve glycemic control and lower serum cholesterol (if processing has not attenuated gel-forming capacity); readily fermented [gas formation, energy harvest (calorie uptake) from fermentation by-products]; does not retain its gelled nature throughout the large bowel, so cannot act as a stool normalizer.
4. Soluble viscous/gel-forming, non-fermented (e.g., psyllium): dissolves in water; forms a viscous gel; increases chyme viscosity to improve glycemic control and lower serum cholesterol; not fermented [no gas production,

no appreciable calorie harvest from fermentation by-products (weight control)]; retains gelling capacity throughout the large bowel that provides a stool normalizing effect (softens hard stool in constipation, firms loose/liquid stool in diarrhea).

8.2 SOLUBILITY, VISCOSITY, AND GEL FORMATION

Fiber supplements from carbohydrates are polymers of sugar molecules (monomers) linked together by bonds that resist degradation by digestive enzymes in the upper gastrointestinal tract. Solubility refers to the ability of fiber supplements to dissolve in water. Fibers that readily dissolve in water are considered water soluble, whereas insoluble fibers may disperse, float, or sink in water, but do go into solution and have no water-holding capacity or appreciable impact on viscosity (e.g., wheat bran). Many soluble fibers also do not appreciably alter viscosity or form a gel when dissolved in water, and these soluble fibers are referred to as "non-viscous" (e.g., inulin, wheat dextrin) [17]. Some soluble fibers increase the viscosity of a solution without forming a gel (e.g., methylcellulose), while others have the added ability to exhibit gel formation (e.g., guar gum, β-glucan, psyllium) [17]. The degree of "thickening" depends on both the chemical composition and concentration of the polysaccharide [17]. The capacity to form a gel is dependent on the ability of adjacent fibers to form cross-links, creating a three-dimensional network that can entrap water and behave like a solid (visco-elastic gel).

Fiber supplements have unique characteristics based on the types of sugars that they are made of, and the way in which the polymer chains interact with one another (e.g., straight chain versus highly branched chain). A straight-chain or linear polymer consists of a long string of carbon–carbon bonds between sugar molecules (Figure 8.1). The longer the straight chain, the greater the effect the fiber can have on viscosity when hydrated (Figure 8.2). In contrast, polymers with multiple branches at irregular intervals along the polymer chain are called branched polymers

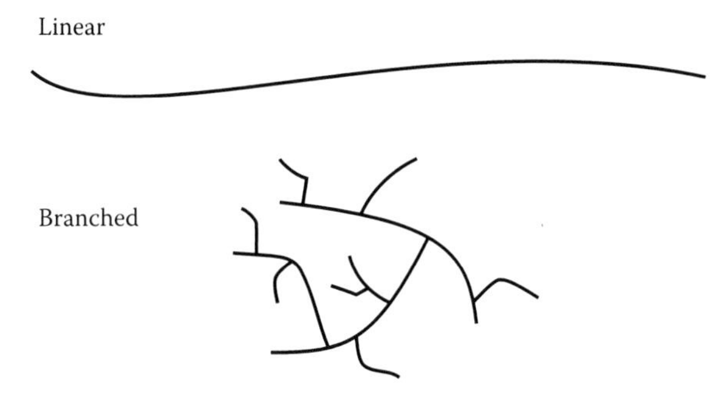

FIGURE 8.1 Linear versus branched polymers. This shows drawings representing linear and branched polysaccharides. Long-chain linear polymers (top) can have a similar molecular weight to highly branched polymers (bottom), but the relative effect on viscosity is much greater for linear polymers than for branched polymers. (From John D. Keller, Jr., Keller Konsulting LLC, Freehold, NJ. With permission.)

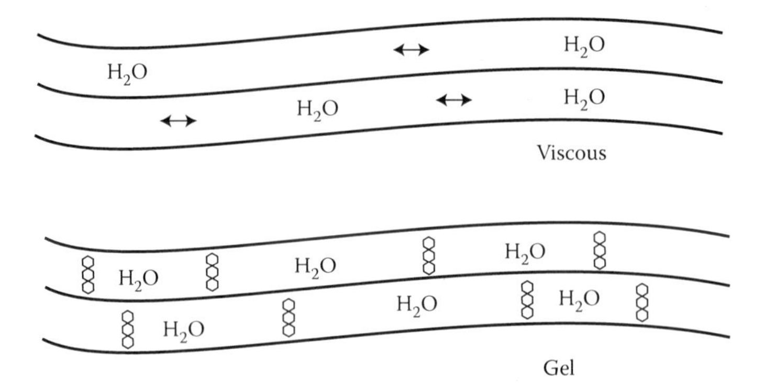

FIGURE 8.2 Viscous and gel-forming linear polymers. This shows drawings representing viscous linear polymers (top) and gel-forming linear polymers (bottom). Long-chain linear polymers orient parallel to adjacent fibers and increase viscosity in a concentration-dependent manner. Some long-chain linear polymers also can form cross-links that create a gel in a concentration-dependent manner. (Drawings recreated with permission from John D. Keller, Jr., Keller Konsulting LLC, Freehold, NJ. With permission.)

(Figure 8.1). The irregular branches make it difficult for the polymer molecules to pack in a regular array and, therefore, highly branched polymers have little effect on viscosity. Viscosity is a function of the volume of a molecule as it rotates in water (effective hydrodynamic size). The volume "swept out" by a fully extended linear fiber is much greater than a fiber with an equal number of sugar units (same molecular weight) but with a "bush-like," highly branched configuration (Figure 8.1). As the volume occupied by a polymer molecule is a function of the radius-cubed, even a small increase in effective hydrodynamic size can translate into a large increase in viscosity. Straight chain viscous polymers that have the added ability to form cross-links with adjacent polymers also can form a gel (behave as a visco-elastic solid) (Figure 8.2). Both viscosity and gel formation are concentration-dependent phenomena. Gel-formation is an important driver of several metabolic health benefits for dietary fiber supplements, including cholesterol lowering, improved glycemic control, weight control and stool normalization (soften hard stool in constipation and firm loose/liquid stool in diarrhea). Note that molecular weight is often used as a correlate of viscosity and/or gel-formation, but this is not always accurate unless one is comparing within the same fiber (e.g., high molecular weight β-glucan versus low molecular weight β-glucan). Correlating molecular weight and viscosity across fiber types can lead to an erroneous conclusion if one fiber type is linear and one is highly branched. As described above, a linear polymer can have a significant effect on viscosity proportionate to its molecular weight (e.g., β-glucan), whereas a highly branched "bush-like" polymer (Figure 8.1) with a similar molecular weight may have little/no significant effect on viscosity (e.g., wheat dextrin, inulin).

A recent study [17] quantified the viscosity of select dietary fibers (soluble and insoluble) at various concentrations. The results showed that the viscosity of all fiber solutions was concentration-dependent and shear rate-dependent. Insoluble fibers (rice bran, soy hulls, and wood cellulose) exhibited the lowest viscosities ("non-viscous"), whereas soluble viscous, gel-forming fibers (guar gum, psyllium, and xanthan gum) exhibited the highest viscosities [17]. Guar gum, psyllium, and oat bran (all soluble fibers) were highly viscous, gel-forming fibers indicating a potential for these fibers to exhibit blood glucose and cholesterol lowering benefits in man. In contrast, wheat bran, rice bran, and wood cellulose (all insoluble fibers), under conditions simulating the small intestine, did not exhibit an ability to raise viscosity or form a gel, indicating that these fibers would not be expected to have a significant effect on blood glucose and cholesterol lowering. Note that there are only two fiber supplements that are recognized by the United States FDA for reducing the risk of cardiovascular disease by lowering serum cholesterol: β-glucan (from oats and barley) and psyllium [22]. Both are soluble, gel-forming fibers. As the following sections will demonstrate, when assessing viscosity/gel-forming-dependent health benefits like cholesterol lowering and improved glycemic control, insoluble fiber (e.g., wheat bran), low viscosity soluble fiber (acacia gum/gum Arabic, low molecular weight β-glucan), and non-viscous soluble fibers (e.g., wheat dextrin, inulin) have no appreciable effect on viscosity/gel-dependent health benefits, and can be/have been used as negative controls (placebo) in these studies [16,21,23–25].

8.2.1 Fermentation

By definition, fiber supplements must be resistant to digestion in the stomach and small intestine, arriving in the proximal large intestine (cecum) relatively intact. The large intestine is home for 10^{11}–10^{12} bacteria per milliliter, approximately 10-times the number of cells in the human body [26,27]. These bacteria are capable of feeding on most fiber supplements to varying degrees. The terms "fermentable" and "non-fermentable" are used to describe whether a fiber supplement can be degraded (fermented) by the bacteria residing in the intestines. Some fiber supplements are readily fermented (e.g., inulin, wheat dextrin, β-glucan, guar gum), some are only partially/poorly fermented (e.g., wheat bran), and some are not fermented (e.g., methylcellulose, psyllium). Non-fermented and poorly fermented fiber supplements pass through the gastrointestinal tract largely unchanged. Readily fermented fiber supplements can be rapidly degraded by bacteria in the proximal large bowel, and the bacteria can use the degradable fiber as an energy source, leading to an increased biomass. Byproducts of fermentation include short-chain fatty acids (SCFAs; acetate, propionate, and butyrate) and gas [28]. Butyrate provides a preferred energy source for colonic mucosal cells. SCFAs also can be absorbed by the large intestine, providing harvested energy as a calorie source for the host. It is important to note that this energy harvest by the host means that many fiber supplements are not calorie-free, which may affect their ability to provide a long-term weight benefit.

Intestinal gas produced by fermentation is eliminated from the bowel by one of two mechanisms: it is absorbed into the blood stream and exhaled by the lungs, objectively measured in a breath gas analysis; or it is expelled as flatulence, objectively assessed by volume and content of expelled gas, and subjectively assessed as frequency of episodes and odor [29,30]. The vast majority of gases in the human gut are nitrogen (N_2), oxygen (O_2), hydrogen (H_2), carbon dioxide (CO_2), and methane

(CH_4) [29,31]. These gases are odorless and comprise more than 99% of intestinal gas. The unpleasant odors that can accompany intestinal gas are the result of trace gases that contain sulfur, such as hydrogen sulfide (H_2S) [29]. In the intestines, frequent low amplitude, rapidly propagating contractions propel gas toward the anus more rapidly than higher viscosity substrates like solid stool, which is propelled by infrequent (approximately six per day) high amplitude propagating contractions [32]. Consistent with the high frequency, low amplitude and high rate of propagation of these small, rapidly propagating contractions, gas can transit the entire gastrointestinal tract in less than 1 h [32]. In contrast, solids may take 1–2 days. Flatulence episodes also occur far more frequently (14/day) [32,33] than bowel movements (1–2 per day), consistent with their relative speed of transport through the gut.

Much of what is known about the relative degree of fermentation of various fibers has been gleaned from *in vitro* testing. *In vitro* testing is used as a model, designed as an inexpensive and rapid method to predict what *could* happen in the human intestinal tract. As with all models, however, the technique has limitations. For instance, for many years psyllium has been considered fermentable based on *in vitro* techniques for assessing fermentation [34–36]. There is a significant discrepancy, however, between *in vitro* data and human (clinical) experience with psyllium. Psyllium, a soluble viscous, gel-forming fiber, can be fermented under *in vitro* test conditions because samples are diluted and homogenized with a high-speed mechanical blender [34–36]. Exposure of the hydrated/gelled psyllium to the rapid shearing forces of a high-speed blender will destroy the physical structure of the gel matrix, artificially rendering psyllium fermentable by destroying the steric hindrance that would otherwise physically impede enzymatic degradation (steric protection). In contrast to the *in vitro* results, there are five published, well-controlled clinical studies, which show that psyllium is not fermented in the human gut [37–41]. The five clinical studies assessed the fermentation of psyllium versus a negative control (placebo), a positive control (lactulose), and/or comparative fibers (e.g., methylcellulose, guar gum, pectin, cellulose) using assessments for both of the mechanisms by which the gut handles gas: breath gas analysis that assesses intestinal gas that has been absorbed into the blood stream and expelled via the lungs, and flatulence, which assesses gas expelled via the anus [37–41]. For example, a randomized, blinded, two-period cross-over design study assessed a high-dose of psyllium (18 g/day) versus placebo for breath gas production (accepted marker for degree of fermentation) [41]. The study showed that breath hydrogen was directionally higher for placebo (38.6 ml/h) than for the high-dose psyllium (23.8 ml/h). There was no significant difference in bacterial dry mass for either test product (indicative of no increase in biomass due to fermentation), and there was no difference in reported symptoms, though the mean score for flatulence was directionally higher for placebo (9.3) than for psyllium (6.1) [41]. Another study, a randomized, blinded, three-way cross-over design assessing high doses of guar gum (20 g/day), psyllium (20 g/day), and control (polysaccharide-free diet), showed that guar gum was readily fermented compared to placebo, but psyllium was not fermented [37]. Assessments of breath methane were identical for psyllium (20 ppm) and placebo (20 ppm), but significantly higher for guar gum (37 ppm). Additionally, serum acetate increased significantly for guar gum, but decreased versus baseline for both psyllium and placebo [37]. In a third study, a double-blind, randomized, placebo-controlled design with 108 subjects who believed their "gas" symptoms (increased flatulence and bloating) were caused by ingestion of fiber, subjects were given doses of placebo 10 g, psyllium 3.4 g, methylcellulose 2 g, or lactulose 5 g (readily fermented) [39]. The lactulose group passed gas significantly more often than did the psyllium or methylcellulose groups ($p < 0.01$). Psyllium was not different from baseline or placebo for passing gas, or any other symptom [39]. Another study included 25 healthy volunteers and assessed the effects of diets supplemented with 10 g psyllium, methylcellulose, or lactulose versus placebo for reports of "gaseous" symptoms, including number of flatulence episodes, impression of increased rectal gas, and abdominal bloating [38]. Five of the subjects were also assessed for breath hydrogen excretion. The results showed that participants passed gas an average of 10 times per day during the placebo period. A significant increase in gas passages (19 times/day) and a subjective impression of increased rectal gas were reported with lactulose, but not with either of the two fiber preparations. Breath hydrogen excretion did not increase after ingestion of either of the fiber supplements. In contrast, a significant ($p < 0.05$) increase in feelings of abdominal bloating, which subjects perceived as "excessive gas", was reported with lactulose and both fiber supplements. The authors concluded that clinicians should distinguish between excessive rectal gas, which indicates excessive gas production, and feelings of bloating, which are usually unrelated to excessive gas production [38]. They recommended that treatment of excessive rectal gas consists of limiting the supply of fermentable substrates to the colonic bacteria (e.g., fermentable fibers). Symptoms of bloating without evidence of excessive rectal gas may be indicative of IBS [38]. Considering together, five clinical studies provided congruent results: objective measures of breath gas, and subjective assessments of flatulence episodes (the two mechanisms by which gas is handled in the large bowel), showed that psyllium did not increase intestinal gas. Two of these studies also assessed SCFA production [37,41]. The first study, in which subjects were fed a low fiber diet (6 g dietary fiber/day and 1–2 g resistant starch/day), showed that three of six SCFAs increased with psyllium consumption [41]. The study also showed significant increases in arabinose and xylose (the sugars that comprise psyllium), recovered in a highly polymerized form, confirming that the psyllium gel transited the large bowel intact. In contrast to the first study, the second study, in which subjects were fed a polysaccharide-free diet, showed no increase in SCFAs with psyllium dosing, supporting that psyllium is not fermented in the large bowel [37]. The SCFA increase noted in the first study was likely due to residual nutrients captured in the gel matrix and carried into the large bowel, but the amount was insufficient to be detected on breath gas analysis [37]. On the basis of these five published clinical assessments of gas production and SCFA production, it is reasonable to conclude that the psyllium gel remains intact throughout the large bowel, and is not fermented in the human gut. The data further support that *in vitro* assessments of fermentation may not always be predictive of the human experience for gel-forming fibers.

An emerging area of research is exploring the effects of fermentable fibers, some of which are prebiotics that can provide a preferred food source for specific "healthy" bacteria (typically lactic acid-producing bacteria like bifidobacteria and lactobacilli), thereby increasing the number of these bacterial species present in the large bowel [42]. A "prebiotic" has been defined as "a selectively fermented ingredient that allows specific changes in the composition and/or activity in the intestinal microflora that confers benefits upon host well-being and health" [42]. While this continues to be an area of emerging science, regulatory bodies do not yet recognize a correlation between increasing the numbers of specific gut bacteria and a clinically meaningful health benefit. The European Food Safety Authority concluded that the available clinical evidence does not establish that increasing numbers of gastrointestinal microorganisms is a beneficial physiological effect [43]. The panel further concluded that a cause and effect relationship has not been established between the consumption of prebiotics and a beneficial physiological effect related to increasing numbers of gastrointestinal microorganisms [43]. Similarly, the Dietary Guidelines for Americans 2010 Committee (DGAC) conducted a review that included prebiotics [44]. Though the DGAC believed that gut microflora play a role in health, and investigation of the gut microflora is an important emerging area of research, they concluded that there was insufficient evidence to make dietary recommendations for Americans regarding prebiotics.

8.3 PHYSICAL EFFECTS OF FIBER SUPPLEMENTS IN THE STOMACH

Anatomically, the stomach is divided into four regions (cardiac, fundus, corpus, and pyloric antrum), but functionally the stomach has only two regions: proximal (storage) and distal (antral pump) [5]. The proximal region of the stomach has rugae, accordion-like folds that can relax and stretch to accommodate a meal (Figure 8.3). When stretched (filled), the proximal stomach exerts a tonic contraction that gradually forces food into the distal portion of the stomach, where rugae give way to a smooth-walled, muscular tube called the gastric antrum (upper right corner of

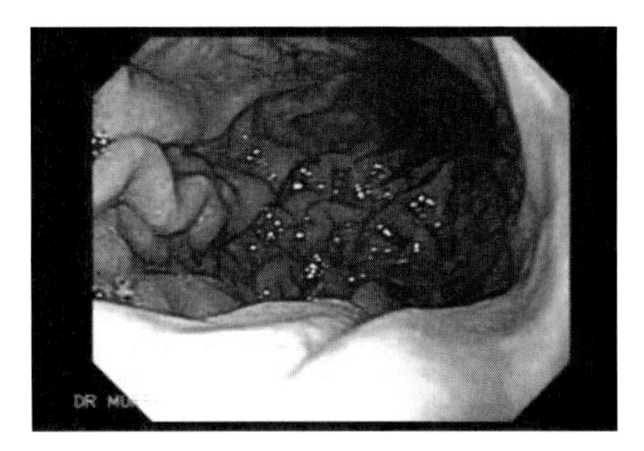

FIGURE 8.3 Endoscopic view of rugae in the proximal stomach. This is an endoscopic view of the proximal stomach. Note the mucosal folds (rugae) that allow for expansion of the proximal stomach to accommodate a meal. During the fed state, after relaxing to accommodate the meal, the proximal stomach provides tonic pressure to gradually push food toward the distal stomach. In the upper right corner of this endoscopic view, the rugae give way to a smooth-walled muscular tube (antrum), known as the "antral pump." (Reprinted with permission from Julio Murra-Saca, Chief of Department of Gastroenterology, Hospital Centro de Emergencias; El Salvador Atlas of Gastrointestinal Video Endoscopy.)

Figure 8.3). In the gastric antrum, phasic waves of contraction, known as the "antral pump," start in mid-stomach and move as a ring of contraction toward the duodenum (Figure 8.4), driving discreet boluses of gastric contents toward the pyloric sphincter [5]. The pyloric sphincter, which is normally closed (Figure 8.4a), acts at the primary gate for controlling the rate of gastric emptying. During the fed state (food in the stomach), the pyloric sphincter transiently opens (only 1–2 mm) at the beginning of an antral wave of contraction, and the progressive wave of contractions forces small boluses of liquid and small food particles (less than 2 mm) through the pyloric sphincter, into the duodenum [45]. Partially through the antral contraction, the pyloric sphincter closes, blocking the exit of gastric contents and causing pressure to build between the advancing wave of contraction and the closed pyloric sphincter. The trapped digesta is forced to "back-extrude" through the advancing fist-like wave of contraction (Figure 8.4b). This back extrusion under pressure is the grinding action of the stomach, mechanically shearing large food particles into smaller ones, and mixing food with gastric acid and pepsin (an enzyme that degrades proteins into peptides). The rate of gastric emptying is controlled by several factors, including caloric density (low calorie digesta empties faster than high calorie digesta) and meal composition (liquids empty faster than solids; low viscosity empties faster than high viscosity) [5]. The first line (immediate) control of gastric emptying is the small size of the pyloric sphincter opening (1–2 mm). A secondary control mechanism is the feedback mechanism between the duodenum and stomach that senses caloric density. A more delayed mechanism that affects the rate of gastric emptying is the "ileal brake" phenomenon. Nutrients are normally absorbed early in the small bowel. If nutrients are captured in the gel-matrix of a viscous, gelling fiber, they can be

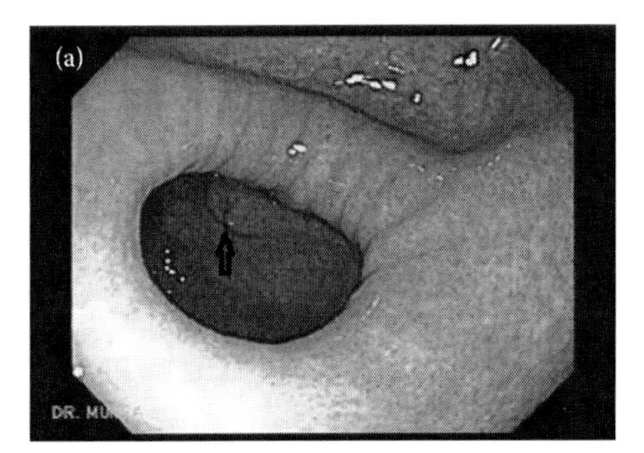

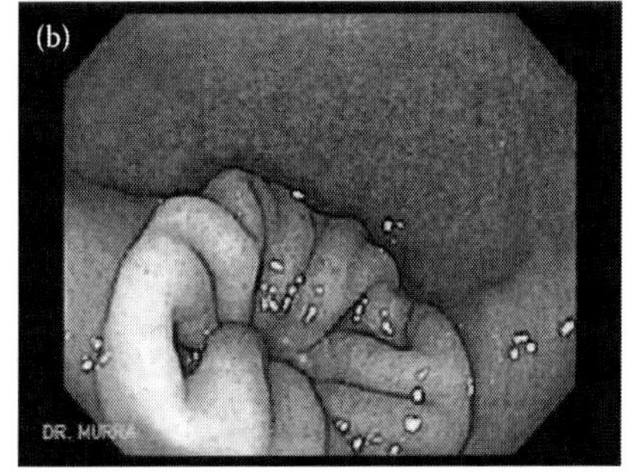

FIGURE 8.4 Endoscopic view of a peristaltic wave of contraction in the gastric antrum. This shows two endoscopic views of the distal stomach (antrum). (a) A wave-like contraction can be seen moving toward the pyloric sphincter. Early in the contraction, which is not yet lumen-occluding, the pyloric sphincter is open (1–2 mm) to allow liquids and small food particles to exit the stomach under low pressure. Mid-way through the contraction, the sphincter closes (arrow). As the peristaltic wave of contraction progresses, it becomes lumen-occluding, and gastric contents become trapped between the closed pyloric sphincter and the "fist-like" wave of contraction (b), which provides the grinding action of the stomach. (Reprinted with permission from Julio Murra-Saca, Chief of Department of Gastroenterology, Hospital Centro de Emergencias; El Salvador Atlas of Gastrointestinal Video Endoscopy.)

delivered to the distal ileum where nutrients are not usually present, stimulating a cascade of feedback mechanisms that slow gastric emptying and small bowel transit to reduce/prevent loss of nutrients to the large bowel, and release peptides that have several metabolic effects important to glycemic control (discussed in the section on small bowel effects) [5].

Published data on the effects of fiber supplements on gastric emptying show mixed results, which may be due in large part to the different methods used to assess gastric emptying. For example, if a soluble viscous/gel-forming fiber is added to a liquid test meal (e.g., glucose tolerance test), the increased viscosity provided by a gel-forming fiber would tend to slow the rate of gastric emptying [46]. In contrast, if a viscous soluble fiber is added to a solid test meal, the apparent rate of gastric emptying may not be significantly altered. For example, guar gum slows gastric emptying to a greater extent when given with a liquid meal than with a solid meal [47]. Additional studies show that guar gum and psyllium, both soluble viscous/gel-forming fibers, had no significant effect on gastric emptying when combined with a solid test meal [48] or a semi-solid test meal [49]. The observable effects of a fiber supplement on gastric emptying may also be tied to the duration of the dosing period in the study. Most studies assess gastric emptying after a single dose of fiber. A longer-term study assessed the effects of sustained fiber ingestion on gastric emptying in healthy volunteers placed on a low-fiber (3 g) diet for 2 weeks, followed by 4 weeks of an isocaloric diet supplemented with 20 g/day of either apple pectin (soluble viscous fiber) or cellulose (insoluble fiber used as a placebo) [50]. At the conclusion of each test period, subjects ingested a technetium-labeled low-fiber test breakfast. The study showed that gastric emptying was prolonged approximately two-fold after pectin supplementation ($p < 0.005$), but cellulose supplementation did not alter the rate of gastric emptying. Taken together, these data show that fiber supplements can have an effect on the rate of gastric emptying, but the outcome may be significantly affected by the study techniques employed, and the duration of the study. It should also be noted that a fiber-induced change in the rate of gastric emptying is a *mechanism* that could be a contributing factor associated with a health benefit, but an alteration in the rate of gastric emptying should not be construed as direct evidence of a clinically meaningful health benefit.

The above studies assessed an early or "immediate" effect on gastric emptying, which is primarily a function of restricted flow through the small (1–2 mm) opening in the pyloric sphincter, and calorie density (duodenal feedback). Another technique that has been used to assess the rate of gastric emptying is time to peak excretion in a 13-C breath-gas analysis. In a cross-over study, a labeled (13-C) liquid test meal (200 mL) was administered alone (control) or with 6, 12, or 18 g of psyllium fiber (soluble viscous, gel-forming, non-fermented fiber) [51]. Breath samples collected over a 4-h period showed a statistically significant, dose-dependent increase in time to peak excretion (54.5 min for control to 93.3 min for 18 g of psyllium), which was interpreted as a dose-dependent delay in gastric emptying. What is unclear, however, is the degree to which this delay in absorption is directly attributable to gastric emptying versus a viscosity-dependent delay in nutrient absorption in the small bowel. Also, note that psyllium *slowed* absorption of the liquid test meal/label, but did not change the *total* absorption of nutrients/label (assessed as area under the curve). In an earlier study that assessed the effects of the pectin (15 g) on gastric emptying and blood glucose concentration, the viscous soluble fiber slowed gastric emptying when added to both liquid and solid test meals, but only affected peak postprandial glucose concentration with the liquid test meal [52]. This suggests that the observed immediate (first hour) delay in gastric emptying with both test meals was not the mechanism driving the immediate (first hour) change observed in postprandial glucose, which was observed only with the liquid test meal. The data suggest that pectin increased the viscosity of chyme in the small bowel, thereby slowing nutrient absorption. Similarly, a placebo-controlled study that assessed the effects of psyllium (7.4 g) on gastric emptying, feelings of hunger and energy intake in 14 normal volunteers, showed that there was no psyllium-induced delay in gastric emptying, yet feelings of hunger and measures of energy intake were significantly lower with psyllium versus placebo (13 and 17% lower, respectively; $p < 0.05$) [53]. Postprandial increases in serum glucose, triglycerides, and insulin concentrations were also lower with psyllium versus placebo ($p < 0.05$). Considered together, these data support that, while a delay in gastric emptying could be a mechanism that supports a health benefit like improved glycemic control, it is apparent that a mechanism other than delayed gastric emptying is exerting a significant effect on viscous/gel-forming fiber-induced increases in satiety, decreases in energy intake, and decreases in postprandial measures of blood glucose. In conclusion, the data on the effects of fiber supplements on gastric emptying can vary depending on the study techniques used, and are not always well-correlated with a measurable health benefit.

8.4 PHYSICAL EFFECTS OF FIBER SUPPLEMENTS IN THE SMALL INTESTINE

8.4.1 Importance of Gel-Formation in the Small Intestine

The small intestine is approximately 7 meters long and divided anatomically into 3 regions: duodenum, jejunum, and ileum. The mucosa of the small intestine is studded with millions of small villi (Figure 8.5), each covered with approximately 1000 microvilli per 0.1 micron^2, making the small intestine the largest body surface exposed to the outside world (approximately 250 m^2, roughly the size of a tennis court) [5,54]. Delivery of acidic nutrients into the duodenum (proximal small bowel) stimulates the gall bladder to contract and release bile, and stimulates pancreatic secretion (inorganic = water, bicarbonate and electrolytes; organic = digestive enzymes). The total quantity of fluid absorbed by the small bowel each day is a combination of fluids consumed (about 1.5 L/day) and the digestive juices secreted (about 6 to 7 L/day). In the fed state, the motor activity of the small bowel predominantly consists of segmental (mixing) contractions [5,54]. These segmental contractions mix chyme back and forth, exposing food particles to digestive enzymes and bile, and facilitating exposure of digested nutrients to the absorptive brush border of the mucosa for absorption. Chyme, the liquid contents of the small intestine, is normally very low in viscosity, and is easily mixed with digestive enzymes for degradation and absorption of nutrients. The very large surface area of the mucosa results in efficient absorption of nutrients, which normally occurs early in the proximal

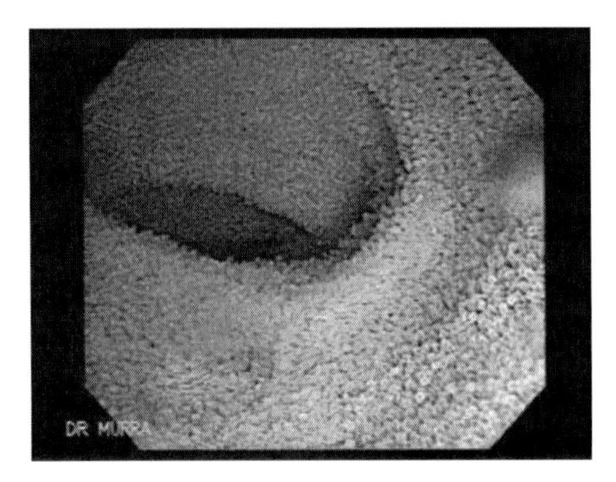

FIGURE 8.5 Endoscopic view of the mucosal villi of the small intestine. This shows an endoscopic view of the mucosa of the small intestine. Note that the mucosa is studded with millions of small villi, each covered with approximately 1000 microvilli per 0.1 micron^2. The large surface area of the small intestine (roughly the size of a tennis court) allows for efficient absorption of nutrients, which is normally accomplished early in the proximal regions of the small bowel. (Reprinted with permission from Julio Murra-Saca, Chief of Department of Gastroenterology, Hospital Centro de Emergencias; El Salvador Atlas of Gastrointestinal Video Endoscopy.)

small bowel (Figure 8.6) [5,54]. Introduction of insoluble fiber (e.g., wheat bran) or soluble non-viscous fiber (e.g., inulin, wheat dextrin) has no significant effect on the rate of nutrient absorption in the small bowel. In contrast, introduction of a soluble, viscous, gel-forming fiber (e.g., guar gum, psyllium, high molecular weight β-glucan) significantly increase the viscosity of chyme in a dose-dependent manner, which slows the mixing of chyme and slows the interactions of digestive enzymes with nutrients. This results in a slowing of the degradation of complex nutrients into simple, absorbable components, all of which slows the absorption of glucose and other nutrients (Figure 8.6) [5]. This slowing of nutrient degradation and absorption also can lead to delivery of nutrients to the distal ileum, where nutrients are not normally present (Figure 8.6). Nutrients in the distal ileum stimulate mucosal receptors to initiate several metabolic responses, one of which is the release of glucagon-like peptide 1 (GLP-1) into the blood stream. GLP-1 is a short-lived (approximately 2-min half-life) peptide that significantly decreases appetite, increases insulin secretion, decreases glucagon-secretion [a peptide that stimulates glucose production in the liver], increases pancreatic β-cell growth (cells that produce insulin), improves insulin production and sensitivity, and slows gastric emptying and small bowel transit via a feedback loop called the "ileal brake" phenomenon [5]. Considered together, the viscosity/gel-related mechanisms for improved glycemic control include: lowering of the glycemic index of ingested foods, increasing the viscosity of chyme to slow glucose absorption and starch degradation in the small bowel, and hormonal responses to delayed nutrient absorption [18,56–58]. All of these phenomena lead to a viscosity/gel-dependent improvement in glycemic control for patients with type 2 diabetes, and those at risk for developing the disease (e.g., metabolic syndrome) [5,18,59–65].

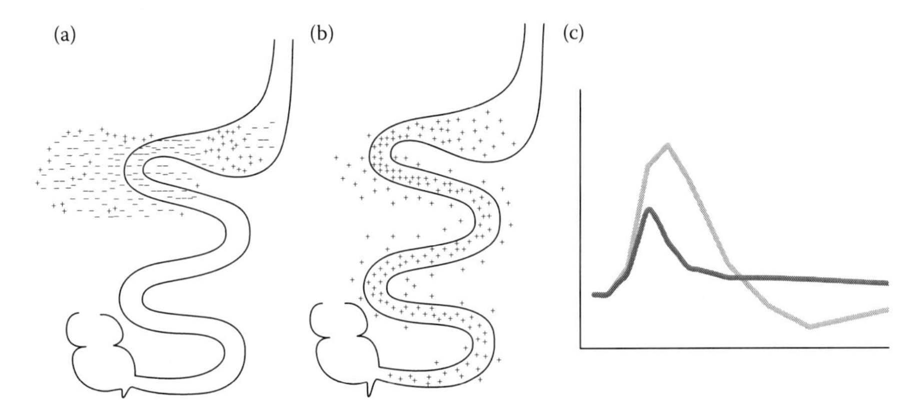

FIGURE 8.6 Absorption of nutrients in the small bowel is delayed by viscous fiber. This shows diagrams of nutrient absorption in the small bowel. Nutrients normally absorb very early in the proximal small bowel (a). Introduction of a viscous, gel-forming fiber (e.g., guar gum, psyllium, high molecular weight β-glucan) can delay nutrient absorption to more distal regions of the small bowel (b). Respective blood glucose concentrations reflect the rate of absorption in the small bowel (c). Rapid nutrient absorption (c: gray line, corresponds with (a)) is reflected by the higher peak concentration of blood glucose followed by a transient hypoglycemic trough below baseline. With the introduction of a viscous, gel-forming soluble fiber, the delay in nutrient absorption (c: black line, corresponds with (b)) results in an attenuation of glucose excursions: lower peak concentration of blood glucose, and attenuated hypoglycemic trough. The viscous/gel-forming fiber-related delay in nutrient absorption does not result in a significant difference in total nutrient absorption. (Drawings recreated with permission from Thomas Wolever, Ph.D, University of Toronto.)

Another health benefit of fiber associated with small bowel absorption is the lowering of elevated serum cholesterol concentrations, specifically low-density lipoprotein (LDL)-cholesterol. An example of this viscosity/gel-related effect is shown in a double-blind, parallel-design, multicenter clinical study that randomly assigned 386 subjects to receive cereal containing wheat fiber (negative control) or one of three oat bran cereals (high, medium, and low viscosity), equaling 3–4 g of β-glucan daily [23]. The viscosity of the cereals was altered by the degree of processing (heat and pressure) to which the fiber was exposed while making the cereal. The results showed that cholesterol lowering was highly correlated with the viscosity of the gel-forming fiber: high viscosity was correlated with significant cholesterol lowering; low viscosity was correlated with diminished cholesterol lowering. The study clearly demonstrated that the physiochemical properties of oat β-glucan were altered by processing, and the degree to which a fiber is processed before marketing should be considered when assessing the cholesterol-lowering ability of an oat-containing product. It should be noted that this study was performed with a gel-forming fiber, and the altered viscosity of the gel-forming fiber was correlated with efficacy. This does not, however, imply that simple viscosity, without gel-formation, is highly correlated with cholesterol lowering. This observation was highlighted in a placebo-controlled, randomized, parallel study of 105 patients with hypercholesterolemia that assessed the cholesterol-lowering effects of a high viscosity, gel-forming soluble fiber (psyllium) versus a viscous but non-gel-forming soluble fiber (methylcellulose) and a synthetic soluble viscous fiber (calcium polycarbophil) dosed three times a day for 8 weeks [66]. The results showed that LDL-cholesterol concentrations versus placebo were significantly lower for the gel-forming psyllium treatment group (−8.8%, $p = 0.02$), but the non-gel-forming methylcellulose and calcium polycarbophil failed to show a significant reduction in LDL-cholesterol [66]. It should be noted that raw polycarbophil is a gel-forming synthetic fiber, but the commercially available version is a calcium salt, a formulation intended to prevent gel-formation with swallowing (reduction in the risk for choking). This formulation depends on the assumption that the calcium will dissociate from the polycarbophil in the gut, allowing it to form a gel. A preclinical study, however, showed that while raw polycarbophil had a significant stool softening effect, the calcium polycarbophil formulation was not different from placebo [67]. Both the clinical cholesterol-lowering study and the preclinical stool softening study support that the calcium does not significantly dissociate from the polycarbophil in the gut, leaving the fiber inactive (non-gel-forming). Another example of the importance of gelling is raw guar gum, which is a highly viscous, gel-forming soluble fiber with proven viscosity/gel-related health benefits. The commonly marketed version of guar gum, however, is a "partially hydrolyzed guar gum" (PHGG) which, depending on the degree of hydrolysis, is non-gel-forming to improve palatability ("dissolves completely in water with no viscosity"). This non-viscous version will not provide the viscosity/gel-dependent health benefits associated with the original, gel-forming raw guar gum [68]. Considered together, these observations emphasize the importance of being cognizant of not only the specific fiber types that exhibit characteristics closely associated with specific health benefits, but also the degree of processing to which the final marketed products have been exposed. For a simple and reasonable test to determine if a fiber supplement can provide viscosity/gel-related health benefits, stir a single dose of the marketed product (usually 2–4 g fiber) into 120 mL of water, and let it sit for 15 min. If the fiber supplement does not readily dissolve in the water, then form a viscous gel within the allotted time, it is unlikely to have a clinically meaningful effect on cholesterol lowering, improved glycemic control, appetite control, or other viscosity/gel-related health benefits.

8.5 SMALL INTESTINE: CLINICAL DATA SUPPORT AN "IMPROVED GLYCEMIC CONTROL" HEALTH BENEFIT FOR GEL-FORMING SOLUBLE FIBER SUPPLEMENTS

There are two primary methods to assess the effects of fiber supplements on glycemic control. The first is an acute test on postprandial blood glucose concentrations (glucose tolerance test) in which a glucose load (e.g., 50 g glucose solution) is administered alone or with a fiber supplement (Figure 8.6). Blood glucose concentrations are drawn at frequent, pre-determined intervals over a few hours to assess the rate of glucose absorption. Glucose is normally rapidly absorbed, resulting in a relatively fast rise in blood glucose leading to a high peak concentration, followed by a relatively rapid decline, with a transient excursion below the baseline level (Figure 8.6a and c). This transient hypoglycemia is due to a rapid rise in insulin, which tends to stay elevated past the point where the blood glucose concentration has returned to baseline, resulting in transient hypoglycemia. It has been established for over three decades that the viscosity of a gel-forming dietary fiber is highly correlated with reducing postprandial glucose and insulin serum concentrations. In a study published in 1978 [68], volunteers underwent glucose (50 g) tolerance tests with and without the addition of several fiber supplements, including guar gum. Native guar gum is a highly viscous, gel-forming fiber, and it was effective in significantly lowering both postprandial blood glucose and insulin concentrations. This beneficial response, however, was abolished when the guar gum was hydrolyzed (to a non-viscous form). The study showed that a reduction in postprandial blood glucose was highly correlated with viscosity ($r = 0.926$; $p < 0.01$), and a slowing of mouth-to-cecum transit time ($r = 0.885$; $p < 0.02$). This means that high viscosity, gel-forming fiber supplements (e.g., psyllium, high molecular weight β-glucan, raw guar gum) can provide a clinically meaningful effect on elevated blood glucose, but non-viscous soluble fiber supplements (e.g., wheat dextrin, inulin) do not alter viscosity or provide a clinically meaningful glycemic benefit [4,5]. Note that the study above [68] was conducted with a gel-forming fiber, and the results stem from alteration of the viscosity of this gel-forming fiber. These data should not be construed to support a health benefit for viscosity alone, without cross-linking of fiber molecules to form a gel. All of the fiber supplements shown to improve glycemic control in patients with type 2 diabetes are gel-forming fibers.

Patients with type 2 diabetes have an impaired sensitivity to insulin and/or a decreased insulin output, resulting in an exaggerated elevation in peak postprandial glucose concentrations. An effective fiber supplement will delay glucose absorption, lowering the peak blood glucose concentration and attenuating the hypoglycemic excursion below baseline without significantly affecting total nutrient absorption (area under the curve; Figure 8.6b and c). Note that postprandial glucose studies should only be considered as a diagnostic tool for assessing patients at risk for diabetes, and a mechanistic tool for assessing the acute effects of fiber on glucose absorption. These single-meal studies do not necessarily predict a longer-term metabolic health benefit, such as improving glycemic control in type 2 diabetes. For example, acute postprandial studies of the effects of viscous fiber can show an attenuation of peak postprandial blood glucose concentrations in healthy subjects with normal glycemic control [69–72], while longer-term studies (weeks or months) do not show a reduction in the already normal blood glucose concentration of healthy subjects with normal glycemic control [73–75]. Fiber supplements will not cause hypoglycemia in healthy subjects or subjects with compromised glycemic control because suppression of glucagon by GLP-1 does not occur at hypoglycemic levels (feedback mechanism) [5]. The longer-term effects of an effective soluble viscous, gel-forming fiber on fasting blood glucose concentrations are proportional to baseline glycemic control: no significant effect on normal blood glucose concentrations in healthy subjects [73–75], a moderate effect in patients with pre-diabetes and metabolic syndrome [e.g., −19.8 mg/dL for psyllium 3.5 g bid; −9 mg/dL for guar gum 3.5 g bid] [76] and a larger effect in patients with type 2 diabetes (e.g., psyllium, −35.0 mg/dL [77] to −89.7 mg/dL [78]).

Recall that nutrients are normally absorbed early in the small bowel. Delaying the degradation and absorption of nutrients in the small bowel, leading to release of metabolically active peptides from the distal ileum, is a viscosity/gel-driven phenomenon that is not exhibited by insoluble fiber supplements (e.g., wheat bran). Similarly, there is a paucity of clinical data supporting that marketed soluble non-viscous fiber supplements (e.g., inulin, wheat dextrin), or marketed soluble viscous, non-gel forming fiber supplements (e.g., methylcellulose) exhibit a clinically meaningful, long-term effect on glycemic control at physiologic doses. To appropriately assess the long-term benefits of a soluble viscous/gel-forming fiber in subjects with impaired glycemic control, studies should include multiple daily pre-meal doses of a fiber supplement (so the fiber becomes mixed with the meal), and the assessment period should be two or more months to allow for a meaningful assessment of hemoglobin-A1c (HbA1c). HbA1c is a form of hemoglobin that becomes glycated over time, reflecting average plasma glucose concentrations over several months. As average blood glucose increases, the fraction of glycated hemoglobin increases, serving as a marker for elevated blood glucose exposure over the previous several months. Numerous multi-month clinical studies have demonstrated that consumption of a soluble, viscous/gel-forming fiber (e.g., psyllium, raw guar gum, high molecular weight β-glucan) before meals can improve glycemic control (lowers fasting blood glucose, insulin, and HbA1c concentrations) in subjects at risk for type 2 diabetes (e.g., metabolic syndrome) and in patients being treated for type 2 diabetes [4,5,23,76–89].

An example of a gel-forming fiber demonstrating long-term improved glycemic control is a double-blind, placebo-controlled clinical study designed to evaluate the effects of two doses of psyllium on fasting blood glucose and HbA1c in 37 patients already being treated (prescription hypoglycemic medications) for type 2 diabetes mellitus [82]. In this study, patients were randomly assigned to one of three treatment groups: a relatively low dose of psyllium (3.4 g twice a day), a higher dose psyllium (6.8 g twice a day), or placebo. All doses were consumed just prior to breakfast and dinner, to allow for mixing with food. The study was 20 weeks in duration (8 weeks baseline, 12 weeks treatment). Results show that psyllium treatment provided a statistically significant ($p < 0.05$) lowering of fasting blood glucose concentrations (versus placebo) at treatment weeks 4, 8, and 12 (Figure 8.7a) that was directionally dose-responsive (Figure 8.7a). The results were similar for HbA1c (Figure 8.7b). Note that the improvement in glycemic control observed with both doses of psyllium was above that already conferred by a restricted diet (all patients) and a stable dose of a sulfonylurea (81.1% of patients) [82].

In summary, when considered across studies, the effects of a viscous, gel-forming fiber supplement (e.g., raw guar gum, psyllium, high molecular weight β-glucan) on glycemic control are heavily influenced by the baseline fasting blood glucose concentrations (e.g., degree of loss of glycemic control): no effect on normal fasting blood glucose concentrations, a moderate effect on moderately elevated fasting blood glucose concentrations, and a markedly greater effect in patients with significantly elevated fasting blood glucose concentrations. It is important to note that consumption of viscous, gel-forming fiber supplements will not cause blood glucose concentrations to drop below normal limits (hypoglycemia), because the suppression of glucagon by GLP-1 does not occur at hypoglycemic levels. When initiating an effective fiber therapy in patients already being treated for diabetes with prescription drugs, however, it is important to monitor blood glucose concentrations, as an

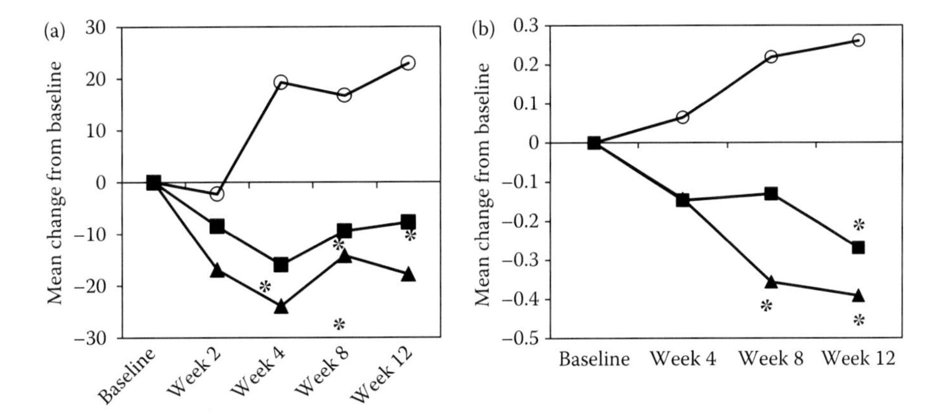

FIGURE 8.7 Psyllium lowers fasting blood glucose and HbA1c in patients with type 2 diabetes. (a) A graph of fasting blood glucose concentration (mg/dL) as a response to treatment. Both doses of psyllium significantly ($p < 0.05$) lowered fasting blood glucose compared to placebo at weeks 4, 8, and 12 (placebo = circle; psyllium 3.4 g BID = square; psyllium 6.8 g BID = triangle). (b) A graph of HbA1c (%) as a response to treatment. Pysllium 6.8 g BID significantly ($p < 0.05$) lowered HbA1c compared to placebo at week 8, and both doses of psyllium significantly ($p < 0.05$) lowered HbA1c compared to placebo at week 12 (placebo = circle; psyllium 3.4 g BID = square; psyllium 6.8 g BID = triangle). (Reprinted with permission from Feinglos, M. et al. 2013. *Bioact Carbohydr Diet Fibre.* 1, 156–161.)

effective gel-forming fiber co-therapy may decrease the required doses of the prescription hypoglycemic drugs. Insoluble fiber (e.g., wheat bran), soluble non-viscous fiber (e.g., inulin, wheat dextrin), and soluble viscous non-gel forming fiber (e.g., methylcellulose) have no significant glycemic benefit, and have been used as placebo controls in clinical studies of soluble viscous, gel-forming fibers.

8.5.1 Small Intestine: Reduced Risk of Cardiovascular Disease by Lowering Serum Cholesterol

It is well established that reducing serum LDL-cholesterol concentration reduces the risk of coronary artery disease [90]. It had been estimated that a 1% reduction in LDL-cholesterol reduces the risk of coronary artery disease by 1.2–2.0% [91]. It is also well-established that a soluble viscous, gel-forming fiber can lower serum total- and LDL-cholesterol, and the degree of cholesterol lowering is highly correlated with the viscosity of the gel-forming fiber: high viscosity is correlated with significant cholesterol lowering; low viscosity is correlated with diminished/no appreciable cholesterol lowering [23]. Clinical studies have shown that the viscosity of a gel-forming fiber is actually a better predictor of cholesterol lowering efficacy than the quantity of fiber consumed [24]. The primary mechanism by which soluble gel-forming fibers lower serum cholesterol is by trapping and eliminating bile. Bile is secreted by the liver (normally 600–1000 mL/day) to emulsify large fat particles into many small particles for digestion by lipase enzymes and absorption across the mucosa [54]. Bile is normally recovered in the distal ileum and recycled, potentially several times within a single meal. When bile is trapped in a gel-forming fiber and eliminated via stool, the liver must produce more bile to meet digestive needs. Cholesterol is a component of bile, and the liver uses serum stores of cholesterol to generate more bile, effectively lowering serum LDL-cholesterol and total-cholesterol, without affecting HDL cholesterol [92].

To assess the importance of viscosity/gel-formation for cholesterol lowering, a clinical study in 26 patients with hypercholesterolemia compared the cholesterol-lowering effects of a medium-viscosity blend of gel-forming fibers (psyllium, pectin, guar gum, and locust bean gum) compared with an equal amount of low-viscosity gum Arabic (Acacia gum, highly branched) [93]. The fibers were consumed in a beverage three times daily (5 g/serving) for 4 weeks. Diet, exercise, and body weight were held constant. The medium-viscosity gel-forming blend exhibited a 10% reduction in total cholesterol ($p < 0.01$) and a 14% reduction in LDL-cholesterol ($p < 0.001$), with no significant change in HDL or triglycerides. In contrast, the low-viscosity gum Arabic-treated group showed no change in any plasma lipid characteristics [93]. A second publication with 4 studies (duration 4–12 weeks) explored the plasma lipid-lowering effects of a variety of soluble dietary fibers [94]. The studies were randomized, double-blind, placebo-controlled trials involving men and women with hyperlipidemia (plasma cholesterol >200 mg/dL). Low viscosity gum Arabic (acacia gum) consumed for 4 weeks as the sole fiber source (15 g/day) or the primary fiber source in a soluble fiber blend (17 g/day; 56% acacia gum) did not produce a significant lipid-lowering effect versus placebo. In contrast, 15 g/day of a medium-viscosity blend of soluble fibers (psyllium, pectin, guar gum, and locust bean gum) consumed for 4 weeks yielded significant reductions in total cholesterol (8.3%) and LDL-cholesterol (12.4%)($p < 0.001$) that were comparable to 10 g/day high-viscosity raw guar gum. Note that the lipid-lowering benefit of the medium viscosity blend of soluble fibers (psyllium, pectin, guar gum, and locust bean gum) showed a dose-response effect for reducing LDL-cholesterol: placebo +0.8%; 5 g/day—5.6%; 10 g/day—6.8%, and 15 g/day—14.9% (all doses $p < 0.01$ versus placebo). The effects of the soluble viscous/gel-forming fibers on plasma lipids were similar in both men and women. The authors concluded that the findings support the usefulness of soluble viscous/gel-forming fibers as a cholesterol lowering therapy, but cautioned against ascribing cholesterol lowering benefits solely on a classification of solubility [94]. As with improved glycemic control, viscosity/gel-formation is a key driver of efficacy for lowering cholesterol in patients with hyperlipidemia.

Low viscosity fiber supplements (gum Arabic/acacia gum), non-viscous fiber supplements (e.g., inulin, wheat dextrin) and viscous non-gel forming fiber supplements (e.g., methylcellulose) will not exhibit a significant cholesterol-lowering benefit [23,66,93–95]. In contrast, viscous, gel-forming fiber supplements (e.g., psyllium, pectin, guar gum, locust bean gum) will exhibit a significant cholesterol lowering benefit if the final processing of the marketed product has not significantly altered the viscosity/gelling capacity of the raw fiber [4,5,23,24,66,73,76–78,96–98]. For example, two clinical studies investigated the effects of β-glucan from oat bran, either baked into bread and cookies (study 1), or provided as a raw fiber in orange juice (study 2), on serum cholesterol in 48 subjects with hypercholesterolemia [87].

In study 1, subjects completed a 3-week baseline with control bread and cookies rich in wheat fiber (insoluble, no effect on cholesterol) followed by a 4-week treatment period where they were randomly assignment to remain on the control fiber products (placebo), or switch to bread and cookies enriched with β-glucan (5.9 g/day). The β-glucan baked into bread and cookies had no effect on serum LDL-cholesterol as compared to the control fiber. In contrast, study 2 provided a lower dose of β-glucan (5 g/day) in orange juice, which significantly decreased LDL-cholesterol versus the wheat fiber control ($p < 0.001$). The authors concluded that food matrix, food processing, or both, could adversely affect the cholesterol-lowering efficacy of β-glucan [87]. This emphasizes the importance of recognizing that not all marketed fiber supplements will provide the clinical efficacy of the original raw fiber.

As mentioned above for glycemic control, it is not only important to recognize the specific fiber in a supplement to understand its potential health benefits, but also the degree and type of processing the raw fiber has been exposed to in preparing the marketed product. As discussed previously, the cholesterol-lowering effectiveness of β-glucan depends on its ability to retain its gelling nature, significantly increase the viscosity of chyme, and trap/eliminate bile. The viscosity/gelling nature of β-glucan, in turn, is determined by its molecular weight (chain length), which can be influenced by methods of processing and storage of the final fiber product [23]. High and medium molecular weight cereals significantly lowered serum LDL-cholesterol (high viscosity > medium viscosity) versus wheat bran, while low molecular weight β-glucan (low viscosity) failed to show a significant difference versus wheat bran. Also remember that within a given viscous/gel-forming fiber (e.g., β-glucan), molecular weight correlates with viscosity. It is across fiber comparisons of molecular weight that may *not* be predictive of viscosity (straight chain versus highly branched). Considered together, these studies support that the cholesterol lowering benefit of fiber supplements is proportional to the viscosity of gel-forming fibers. The higher the viscosity of a marketed gel-forming fiber supplement product when hydrated, the greater the potential cholesterol lowering benefit. Again, the simple test referred to previously can be conducted to predict the potential cholesterol-lowering benefit of a fiber supplement.

As with glycemic control, the potential for a cholesterol lowering benefit is also highly influenced by the baseline cholesterol level: soluble viscous, gel-forming fibers have no appreciable effect on cholesterol concentrations in healthy subjects with normal cholesterol concentrations, but exhibit a progressively greater benefit as baseline cholesterol exceeds normal concentrations. Also, as observed with improved glycemic control, the cholesterol-lowering benefit of soluble viscous, gel-forming fiber supplements is observed in addition to the benefits conveyed by the prescription drugs in patients already being treated for hyperlipidemia. Eight clinical studies have shown that psyllium (gel-forming fiber) enhanced the cholesterol lowering benefit of prescription drugs when dosed as a co-therapy to statin drugs (class of drugs used to lower cholesterol levels by inhibiting the enzyme HMG-CoA reductase) or bile sequestrants (bind bile in the gastrointestinal tract to prevent its re-absorption) [96–104]. Also, as with improved glycemic control, a soluble viscous gel-forming fiber supplement can lower the required dose of a prescription statin drug. In a 12-week randomized, double-blind study including 68 patients with hyperlipidemia, a low dose of simvastatin (10 mg) combined with psyllium (15 g/day) was superior to the low dose of simvastatin alone (–63 mg/dL versus –55 mg/dL, respectively; $p = 0.03$), and identical to a high dose of simvastatin (20 mg, –63 mg/dL) for lowering elevated serum LDL-cholesterol concentration [99].

8.5.2 Small Intestine: Effectiveness of Fiber Supplements on Satiety and Weight Loss

The Center for Disease Control has declared obesity an epidemic in the United States [105]. More than one-third of United States adults (35.7%) are obese, and obesity-related conditions include heart disease, stroke, type 2 diabetes, and certain types of cancer [105]. The estimated annual medical cost of obesity in the U.S. was $147 billion in 2008 [105]. Observational studies have shown an inverse association between body weight and high intakes of dietary fiber (e.g., replacement), and a high-level of dietary fiber consumption can reduce the risk for gaining weight or developing obesity by approximately 30% [106–108]. Early clinical studies dosed fiber supplements to facilitate weight loss [109,110]. Epidemiologic studies show that diets high in fiber and whole grains are associated with lower body weight, and prevention of weight gain, compared to diets low in fiber and whole grains [111,112]. As discussed in previous sections, however, care must be taken when attributing health benefits to "fiber supplements" in general, as they reflect a heterogeneous group of fibers sources that differ in their physicochemical properties, and ability to affect appetite and energy intake [113–116]. It is also important to understand the terminology, for while "satiation" and "satiety" are often used interchangeably, their actual meaning is different. Satiation is your reaction during a meal that causes you to stop eating a given meal. Satiety is the response to availability of nutrients from food consumed, that is being/has been digested. So claims relative to "feel full longer" and "helps you feel less hungry between meals" are related to satiety. A recent comprehensive review of available clinical data concluded that resistant starch (soluble, non-viscous, fermentable) (e.g., wheat dextrin) had no significant effect on satiety or weight loss at physiologic doses [117]. A year-long study in 97 adolescents has been quoted as demonstrating weight loss for a "prebiotic" fiber supplement (soluble, non-viscous, fermentable), but a closer look at the data shows that the prebiotic fiber group (8 g/day) was not different from baseline for body mass index (BMI) [118]. The study appeared to show a favorable result because there was a significant increase in BMI in the control group (fed maltodextrin, readily digested/absorbed as glucose), so at best an argument could be made that the prebiotic fiber was a healthier option than the maltodextrin substitute, but the data do not support a claim for weight loss [118].

In contrast to non-viscous, fermentable fiber supplements (e.g., inulin, wheat dextrin), soluble viscous, gel-forming fibers, such as guar gum, pectin, and psyllium, have been shown to increase satiety and reduce subsequent energy intake [119–121]. A well-cited experiment on fiber-induced satiety demonstrated that apples were significantly more satiating than fiber-free apple juice, even though the juice provided the same level of carbohydrate as the apples [122]. Pectin, the soluble viscous, gel-forming fiber present in apples, has been shown to delay gastric emptying and increase satiety [123]. Soluble, viscous, gel-forming fibers can influence satiety by several mechanisms mentioned previously, including delayed degradation and absorption of nutrients in the small bowel, leading to a "sustained" delivery of nutrients, and delivery of nutrients to the distal ileum with subsequent stimulation of feedback mechanism like the "ileal brake" phenomenon and decreased appetite [4,5,114–116]. Some studies of the effects of gel-forming fiber on satiety used either an insoluble fiber or a soluble non-viscous fiber as a negative control, supporting the assertion that the effect on satiety for fiber supplements is proportional to viscosity/gel-formation [21,23–25,119,124]. Satiety often is assessed in short-term clinical studies as a tool or mechanism for predicting the potential for weight-loss effects, but the end therapeutic goal is weight loss (or prevention of weight re-gain). Showing a long-term (e.g., 6-months or longer) reduction in body weight in a clinical study, however, can be much more challenging than a short-term difference in satiety. A review of the effects of fiber supplements on weight loss [125] identified 17 placebo-controlled clinical studies. In most studies, subjects were maintained on energy-restricted diets, and fiber supplements (mostly insoluble fiber) were provided three times daily before meals. Fiber supplement intake ranged from 4.5 to 20 g/day. Results show that only 1 of 17 studies provided evidence of weight loss greater than placebo [125].

One factor that may not have been considered in previous weight loss studies is the degree of fermentation of the fiber supplements tested. Fermentation of a fiber supplement releases nutrients into the gut that are absorbed into the blood stream, so fermentable fibers are not calorie free. A 6-month study compared objective measures of health benefits for a viscous, gel-forming, non-fermented fiber (psyllium) versus a less viscous, readily fermented fiber (PHGG) [76]. This randomized, controlled, 6-month study included 141 patients with metabolic syndrome maintained on a restricted diet alone (negative control) or the restricted diet supplemented with psyllium or PHGG (both dosed 3.5 g twice a day with breakfast and dinner). The control group (restricted diet alone) showed a gradual loss in weight over the first 4 months, followed by a gradual weight re-gain. After 2 months, the guar gum treatment group showed a marked weight reduction (–2.4 kg versus baseline), but this reversed to weight re-gain over the following 4 months (Figure 8.8). In contrast, the psyllium treatment group showed gradual and continued weight loss across the 6-month test period. At 6 months, weight loss for the psyllium treatment group was –3.3 kg versus baseline, –2.1 kg versus placebo, and –1.76 kg versus guar gum ($p < 0.01$ for all 3 comparisons; Figure 8.8) [76]. The data suggest that two fiber characteristics, high viscosity/gel-forming, and non-fermented, played key roles in the greater long-term weight loss observed in the psyllium treatment group. This study also emphasizes the importance of longer-term studies. The conclusions drawn from this study would be quite different had it stopped at 2 or 4 months, potentially affecting the clinical advice offered to patients/clients, and their future success in weight loss/maintenance programs [76].

8.5.3 Small Intestines: Effectiveness of Fiber Supplements in Metabolic Syndrome

According to the International Diabetes Federation, Metabolic Syndrome is defined as a cluster of the most dangerous heart attack risk factors: diabetes and raised

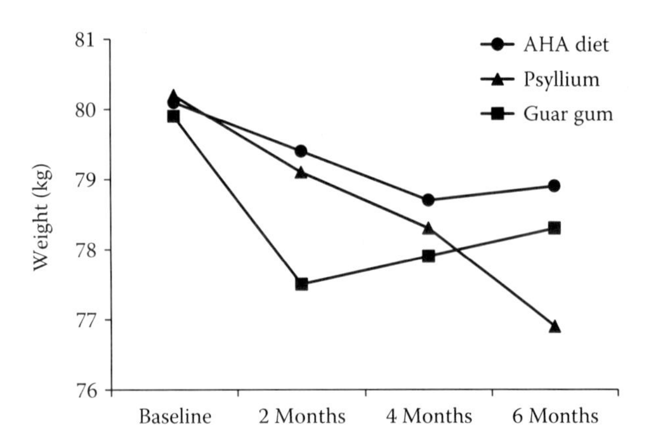

FIGURE 8.8 Both viscosity and fermentation affect fiber supplement-related weight loss efficacy. In a 6-month study in patients with Metabolic Syndrome, a restricted diet alone showed a modest weight loss over 4 months, followed by weight re-gain. In addition to the restricted diet, psyllium (3.5 g twice a day), a viscous, gel-forming, non-fermented fiber supplement, showed sustained weight loss over a 6-month study [76]. In contrast, PHGG, a less viscous readily fermented fiber at the same dose and restricted diet, showed a marked weight loss followed by weight re-gain. The data support that clinical studies assessing weight loss should be at least 6 months in length. The data further support that psyllium (viscous, gel-forming, not fermented), in conjunction with a healthy diet, is more effective for long-term weight loss than a healthy diet alone, or a healthy diet with a less viscous, fermented fiber (PHGG). (Figure recreated with permission from McRorie J, Fahey G. 2013. *Clin Nurs Stud.* 1(4), 82–92.)

fasting plasma glucose, abdominal obesity, high cholesterol, and high blood pressure [126]. The Federation also states that people with metabolic syndrome are twice as likely to die from, and three times as likely to have, a heart attack or stroke compared with patients without the syndrome, and have a five-fold greater risk of developing type 2 diabetes [126]. It was estimated that 1/4 of adults worldwide have Metabolic Syndrome [126]. Given the growing evidence that soluble viscous, gel-forming fiber supplementation improves indices related to insulin resistance [78,81,127,128], cholesterol lowering, improved glycemic control and weight loss, all risks associated with metabolic syndrome, it is reasonable to predict that viscous/gel-forming fibers will also show efficacy in attenuating objective clinical measures of Metabolic Syndrome. In the same 6-month study mentioned above, the investigators assessed the clinical benefits of two soluble viscous fibers in 141 patients with metabolic syndrome [76]. Patients were fed an American Heart Association step-2 diet alone (control), or the same diet supplemented with psyllium or guar gum (both dosed at 3.5 g twice a day with breakfast and dinner). After 6 months of treatment, both psyllium and guar gum treatment groups showed significant improvement in BMI (–7.2% versus –6.5%), fasting plasma glucose (–27.9% versus –11.1%), fasting plasma insulin (–20.4% versus –10.8%), HbA1c (–10.4% versus –10.3%), and LDL cholesterol (–7.9% versus –8.5%), respectively [76]. Only the psyllium group exhibited a significant improvement in plasma triglyceride concentration (–13.3%) and systolic (–3.9%) and diastolic (–2.6%) blood pressure. At the conclusion of the study, 12.5% of patients in the psyllium group no longer qualified for a diagnosis of Metabolic Syndrome, versus 2.1% of patients in the guar gum group and 0% of patients in the diet-alone group [76]. Considered together, these data support that a soluble viscous, gel-forming fiber supplement can be an effective co-therapy for treating Metabolic Syndrome.

8.6 PHYSICAL EFFECTS OF FIBER SUPPLEMENTS IN THE LARGE INTESTINE

The large intestine is comprised of the cecum (most proximal portion, receives liquid residue from ileum), the colon (ascending, transverse, descending, and sigmoid), the rectum, and the anus. The large bowel exhibits a series of chambers known as "haustrations" (Figure 8.9), and a triangular appearance duc to the three strips of longitudinal muscle known as "taenia coli" (Figure 8.9) [5,54]. Approximately 1500 mL of liquid residue arrives in the large intestine daily. Normally, over 90% of the water and electrolytes that arrive in the cecum are absorbed by the large intestine, eventually resulting in formed stool. The motor events of the large intestine are approximately 95% segmental ("mixing" waves) that facilitate the absorption of water and electrolytes, while the remaining approximately 5% are propagating contractions (peristalsis) [129]. Propagating contractions in the large bowel occur across a wide range of amplitudes and propagating rates, where amplitude is inversely proportional to propagation rate (high amplitude = slowly propagating; low amplitude = rapidly propagating) [129]. The rate of propagation is also proportional to

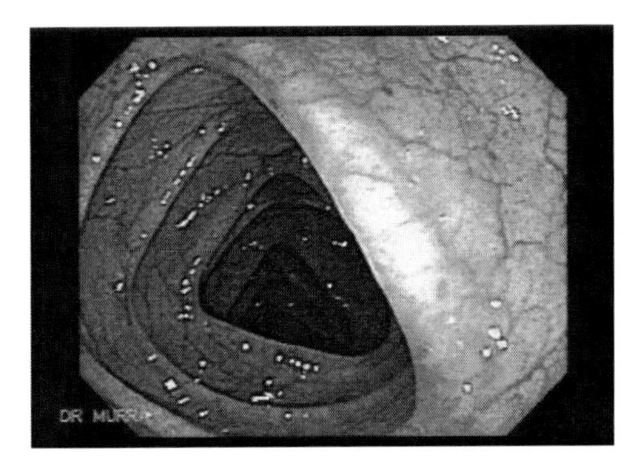

FIGURE 8.9 Endoscopic view of the large intestine. This is an endoscopic view of the large intestine. As opposed to the millions of villi that stud the mucosa of the small intestine (Figure 8.5), the mucosa in the large intestine is relatively smooth (no villi, smaller surface area), but still highly vascular. Note the segmented appearance (haustra) of the large bowel, and the triangular appearance of each chamber resulting from the three strips of longitudinal muscle (taenia coli) on the surface of the large bowel. (Reprinted with permission from Julio Murra-Saca, Chief of Department of Gastroenterology, Hospital Centro de Emergencias; El Salvador Atlas of Gastrointestinal Video Endoscopy.)

the frequency of the specific wave types (slowly propagating = few per day; rapidly propagating = many per day) [129]. The two proportionalities provide a wide range of propagating contractions. At one extreme, high amplitude (>100 mm Hg), slowly propagating (≤1 cm/s) contractions are infrequent (≤6/day) lumen-occluding events that propel all large bowel contents (gas, liquids, soft to hard stool) toward the anus. At the other extreme, low amplitude (10 mm Hg), rapidly propagating (≥10 cm/s) contractions are frequent events (≥30/day) that act like a "squeegee" to propel gas more rapidly than all other gut contents. There are also "medium amplitude/propagating rate" contractions that populate the middle of the range, between extremes [5,54,129–132].

When considered in light of the different viscosities present in the large bowel (e.g., gas, liquid/loose/soft/formed/hard stool), the rate of transit through the large intestine is a function of the frequency and amplitude/rate of propagating contractions versus the viscosity of the substrate [129]. For example, gas is propelled by all propagating contractions, from infrequent high amplitude slowly propagating contractions (HAPCs) that are lumen-occluding events that propel all contents, to frequent low amplitude, rapidly propagating contractions that propel only gas, making gas the most rapidly propelled substrate in the gut. Gas can transit the entire gastrointestinal tract in less than 1 h (flatulence approximately 14 episodes/day) [5,129]. Liquid stool is propelled by all but the smallest/fastest propagating contractions that propel only gas, resulting in rapid transit through the large bowel (e.g., diarrhea) and the potential for multiple bowel movements a day [5]. In contrast, formed or hard stool is only propelled by infrequent HAPCs, and transit through the chambered large bowel can require days (approximately one bowel movement/day) [5]. This is why fiber that retains its gel-forming nature and exerts a significant stool softening (water-holding) effect can result in faster transit and more frequent bowel movements, which can provide clinical relief from constipation.

8.6.1 Large Bowel Effects: Fiber Benefits in Patients with Constipation and Diarrhea

The laxative effects of fiber can be driven by several different physicochemical properties of fiber. Despite the lack of water-holding capacity, insoluble fiber (e.g., wheat bran) can increase fecal mass and colonic transit rate by mechanical stimulation (irritation) of gut mucosa, inducing secretion and peristalsis [4,5,67,130]. The importance of this effect was illustrated in an early study comparing the laxative efficacy of wheat bran, ground to varying particle sizes, with that of inert plastic particles, cut in size to match the different wheat bran particles. Note that plastic particles are not fermented and have no water-holding capacity [133]. The laxative effect of the wheat bran was comparable to that of the plastic particles: a greater laxative effect was associated with larger particles, while no laxative effect was observed with fine particles. A subsequent investigation confirmed that the stimulatory effect of particles in the intestinal lumen depends on both particle size and shape, with large coarse (gritty) particles having a greater laxative benefit than fine, smooth particles [134]. Thus, insoluble fiber can provide a laxative benefit, but only if the fiber supplement provides large, coarse particles. Highly processed, finely ground insoluble fiber (e.g., whole wheat flour) will not provide a significant laxative benefit. Further, with no water-holding capacity and no gel-forming capacity, insoluble fiber supplements cannot be of benefit for attenuating loose/liquid stools in diarrhea. The mucosal stimulating/irritating effect of insoluble particles could actually make symptoms of diarrhea worse [135].

Soluble non-viscous, readily fermented fiber supplements (e.g., wheat dextrin, inulin) dissolve in water with no appreciable change to viscosity, and are readily fermented in the large bowel, resulting in dose-dependent gas production and an increase in flatulence, but without a significant laxative benefit at physiologic doses [4,5,136–138]. Similarly, viscous soluble fibers that are readily fermented (e.g., β-glucan, guar gum) will also result in a dose-dependent increase in gas formation, leading to a potential increase in flatulence, but fermentation of the fiber results in loss of viscosity and water-holding capacity, resulting in a no appreciable laxative benefit at physiological doses [37,40,60].

There are few studies on the effects of readily fermented fibers on diarrhea in adults. A study of antibiotic-induced diarrhea had patients consume oligofructose (12 g/day) while taking a broad-spectrum antibiotic for 7 days, followed by another 7 days of the prebiotic therapy (after stopping the antibiotic therapy) [139]. The study showed that the readily fermented fiber was not different from placebo for the incidence of diarrhea, *Clostridium difficile* infections, or hospital stays. Another study assessed the risk of developing traveler's diarrhea, and reported that consumption of fructooligosaccharides (10 g/day) for a 2-week pre-travel period, and continued during the 2-week travel period to destinations of medium and high risk, had no effect on the prevention of traveler's diarrhea [140]. Another study of traveler's diarrhea was a placebo-controlled, randomized, double blind of parallel design in 159 healthy volunteers who traveled for minimum of 2 weeks to a country of low or high risk for travelers diarrhea [141]. In this study, a novel galactooligosaccharide (GOS; 5.5 g/day) was compared to placebo (maltodextrin), and the results showed significant improvement with GOS versus control for the incidence ($p < 0.05$) and duration ($p < 0.05$) of travelers diarrhea. While prebiotics remain an area of emerging science, and there is a rationale for the use of soluble, non-viscous, readily fermented fibers in the prevention of infectious diseases, the totality of clinical data for currently marketed non-viscous, readily fermented fiber supplements is mixed at best, and does not readily support a clinically meaningful benefit in attenuating symptoms of constipation or diarrhea at physiologic doses.

For a fiber supplement to be beneficial in attenuating both constipation and diarrhea, it should have high water-holding capacity, and retain its gelled, visco-elastic nature throughout the large bowel. In other words, it should be a gel-forming fiber that is not fermented. Most soluble viscous, gel-forming fiber supplements (e.g., guar gum, Acacia gum, β-glucan from oats and barley) are readily fermented in the large bowel, resulting in a loss of their gelled nature, leading to no significant benefit for improving symptoms of constipation or diarrhea [4,5,60]. In contrast to the other fiber supplements discussed above (poorly fermented insoluble fiber, readily fermented soluble non-viscous fibers, and readily fermented soluble viscous fibers), a fourth fiber category exists that is soluble, viscous, gel-forming, and non-fermented. This fiber category (i.e., psyllium) maintains its gelled state/

water-holding capacity throughout the large bowel [67]. Consumption of a gel-forming, non-fermented fiber with high water-holding capacity results in a dose-related formation of high moisture, soft, bulky stools [67,142–144], without an increase in gas production or flatulence [37–41]. Further, a fiber that retains its gel/water-holding capacity throughout the large bowel provides a dichotomous, "stool normalizing" effect: it decreases the viscosity of hard stool in constipation (softer stool, increased transit rate, improved bowel movement frequency) [144], and improves the viscosity of loose/liquid stool in diarrhea (firmer stool, slower transit rate, less frequent bowel movements) [145–147]. Stool consistency is highly correlated with stool water content, and a relatively small change in stool water content (e.g., an increase of 5% water content) can lead to a relatively large stool softening effect (five-fold difference in stool viscosity) [67]. In a randomized, double-blind, clinical study, 170 patients with chronic idiopathic constipation underwent 2 weeks of therapy with either a gel-forming, non-fermented fiber (psyllium, 5.1 g twice daily) or a marketed stool softener, docusate sodium (100 mg twice daily) [144]. Results show that psyllium was superior to docusate for increasing stool water content ($p = 0.007$) and the frequency of bowel movements ($p = 0.02$) [144]. The stool softening effect of psyllium gradually increased over the treatment period, suggesting that the stool softening benefit would not be lost with long-term daily dosing. The American College of Gastroenterology Chronic Constipation Task Force systematically reviewed the available clinical evidence regarding the use of fiber supplements in chronic constipation, and concluded that there was insufficient clinical evidence to support a recommendation for calcium polycarbophil, methylcellulose, or bran, but concluded that psyllium was the only fiber supplement with sufficient clinical evidence to support a recommendation for treatment of chronic constipation (Grade B recommendation) [148]. Clinical studies have also documented the beneficial effects of psyllium in attenuating symptoms in diarrhea, including reducing the frequency of bowel movements and improving stool form in chronic diarrhea [147,149], lactulose-induced diarrhea [150], Crohn's disease [151], and phenolphthalein-induced diarrhea [146]. Taken together, the clinical data support that two fiber supplements can provide a significant health benefit for constipation (e.g., insoluble bran of sufficient coarseness, and psyllium), where as only one fiber supplement (psyllium) has been shown to act as a stool normalizer, softening hard stool in constipation and firming loose/liquid stool in diarrhea [5].

8.6.2 Large Bowel Effects: Fiber Benefits in Patients with Irritable Bowel Syndrome

Another potential area of benefit for fiber supplements is a functional bowel disorder known as IBS. IBS is manifested by chronic, recurring abdominal discomfort/pain often associated with disturbed bowel habit, but in the absence of structural abnormalities that would account for the symptoms [152]. In addition to abdominal discomfort/pain, typical symptoms can include sensations of distension, cramping, bloating, flatulence, and changes in stool form and frequency. The use of dietary fiber is frequently recommended to normalize bowel function and reduce pain in patients with IBS, but, as discussed above, not all fiber supplements are equal in clinically-demonstrated efficacy [153–155]. A randomized 12-week clinical study in a primary care setting included 275 patients (aged 18–65 years) with IBS, and assessed the effectiveness of a soluble fiber supplement (psyllium 10 g), an insoluble fiber supplement (wheat bran 10 g), or placebo (rice flour) in two daily doses taken with meals [154]. The primary end point was adequate symptom relief, analyzed after 1, 2, and 3 months of treatment to assess both short-term and sustained effectiveness. Results showed that the proportion of responders was significantly greater in the psyllium group than in the placebo group, and bran was not different from placebo. After three months of treatment, symptom severity in the psyllium group was reduced by 90 points, compared with 49 points in the placebo group ($p = 0.03$). Again, the bran group was not different from placebo. The authors concluded that "psyllium offers benefits in patients with IBS in primary care" [154]. A recent (2013) comprehensive review on the effects of fiber in functional bowel disorders assessed a wide range of products, including oligosaccharides, pectin, guar gum, oats, inulin, psyllium, wheat bran, flax seed, cellulose, and methylcellulose [155]. The authors determined that knowing the relative degree to which a fiber is fermented is of clinical importance when making a recommendation [155]. The byproducts of fermentation can affect gastrointestinal function and sensation, and rapid gas production can lead to increased flatulence and other gastrointestinal symptoms. The authors concluded that a recommendation for psyllium was best supported by the available clinical evidence [155], and a subsequent published letter to the editor [156] further clarified the clinical data supporting that psyllium is not fermented in the gut. An earlier systematic review, conducted by the American College of Gastroenterology Task Force on IBS, also concluded that psyllium was effective for IBS, and assigned it a conditional recommendation [153].

In contrast, in a meta-analysis of five studies that compared insoluble bran with either a low fiber diet or placebo, bran failed to improve overall IBS symptoms [157]. Insoluble fibers, including wheat bran and corn bran, are not recommended for routine use in patients with IBS. Not only have these insoluble fibers not demonstrated efficacy over placebo in this setting, some studies also suggest that bran, with its mechanical stimulation/irritation of the gut mucosa, may worsen IBS symptoms [135,158]. A few studies have assessed the efficacy of soluble non-viscous, readily fermented fibers in adult patients with IBS. One study [159] assessed the effects of a 20 g dose of a readily fermented fructooligosaccharide, and found that after 4–6 weeks on treatment, IBS symptoms became markedly worse versus placebo. With continued dosing (out to 12 weeks), an apparent adaptation occurred, and symptoms returned to a level not significantly different from placebo. A reasonable conclusion is that large doses of any fermentable fiber should not be recommended to patients with IBS. A second study found that a more modest dose (6 g/day) of oligofructose had no effect on IBS symptoms [160]. A third study again assessed a relatively modest dose of fermentable short chain fructooligosaccharides (5 g/day for 6 week) in patients with IBS symptoms, and showed a statistically significant improvement in symptoms versus placebo, but less than half of the 105 randomized subjects were included in the per-protocol analysis, and no intent-to-treat analysis was provided for efficacy [161]. A fourth study assessed the effects of 6 weeks of treatment with a trans-galactooligosaccharide at two dose levels (3.5 or 7 g/day) versus placebo, and found that the lowest dose significantly improved bloating, flatulence, and abdominal pain, while the 7 g dose did not improve any of these three symptoms of IBS [162]. Considered together, these data support that insoluble fiber supplements (e.g., wheat bran, corn bran) and fermentable fiber supplements (e.g., inulin, wheat dextrin, polydextrose, Acacia, maltodextrin, guar gum) should not be recommended for patients with IBS. A gel-forming, non-fermentable fiber supplement (i.e. psyllium) that acts as a stool normalizer (softens hard stool in constipation, firms loose/liquid stool in diarrhea) is well-suited for patients with IBS, and was recommended in both a recent review in the *American Journal of Gastroenterology* [155], and by the American College of Gastroenterology Task Force on IBS [153].

8.7 WHY FIBER SUPPLEMENTS CAN CAUSE GASTROINTESTINAL SYMPTOMS, AND HOW TO AVOID SYMPTOMS TO FACILITATE LONG-TERM COMPLIANCE

8.7.1 Discomfort and Cramping Pain

Sensations of slight discomfort to cramping pain may be associated with an increase in consumption of dietary fiber, particularly if the patient is constipated and a fiber supplement is initiated at a relatively high dose [4,5]. Lower intestinal symptoms can be replicated by passive stretch of the bowel wall via stepwise inflation of a balloon in the colon and rectum, generating sensations ranging from vague awareness to severe cramping pain with increasing intra-luminal pressure [163–165]. This suggests that the term "cramping pain" is actually a misnomer, as the term "cramping" implies spastic bowel wall contraction. Sensations including slight discomfort, the urge to defecate, and cramping pain, are also strongly correlated with HAPCs [4,5,163,165], suggesting that physiologic colonic motor events give rise to these sensations. Studies conducted with healthy subjects demonstrated that sensations of cramping pain were associated with the passage of formed stool followed by loose/liquid stool, objectively characterized as a high "stool viscosity ratio" (highest viscosity stool value divided by the lowest viscosity stool value in a given day) [166]. In the large bowel, HAPCs (peristalsis) have been correlated with mass movements, propelling luminal contents toward the rectum [32,166,167].

8.7.2 Stool Form and Cramping Pain—A Collision of Divergent Viscosities

When stool is formed, and of similar consistency (Figure 8.10), it resists significant deformation, so the forces associated with the propelled stool remain axial, and no significant bowel wall distention is generated. In normal individuals, this propulsion is not typically perceived unless it causes stool to fill the rectum, stimulating an urge to defecate [4,5,166]. In contrast, if a propagating contraction causes a bolus of lower-viscosity stool to collide with more distal formed stool (Figure 8.11), acute dilation of the bowel wall can occur, stretching mechanoreceptors, and causing sensations from discomfort to cramping pain. The discomfort/pain would be transient,

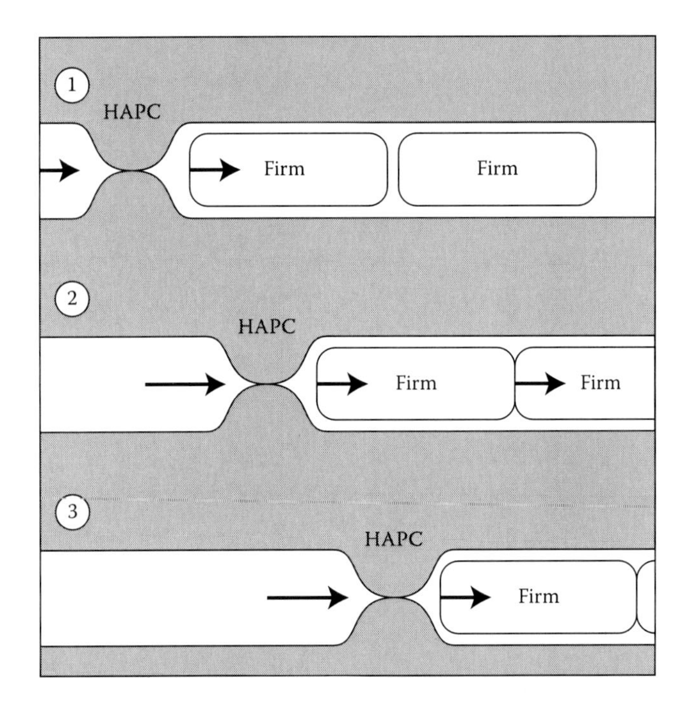

FIGURE 8.10 Stool of similar (firm) consistency does not stress the bowel wall. A model for the transit of firm digesta/stool [167]. Frame 1, high-amplitude propagating contraction (HAPC) propels stool toward the rectum. Frames 2 and 3, an HAPC propels formed stool against more distal formed stool. Both segments of stool are of sufficient viscosity to resist deformation, so the forces remain axial and no significant bowel wall distension is generated. In normal individuals, this propulsion would not be perceived until the stool filled the rectum, stimulating an urge to defecate. (Reprinted with permission from Chutkan R et al. 2012. *J Am Acad Nurse Pract.* 24, 476–487.)

occurring with the frequency of propagating contractions and relieved with a bowel movement. Such a bowel movement would consist of formed stool followed by loose/liquid stool. Given the importance of minimizing GI symptoms to improve adherence with a new fiber therapy, taking steps to keep the stool viscosity ratio low is an important consideration. For non-constipated subjects, this entails starting a new fiber supplement gradually, initiating dosing at no more than 3 or 4 g/day the first week, then increasing by one daily dose each subsequent week until 3–4 doses of the supplement per day is achieved (about 10–15 g/day). For constipated patients, any introduction of a new fiber regimen carries a significant risk of cramping pain unless the hard stool present in the distal large bowel is eliminated before initiation of a fiber supplement. A reasonable suggestion is to first clear the hard stool from the bowel with a significant dose of an osmotic laxative (e.g., polyethylene glycol). The ensuing cramping pain and potential loose stool following evacuation of the hard stool will be associated with the osmotic laxative, not a fiber supplement. Once the hard stool is cleared, gradually introduce a new fiber supplement as above. This may improve long-term compliance with a new fiber supplement.

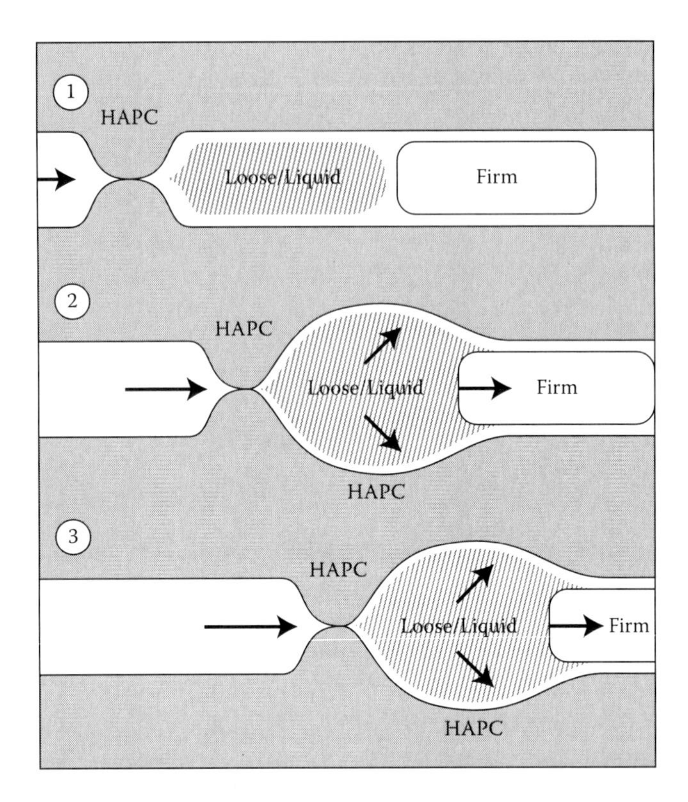

FIGURE 8.11 Acute bowel wall distention with disparate stool viscosities. A model for the transit of low-viscosity digesta [167]. Frame 1, an HAPC propels soft stool toward the rectum. Frames 2 and 3, an HAPC propels soft stool against more distal firm stool. The soft stool is readily deformable, and the forces are no longer axial but extend radially (oblique arrows), causing acute GI symptoms. The symptoms (e.g., cramping pain) would be intermittent with the frequency of HAPCs and relieved by a bowel movement. (Reprinted with permission from Chutkan R et al. 2012. *J Am Acad Nurse Pract.* 24, 476–487.)

8.8 CONCLUSIONS

Despite the general consensus that fiber is "good for you," each specific health benefit attributed to dietary fiber is associated with specific fiber characteristics, so it is important to have a good understanding of the fiber characteristics that provide each health benefit (Table 8.1). Insoluble fiber (e.g., wheat bran) has been shown to have a laxative benefit by mechanical stimulation/irritation of the intestinal mucosa, but only if the fiber particles are of sufficient "grittiness." Soluble non-viscous fiber supplements (e.g., inulin, wheat dextrin, polydextrose, maltodextrin) are readily fermented, and whereas these fibers are part of an emerging science (e.g., prebiotics) with a plethora of data showing significant and potentially beneficial effects on the gut microbiome, there is only limited reproducible, well-controlled clinical data demonstrating a clinically meaningful health benefit at physiologic doses for these marketed fiber supplements. In contrast, there are numerous well-controlled clinical

TABLE 8.1
Clinically Demonstrated Health Benefits Associated with Common Fiber Supplements

	No Water-Holding Capacity			Water-Holding Capacity			
	Insoluble	Soluble, Non-Viscous		Soluble Viscous	Soluble Gel-Forming		
	Wheat Bran	**Wheat Dextrin**	**Inulin**	**Methylcellulose**	**Partially Hydrolyzed Guar Gum**	**β-glucan**	**Psyllium**
Source	Wheat	Chemically treated wheat	Chicory root	Chemically treated wood pulp	Guar Beans	Oats, Barley	Seed husk, Plantago ovata
Degree of fermentation	Poorly fermented	Readily fermented	Readily fermented	Non-fermented	Readily fermented	Readily fermented	Non-fermented
Cholesterol lowering					+/–[b]	+[c]	+
Improved glycemic control					+/–[b]	+[c]	+
Satiety						+[c]	+
Weight loss							+
Constipation/Stool softener	+[a]			+/–[d]			+
Diarrhea/Stool normalizer							+
Irritable bowel syndrome (IBS)							+

[a] If particle size is sufficiently large/coarse.

[b] The efficacy of PHGG depends on the degree to which it has been hydrolyzed. If a marketed product has little/no viscosity when mixed with water (as described above), then it will not exhibit significant gel-dependent health benefits.

[c] Typically marketed in fiber bars or cereals, requiring pressure and/or heat to make the final product, potentially reducing gel-forming capacity.

[d] Methylcellulose has an OTC indication for treatment of occasional constipation, but the American College of Gastroenterology determined that methylcelluose had insufficient clinical data to recommend it for treatment of chronic constipation.

studies demonstrating viscosity/gel-dependent health benefits associated with small bowel function, including cholesterol lowering and improved glycemic control. The greater the viscosity/gel-forming capacity exhibited by a soluble fiber, the greater the potential health benefit. Highly viscous, gel-forming fiber supplements (e.g., high molecular weight β-glucan, raw guar gum, psyllium) have been shown clinically to lower serum LDL-cholesterol concentrations in patients with hyperlipidemia, and improve glycemic control in patients with Type 2 Diabetes and Metabolic Syndrome. Both the cholesterol lowering and improved glycemic control benefits are observed in addition to the effects already conveyed by prescription drugs to treat hyperlipidemia and hyperglycemia, demonstrating that viscous/gel-forming fiber supplements can provide an effective co-therapy in patient care. It is important to note that viscosity/gel-dependent health benefits can be lost if a marketed fiber supplement is modified to improve palatability by reducing viscosity (e.g., PHGG), or exposed to extrusion pressure/heat to form the marketed product (e.g., extruded cereal products). A gel-forming fiber supplement can also provide a satiety benefit, as well as a weight loss/weight maintenance benefit, both of which appear dependent on gel-forming capacity and being non-fermented.

For lower gastrointestinal benefits, such as attenuating symptoms in constipation, diarrhea, and IBS, an ideal fiber supplement would be a non-fermented, gel-forming fiber that retains its gelling capacity throughout the large bowel (Table 8.1). Insoluble fiber supplements can be effective for constipation if particles are sufficiently large/coarse, but insoluble fiber supplements should not be recommended for treating diarrhea or IBS due to the mucosa stimulating/irritating mechanism of action that could make symptoms worse. Soluble fiber supplements that are readily fermented, whether non-viscous (e.g., inulin, wheat dextrin, polydextrose, maltodextrin) or viscous (e.g., guar gum, β-glucan), can increase gas/flatulence and bacterial biomass, and provide calories to the host due to fermentation, but have no appreciable laxative effect at physiologic doses. In contrast, a non-fermented fiber that maintains its gel throughout the large bowel (i.e., psyllium) has been shown clinically to meet this definition, acting as a stool normalizer: more effective than the market-leading stool softener for softening hard stool and decreasing symptoms in patients with chronic constipation; effective for firming loose/liquid stools and decreasing symptoms in patients with diarrhea. Psyllium is also the only fiber supplement recommended by the American College of Gastroenterology for treating both chronic constipation and IBS. To decrease the potential for unwanted symptoms associated with starting a new fiber supplement regimen, it is recommended to begin at a relatively low dose, and gradually increase the dose over several weeks. Constipated patients should be encouraged to eliminate hard stools with an osmotic laxative before beginning a new fiber therapy.

Relying on an ingredient name of the raw fiber (e.g., guar gum, oat bran) can be misleading if the marketed supplement no longer provides the same viscosity/gel-forming capacity as the raw fiber. FDA does not require any clinical data on the final marketed product to support a claim for "a good source of fiber". A simple test to predict the potential health benefits of a fiber supplement is to mix a single dose of fiber supplement in a glass of water (usually 2–4 g of fiber; added to 120 mL water), and let it stand for 15 min. If the supplement dissolves in water, then forms a visco-elastic gel, it should provide clinically meaningful, gel-dependent health benefits (e.g., cholesterol lowering, improved glycemic control, satiety/weight loss). If a supplement does not form a gel, it is unlikely to provide these clinically meaningful health benefits. This test is obviously not practical for fiber supplements marketed as fiber bars, yogurts, cereals, or "gummy" dose forms. The vast majority of these products contain a soluble, non-viscous, readily fermented fiber, so the test is not needed, as it has already been established that this category of fiber supplement does not have clinical data supporting health benefits. Note that, for "gummy" fiber supplements, the fiber (e.g., inulin) is non-viscous. The "gum" is a digestible gelatin.

Finally, read the label for the fiber ingredient(s), not the advertising on the marketed product, to determine what fiber source is being provided, and at what dose. Determine if there exists significant clinical evidence to support a health benefit for the raw fiber, and then consider the form of the marketed fiber product, and how processing may have diminished the health benefit(s) of the raw fiber. Be aware that the label claims on a fiber product may not represent the fiber. A product labeled "fiber weight management" may contain one or more fibers that have no supporting clinical data for weight loss or weight maintenance. Several products claim "non-thickening" as a desirable trait, with names implying a health benefit, yet they contain a soluble non-viscous, fermentable fiber with no supporting clinical evidence that the marketed product delivers a health benefit. As discussed above, formulation and processing can affect final product efficacy, so it may not be appropriate to assume that products with the fiber will deliver the same benefits. While one product may have numerous well-controlled clinical studies on the marketed product itself, others with the same active, but a potentially different formulation, may have no clinical support yet make the same health claims. Generic drugs are required to demonstrate bioequivalence and gain regulatory approval before being marketed, but fiber supplements have no similar requirements, so fiber products can make claims without clinical support for their formulation. Not all fiber supplements are equal.

8.8.1 Examples of Commonly Marketed Fiber Supplements

Acacia gum (gum Arabic) is a tree exudate collected for centuries by hand from Acacia trees across the Sahelian belt of Africa (North of the equator). The gum oozes from stems and branches of the trees when subjected to stress, including removing sections of bark with an ax. Acacia readily dissolves in water, and the highly branched structure gives rise to a low hydrodynamic volume that yields a low viscosity. A 30% solution of Acacia gum has a lower viscosity than a 1% solution of xanthan gum. Acacia gum is readily fermented by bacteria in the gut, and is part of an emerging area of science related to the microbiome and prebiotics.

Guar gum is a soluble, readily fermented, highly viscous/gel-forming fiber derived from the Indian cluster bean (*Cyanopsis tetragonolopus*). To make the high viscosity gel more palatable as a dietary supplement, raw guar gum is hydrolyzed to a less viscous or non-viscous marketed product known as PHGG. The chain length of hydrolyzed guar gum can vary greatly, affecting the viscosity of the fiber supplement. While the high viscosity gel of raw guar gum is effective for both cholesterol lowering and improved glycemic control, partial hydrolysis will attenuate both the viscosity and the health benefits of guar gum. The degree of hydrolysis, and the resulting loss of gel-forming capacity, influence whether the marketed product will provide measurable health benefits.

Inulin is a naturally occurring fructose polymer (fructan) found in plants such as chicory root, onions, and Jerusalem artichoke. Inulin is well tolerated at doses less than 10 g/day, but may cause flatulence and other gastrointestinal symptoms at higher doses. The number of fructose units found in a given product can vary from 3 to 60 (note that fructans with a degree of polymerization less than 10 are called oligofructose). Inulin readily dissolves in water, and is readily fermented by bacteria in the gut.

Maltodextrin is a polymer of D-glucose units connected in chains of variable length. Maltodextrin is normally easily digested and absorbed as glucose. It can be purposefully converted to a resistant starch by rearrangement of starch or hydrolyzed starch from the normal *alpha*-1,4-glucose linkages (easily digested) to random 1,2-, 1,3-, and 1,4-*alpha* or *beta* linkages. Since the human digestive system effectively digests only *alpha*-1,4-linkages, the other linkages render the molecules "resistant" to digestion, hence resistant starch. Maltodextrin is soluble, non-viscous and readily fermented.

Methylcellulose is chemically treated (methyl chloride) cellulose, harvested from wood pulp. Cellulose is normally an insoluble fiber, but by treating the wood pulp with methyl chloride, the cellulose becomes soluble. While marketed as a bulk-forming laxative, with a caution not to use the product for more than 1 week unless directed by a doctor, the product might be recommended as a fiber supplement, so it was mentioned here. Methylcellulose is both soluble and viscous, but does not form a gel, so it does not significantly lower cholesterol, improve glycemic control, or exhibit other health benefits associated with gel-forming fibers.

Oat bran is a mixture of insoluble fiber and soluble fiber. The insoluble portion of oat bran has the potential to exhibit a laxative effect if the particle size of the marketed product has remained sufficiently large/coarse, and the dose is sufficiently large. The soluble viscous, gel-forming portion (β-glucan) can exhibit both a cholesterol-lowering effect in hyperlipidemia and improved glycemic control in type 2 diabetes, but only if processing has not destroyed the gel-forming capacity of the β-glucan. Recall the study above that assessed the cholesterol-lowering efficacy of cereals exposed to three different levels of heat and pressure during the extrusion process, and showed that with increasing heat/pressure, viscosity/gel-forming capacity was lost. β-glucan (3 g/day, about 1 1/2 cups of oatmeal) has FDA approval to claim a reduced risk of cardiovascular disease by lowering elevated serum cholesterol, but there is no specification for minimal gel-forming capacity. While oatmeal is obviously high in viscosity/gel-forming capacity, extruded cereals (e.g., heat/pressure extruded into specific shapes) and baked products may not retain a significant gelling capacity, yet can still make a health claim based on β-glucan. It is important to consider the degree of processing for a marketed product when considering potential for health benefits.

Polydextrose is a synthetic, indigestible glucose polymer that is soluble, non-viscous and readily fermented by the bacteria in the gut. The highly branched structure of polydextrose gives rise to a low hydrodynamic volume, which yields little effect on viscosity. Polydextrose is part of an emerging area of science related to the microbiome of the gut.

Psyllium, the seed husk of the Plantago plant, is a naturally occurring soluble viscous, gel-forming fiber that is not fermented by bacteria in the gut, so it retains its gelled nature throughout the digestive tract. Numerous well-controlled, randomized clinical studies show psyllium significantly lowers serum cholesterol in patients with hyperlipidemia, and reduces both fasting blood glucose concentrations and HbA1c in patients with Type 2 Diabetes and pre-diabetes (e.g., Metabolic Syndrome). As psyllium is not fermented and retains its gel throughout the large bowel, it acts as a stool normalizer, softening hard stool in constipation, firming loose/liquid stool in diarrhea, and reducing associated symptoms in both constipation and diarrhea. Psyllium is the only fiber recommended by the American College of Gastroenterology for improving symptoms of chronic constipation, and also is recommended for treating symptoms in patients with IBS.

Wheat dextrin is a soluble, non-viscous fiber formed by heating wheat starch (normally readily digested/absorbed in the small bowel) at high temperature, followed by enzymatic (amylase) treatment to form a resistant starch. Wheat dextrin is readily fermented in the large bowel, and does not form a gel, so it does not significantly lower cholesterol, improve glycemic control, or exhibit other health benefits associated with gel-forming fibers.

REFERENCES

1. Institute of Medicine, Food and Nutrition Board. 2002. Dietary reference intakes: Energy, carbohydrates, fiber, fat, fatty acids cholesterol, protein and amino acids. Washington, DC: National Academies Press.
2. Panel on Macronutrients, Panel on the Definition of Dietary Fiber, Subcommittee on Upper Reference Levels of Nutrients, Subcommittee on Interpretation and Uses of Dietary Reference Intakes, and the Standing Committee on the Scientific Evaluation of Dietary Reference Intakes. 2002/2005. Dietary reference intakes for energy, carbohydrate, fiber, fatty acids, cholesterol, protein, and amino acids. Washington, DC, USA: The National Academies Press.
3. Slavin JL. 2008. Position of the American Dietetic Association: Health implications of dietary fiber. *J Am Diet Assoc*. 108, 1716–1731.
4. Chutkan R, Fahey G, Wright W, McRorie J. 2012. Viscous versus non-viscous soluble fiber supplements: Mechanisms and evidence for fiber-specific health benefits. *J Am Acad Nurse Pract*. 24, 476–487.
5. McRorie J, Fahey G. 2013. A review of gastrointestinal physiology and the mechanisms underlying the health benefits of dietary fiber: Matching an effective fiber with specific patient needs. *Clin Nurs Stud.* 1(4), 82–92.
6. Klosterbuer A, Roughead Z, Slavin J. 2011. Benefits of dietary fiber in clinical nutrition. *J Nutr Clin Pract.* 26(5), 625–635.
7. U.S. Department of Agriculture (n.d.). Choose My Plate/Vegetables. Available at: http://www.choosemyplate.gov/food-groups/vegetables.html (accessed on March 11, 2015).
8. Reicks M, Jonnalagadda S, Albertson AM, Joshi N. 2014. Total dietary fiber intakes in the US population are related to whole grain consumption: Results from the National Health and Nutrition Examination Survey 2009 to 2010. *Nutr Res*. 34(3), 226–234.
9. Slavin J, Green H. 2007. Dietary fiber and satiety. *Nutr Bull*. 32, 32–42.

10. Dietary Reference Intakes for energy, carbohydrate, fiber, fat, fatty acids, cholesterol, protein, and amino acids. 2002/2005 and Dietary Reference Intakes for water, potassium, sodium, chloride, and sulfate 2005. http://www.nal.usda.gov/fnic/DRI/DRI_Energy/energy_full_report.pdf
11. U.S. Department of Health and Human Services; U.S. Department of Agriculture. 2010. Dietary Guidelines for Americans. Washington, DC, USA: Government Printing Office.
12. Slavin JL. 2005. Dietary fiber and body weight. *Nutrition* 21, 411–418.
13. Rimm EB, Ascherio A, Giovannucci E, Spiegelman D, Stampfer MJ, Willett WC. 1996. Vegetable, fruit, and cereal fiber intake and risk of coronary heart disease among men. *J Am Med Assoc.* 275, 447–451.
14. Mozaffarian D, Kumanyika SK, Lemaitre RN, Olson JL, Burke GL, Siscovick DS. 2003. Cereal, fruit, and vegetable fiber intake and the risk of cardiovascular disease in elderly individuals. *J Am Med Assoc.* 289, 1659–1666.
15. Wolever TM. 2013. Is glycaemic index (GI) a valid measure of carbohydrate quality? *Eur J Clin Nutr.* 67(5), 522–531.
16. A Report of the Panel on Macronutrients Subcommittees on Upper Reference Levels of Nutrients Interpretation Uses of Dietary Reference Intakes Standing Committee on the Scientific Evaluation of Dietary Reference Intakes. 2005. In: Dietary Reference Intakes for energy, carbohydrate, fiber, fat, fatty acids, cholesterol, protein, and amino acids (macronutrients). Washington, DC, USA: The National Academies Press. http://www.nap.edu/catalog/10490/dietary-reference-intakes-for-energy-carbohydrate-fiber-fat-fatty-acids-cholesterol-protein-and-amino-acids-macronutrients.
17. Dikeman C, Fahey G. 2006. Viscosity as related to dietary fiber: A review. *Crit Rev Food Sci Nutr.* 46, 649–663.
18. Guillon F, Champ MM. 2002. Carbohydrate fractions of legumes: Uses in human nutrition and potential for health. *Br J Nutr.* 88 (Suppl 3), S293–S306.
19. Morris ER, Cutler AN, Ross-Murphy DA, Rees DA, Price J. 1981. Concentration and shear rate dependence of viscosity in random coil polysaccharide solutions. *Carbohydr Polym.* 1, 5–21.
20. Anderson JW. 2009. All fibers are not created equal. *J Med.* 2, 87–91.
21. Kim J, Cha YJ, Lee KH, Park E. 2013. Effect of onion peel extract supplementation on the lipid profile and antioxidative status of healthy young women: A randomized, placebo-controlled, double-blind, crossover trial. *Nutr Res Pract.* 7(5), 373–379.
22. Code of Federal Regulations, Title 21: http://www.accessdata.fda.gov/scripts/cdrh/cfdocs/cfcfr/CFRSearch.cfm?fr=101.81.
23. Wolever T, Tosh S, Gibbs A et al. 2010. Physicochemical properties of oat β-glucan influence its ability to reduce serum LDL cholesterol in humans: A randomized clinical trial. *Am J Clin Nutr.* 92, 723–732.
24. Vuksan V, Jenkins AL, Rogovik AL, Fairgrieve CD, Jovanovski E, Leiter LA. 2011. Viscosity rather than quantity of dietary fibre predicts cholesterol-lowering effect in healthy individuals. *Br J Nutr.* 106, 1349–1352.
25. Schwartz SE, Levine RA, Singh A, Scheidecker JR, Track NS. 1982. Sustained pectin ingestion delays gastric emptying. *Gastroenterology.* 83(4), 812–817.
26. Whitman WB, Coleman DC, Wiebe WJ. 1998. Prokaryotes: The unseen majority. *Proc Natl Acad Sci USA.* 95, 6578–6583.
27. Ley RE, Peterson DA, Gordon JI. 2006. Ecological and evolutionary forces shaping microbial diversity in the human intestine. *Cell.* 124, 837–848.
28. Cummings JH, Macfarlane GT, Englyst HN. 2001. Prebiotic digestion and fermentation. *Am J Clin Nutr.* 73(Suppl 2), 415S–420S.
29. Suarez FL, Levitt MD. 2000. An understanding of excessive intestinal gas. *Current Gastroenterology Reports.* 2, 413–419.

30. Suarez FL, Furne JK, Springfield JR, Levitt MD. 1998. Identification of gases responsible for the odor of human flatus and evaluation of a device purported to reduce this odor. *Gut*. 43, 100–104.
31. Levitt MD. 1971. Volume and composition of human intestinal gas determined by means of an intestinal washout technique. *N Engl J Med*. 284, 1394–1398.
32. McRorie J, Greenwood-Van Meerveld B, Rudolph C. 1998. Characterization of propagating contractions in the proximal colon of ambulatory mini pigs. *Dig Dis Sci*. 43(5), 957–963.
33. Levitt M. 1979. Follow-up of a flatulent patient. *Dig Dis Sci*. 24(8), 652–654.
34. Campbell J, Fahey G. 1997. Psyllium and methylcellulose fermentation properties in relation to insoluble and soluble fiber standards. *Nutr Res*. 17, 619–629.
35. Kaur A, Rose D, Rumpagaporn P et al. 2011. *In vitro* batch fecal fermentation comparison of gas and short-chain fatty acid production using "slowly fermentable" dietary fibers. *J Food Sci*. 76, H137–H142.
36. Timm D, Stewart M, Hospattankar A et al. 2010. Wheat dextrin, psyllium, and inulin produce distinct fermentation patterns, gas volumes, and short-chain fatty acid profiles *in vitro*. *J Med Food*. 13, 961–966.
37. Wolever T, ter Wal P, Spadafora P et al. 1992. Guar, but not psyllium, increases breath methane and serum acetate concentrations in human subjects. *Am J Clin Nutr.* 55, 719–722.
38. Levitt MD, Furne J, Olsson S. 1996. The relation of passage of gas and abdominal bloating to colonic gas production. *Ann Intern Med*. 124, 422–424.
39. Zumarraga L, Levitt M, Suarez F. 1997. Absence of gaseous symptoms during ingestion of commercial fibre preparations. *Aliment Pharmacol Ther*. 11, 1067–1072.
40. Wolever T, Robb P. 1992. Effect of guar, pectin, psyllium, soy polysaccharide and cellulose on breath hydrogen and methane in healthy subjects. *Am J Gastroenterol*. 87, 305–310.
41. Marteau P, Flourié B, Cherbut C et al. 1994. Digestibility and bulking effect of ispaghula husks in healthy humans. *Gut*. 35, 1747–52.
42. Roberfroid M. 2007. Prebiotics: The concept revisited. *J Nutr*. 137, 830S–837S.
43. Scientific opinion on the substantiation of health claims related to various food(s)/food constituents(s) and increasing numbers of gastro-intestinal microorganisms (ID 760, 761, 779, 780, 779, 1905), and decreasing potentially pathogenic gastro-intestinal microorganisms (ID 760, 761, 779, 780, 779, 1905) pursuant to Article 13(1) of Regulation (EC) No 1924/2006).
44. Department of Agriculture. Carbohydrates (Dietary Guidelines for Americans), 2010. Available at: http://www.cnpp.usda.gov/Publications/DietaryGuidelines/2010/DGAC/Report/D-5-Carbohydrates.pdf (accessed on October 6, 2011).
45. Meyer J, Ohashi H, Jehn D, Thompson J. 1981. Size of liver particles emptied from the human stomach. *Gastroenterology*. 80, 1489–1496.
46. Holt S, Heading RC, Carter DC, Prescott LF, Tothill P. 1979. Effect of gel fibre on gastric emptying and absorption of glucose and paracetamol. *Lancet*. 24;1(8117), 636–639.
47. Todd PA, Benfield P, Goa KL. 1990. Guar gum a review of its pharmacological properties, and use as a dietary adjunct in hypercholesterolaemia. *Drugs*. 39, 917–928.
48. Bianchi M, Capurso L. 2002. Effects of guar gum, psyllium and microcrystalline cellulose on abdominal symptoms, gastric emptying, orocaecal transit time and gas production in healthy volunteers. *Dig Liver Dis*. 34 (Suppl 2), S129–S133.
49. van Nieuwenhoven M, Kovacs E, Brummer R, Westerterp-Plantenga M, Brouns F. 2001. The effect of different dosages of guar gum on gastric emptying and small intestinal transit of a consumed semisolid meal. *Am Coll Nutr*. 20(1), 87–91.
50. Schwartz SE, Levine RA, Singh A, Scheidecker JR, Track NS. 1982. Sustained pectin ingestion delays gastric emptying. *Gastroenterology*. 83(4), 812–817.

51. Kawasaki N, Suzuki Y, Urashima M, Nakayoshi T, Tsuboi K, Tanishima Y, Hanyu N, Kashiwagi H. 2008. Effect of gelatinization on gastric emptying and absorption. *Hepatogastroenterology*. 55(86–87), 1843–1845.
52. Sandhu KS, el Samahi MM, Mena I, Dooley CP, Valenzuela JE. 1987. Effect of pectin on gastric emptying and gastroduodenal motility in normal subjects. *Gastroenterology*. 92(2), 486–492.
53. Rigaud D, Paycha F, Meulemans A, Merrouche M, Mignon M. 1998. Effect of psyllium on gastric emptying, hunger feeling and food intake in normal volunteers: A double blind study. *Eur J Clin Nutr*. 52(4), 239–245.
54. Guyton A, Hall J. 2006. *Textbook of Medical Physiology*, 11th edition. Philadelphia, PA: Elsevier Inc., Unit XII, Chapters 62–66.
55. Lobo D, Hendry P, Rodrigues G, Marciani L, Totman J, Wright J, Preston T, Gowland P, Spiller R, Fearon K. 2009. Gastric emptying of three liquid oral preoperative metabolic preconditioning regimens measured by magnetic resonance imaging in healthy adult volunteers: A randomized double-blind, crossover study. *Clin Nutr*. 28, 636–641.
56. Bergmann JF, Chassany O, Petit A, Triki R, Caulin C, Segrestaa JM. 1992. Correlation between echographic gastric emptying and appetite: Influence of psyllium. *Gut*. 33, 1042–1043.
57. Jenkins DJ, Wolever TM, Taylor RH et al. 1981. Glycemic index of foods: A physiological basis for carbohydrate exchange. *Am J Clin Nutr.* 34, 362–366.
58. Morris, ER, Cutler, AN, Ross-Murphy, DA, Rees, DA, and Price, J. 1981. Concentration and shear rate dependence of viscosity in random coil polysaccharide solutions. *Carbohydr Polym*. 1, 5–21.
59. Schirra J, Goke B. 2005. The physiological role of GLP-1 in human: Incretin, ileal brake or more? *Regul Pept*. 128, 109–115.
60. Dikeman C, Murphy M, Fahey G. 2006. Dietary fibers affect viscosity of solutions and simulated human gastric and small intestine digesta. *J Nutr*. 136, 913–919.
61. Jenkins D, Wolever T, Taylor R, Barker H, Fielden H, Baldwin J, Bowling A, Newman H, Jenkins A, Goff D. 1981. Glycemic index of foods: A physiological basis for carbohydrate exchange. *Am J Clin Nutr*. 34, 362–366.
62. Wolever T, Jenkins D. 1986. The use of the glycemic index in predicting the blood glucose response to mixed meals. *Am J Clin Nutr*. 43, 167–172.
63. Maljaars P, Peters H, Mela D, Masclee A. 2008. Ileal brake: A sensible food target for appetite control. A review. *Physiol Behav*. 95, 271–281.
64. Holst J, Deacon C, Vilsbøll T, Krarup T, Madsbad S. 2008. Glucagon-like peptide-1, glucose homeostasis and diabetes. *Trends Mol Med*. 14, 161–168.
65. Maljaars P, Peters H, Kodde A, Geraedts M, Troost F, Haddeman E, Masclee A. 2011. Length and site of the small intestine exposed to fat influences hunger and food intake. *Br J Nutr*. 106, 1609–1615.
66. Anderson JW, Floore TL, Geil PB, O'Neal DS, Balm TK. 1991. Hypocholesterolemic effects of different bulk-forming hydrophilic fibers as adjuncts to dietary therapy in mild to moderate hypercholesterolemia. *Arch Intern Med*. 151(8), 1597–1602.
67. McRorie J, Pepple S, Rudolph C. 1998. Effects of fiber laxatives and calcium docusate on regional water content and viscosity of digesta in the large intestine of the pig. *Dig Dis Sci*. 43(4), 738–745.
68. Jenkins D, Wolever T, Leeds A et al. 1978. Dietary fibres, fibre analogues, and glucose tolerance: Importance of viscosity. *Br Med J*. 1, 1392–1394.
69. Jarjis H, Blackburn N, Redfern J, Read N. 1984. The effect of ispaghula (Fybogel and Metamucil) and guar gum on glucose tolerance in man. *Br J Nutr.* 51, 371–378.
70. Wolever T, Vuksan V, Eshuis H, Spadafora P, Peterson R, Chao E, Storey M, Jenkins D. 1991. Effect of method of administration of psyllium on glycemic response and carbohydrate digestibility. *J Am Coll Nutr*. 10, 364–371.

71. Cherbut C et al. 1994. Digestibility and bulking effect of ispaghula husks in healthy humans. *Gut.* 35, 1747–1752.
72. Sierra M, García JJ, Fernández N, Diez MJ, Calle AP. 2002. Therapeutic effects of psylliumin type 2 diabetic patients. *Eur J Clin Nutr.* 56(9), 830–842.
73. Anderson J, Zettwoch N, Feldman T, Tietyen-Clark J, Oeltgen P, Bishop C. 1988. Cholesterol-lowering effects of psyllium hydrophilic mucilloid for hypercholetserolemic men. *Arch Intern Med.* 148, 292–296.
74. Bell LP, Hectorne K, Reynolds H, Balm TK, Hunninghake DB. 1989. Cholesterol-lowering effects of psyllium hydrophilic mucilloid. Adjunct therapy to a prudent diet for patients with mild to moderate hypercholesterolemia. *JAMA.* 261(23), 3419–3423.
75. Levin EG, Miller VT, Muesing RA, Stoy DB, Balm TK, LaRosa JC. 1990. Comparison of psyllium hydrophilic mucilloid and cellulose as adjuncts to a prudent diet in the treatment of mild to moderate hypercholesterolemia. *Arch Intern Med.* 150(9), 1822–1827.
76. Cicero AFG, Derosa G, Bove M et al. 2010. Psyllium improves dyslipidemaemia, hyperglycaemia and hypertension, while guar gum reduces body weight more rapidly in patients affected by metabolic syndrome following an AHA Step 2 diet. *Mediterr J Nutr Metab.* 3, 47–54.
77. Rodriguez-Moran M, Guerrero-Romero F, Laczano-Burciaga L et al. 1998. Lipid- and glucose-lowering efficacy of plantagopsyllium in type II diabetes. *J Diab Complicat.* 12, 273–278.
78. Ziai S, Larijani B, Akhoondzadeh S et al. 2005. Psyllium decreased serum glucose and glycosylated hemoglobin significantly in diabetic outpatients. *J Ethnopharmacol.* 102, 202–207.
79. Dall'Alba V, Silva FM, Antonio JP, Steemburgo T, Royer CP, Almeida JC, Gross JL, Azevedo MJ. 2013. Improvement of the metabolic syndrome profile by soluble fibre-guar gum-in patients with type 2 diabetes: A randomised clinical trial. *Br J Nutr.* 110(9), 1601–1610.
80. Gupta RR, Agrawal CG, Singh GP et al. 1994. Lipid-lowering efficacy of psyllium hydrophilic mucilloid in non-insulin dependent diabetes mellitus with hyperlipidemia. *Ind J Med Res.* 100, 237–241.
81. Anderson J, Allgood L, Turner C, Oelgten P, Daggy B. 1999. Effects of psyllium on glucose and serum lipid responses in men with type 2 diabetes and hypercholesterolemia. *Am J Clin Nutr.* 70, 466–473.
82. Feinglos M, Gibb R, Ramsey D, Surwit R, McRorie J. 2013. Psyllium improves glycemic control in patients with type-2 diabetes mellitus. *Bioact Carbohydr Diet Fibre.* 1, 156–161.
83. Tosh SM. 2013. Review of human studies investigating the post-prandial blood-glucose lowering ability of oat and barley food products. *Eur J Clin Nutr.* 67(4), 310–317.
84. Sartore G, Carlström S, Scherstén B. 1981. Dietary supplementation of fibre (Lunelax) as a means to reduce postprandial glucose in diabetics. *Acta Med Scand Suppl.* 656, 51–53.
85. Karmally W, Montez M, Palmas W, Martinez W, Branstetter A, Ramakrishnan R, Holleran S, Haffner S, Ginsberg H. 2005. Cholesterol-lowering benefits of oat-containing cereal in Hispanic Americans. *J Am Diet Assoc.* 105, 967–970.
86. Keogh G, Cooper G, Mulvey T, Mcardle B, Coles G, Monro J, Poppitt S. 2003. Randomized controlled cross-over study of the effect of a highly β-glucan-enriched barley on cardiovascular disease risk factors in mildly hypercholesterolemic men. *Am J Clin Nutr.* 78, 711–718.
87. Kerkhoffs D, Hornstra G, Mensick R. 2003. Cholesterol-lowering effect of β-glucan from oat bran in mildly hypercholesterolemic subjects may decrease when β-glucan is incorporated into bread and cookies. *Am J Clin Nutr.* 78, 221–227.

88. Naumann E, Van Rees A, Onning G, Oste R, Wydra M, Mensick R. 2006. β-glucan incorporated into a fruit drink effectively lowers serum LDL-cholesterol concentrations. *Am J Clin Nutr*. 83, 601–605.
89. Beer M, Arrigoni E, Amado R. 1995. Effects of oat gum on blood cholesterol levels in healthy young men. *Eur J Clin Nutr*. 49, 517–522.
90. Delahoy PJ, Magliano DJ, Webb K, Grobler M, Liew D. 2009. The relationship between reduction in low-density lipoprotein cholesterol by statins and reduction in risk of cardiovascular outcomes: An updated meta-analysis. *Clin Ther*. 31, 236–244.
91. Katan MB, Grundy SM, Jones P, Law M, Miettinen T, Paoletti R; Stresa Workshop Participants. 2003. Efficacy and safety of plants tanols and sterols in the management of blood cholesterol levels. *Mayo Clin Proc*. 78(8), 965–978.
92. Gunness P, Gidley M. 2010. Mechanisms underlying the cholesterol-lowering properties of soluble dietary fibre polysaccharides. *Food Funct*. 1, 149–155.
93. Jensen C, Spiller G, Gates J, Miller A, Whittam J. 1993. The effect of acacia gum and a water-soluble dietary fiber mixture on blood lipids in humans. *J Am Coll Nutr*. 12(2), 147–154.
94. Haskell WL, Spiller GA, Jensen CD, Ellis BK, Gates JE. 1992. Role of water-soluble dietary fiber in the management of elevated plasma cholesterol in healthy subjects. *Am J Cardiol*. 69(5), 433–439.
95. Brownawell AM, Caers W, Gibson GR, Kendall CW, Lewis KD, Ringel Y, Slavin JL. 2012. Prebiotics and the health benefits of fiber: Current regulatory status, future research, and goals. *J Nutr*. 142(5), 962–974.
96. Shrestha S, Volek JS, Udani J, Wood RJ, Greene CM, Aggarwal D, Contois JH, Kavoussi B, Fernandez ML. 2006. A combination therapy including psyllium and plant sterols lowers LDL cholesterol by modifying lipoprotein metabolism in hypercholesterolemic individuals. *J Nutr*. 136(10), 2492–2497.
97. Shrestha S, Freake H, McGrane M, Volek J, Fernandez M. 2007. A combination of psyllium and plant sterols alter lipoprotein metabolism in hypercholesterolemic subjects by modifying the intravascular processing of lipo proteins and increasing LDL uptake. *J Nutr.* 137(5), 1165–1170.
98. Neal G, Balm T. 1990. Synergistic effects of psyllium in the dietary treatment of hypercholesterolemia. *South Med J*. 83, 1131–1137.
99. Moreyra AE, Wilson AC, Koraym, A. 2005. Effect of combining psyllium fiber with simvastatin in lowering cholesterol. *Arch Int Med*. 165, 1161–1166.
100. Maciejko JJ, Brazg R, Shah A, Patil S, Rubenfire M. 1994. Psyllium for the reduction of cholestyramine-associated gastrointestinal symptoms in the treatment of primary hypercholesterolemia. *Arch Fam Med*. 3, 955–960.
101. Spence J, Huff M, Heidenheim P et al. 1995. Combination therapy with colestipol and psyllium mucilloid in patients with hyperlipidemia. *Ann Int Med*. 123, 493–499.
102. Agrawal A, Tandon M, Sharma, P. 2007. Effect of combining viscous fibre with lavastatin on serum lipids in normal human subjects. *Int J Clin Pract*. 61, 1812–1818.
103. Jayaram S, Prasad HB, Sovani VB, Langade DG, Mane PR. 2007. Randomised study to compare the efficacy and safety of is apgol plus atorvastatin versus atorvastatin alone in subjects with hypercholesterolaemia. *J Indian Med Assoc*. 105(3), 142–145.
104. Roberts D, Truswell A, Bencke A, Dewar H, Farmakalidis E. 1994. The cholesterol-lowering effect of a breakfast cereal containing psyllium fibre. *Med J Aust*. 161, 660–664.
105. CDC. Overweight and Obesity. Available at http://www.cdc.gov/obesity/data/adult.html (accessed on March 11, 2015).
106. Anderson J, Baird P, Davis R et al. 2009. Health benefits of dietary fiber. *Nutr Rev.* 67, 188–205.

107. Du H, van der ADL, Boshuizen HC et al. 2010. Dietary fiber and subsequent changes in body weight and waist circumference in European men and women. *Am J Clin Nutr.* 91, 329–336.
108. Liu S, Willett WC, Manson JE, Hu FB, Rosner B, Colditz G. 2003. Relation between changes in intakes of dietary fiber and grain products and changes in weight and development of obesity among middle-aged women. *Am J Clin Nutr.* 78, 920–927.
109. Duncan LJP, Rose K, Meikeljohn AP. 1960. Phenmetrazine hydrochloride and methylcellulose in the treatment of "refractory" obesity. *Lancet* 1, 1262–1265.
110. Yudkin J. 1959. The causes and cure of obesity. *Lancet* 2, 1135–1138.
111. Davis J, Hodges V, Gillham M. 2006. Normal-weight adults consume more fiber and fruit than their age- and height-matched overweight/obese counterparts. *J Am Diet Assoc.* 106, 833–840.
112. Tucker L, Thomas K. 2009. Increasing total fiber intake reduces risk of weight and fat gains in women. *J Nutr.* 139, 576–581.
113. Blackwood AD, Salter J, Dettmar PW, Chaplin MF. 2000. Dietary fibre, physicochemical properties and their relationship to health. *J R Soc Promot Health.* 120, 242–247.
114. Howarth N, Saltzman E, Roberts S. 2001. Dietary fiber and weight regulation. *Nutr Rev.* 59, 129–139.
115. Pereira M, Ludwig D. 2001. Dietary fiber and body-weight regulation: Observations and mechanisms. *Pediatr Clin North Am.* 48, 969–980.
116. Slavin J. 2005. Dietary fiber and body weight. *Nutrition.* 21, 411–418.
117. Higgins J. 2014. Resistant starch and energy balance: Impact on weight loss and maintenance. *Crit Rev Food Sci Nutr.* 54, 1158–1166.
118. Abrams S, Griffin I, Hawthorne K, Ellis KJ. 2007. Effect of prebiotic supplementation and calcium intake on body mass index. *Pediatr.* 151(3), 293–298.
119. Wanders A, van den Borne J, de Graaf C, Hulshof T, Jonathan M, Kristensen M et al. 2011. Effects of dietary fibre on subjective appetite, energy intake and body weight: A systematic review of randomized controlled trials. *Obes Rev.* 12, 724–739.
120. Archer B, Johnson S, Devereux H, Baxter A. 2004. Effect of fat replacement by inulin or lupin-kernel fibre on sausage patty acceptability, post-meal perceptions of satiety and food intake in men. *Br J Nutr.* 91, 591–599.
121. Tiwary C, Ward J, Jackson B. 1997. Effect of pectin on satiety in healthy US army adults. *J Am Coll Nutr.* 16, 423–428.
122. Haber GB, Heaton KW, Murphy D, Burroughs LF. 1977. Depletion and disruption of dietary fibre. Effects on satiety, plasma-glucose, and serum-insulin. *Lancet.* 2, 679–682.
123. Di Lorenzo C, Williams C, Hajnal F, Valenzuela J. 1988. Pectin delays gastric emptying and increases satiety in obese subjects. *Gastroenterology.* 95(5), 1211–1215.
124. Wanders AJ, Jonathan MC, van den Borne JJ, Mars M, Schols HA, Feskens EJ et al. 2013. The effects of bulking, viscous and gel-forming dietary fibers on satiation. *Br J Nutr.* 109, 1330–1337.
125. Anderson JW. 2008. Dietary fiber and associated phytochemicals in prevention and reversal of diabetes. In: Pasupuleti VK, Anderson JW, eds. *Nutraceuticals, Glycemic Health and Type 2 Diabetes.* Ames, IA: Blackwell Publishing Professional, 111–142.
126. Alberti G, Zimmet P, Shaw J, Grundy S. 2006. The IDF Worldwide Definition of the Metabolic Syndrome. International Diabetes Federation. Available at: http://www.idf.org/metabolic-syndrome (accessed on March 11, 2015).
127. Pastors JG, Blaisdell PW, Balm TK, Asplin CM, Pohl SL. 1991. Psyllium fiber reduces rise in postprandial glucose and insulin concentrations in patients with non-insulin-dependent diabetes. *Am J Clin Nutr.* 53(6), 1431–145.

128. Sierra M, Garcia JJ, Fernández N, Diez MJ, Calle AP, Sahagún AM. 2001. Effects of ispaghula husk and guar gum on postprandial glucose and insulin concentrations in healthy subjects. *Eur J Clin Nutr.* 55(4), 235–243.
129. McRorie J, Greenwood-Van Meerveld B, Rudolph C. 1998. Characterization of propagating contractions in the proximal colon of ambulatory mini pigs. *Dig Dis Sci.* 43(5), 957–963.
130. Greenwood-Van Meerveld B, Neeley D, Tyler K, Peters L, McRorie J. 1999. Comparison of effects on colonic motility and stool characteristics associated with feeding olestra and wheat bran to ambulatory mini-pigs. *Dig Dis Sci.* 44(7), 1282–1287.
131. Bassotti G, Crowell M, Whitehead W. 1993. Contractile activity of the human colon: Lessons from 24 hour studies. *Gut.* 34, 129–133.
132. Bassotti G, Germani U, Morelli A. 1996. Flatus-related colorectal and anal motor events. *Dig Dis Sci.* 41(2), 335–338.
133. Tomlin J, Read N. 1988a. Laxative properties of indigestible plastic particles. *Br Med J.* 297, 1175–1176.
134. Lewis SJ, Heaton KW. 1999. Roughage revisited: The effect on intestinal function of inert plastic particles of different sizes and shapes. *Dig Dis Sci.* 44, 744–748.
135. Francis CY, Whorwell PJ. 1994. Bran and irritable bowel syndrome: Time for reappraisal. *Lancet.* 344(8914), 39–40.
136. Grabitske HA, Slavin JL. 2009. Gastrointestinal effects of low-digestible carbohydrates. *Crit Rev Food Sci Nutr.* 49, 327–360.
137. Olesen M, Gudmand-Hoyer E. 2000. Efficacy, safety, and tolerability of fructooligosaccharides in the treatment of irritable bowel syndrome. *Am J Clin Nutr.* 72, 1570–1575.
138. Suarez F, Springfield J, Furne J, Lohrmann T, Kerr P, Levitt M. 1999. Gas production in humans ingesting a soybean flour derived from beans naturally low in oligosaccharides. *Am J Clin Nutr.* 69, 135–139.
139. Lewis S, Burmeister S, Cohen S et al. 2005. Failure of dietary oligo-fructose to prevent antibiotic-associated diarrhoea. *Aliment Pharmacol Ther.* 21, 469–477.
140. Cummings JH, Christie S, Cole TJ. 2001. A study of fructo-oligosaccharides in the prevention of travellers' diarrhoea. *Aliment Pharmacol Ther.* 15, 1139–1145.
141. Drakoularakou A, Tzortzis G, Rastall RA, Gibson GR. 2010. A double-blind, placebo-controlled, randomized human study assessing the capacity of a novel galacto-oligosaccharide mixture in reducing travellers' diarrhoea. *Eur J Clin Nutr.* 64(2), 146–152.
142. Tomlin J, Read N. 1988b. A comparative study of the effects on colon function caused by feeding ispaghula husk and polydextrose. *Aliment Pharmacol Ther.* 2(6), 513–519.
143. Marlett JA, Kajs TM, Fischer MH. 2000. An unfermented gel component of psyllium seed husk promotes laxation as a lubricant in humans. *Am J Clin Nutr.* 72, 784–789.
144. McRorie J, Daggy B, Morel J, Diersing P, Miner P, Robinson M. 1998. Psyllium is superior to docusate sodium for treatment of chronic constipation. *Aliment Pharmacol Ther.* 12, 491–497.
145. Singh B. 2007. Psyllium as a therapeutic and drug delivery agent. *Int J Pharm.* 334, 1–14.
146. Eherer A, Santa Ana C, Fordtran J. 1993. Effect of psyllium, calcium polycarbophil, and wheat bran on secretory diarrhea induced by phenolphthalein. *Gastroenterology.* 104, 1007–1012.
147. Qvitzau S, Matzen P, Madsen P. 1988. Treatment of chronic diarrhoea: Loperamide versus ispaghula husk and calcium. *Scand J Gastroenterol.* 23, 1237–1240.
148. Brandt LJ, Prather CM, Quigley EM, Schiller LR, Schoenfeld P, Talley NJ. 2005. Systematic review on the management of chronic constipation in North America. *Am J Gastroenterol.* 100, S5–S22.
149. Wenzl HH, Fine KD, Schiller LR et al. 1995. Determinants of decreased fecal consistency in patients with diarrhea. *Gastroenterol.* 108, 1729–1738.

150. Washington N, Harris M, Mussellwhite A, Spiller R. 1998. Moderation of lactulose-induced diarrhea by psyllium: Effects on motility and fermentation. *Am J Clin Nutr*. 67, 317–321.
151. Fujimori S, Tatsuguchi A, Gudis K et al. 2007. High dose probiotic and prebiotic cotherapy for remission induction of active Crohn's disease. *J Gastroenterol Hepatol.* 22, 1199–1204.
152. Spiller R, Aziz Q, Creed F et al. 2007. Guidelines on the irritable bowel syndrome: Mechanism and practical management. *Gut*. 56, 1770–1798.
153. Brandt LJ, Chey WD, Foxx-Orenstein AE et al. 2009. American College of Gastroenterology Task Force on IBS. An evidence-based systematic review on the management of irritable bowel syndrome. *Am J Gastroenterol*. 104(Suppl 1), S1–S35.
154. Bijkerk CJ, Muris JWM, Knottnerus JA, Hoes AW, De Wit NJ. 2004. Systematic review: The role of different types of fibre in the treatment of irritable bowel syndrome. *Aliment Pharmacol Ther.* 19, 245–251.
155. Eswaran S, Muir J, Chey W. 2013. Fiber and functional gastrointestinal disorders. *Am J Gastroenterol.* 108, 718–727.
156. McRorie, J. 2013. Clinical data support that psyllium is not fermented in the gut. Letter to the Editor, *Am J Gastroenterol.* 108(9), 1541.
157. Ford AC, Talley NJ, Spiegel BM et al. 2008. Effect of fibre, antispasmodics, and peppermint oil in the treatment of irritable bowel syndrome: Systematic review and meta-analysis. *Br Med J.* 337, a2313.
158. Thompson WG. 1994. Doubts about bran. *Lancet*. 344, 3.
159. Olesen M, Gudmand-Hoyer E. 2000. Efficacy, safety, and tolerability of fructo-oligosaccharides in the treatment of irritable bowel syndrome. *Am J Clin Nutr*. 72, 1570–1575.
160. Hunter JO, Tuffnell Q, Lee AJ. 1999. Controlled trial of oligo-fructose in the management of irritable bowel syndrome. *J Nutr*. 129, 1451S–1453S.
161. Paineau D, Payen F, Panserieu S et al. 2008. The effects of regular consumption of short-chain fructo-oligosaccharides on digestive comfort of subjects with minor functional bowel disorders. *Br J Nutr.* 99, 311–318.
162. Silk DBA, Davis A, Vulevic J et al. 2009. Clinical trial: The effects of a trans-galactooligosaccharide prebiotic on faecal microbiota and symptoms in irritable bowel syndrome. *Aliment Pharmacol Ther.* 29, 508–518
163. Lembo T, Munakata J, Naliboff B, Fullerton S, Mayer E. 1997. Sigmoid afferent mechanisms in patients with irritable bowel syndrome. *Dig Dis Sci.* 42, 1112–1120.
164. Serra J, Azpiroz F, Malagelda J. 1995. Perception and reflex responses to intestinal distention in humans are modified by simultaneous or previous stimulation. *Gastroenterology*. 109, 1742–1749.
165. Zighboim J, Talley N, Phillips S, Harmsen W, Zinmeister A. 1995. Visceral perception in irritable bowel syndrome. *Dig Dis Sci.* 40, 819–827.
166. McRorie J, Zorich N, Riccardi K, Bishop L, Filloon T, Wason S, Giannella R. 2000. Effects of olestra and sorbitol consumption on objective measures of diarrhea: Impact of stool viscosity on common gastrointestinal symptoms. *Regul Toxicol Pharmacol.* 31(1), 59–67.
167. Crowell M, Bassotti G, Cheskin L, Schuster M, Whitehead W. 1991. Method for prolonged ambulatory monitoring of high-amplitude propagated contractions from colon. *Am J Physiol*. 261, G263–G268.

9 Mechanisms of Docosahexaenoic Acid (DHA) in Neurodevelopment and Brain Protection

Christopher M. Butt and Norman Salem, Jr.

CONTENTS

9.1 INTRODUCTION

Converging evidence from multiple preclinical models suggests that the omega-3 long-chain polyunsaturated fatty acid (LC-PUFA), docosahexaenoic acid (DHA; 22:6n-3), supports nervous system health and function after mechanical damage. Much of this evidence has been acquired from therapeutic approaches attempting to mitigate traumatic brain injury (TBI) or spinal cord injury (SCI) with DHA or other LC-PUFAs. Such findings from multiple approaches are encouraging because only a few compounds have been shown to be clinically effective in treating nervous system damage (e.g., progesterone). Alternatively, it may be that receptor-directed, therapeutic approaches may not be the best way to improve outcomes after nervous system injury because a myriad of cell damage pathways are activated by TBI and SCI. Accordingly, multiple pathways for the protective effects of DHA in TBI and SCI have been proposed, and it may be that pleiotropic approaches (Stein, 2013), such as that with DHA, could prove more effective than receptor-directed drugs. However, the recent findings for DHA as a potential therapeutic for TBI and SCI (see Michael-Titus and Priestley, 2014 for review) have not fully accounted for the important roles that DHA plays, as a nutrient for nervous system development and homeostasis. This chapter discusses how the developmental requirements and functions of DHA may provide further explanations for the benefits of DHA after nervous system injury.

Mechanical injury involving the brain or spinal cord is the leading cause of neurological injury and trauma-related morbidity and death in the US. Worldwide, at least 10 million cases of TBI occur annually (Risdall and Menon, 2011), and at least 150,000 cases of SCI also happen each year (Tuszynksi et al., 2007). Nearly 80% of individuals seen for closed-head injuries are treated and released by emergency departments. However, these patients might still suffer from post-concussion syndrome (PCS), which can include headache, dizziness, fatigue, increased sensitivity to light or sound, and altered emotional, behavioral, cognitive, and motor functions (Bohnen et al., 1991; Learoyd and Lifshitz, 2012; Lidvall et al., 1974; McAllister, 1992; Rutherford et al., 1979).

Multiple lines of evidence from preclinical studies indicate that DHA and other LC-PUFAs (e.g., eicosapentaenoic acid; EPA; 20:5n-3) may reduce the impacts of nervous system injury. These studies have been reviewed in detail elsewhere (Michael-Titus and Priestley, 2014), and they indicate that DHA intake must be at adequate levels before an injury, or that DHA must be administered sometime soon after an injury occurs for any benefits to be conferred. DHA, EPA, or their metabolites have shown protective benefits in models of brain injury (Mills et al., 2011; Wu et al., 2014), in models of spinal cord (Hall et al., 2012; Paterniti et al., 2014) and peripheral nervous system (PNS) injury (Gladman et al., 2012), in models of stroke (Belayev et al., 2011), and in models of age-related neurodegenerative disorders such as Alzheimer's disease (AD; Calon, 2011; Green et al., 2007). These findings support the assertion that sufficient LC-PUFA intake may provide its benefits by acting on elements that are common to all of these conditions/injuries that induce damage to the nervous system.

9.2 RECOMMENDED DHA INTAKES

There are four primary sources of DHA that are found in nature. The best source of preformed DHA is marine algae. Algae such as *Crypthecodinium conii* and *Schizochytrium* naturally produce DHA at levels up to ~45% of the oil that is contained in the storage vesicles of these microorganisms (Fedorova-Dahms et al., 2014). The reason that fish oil contains DHA and other LC-PUFAs is due to the fish consuming the marine algae. The concentration of DHA in the fish oil is dependent on the diet of the fish, and seasonal variations in the lipid compositions of fish oil are accordingly common (Bandarra et al., 1997; Bell et al., 1985; Shirai et al., 2002a, b). The livers of land animals can also make DHA from omega-3 precursors such as α-linolenic acid (ALA; 18:3n-3), but the efficiency of this process is species dependent. For example, rats convert about 5% of ingested ALA to DHA (Lin and Salem, 2007), while the ALA-to-DHA conversion rate in humans is significantly less efficient (0.1%; Lin et al., 2010; Pawlosky and Salem, 2004; Plourde and Cunnane, 2007). The most common source for DHA intake is mother's milk. Human breast milk can contain DHA up to

1.4% of total fatty acids (FA), but such levels are highly dependent on the mother's marine food consumption (Brenna et al., 2007) and other health factors, such as the number of pregnancies a mother has had (Morse et al., 2012).

DHA is necessary for optimal brain development (Innis, 2008; McNamara and Carlson, 2006). The DHA intake that is generally recommended for infants is near to that found in human milk, and this recommendation is supported by randomized, controlled clinical trials (RCTs). For example, the addition of DHA to infant formula improves visual acuity and mental performance later in life (Hoffman et al., 2009), and these benefits are most often noted when the formulas contain DHA near its average worldwide concentration in human milk (0.32% of total FA; Brenna et al., 2007). Some RCTs have tested whether DHA levels above 0.32% confer greater benefits to developing infants (Birch et al., 2010; Makrides et al., 2009). These studies found that a minimum DHA concentration of ~0.32% is necessary for proper brain development and that some individuals could benefit from higher DHA concentrations, particularly preterm infants. However, the recommendations of the World Association of Perinatal Medicine, the Early Nutrition Academy, and the Child Health Foundation remain appropriately conservative and are based on the LC-PUFA levels used in successful clinical studies. Accordingly, the recommended levels (0.2%–0.5% of total FA; Koletzko et al., 2008) represent the global averages observed in human milk (Brenna et al., 2007).

Recommended DHA intakes for older children and adults are still developing. These recommendations are typically in the conservative range of 500–1000 milligrams per day (European Food Safety Authority, 2012; Gebauer et al., 2006), and some are simplified further into the number of servings of fatty fish per week because, as alluded to above, some fish are excellent sources of DHA (Gebauer et al., 2006). For example, consumption of 0.5–3 servings of unfried fish per week has been associated with decreased risk of stroke (Bouzan et al., 2005; He et al., 2002; Larsson and Orsini, 2011; Virtanen et al., 2008; Wang et al., 2006). However, as with the infant formula recommendations, some data support DHA intakes that are significantly higher.

9.3 DELIVERY OF DHA TO THE NERVOUS SYSTEM

Once LC-PUFAs have been introduced to the body, they are delivered to the nervous system through several pathways. This section focuses on DHA for simplicity as other LC-PUFAs are likely provided to the nervous system in similar fashions (Ouellet et al., 2009). Pharmacokinetic data suggest that the adult human brain needs to replace ~4 mg of the DHA that it metabolizes each day (Umhau et al., 2009). The intake necessary to accomplish this replacement is a subject of controversy because the absorption, processing, and trafficking of DHA to the central nervous system is complex. Like other LC-PUFAs, DHA is processed into its free FA, unesterified form by lipases in the gut before it can be absorbed by the small intestine. The small intestine then assembles and packages DHA-containing triacylglycerols (TAGs) into chylomicrons. Liver enzymes process the chylomicrons to DHA-TAGs, DHA-phosphatidylcholine (PC), unesterified DHA, and DHA-lysophosphatyidylcholine (LPC). DHA-TAGs and DHA-PC are then bound to low-density lipoprotein (LDL), while unesterified DHA and DHA-LPC are bound by serum albumin (Brossard et al., 1996). LDL and albumin carry DHA in its various forms throughout the bloodstream at a total concentration of about 5% of the orally ingested dose (Lemaitre-Delaunay et al., 1999). Monkey and rodent data suggest that approximately 0.5% of the unesterified DHA in the plasma reaches the brain (Polozova and Salem, 2007; Umhau et al., 2009). These data further suggest that a 1 g oral dose of DHA will result in only 250 μg being delivered to the brain in a naïve individual (16× below what is needed). However, the body processes DHA as an essential nutrient (not a drug), and no individual completely lacks DHA. Moreover, the existing data indicate that DHA deficiencies exist and that supplementation can result in optimal DHA levels in the brain.

It is accepted that unesterified DHA will freely cross the blood–brain barrier (BBB) interface through a non-saturable mechanism, even at low equilibrium concentrations (Ouellet et al., 2009; Vandal et al., 2014). The dissociations of unesterified DHA and DHA-LPC from albumin near the BBB clearly serve as a DHA source. However, endothelial lipase, which is anchored on the luminal surface of capillaries, also likely helps to ensure a consistently available supply of DHA to the brain (Chen and Subbaiah, 2013). This enzyme cleaves FAs from LC-PUFA-TAGs and LC-PUFA-PC that are bound to LDL. Interestingly, the lipase can also serve as a molecular bridge between LDL in the plasma and LDL receptors on the capillary surface (Goti et al., 2002), thus providing another potential mechanism for the internalization of DHA into the brain's epithelium. The mechanisms of endothelial lipase are saturable, and they are distinct from the passive diffusion of FA across the BBB. However, they also provide regulatory checkpoints for FA flux across the BBB (Chen and Subbaiah, 2013; Young and Zechner, 2013) along with other carrier proteins. Other carrier proteins include plasma membrane FA-binding proteins (FABPs), FA transporters, and FA-transport protein (Abumrad et al., 1999; Veerkamp et al., 2000). The brain-specific FABPs and apolipoprotein E (ApoE) are of particular interest as they have been implicated in both brain development and brain injury.

Upon transport to the glia that interact directly with the epithelial cells, PUFAs are carried by the brain FABPs and ApoE. Three brain FABPs have been identified thus far (FABP-3, -5, and -7), and they have different developmental expression profiles. Each FABP subtype also has differential selectivity for the various types of FAs. FABP-3 selectively binds arachidonic acid (ARA; 20:4n-6) and oleic acid (18:1n-9). FABP-5 has its highest affinity for saturated FAs like stearic acid (18:0), while the ligand preferences of FABP-7 are for DHA, EPA, and oleic acid (Liu et al., 2010). Similarly, ApoE is an important brain-specific lipoprotein that astrocytes use to transport FAs to the neurons. The ApoE4 isoform is significantly less efficient at carrying DHA than the ApoE2 and ApoE3 isoforms (Vandal et al., 2014). Interestingly, ApoE4 is associated with greater rates of Alzheimer's disease (Barberger-Gateau et al., 2011) and worse outcomes after TBI (Mahley and Huang, 2012; Zhou et al., 2008), and brain FABPs have been proposed as plasma biomarkers for brain injury (Chan et al., 2005). Overall, these lipid binding proteins serve to solubilize FAs in the cytosolic space and to carry the FAs to their target locations in the brain.

Regardless of the source, the incorporation of DHA and other LC-PUFAs into the plasma, red blood cells, and nervous tissue is saturable. For example, consumption of 1 g of DHA per day results in a plateau of DHA in the plasma at 8% of total FA after only 1 month. The incorporation of DHA into red blood cells is similar, but it is slower in that plateau levels of 8%–9% of total FA requires 4–6 months to occur. Interestingly, supplementation of the DHA precursor ALA does not change DHA levels in the human bloodstream. Similarly, supplementation with EPA, which can be interconverted to DHA, only changes EPA levels in the blood (Arterburn et al., 2006; Brenna et al., 2009). The lack of effect of both DHA precursors on DHA levels could be due to several possibilities. First, the production of DHA from its ALA precursor has an efficiency of only 0.1% in humans (Lin et al., 2010; Pawlosky and Salem, 2004; Plourde and Cunnane, 2007), possibly because a large proportion of ALA is oxidized (Burdge et al., 2002; Lin and Salem, 2007), and dietary background can influence conversion rates. Dietary EPA and DHA reduce the conversion of ALA to DHA by 70% (Pawlosky et al., 2003). Furthermore, dietary linoleic acid (LA; 18:2n-6) competitively inhibits the Δ^6 desaturase important for ALA conversion and reduces omega-3 accumulation by up to 70% (Emken et al., 1994). Thus, the shift in Western diets to high LA intakes (~15 g/day) and low ALA intakes (~1.5 g/day) likely plays a role in reducing the omega-3 status in Westerners (Blasbalg et al., 2011).

The findings described above support the assertion that consumption of preformed DHA is the most effective way for humans to attain DHA sufficiency (Brenna et al., 2009). When they are coupled with the high correlation between the FA status in the blood with that in the brain of non-human primates (Sarkadi-Nagy et al., 2003), and with findings that FA levels in the cerebrospinal fluid are directly related to plasma FA levels in humans (Freund-Levi et al., 2014), it is likely that low omega-3 status in human blood also translates to low omega-3 status in human brain. This circumstance may explain why most successful RCTs using DHA in adult humans have provided 900–4000 mg of DHA per day for at least 3–6 months. Such studies have demonstrated clinical improvements in mild cognitive impairment (Yurko-Mauro et al., 2010) and cardiovascular measures (Ryan et al., 2009).

An outside observer may perceive confusion in the literature over omega-3 intake and its resulting deposition in target organs. This circumstance is largely due to differences in analytical methodology (total FA vs. phospholipids vs. unesterified FA) and presentation (percent total FA vs. milligrams per liter vs. nanograms per gram, etc.). Simplification and interpretation of all these data are possible. For example, DHA-phospholipids contain ~80% of the total DHA concentration in human plasma (Brossard et al., 1996). The DHA-phospholipids in unsupplemented human plasma is about 60 mg/L (Rusca et al., 2009) or 4% of total FAs (Arterburn et al., 2006). These data indicate that the total DHA content in the plasma is 80 mg/L on average in a DHA-deficient individual and that 400 mg of DHA is circulating in the bloodstream (5 L) at any given moment.

The average unesterified DHA content in the unsupplemented human brain is ~110 nmol/g and is associated with a total DHA brain content of ~10 μmol/g (Astarita et al., 2010; Igarashi et al., 2011). While the unesterified pool is a very small fraction of the total, measurements of the unesterified pool allow for the best approximation of DHA pharmacokinetics at the BBB. The 110 nmol/g of unesterified DHA in the brain translates to a total of 54.2 mg of unbound DHA in the brain and 13.6% bioavailability from the blood when the weights of DHA (328.5 g/mol) and the average brain

(1500 g) are taken into account. Thus, at equilibrium in unsupplemented individuals on a Western diet, taking in 100 mg or less of dietary DHA per day, the oral bioavailability of DHA to the brain is about 680 μg/day (100 mg × 0.05 [Lemaitre-Delaunay et al., 1999] × 0.136) with the brain consuming ~4 mg/day (Umhau et al., 2009). Mechanisms clearly exist to maintain this unsupplemented equilibrium (Emken et al., 1994; Farooqui et al., 2004; Pawlosky et al., 2003; Orr et al., 2013), otherwise the brain's pool of DHA would be in a constant state of decline, which it can be in cases of liver toxicity (Astarita et al., 2010; Umhau et al., 2013). Nonetheless, such circumstances are less than ideal, particularly when unsupplemented brains from Alzheimer's patients have about 65–95 nmol/g of unesterified DHA, which is a relatively small difference from normal controls (110 nmol/g), albeit a significant one (Astarita et al., 2010; Igarashi et al., 2011).

Supplementation of Alzheimer's patients can improve their omega-3 status and biomarkers of the condition (Freund-Levi et al., 2013), but potential problems with DHA processing in Alzheimer's disease (Vandal et al., 2014) may contribute to an overall lack of effect of DHA supplementation after clinical diagnosis (Quinn et al., 2010). It is therefore interesting that some Alzheimer's biomarkers (e.g., tau, low DHA status, ApoE4 status) are also associated with poor outcomes after TBI (Mahley and Huang, 2012; Mills et al., 2010; Zhou et al., 2008).

The situation is better for individuals that consume adequate dietary levels of DHA. Just 1 month of consuming at least 1 g of DHA/day significantly increases the total DHA status in the blood (138 mg/L or 8%–10% of total FA; Rusca et al., 2009; Arterburn et al., 2006; 690 mg total). Based on non-human primate studies, this level of supplementation results in a plateau that represents a 140% increase of total DHA in the brain (from 10% total FAs to 14% total FAs; Sarkadi-Nagy et al., 2003). These findings suggest that at equilibrium the unesterified DHA content in the brains of DHA-sufficient individuals is on the order of 150 nmol/g (110 nmol/g [Astarita et al., 2010; Igarashi et al., 2011] × 1.4; 75.9 mg total; 11% blood bioavailability) and that the oral bioavailability of DHA to the brain would be 5.5 mg/day (1000 mg × 0.05 [Lemaitre-Delaunay et al., 1999] × 0.11). These values exceed the brain's daily metabolism of DHA (~4 mg/day; Umhau et al., 2009), and would allow for accumulation to more optimal levels. It should be noted that the above calculations are based on global averages and that significant variation would be encountered readily in any clinical population.

Despite the clinical findings for mild cognitive impairment (Yurko-Mauro et al., 2010; Janssen and Kiliaan, 2014) and the existing preclinical data for DHA's potential role in mitigating nervous system injuries (Michael-Titus and Priestley, 2014), an RCT that investigates DHA in human nervous system injuries has not been completed as of yet. Nonetheless, the Institute of Medicine has taken notice of the preclinical data available for brain and spinal cord injuries, it is promoting nutritional approaches to these injuries, and DHA and other omega-3 FAs are high on the priority list of nutrients of interest (Institute of Medicine, 2011).

9.4 DHA-RELATED MECHANISMS DURING DEVELOPMENT

The importance of DHA during infant brain development is well established and has been reviewed in great detail elsewhere (Carlson, 2009; Innis, 2008; McNamara and

Carlson, 2006). The purpose of this chapter is to link DHA's nutritional and neurodevelopmental mechanisms to how it protects the nervous system from injury. Human brain development has a number of distinct phases that vary in their rate, duration, and occurrence during childhood and adolescence. These phases include: (1) brain cell migration very early in development, (2) neuron growth and axon elongation, (3) synaptogenesis, (4) the critical step of appropriate myelination, and (5) continued plasticity and maintenance of the nervous system in the presence or absence of an injury. DHA interacts with all of the above (or their maintenance), and these developmental roles (McNamara and Carlson, 2006) have implications for its protective role during nervous system injury.

The existing data support the premise that DHA is not merely a membrane component. Indeed, the molecular properties of DHA have organizational effects on membrane structure. These structural changes can affect the efficiency of membrane contact signaling, which results in changes in the function of the neurovascular unit (i.e., neuron, glia, microglia, and blood supply). It is likely that the structural effects of DHA are important to its nutritional value during development as well as its prophylactic protective effects when provided before a nervous system injury. Furthermore, DHA and its metabolites have their own signaling properties that contribute to the therapeutic value of this nutrient after nervous system injury (reviewed by Michael-Titus and Priestley, 2014). Overall, the current knowledge in the field argues that DHA's protective effects stem from its structural and signaling functions during development that ultimately allow for better myelin maintenance and better neuron function during injury or neurodegeneration.

9.4.1 Brain Cell Migration

Brain cell migration starts during the middle of gestation and continues throughout pregnancy (Rakic, 2006), a time period where more than half of the DHA that the brain needs during developmental is accumulated (McNamara and Carlson, 2006). Brain cell migration is characterized by the movement of postmitotic cells that were born near the core of the brain's early structure (i.e., the subventricular zone) to outer layers of the brain, where they eventually organize and resemble the adult brain structure (Rakic, 2006). While not necessarily causal, the lack of DHA during this critical period (e.g., in the case of preterm birth) has been associated with the reduction in size of important brain regions such as the cortex, hippocampus, and amygdala (Peterson et al., 2000) and with attention and learning deficits later in life (McNamara and Carlson, 2006). Similar problems occur in the Reeler mouse, an animal that is ataxic, exhibits reversal of the normal brain layer pattern, and due to its genetic mutation has deficient levels of a protein known as reelin. Interestingly, reelin signaling involves lipids and lipid carriers, it affects cognitive behaviors, brain size, brain layer patterning and neuronal survival (Herz and Chen, 2006), and omega-3 status has been linked to reelin expression in the nervous system (Yavin et al., 2009).

Reelin is a glycoprotein that is secreted into the extracellular matrix. Reelin works through the very low-density lipoprotein receptor (VLDL-R) and the ApoE receptor subtype 2 (ApoE-R2) to regulate migration during development and to regulate synaptic function in the adult brain. Accordingly, altered reelin expression has been detected in autism, schizophrenia, depression, and Alzheimer's disease (Folsom et al., 2013). Furthermore, reelin is upregulated at sites of brain injury (Courtès et al., 2011; Massalini et al., 2009) and PNS injury (Panteri et al., 2006). Reelin is first made by Cajal–Retzus cells in peripheral, less-developed brain tissue that calls for the migration of new neurons to those peripheral layers through reelin signaling. As development proceeds, reelin is then expressed by GABAergic neurons (Rossel et al., 2005) that provide the initial permissive state for synaptogenesis and neuron maturation. The developing brain then switches to using excitatory glutamatergic transmission for synaptogenesis (Akerman and Cline, 2007), and later reelin expression is found in excitatory granule and pyramidal cells as well as glial cells (Folsom et al., 2013).

The expression of reelin seems to be well-coordinated with the developmental shift toward glutamatergic neurotransmission. Presynaptic reelin signaling promotes the stabilization of N-methyl-D-aspartate (NMDA) receptor complexes that respond to glutamate in postsynaptic cells (Herz and Chen, 2006), while interference with GABAergic signaling disrupts the expression of reelin and the maturation of those NMDA-receptor complexes (Melamed et al., 2014). Ultimately, reelin first acts as a promigratory signal via ApoE-R2. When migrating neurons have reached the appropriate brain layer, and reelin levels are presumably high, the reelin serves as an environmental signal via VLDL-R for those neurons to stop migrating (Hack et al., 2007), to mature, and to make synaptic connections (Herz and Chen, 2006).

Reelin expression is subject to environmental and dietary regulation. For example, rodent studies have suggested that prenatal infections can reduce reelin expression in the brain and result in autism- or schizophrenia-like behaviors (Meyer et al., 2008). Similarly, activation of the maternal immune system with lipopolysaccharide (LPS) reduces reelin expression in the brains of the offspring (Ghiani et al., 2011). In contrast, a maternal diet that has sufficient levels of omega-3 FAs affects the offspring in that adequate brain tissue levels of DHA are attained, reelin expression is increased, and newborn neurons migrate properly during the development of the hippocampus and cortex, which are both important for cognitive behaviors (Yavin et al., 2009).

The mechanisms through which DHA promotes reelin expression are not understood (He et al., 2014), but interactions exist in the activities of both molecules that may provide some explanation for how DHA could promote reelin-related processes and how both molecules have protective effects in central nervous system injury. One of the most established functions of DHA is to enable conformational changes of an activated transmembrane protein. This function is due to the physical properties of DHA. The 22 carbons and 6 double bonds found in DHA serve to increase membrane permeability, packing volume, deformability, and disorder. These increases allow for greater space in the membrane for a protein to undergo conformation changes after activation (Gawrisch et al., 2008; Niu et al., 2004). As examples, fluorescent resonant energy transfer (FRET) is two-fold more efficient in DHA membranes (Stillwell et al., 2005), and the activity of rhodopsin, the classical model for transmembrane G-protein coupled receptors, is increased by the presence of DHA in the membrane (Niu et al., 2004; Polozova and Litman, 2000; Salem et al., 2001). Accordingly, as the percentage of DHA in the retina increases, the sensitivity of the retinal response also increases (Jeffrey et al., 2001; Weisinger et al., 1999). It is therefore likely, although not tested thoroughly in a case-by-case manner, that the activities of many other transmembrane receptors, such as those for reelin, are also enhanced by the physical properties of DHA in the membrane. Such is indeed the case with regards to the translocation and activity of phosphatidylinositol-3-kinase (PI3K). Interestingly, substitution of DHA with docosapentaenoic acid (DPA; 22:5n-6), which has only 1 less double bond than DHA, results in reduced PI3K activity (Akbar et al., 2005) and reduced rhodopsin activity (Mitchell et al., 2012; Niu et al., 2004).

Reelin signaling (Folsom et al., 2013) and DHA actions on the cell membrane (Akbar et al., 2005) both increase the activity of the PI3K cascade. Activation of this cascade involves protein kinase B (also known as AkT) and subsequent inhibition of glycogen synthase kinase (GSK3β; Folsom et al., 2013), inhibition of caspase-3 (Akbar et al., 2005), and activation of the mammalian target of rapamycin (mTOR; Narayanan et al., 2009). These AkT activities promote structural plasticity, neuron survival, and growth, respectively.

GSK3β inhibits glycogen production and phosphorylates tau, an important microtubule-associated protein. Thus, when GSK3β is inhibited by AkT, glucose uptake and storage are increased, and the stabilizing effects of tau on microtubule dynamics are reduced. These actions would explain to some extent how reelin and omega-3 sufficiency have a promigratory effect (Yavin et al., 2009) by decreasing the rigidity of the microtubule cytoskeleton in an actively migrating cell (Llorens-Marìtin et al., 2014). Hyperphosphorylation of tau and poor glucose utilization by the brain are hallmarks of Alzheimer's disease, and these circumstances are presumably associated with GSK3β activity (Medhi and Chakrabarty, 2013), so it is consistent that appropriate insulin signaling also inhibits GSK3β (Sutherland et al., 1993). Altered glucose metabolism (Giza and Hovda, 2001) and hyperphoshorylation of tau can also occur after multiple types of brain injury (Lee et al., 2013; Ojo et al., 2013; Pluta et al., 2011). The findings that upregulated reelin enhances the migration of progenitor cells to injury sites (Courtès et al., 2011; Massalini et al., 2009) that deficiency in either reelin or omega-3 FA intake are correlated with worse outcomes after nervous system injury (Lorenzetto et al., 2008; Massalini et al., 2009; Mills et al., 2011; Won et al., 2006; Wu et al., 2004, 2011) and that the signaling pathways of both reelin and DHA can reduce the phosphorylation of tau (Calon and Cole, 2007; Matsuki et al., 2012), strongly suggest that reelin and DHA share the AkT/GSK3β pathway and that the two may work together. In concert, the two could promote the brain cell migration that occurs during development and when brain tissue has been injured in some way, with both processes requiring new neurons and other support cells for growth or repair. Low reelin concentrations from remote target sites likely provide the initial migratory signal, while higher local concentrations of reelin at the target sites serve as the stop signal (Folsom et al., 2013; Hack et al., 2007; Rossel et al., 2005). Meanwhile, DHA would serve as a membrane component in newly born cells, provide greater flexibility to their membranes (Gawrisch et al., 2008; Niu et al., 2004; Stillwell et al., 2005), augment the activity of the AkT pathway, and enhance the promigratory state of the cells overall.

Activation of the AkT pathway also reduces caspase-3 activity (Akbar et al., 2005). Caspase-3 is the "executioner" enzyme that is activated during apoptosis and subsequently cleaves proteins that are essential for cell survival. The AkT pathway inhibits caspase-3 by phosphorylating and inhibiting upstream activator enzymes such as caspase-9 (Snigdha et al., 2012). This allows for cell survival under metabolically stressful conditions that occur during differentiation and migration (Huang et al., 2012) as well as during TBI (Giza and Hovda, 2001), neurodegenerative diseases, and brain ischemia. Furthermore, metabolic stress leads to oxidative stress that can increase the production of neuroprotectins derived from DHA. These neuroprotectins also inhibit caspase-3 by upregulating the expression of prosurvival members of the Bcl-2 family of proteins (Bazan, 2013; Mukherjee et al., 2007). Thus, since DHA and reelin share this prosurvival AkT pathway, another way the two could work together is to maintain the viability of cells that are migrating or have otherwise been stressed by a physical or metabolic insult to the brain.

It is notable that prosurvival signals such as brain-derived neurotrophic factor (BDNF) and nerve growth factor (NGF) increase the production of neuroprotectins (Mukherjee et al., 2007) and also share the activations of the AkT/mTOR pathway (Gururajan and van den Buuse, 2014), the extracellular signal regulated kinase (ERK)/mitogen-activated protein kinase (MAPK)/cyclic AMP response element-binding protein (CREB) pathway (Boneva and Yamashima, 2012) and of Src/Fyn kinase (Bartlett and Wang, 2013) with omega-3 sufficiency (Akbar et al., 2005; Bach et al., 2014; Pan et al., 2009) and reelin (Folsom et al., 2013). These observations are consistent with DHA, or its docosanoid metabolites (Bazan, 2013), also being a trophic factor(s), but the explanations and descriptions of these pathways are more appropriate to the sections on growth, synaptogenesis, and myelination that are found later in this chapter.

9.4.2 Neuron Growth and Axon Elongation

The growth of neurons and the extension of their neurites are necessary for new connections to be made during development, maintenance of connections as the brain grows, and reconfiguration of connections after traumatic injury to the nervous system. During development, neuritogenesis occurs soon after neurons have stopped migrating (Hippenmeyer, 2014). The neurites then differentiate into dendrites that receive information and axons that transmit information. Since progenitor cells are called to sites of injured brain tissue (Courtès et al., 2011; Massalini et al., 2009), it is possible that similar events occur to some extent after nervous system injury. Findings consistent with this assertion, such as axon sprouting, have been reported after experimental SCI and after seizure activity in the brain (Perederiy and Westbrook, 2013). Regardless of whether the context is development or injury, the process of neuritogenesis requires the accumulation of new lipids to accommodate the increased surface area of the membranes of a growing neuron (Futerman and Banker, 1996). It also involves pro-growth mechanisms that are engaged by growth factors and signaling actions by the lipids, such as DHA, that help build the neuronal membranes.

Supplementation of neuronal cultures with exogenous DHA increases the extension of neurites in those cultures. Similar findings have been reported in cells derived from the hippocampus of the central nervous system (Calderon and Kim, 2007) and in cells derived from the dorsal root ganglia of the PNS (Robson et al., 2010). These two regions are of particular interest as they are typically affected in cases of TBI and SCI, respectively.

As DHA is accumulated into a growing membrane, it assists with membrane structure organization, enhances the function of some membrane proteins, and acts as a signal itself. For example, DHA plays a role in the formation of lipid raft membrane domains. Lipid rafts are characterized by the increased presence of cholesterol, caveolin, and sphingomyelin that provide a more rigid membrane structure. The presence of DHA in a membrane "pushes" cholesterol into the raft domains. In the case of phospholipase D, this action can lead to the enzyme moving into the DHA/non-raft domains and allow for greater enzyme activity (Shaikh et al., 2004) by reducing steric hindrance on the enzyme and facilitating the conformational changes (via DHA's membrane disordering effects) needed for that activity. These effects of DHA on phospholipase D activity are similar to those on protein kinase C (Stillwell et al., 2005), rhodopsin (Polozova and Litman, 2000), and AkT (Akbar et al., 2005). Such effects on protein activity are likely not universal, but they are intriguing when coupled with the lipid-raft organizing activities of DHA in that they may apply to the function of the reelin receptor complex and other downstream activities of the AkT cascade.

A number of the major extracellular and intracellular proteins involved in neurite extension are associated with lipid rafts. These proteins include integrins, cadherins, and cell adhesion molecules that interact with the extracellular matrix, glutamate receptors that detect neurotransmission, and tau and actin molecules that tether the rafts to the intracellular cytoskeleton. Such lipid rafts are found at the tips of neurites, and neurite guidance and elongation cannot proceed without the polarity imparted by the lipid raft and its connection to the cytoskeleton (Head et al., 2014). Interestingly, cholesterol enrichment into the lipid raft is involved in these elongation and polarization processes (Lingwood et al., 2008). Given that DHA is not concentrated in lipid rafts and can help to enrich lipid rafts with cholesterol (Shaikh et al., 2004), it is tempting to speculate that DHA accumulation during neuron growth/elongation serves to backfill the non-raft domains as a neurite stretches and to organize the lipid rafts into the neurite tips that are binding and interacting with the extracellular environment. Thus, the developmental need for DHA (Moriguchi and Salem, 2003; Fedorova et al., 2009; Ryan et al., 2010) could be partially explained by the disordering actions of DHA on the non-raft domains that allow for increased molecular interactions between the growing neuronal membranes and the extracellular environment. Furthermore, therapies that promote raft organization have been proposed as being potentially beneficial for nervous system injury (Head et al., 2014), and DHA has raft-organizing functions (Shaikh et al., 2004; Stillwell et al., 2005). It therefore follows that DHA has been demonstrated to protect the nervous system from damage in many preclinical studies. Indeed, findings suggest that DHA protects against the loss of intracellular scaffold in models of neurodegeneration (Calon et al., 2004, 2005) are consistent with the observed maintenance of structural integrity after an injury event (Michael-Titus and Priestley, 2014). In contrast, dysregulated or damaged lipid rafts and cytoskeletal scaffolds can lead to dysfunction and/or disease (Bartzokis, 2011).

DHA also modulates pro-growth, cell survival signals that are cascaded through complexes of AkT/mTOR, the retinoid X receptor (RXR; Akbar et al., 2005), or ERK/MAPK/CREB (Boneva and Yamashima, 2012). The mTOR complex is implicated because its activation requires PI3K/AkT, AkT activity is enhanced by DHA (Akbar et al., 2005), and neuritogenesis is reduced when levels/activity of mTOR (Kumar et al., 2005), PI3K, AkT (Jaworski et al., 2005; Tavazoie et al., 2005), or DHA are reduced (Akbar et al., 2005; Calderon and Kim, 2007). Interestingly, inhibitors of the phosphatase and tensin homolog (PTEN) have also been proposed as therapies for SCI that may allow for enhanced neurite growth and reconnection after injury. PTEN normally reduces PI3K activity. Thus, PTEN inhibitors increase AkT cascade activity and its effects on neurite growth. These effects on growth would be particularly import in adult tissue that has lost mTOR activity over time (Liu et al., 2010). The growth occurs because the activated mTOR complex increases the translation of protein synthesis machinery that is needed for growth as well as receptors and other proteins that are associated with synaptogenesis (Gururajan and van den Buuse, 2014).

In contrast to the effects of mTOR on translation, the RXR nuclear receptor complexes engage transcription-related mechanisms that allow for growth and further differentiation. The RXR complexes are of interest because they have selective binding affinity for DHA over other PUFAs. However, questions remain as to whether the micromolar DHA levels needed to bind and activate the RXR transcription factor complex (Lengqvist et al., 2004) are physiologically relevant within the intracellular space. Nonetheless, many citations exist that implicate the activation of the RXR by DHA, heterodimerization of the RXR with the retinoic acid receptor (RAR) or the peroxisomal proliferator agonist receptors (PPAR), and promoted expression of genes for synapse-related proteins (e.g., PSD-95, synaptophysin, and glutamate receptor subunits) and for growth-related proteins (e.g., sonic hedgehog) via the retinoic acid response element (RARE) or other transcription factors (Bazan et al., 2011; van Neerven et al., 2008). Furthermore, some evidence also points to the RXR pathway inducing the phosphorylation of components in the mTOR and ERK/MAPK/CREB pathways (Chen and Napoli, 2008).

The ERK/MAPK/CREB transcription factor pathway is another important way with which DHA, reelin, and lipid rafts interact for increasing the expression of pro-growth and pro-survival signals. As with AkT (Akbar et al., 2005), the presence of DHA in the membrane enhances the translocation and subsequent downstream signaling of ERK (Brand et al., 2008; Florent et al., 2005). Accordingly, ERK signaling increases the expression of BDNF (Boneva and Yamashima, 2012) and of the Bcl-2 prosurvival protein (Pan et al., 2009) after DHA supplementation. Prolonged exposure to DHA and incorporation of it into the membrane seems to be necessary to elicit these protective effects, particularly within the context of ischemic- and neurodegeneration-related damage (Boneva and Yamashima, 2012; Brand et al., 2008; Florent et al., 2006; Pan et al., 2009). However, receptors for unesterified DHA, such as gpr40 (Boneva and Yamashima, 2012; Zamarbide et al., 2014) and gpr120 (Wellhauser and Belsham, 2014) are also connected to the ERK pathway. In light of the recent suggestion that unesterified DHA confers some acute protective effects in the nervous system, DHA in the cell membrane likely serves as an available pool from which cleavage to its unesterified form and/or transformation to other protective docosanoids occurs (Orr et al., 2013). Yet, these findings do not rule-out the membrane translocation effects of DHA on the upstream components of these pathways that have been described (Akbar et al., 2005; Brand et al., 2008).

Reelin is indirectly linked to the ERK pathway via phosphorylation of the NMDA subtype of glutamate receptors by Fyn kinase (Folsom et al., 2013). These events increase the amount of calcium fluxing through the NMDA receptor, which can lead to activation of CREB (Herz and Chen, 2006). Furthermore, Fyn is typically associated with lipid rafts, and, when Fyn is exposed to EPA or DHA, it moves out of the lipid rafts (Aires et al., 2007; Chen et al., 2007; Duraisamy et al., 2007; Yaqoob, 2009). Whether this PUFA-related translocation enhances or inhibits Fyn function in the nervous system is not clear because these observations occurred in transfected HEK-293 cells (Aires et al., 2007), in vascular endothelial cells (Chen et al., 2007), and in T-cells from the immune system (Yaqoob, 2009) where Fyn was associated with increased calcium flux, inhibited inflammatory cascades, and inhibited calcium-related T-cell activation, respectively. This lack of directionality makes it difficult to impart a unified physiological relevance to PUFA effects on lipid raft composition and function. Nonetheless, lipid rafts are clearly dynamic membrane components that can integrate and regulate cell function (Hicks et al., 2012), and their interactions with DHA in the non-raft domains (Shaikh et al., 2004; Stillwell et al., 2005; Teague et al., 2013), as well as how some important membrane proteins may move between the two domains as they function, could become more relevant with greater understanding. It may be a simple extension of better translocation of activated membrane signaling proteins when DHA is present in the membrane, as has been shown for AkT (Akbar et al., 2005) and ERK (Brand et al., 2008).

The current science best supports lipid rafts as concentrators and organizers of pro-growth signals and cytoskeletal components for the migration and elongation of neuronal cells that can be modulated by nutritional lipids and by reelin signaling. However, the clustering of synaptic proteins such as PDS-95, NMDA receptors, non-NMDA glutamate receptors, and receptor tyrosine kinases in lipid rafts (Head et al., 2014) implies that rafts are also important for the generation and maintenance of synapses. It therefore follows that DHA and reelin have correlated modulatory roles for synaptogenesis.

9.4.3 Synaptogenesis

The Hebbian concept of activity-dependent wiring of the brain's circuitry is important not only during development (Debski and Cline, 2002; Katz and Shatz, 1996) but also during rewiring after an injury or similar disruption in connectivity (Perederiy and Westbrook, 2013). Synaptogenic processes require neuronal activity in the forms of action potentials and neurotransmitter release in the presynaptic cell and transduction of the neurotransmitter signal through receptors in the postsynaptic cell. Further activity and protein synthesis is then required on both sides of the synapse for the neurochemical connection to be established and maintained (Chiu and Cline, 2010). Synaptogenesis can be enhanced by DHA (Kim and Spector, 2013), reelin (Herz and Chen, 2006), and properly functioning lipid rafts (Romanelli and Wood,

2008) through the AkT/mTOR mechanism that has already been described, but other mechanisms have also been demonstrated.

Axonal growth cones that transmit signals and the postsynaptic dendrites that receive those signals have similar dynamics for growth and stabilization of the actin cytoskeleton. As such, the AkT/mTOR pathway increases the synthesis of proteins that facilitate the generation of synapses, but these proteins do not necessarily induce synapse formation through activity-dependent mechanisms such as long-term potentiation (LTP). For example, LTP is dependent on the presence of NMDA receptors, but mTOR has primarily been associated with the expression of synaptic scaffold proteins such as PSD-95 as well as proteins needed for protein synthesis and dendrite/axon morphology. This suggests that the mTOR pathway is part of the downstream protein synthesis aspects of synaptogenesis, not the induction phases (Gururajan and van den Buuse, 2014).

In contrast, although DHA, reelin, and lipid rafts enhance the AkT/mTOR pathway, they also employ more direct effects on synaptic protein activity. DHA has mixed effects on glutamatergic synaptic activity. When provided long-term through the diet, it results in increased synapsin expression that is correlated with increased availability of presynaptic glutamate release. Increased neurotransmitter release from presynaptic terminals is consistent with LTP, which is enhanced in tissues derived from DHA-sufficient animals. However, acute applications of unesterifed DHA do not enhance LTP (Cao et al., 2009) even though they potentiate NMDA-receptor responses. This disconnect may be due to the observation that acute DHA applications also reduce the activity of non-NMDA glutamate receptors that are needed to remove the voltage-gated magnesium blockade that is present in NMDA receptors (Nishikawa et al., 1994). These findings are consistent with the suggested differences in the function of esterified vs. unesterified forms of DHA that were recently described (Orr et al., 2013). Furthermore, and as described above, unesterified DHA can activate calcium mobilization and the ERK/CREB pathway to increase the expression of genes related to synaptogenesis by binding to the gpr40 receptor (Yamashima, 2012).

The generation and maturation of synapses and how they are affected by reelin (Folsom et al., 2013; Herz and Chen, 2006), lipid rafts (Head et al., 2014), and beneficial DHA interactions, are very similar to what was described earlier for neuron growth and axon elongation. Reelin increases NMDA-receptor activity that is critical for excitatory synapse formation and maintenance by directing Fyn kinase to phosphorylate the NMDA receptor (Folsom et al., 2013; Herz and Chen, 2006). Lipid rafts serve as clustered signaling platforms that congregate synaptic proteins, receptor complexes, and Fyn kinase along with tethers to the cytoskeleton that ultimately stabilize a synapse (Head et al., 2014). DHA is tightly associated with reelin expression (Yavin et al., 2009), assists with the organization of lipid rafts (Shaikh et al., 2004; Stillwell et al., 2005), and generally increases synaptogenic signaling through multiple pathways (Kim and Spector, 2013). Given the above, the reductions in dopaminergic, serotonergic, and glutamatergic signaling, as well as the associated deficits in learning, memory, and mood, that occur in omega-3- (McNamara and Carlson, 2006) and reelin-deficient animals (Folsom et al., 2013) are consistent with the reduced function and connectivity of synapses that are deficient in both DHA and reelin signaling.

DHA and synapses are lost from brains that have been subjected to injury (Wu et al., 2014) or neurodegeneration (Vandal et al., 2014). Sufficient DHA status improves the resiliency of the nervous system and its synapses to injury (Michael-Titus and Priestley, 2014; Wu et al., 2014) and to neurodegeneration. However, the efficiency of DHA transport to the brain (Vandal et al., 2014) and the bioavailability of DHA (Orr et al., 2013) near the time of such insults are clearly important for the maintenance of existing synapses. The interacting neurodevelopmental mechanisms of DHA sufficiency, reelin signaling, and functional lipid rafts allow for synaptic maintenance at the time of insult, but they also promote new synapses that are less refined than those that have been established during development (Perederiy and Westbrook, 2013). It is notable that manipulation of molecular cascades related to DHA and reelin can allow for new connections and restored function in the difficult environment of injured adult nervous tissue (e.g., Liu et al., 2010). Reports of faster functional recovery from survivable brain trauma when DHA/EPA are supplied are also encouraging (e.g., Lewis et al., 2012; Michael-Titus and Priestley, 2014). However, new synapses that are incorrectly targeted after an insult to the brain are sometimes deleterious in that they can promote post-concussive syndrome, which can include migraines or seizures (Bohnen et al., 1991; Learoyd and Lifshitz, 2012; Lidvall et al., 1974; McAllister, 1992; Rutherford et al., 1979). Alternatively, any new synapses that are produced in the context of diagnosed neurodegenerative disease may not be able to compensate for the damage that has already occurred, which could explain the difficulty in identifying therapies for diseases such as AD (Quinn et al., 2010). These circumstances therefore argue in favor of DHA sufficiency prior to any event that might damage the brain so that appropriate synaptic circuitry is maintained as much as possible.

9.4.4 Myelination

After a synapse is established, the electrical and neurochemical activity of that synapse can become a signal for myelination of its associated axon. Not all axons are destined to be myelinated by oligodendrocytes in the CNS or by Schwann cells in the PNS. Nonetheless, interactions between the neuron, its myelinating cell(s) and signals related to the immune system are necessary for the proper development, maintenance, and repair of nervous system circuitry (Jakovcevski et al., 2009; Lee and Fields, 2009). DHA, reelin, and lipid rafts have likely roles in these processes.

The peak of the omega-3 accumulation rate in the nervous system coincides with the neurodevelopmental onset of myelination (McNamara and Carlson, 2006), and DHA has been reported to normalize myelin in humans who suffer from the demyelination caused by generalized peroxisomal disorders (Martinez and Vazquez, 1998). Peroxisomes are necessary for the production of DHA from its precursors (Lizard et al., 2012). Omega-3 deficient diets have a larger effect on the DHA content of oligodendrocyte membranes and myelin than on most other brain cell membranes. In rats, two generations of omega-3 deficiency results in a 98% loss of DHA from oligodendrocytes and an 86% loss from myelin, while synaptosomes, neurons, and astrocytes lost 73, 71, and 53% of their DHA, respectively (Bourre et al., 1984). Thus,

DHA is a building block for both neurons and oligodendrocytes, and it follows that DHA content increases with neurogenesis and myelination and then decreases with loss of neurons and myelin along with age or damage (Bartzokis, 2011).

Myelinating cells, and the myelin they produce, play important roles in refining the circuitry of the central nervous system and in enabling the propogation of action potentials. For example, artificial knockout of oligodendrocytes during development results in unregulated, mistargeted, and expansive expression of axon guidance molecules and synaptic proteins (Doretto et al., 2011). These findings indicate that it is not merely the correlated firing of two neurons that result in a properly targeted synapse and that oligodendrocytes do more than insulate neurons with myelin. Indeed, myelin-associated glycoprotein (MAG) and myelin oligodendrocyte glycoprotein (MOG) impede axon elongation and are physical obstacles for axon regrowth after injury in adults (Saha et al., 2014), suggesting that one of their functions is to impart an aspect of stability to an established synapse.

Myelination is a highly coordinated process, and DHA can likely interact with its signaling cascades. The electrical and neurochemical activity of a maturing neuron induces the differentiation of myelinating cells that are in the vicinity of the neuron. This axonal activity proceeds to induce the expression of cell adhesion molecules on both the neuron and the myelinating cell. Two of the pivotal cell adhesion molecules that are expressed on neurons at this stage are L1 (Lee and Fields, 2009) and neuregulin (Schulz et al., 2014). L1 is received by the contactin receptor expressed by oligodendrocytes in the CNS and this interaction results in the activation of Fyn kinase and downstream processes that eventually cause the expression of myelin basic protein (MBP; Muller et al., 2013). In the PNS, L1 is necessary for initializing contact between Schwann cells and axons, but neuregulin is also expressed on the extracellular leaflet of PNS axons. The action of neuregulin on Schwann cell receptor, ERBb2, calls for myelin via AkT, and the amount of neuregulin expressed determines the degree and thickness of myelination (Schulz et al., 2014). Similarly, Fyn kinase also regulates the number of myelin sheaths made by oligodendroctyes (Muller et al., 2013) and Schwann cells (Panteri et al., 2006), but the expression of neuregulins and a neuregulin receptor (ErbB4) in the brain suggest that neuregulin also plays a role in myelination by oligodendrocytes. Interestingly, reelin has also been implicated in the degree of myelination (Panteri et al., 2006), and all of the proteins described above that are expressed by myelinating cells are found in lipid rafts (Yang et al., 2004; Muller et al., 2013; White and Kramer-Albers, 2014) much in the same way that Fyn and other receptor complexes are found in the lipid rafts of neurons (Head et al., 2013). Ultimately, the tethering of Fyn to tau on the microtubules in myelinating cells is an important step in transporting and expressing myelin proteins (e.g., MBP and MAG) at the myelin membrane (Muller et al., 2013; White and Kramer-Albers, 2014).

The convergence of signaling pathways that are affected by DHA continues as myelin proteins induce further growth of the axon. MAG is one of the transmembrane signals from myelin to the axon that tells the axon that myelination has commenced. The MAG signal is received by the axon via the p75 neurotrophin receptor. Activation of p75 results in ERK activity (Garcia et al., 2003) that is needed for axon growth and the continuation of appropriate myelination (Ishii et al., 2012). Given the re-engagement of axonal growth processes at this stage, it makes sense that AkT/mTOR also plays a role (Flores et al., 2008). All of these signals seem to culminate in the C-terminus lengthening of neurofilaments with repeated phosphorylation sites. These structural repeats increase the distance between the neurofilaments that run longitudinally down the axon and thereby increase the diameter and radial growth of the axon (Barry et al., 2012). The neurofilaments can be further modified by the action of Fyn (Panteri et al., 2006) and ERK (Garcia et al., 2003) kinases at the repeated neurofilament phosphorylation sites. In contrast, damage to the CNS is associated with decrease in white matter (axon) volume and stability, loss of DHA and other PUFAs (Janssen and Kiliaan, 2014), decrease in neurofilament phosphorylation, and decrease in the expression of MBP (Xiong et al., 2013).

The expression of MBP is the last formal step of myelination, and MBP serves to compact the myelin membrane by interlinking myelin lamella and to organize the membrane into domains of rigidly structured lipids associated with the MBP. The localized expression of MBP in the myelin membrane requires Fyn activation, and phosphorylation of the MBP molecule is needed to fully mature the membrane and to bring MBP into lipid rafts (Baron and Hoekstra, 2010; Lee and Fields, 2009). The organizing functions of Fyn throughout the myelination process (White and Kramer-Albers, 2014), the presence of Fyn and DHA on both sides of the neuron–myelin interface (Bourre et al., 1984; Head et al., 2014; Muller et al., 2013), the interactions of Fyn with DHA signaling (Akbar et al., 2005) and reelin (Folsom et al., 2013), the organizing effects of DHA on lipid rafts (Shaikh et al., 2004; Stillwell et al., 2005), and the correlations of white matter instability with the loss of DHA and nervous system degradation (Janssen and Kiliaan, 2014; McNamara and Carlson, 2006) all point to the likelihood that DHA provides some support to the development and maintenance of myelin. Findings that DHA protects white matter from the damage caused by experimental SCI models also demonstrate the role of DHA in myelin maintenance (Michael-Titus and Priestley, 2014). However, the amount of DHA in myelin is relatively low in comparison to other cell types (Bourre et al., 1984), suggesting that DHA may act on myelin through its actions in the other brain cell types.

9.5 MAINTENANCE OF BRAIN HEALTH

Maintaining the general health of the brain and its myelin is an energetically expensive process. Kinases, phosphatases, and other enzymes are constantly using chemical energy as adenosine triphosphate (ATP) to drive their specific functions and maintain the dynamics of daily brain function. Most of this energy is derived from glucose (110–150 g per day for the adult brain). Ketone bodies and β-oxidation of FAs can also be used as inefficient sources of energy (Henderson, 2008). However, glucose metabolism is altered significantly when nervous system damage occurs. In the case of physical damage, hyperglycolysis occurs in an attempt to make-up for decreased ATP production. This loss of ATP is induced by excess calcium in the cell body that depolarizes the mitochondria that make ATP (Giza and Hovda, 2001). In the case of neurodegeneration, in particular Alzheimer's disease, some evidence points to a loss of brain glucose uptake (Henderson, 2008) and reduced efficiency of lipid delivery to the brain (Vandal et al., 2014). Sufficient intake of DHA has been associated with normalizing the energy imbalances and oxidative stress that occur after TBI, SCI, and ischemia (Michael-Titus and Priestley, 2014; Wu et al., 2014). These observations could be especially important for the myelinating cells of the brain as they consume 2 to 3 times more energy than neurons (Bartzokis, 2011; Connor and Menzies, 1996).

The brain must also protect itself from proinflammatory stressors from the environment. The BBB is the primary defense against environmental stressors, but it can be compromised by trauma, infections, and neurodegenerative diseases such as Alzheimer's (Farkas et al., 2006; Spielman et al., 2014). Even with an intact BBB, some brain regions, such as the olfactory epithelium, are exposed directly to the environment. The olfactory epithelium and the olfactory bulb are also equipped with defensive mechanisms. However, with age and accumulated insults to these tissues, neuroinflammation can ensue and spread to brain areas that are connected to the olfactory system. Furthermore, poor olfaction has been correlated with the development of Alzheimer's. These observations have led to the hypothesis that chronic inflammation can lead to impairments in the axonal cytoskeleton (e.g., neurofibrillary tangles) that are hallmarks of Alzheimer's disease (Krstic et al., 2013). Significant correlations between brain injury, neuroinflammation, and Alzheimer's markers have also been reported (Bailes et al., 2013).

The anti-inflammatory actions of DHA and its docosanoid derivatives have been reviewed in detail elsewhere (Bazan, 2013; Farooqui et al., 2007; Michael-Titus and Priestley, 2014). In brief, injury and neurodegenerative insults induce pro-inflammatory cytokines to be released from the immune cells of the brain (i.e., microglia). Microglia normally take part in synaptic pruning during development and in removing cellular debris. When placed under the long-lasting stimulation of chronic inflammation, microglial activation can be set forth on a positive feedback loop that results in the destruction of healthy brain tissue and further microglial activation. The cytokines released by microglia also cause the breakdown of neuronal membranes, which release proinflammatory arachidonic acid and its metabolites. However, DHA and its metabolites are also released, and their apparent actions of activating PPARγ, inhibiting NFκB, and disrupting lipid raft signaling in immune cells have an important anti-inflammatory effect in the brain. Furthermore, sufficient DHA intake confers neuroprotective effects that are consistent with these anti-inflammatory pathways in models of nervous system injury (Bazan, 2013; Belayev et al., 2011; Gladman et al., 2012; Hall et al., 2012; Michael-Titus and Priestley, 2014; Mills et al., 2011; Paterniti et al., 2014; Wu et al., 2014) and of neurodegeneration (Calon, 2011; Green et al., 2007; Janssen and Kiliaan, 2014). Recently, a mechanism that employs unesterified DHA binding to the gpr120 receptor has also exhibited anti-inflammatory effects, and these actions appear to be independent from AkT, ERK, and PPARγ (Wellhauser and Belsham, 2014).

An interesting side to the chronic inflammation hypothesis of neurodegeneration allows for the introduction of a more global hypothesis that includes the importance and metabolic expense of myelination and its maintenance. Krstic et al. (2013) observed that neurofibrillary tangles followed the olfactory and limbic pathways of the brain. These pathways express reelin, and use reelin to inhibit the hyperphosphorylation of tau by GSK-3β. Furthermore, reelin decreases with age and chronic inflammation (Krstic et al., 2013), and it increases with sufficient DHA intake (Yavin et al., 2009). These findings suggest that environmental and epigenetic factors regulate reelin and its signaling and that somehow restoring reelin expression or reelin signaling may be a key to combating chronic neuroinflammation and its neurodegenerative sequelae (Krstic et al., 2013). DHA sufficiency can fit well with the chronic inflammation hypothesis and its resolution, but the myelin maintenance hypothesis (Bartzokis, 2011) is a better overall fit for what occurs in development, aging, neurodegeneration, and traumatic injury to the nervous system.

Similar to the observation that AD pathology follows reelin-expressing pathways (Krstic et al., 2013), the myelin maintenance model accentuates that AD pathology follows the developmental myelination pattern in reverse. The brain areas that are affected first by AD are the last to be myelinated, and it is this late myelination that makes them vulnerable for several reasons. First, while myelination has given the human brain faster processing, the metabolic demands of oligodendrocytes and myelination make these cells uniquely vulnerable to environmental challenges and genetic defects in lipid processing. Late myelin is thinner and shorter than early myelin and therefore more susceptible to damage (Bartzokis, 2011). Furthermore, white matter integrity is damaged first in neurodegeneration (Goodenowe et al., 2007). Second, the BACE1 and γ-secretase enzymes that regulate neuregulin and axonal diameter are the same ones that produce Aβ. Thus, it is the myelin repair process that secondarily results in the expression of AD biomarkers. Finally, myelin repair slows or halts axonal transport of mitochondria and lipids so that myelin can be repaired. This is exhibited by disinhibition of GSK3β, hyperphosphorylation of tau, axonal swelling, the accumulation of Aβ, and the potential starving and death of neurons for the sake of saving myelin (Bartzokis, 2011). In contrast, DHA sufficiency and its interactions with reelin are associated with Akt activation and subsequent inhibition of GSK3β (Akbar et al., 2005; Folsom et al., 2013), reduced expression of tau, reduced accumulation of Aβ (Calon, 2011; Green et al., 2007), and maintenance of white matter integrity (Janssen and Kiliaan, 2014). These DHA effects are likely due to its signaling roles as well as its importance as an optimized lipid building block of plasma membranes.

9.6 SUMMARY AND CONCLUSIONS

The shared and interacting mechanisms of DHA, reelin, and lipid rafts, and the direction of these mechanisms suggest that the same things that occur during development should also be happening in adult tissue. This is clearly not the case as adult nervous tissue lacks the same degree of plasticity as that of developing tissue. It is this difference that developmental neurobiologists seek to understand so that it can be applied toward efficacious regeneration therapies. If we did have such a complete understanding, it would certainly be applied to the debilitating conditions with which nervous system injury is associated. In the meantime, the research continues, and it suggests that as the human nervous system matures it switches from creating an environment conducive to growth to one that favors generally stable brain circuitry and enough plasticity to form new memories. However, this circuitry requires maintenance, and that maintenance requires energy and the appropriate building blocks.

In many respects, the development and use of myelination to increase the speed of the brain's processing power has been adaptive and has likely contributed to the survival of many species. However, the maintenance of myelin is energetically expensive, and its costs are also realized by reductions in the capabilities of plasticity and repair. For example, humans have relatively large amounts of myelin in comparison to other species, and they arguably have cognitive and evolutionary dominion over the planet that they inhabit. This myelination advantage is also a disadvantage in that the expense of brain and myelin maintenance over time eventually gets overwhelmed by the aging of repair mechanisms, the dysfunction of repair mechanisms due to genetic background, or traumatic injury. Even in normal aging, the brain regions that are myelinated last in development are the first to lose myelin over time. These regions happen to be those that seem to give humans personality and higher cognitive function than other animals, and they also happen to be targeted by Alzheimer's disease, which is essentially accelerated brain aging. Conversely, brain aging has been characterized as the "Alzheimerization" of the brain that results in the relatively slow, but steady, demyelination and disconnection of progressively lower brain centers (Bartzokis, 2011). The system does its best to provide preventative maintenance against the maladaptive loss of brain function, and it appears to utilize developmental mechanisms of growth and plasticity, even if to a different extent, to achieve such repair and maintenance. As this chapter describes, these mechanisms employ reelin, AkT, CREB, neurotransmitter receptors, sensors of cell-to-cell contact, transcription, translation, the cytoskeleton and lipid rafts, many of which functions are altered or enhanced by sufficient levels of DHA.

DHA is one of many of the basic building blocks of the nervous system (e.g., arachidonic acid, tubulin, actin, nucleic acids, cholesterol, etc.), but it is unique in this general list of components in that it is replaceable and not essential for the basic survival of the organism. Levels of docosapentaenoic acid (DPA; 22:5n-6) increase when DHA is lost. The organism survives, but DPA replaces only a certain fraction of DHA function. As the rhodopsin studies demonstrated, the function of transmembrane proteins and receptors may be compromised in the cases of low DHA status since the sufficient presence of DHA was required for the highest level of rhodopsin activity (Polozova and Litman, 2000; Salem et al., 2001). These findings support the assertion that DHA is indeed a building block that not only provides general membrane structure and metabolic energy as a lipid, but it also optimizes membrane structure and provides signaling functions to the cells of the nervous system. If this principal was assumed and applied across the board with regards to the potential of DHA sufficiency being optimal for neuronal function, it would be logical that this principle would also apply to the maintenance of the entire nervous system and its myelinated circuitry.

The notion of optimizing any function of the brain is a matter of context. As pharmaceutical development has demonstrated, too much of an apparently good thing can sometimes be toxic. What is optimal in one subsystem of the nervous system may not be optimal in another, and this may provide some explanation for the plateau of DHA accumulation in the brain (Sarkadi-Nagy et al., 2003). These circumstances also provide rationale for clinical studies and safety studies, some of which have already been performed for DHA. DHA is well-tolerated and has a wide safety window (Lewis and Bailes, 2011). Furthermore, converging data from case studies (e.g., Lewis et al., 2012) and preclinical evidence (Michael-Titus and Priestley, 2014; Bazan, 2013) are encouraging for its potential use in increasing the nervous system's resiliency to and recovery from multiple types of damage.

Clinical researchers should take the lead presented by the Institute of Medicine (2011) and develop RCTs that robustly test the acute and long-term effects of DHA in nervous system injury and neurodegeneration over time. The minimum length of sufficient DHA exposure should be 6 months to allow for brain DHA to accumulate in otherwise deficient individuals (Arterburn et al., 2006). Neurodegeneration should be studied in a longitudinal fashion over years, perhaps decades. Such studies, at a minimum, should seek to correlate DHA status with the rate of conversion to diagnosed neurodegenerative disease and/or outcomes after a traumatic or ischemic event. Trials that compare individuals with sufficient or supplemented DHA status against individuals that remain on an average Western diet should be encouraged strongly, but this encouragement should be balanced with the facts that clinical trials are expensive and are entirely dependent on the level of funding that is available. It is these types of properly designed experiments that will provide definitive answers as to whether sufficient levels of dietary DHA intake protect the human brain from injury, aging, or neurodegeneration to a measurable extent. DHA is ready for this level of scrutiny, and it would be good to know whether, even as adults, we can eat our way to a healthier brain. This may be the case in the context of DHA and mild cognitive impairment (Yurko-Mauro et al., 2010; Janssen and Kiliaan, 2014), but confirmation studies are required. It is now also the time to work toward similar levels of understanding with DHA and any type of brain damage.

REFERENCES

Abumrad N, Coburn C, and Ibrahimi A. 1999. Membrane proteins implicated in long-chain fatty acid uptake by mammalian cells: CD36, FATP and FABPm. *Biochim Biophys Acta* **1441**:4–13.

Aires V, Hichami A, Boulay G, and Khan NA. 2007. Activation of TRPC6 calcium channels by diacylglycerol (DAG)-containing arachidonic acid: A comparative study with DAG-containing docosahexaenoic acid. *Biochimie* **89**:926–937.

Akbar M, Calderon F, Wen Z, and Kim HY. 2005. Docosahexaenoic acid: A positive modulator of Akt signaling in neuronal survival. *Proc Natl Acad Sci USA* **102**:10858–10863.

Akerman CJ and Cline HT. 2007. Refining the roles of GABAergic signaling during neural circuit formation. *Trends Neurosci* **30**:382–389.

Arterburn LM, Hall EB, and Oken H. 2006. Distribution, interconversion, and dose response of n-3 fatty acids in humans. *Am J Clin Nutr* **83**:1467S–1476S.

Astarita G, Jung KM, Berchtold NC, Nguyen VQ, Gillen DL, Head E, Cotman CW, and Piomelli D. 2010. Deficient liver biosynthesis of docosahexaenoic acid correlates with cognitive impairment in Alzheimer's disease. *PLoS One* **5**:e12538.

Bach SA, de Siqueira LV, Muller AP, Oses JP, Quatrim A, Emanuelli T, Vinade L, Souza DO, and Moreira JD. 2014. Dietary omega-3 deficiency reduces BDNF content and activation NMDA receptor and Fyn in dorsal hippocampus: Implications on persistence of long-term memory in rats. *Nutr Neurosci* **17**:186–192.

Bailes JE, Petraglia AL, Omalu BI, Nauman E, and Talavage T. 2013. Role of subconcussion in repetitive mild traumatic brain injury. *J Neurosurg* **119**:1235–1245.

Bandarra NM, Batista I, Nunes ML, Empis JM, Christie WW. 1997. Seasonal changes in lipid composition of sardine (Sardina pilchardus). *J. Food Sci* **62**:40–42.

Barberger-Gateau P, Samieri C, Feart C, and Plourde M. 2011. Dietary omega 3 polyunsaturated fatty acids and Alzheimer's disease: Interaction with apolipoprotein E genotype. *Curr Alzheimer Res* **8**:479–491.

Baron W and Hoekstra D. 2010. On the biogenesis of myelin membranes: Sorting, trafficking and cell polarity. *FEBS Lett* **584**:1760–1770.

Barry DM, Stevenson W, Bober BG, Wiese PJ, Dale JM, Barry GS, Byers NS, Strope JD, Chang R, Schulz DJ et al. 2012. Expansion of neurofilament medium C terminus increases axonal diameter independent of increases in conduction velocity or myelin thickness. *J Neurosci* **32**:6209–6219.

Bartlett TE and Wang YT. 2013. The intersections of NMDAR-dependent synaptic plasticity and cell survival. *Neuropharmacology* **74**:59–68.

Bartzokis G. 2011. Alzheimer's disease as homeostatic responses to age-related myelin breakdown. *Neurobiol Aging* **32**:1341–1371.

Bazan NG. 2013. The docosanoid neuroprotectin D1 induces homeostatic regulation of neuroinflammation and cell survival. *Prostaglandins Leukot Essent Fatty Acids* **88**:127–129.

Bazan NG, Molina MF, and Gordon WC. 2011. Docosahexaenoic acid signalolipidomics in nutrition: Significance in aging, neuroinflammation, macular degeneration, Alzheimer's, and other neurodegenerative diseases. *Annu Rev Nutr* **31**:321–351.

Belayev L, Khoutorova L, Atkins KD, Eady TN, Hong S, Lu Y, Obenaus A, and Bazan NG. 2011. Docosahexaenoic Acid therapy of experimental ischemic stroke. *Transl Stroke Res* **2**:33–41.

Bell MV, Henderson RJ, and Sargent JR. 1985. Changes in the fatty acid composition of phospholipids from turbot (Scophthalmus maximus) in relation to dietary polyunsaturated fatty acid deficiencies. *Comp Biochem Physiol B* **81**:193–198.

Birch EE, Carlson SE, Hoffman DR, Fitzgerald-Gustafson KM, Fu VL, Drover JR, Castaneda YS, Minns L, Wheaton DK, Mundy D et al. 2010. The DIAMOND (DHA Intake And Measurement Of Neural Development) Study: A double-masked, randomized controlled clinical trial of the maturation of infant visual acuity as a function of the dietary level of docosahexaenoic acid. *Am J Clin Nutr* **91**:848–859.

Blasbalg TL, Hibbeln JR, Ramsden CE, Majchrzak SF, and Rawlings RR. 2011. Changes in consumption of omega-3 and omega-6 fatty acids in the United States during the 20th century. *Am J Clin Nutr* **93**:950–962.

Bohnen N, Twijnstra A, Wijnen G, and Jolles J. 1991. Tolerance for light and sound of patients with persistent post-concussional symptoms 6 months after mild head injury. *J Neurol* **238**:443–446.

Boneva NB and Yamashima T. 2012. New insights into "GPR40-CREB interaction in adult neurogenesis" specific for primates. *Hippocampus* **22**:896–905.

Bourre JM, Pascal G, Durand G, Masson M, Dumont O, and Piciotti M. 1984. Alterations in the fatty acid composition of rat brain cells (neurons, astrocytes, and oligodendrocytes) and of subcellular fractions (myelin and synaptosomes) induced by a diet devoid of n-3 fatty acids. *J Neurochem* **43**:342–348.

Bouzan C, Cohen JT, Connor WE, Kris-Etherton PM, Gray GM, Konig A, Lawrence RS, Savitz DA, and Teutsch SM. 2005. A quantitative analysis of fish consumption and stroke risk. *Am J Prev Med* **29**:347–352.

Brand A, Schonfeld E, Isharel I, and Yavin E. 2008. Docosahexaenoic acid-dependent iron accumulation in oligodendroglia cells protects from hydrogen peroxide-induced damage. *J Neurochem* **105**:1325–1335.

Brenna JT, Salem N Jr., Sinclair AJ, and Cunnane SC. 2009. alpha-Linolenic acid supplementation and conversion to n-3 long-chain polyunsaturated fatty acids in humans. *Prostaglandins Leukot Essent Fatty Acids* **80**:85–91.

Brenna JT, Varamini B, Jensen RG, Diersen-Schade DA, Boettcher JA, and Arterburn LM. 2007. Docosahexaenoic and arachidonic acid concentrations in human breast milk worldwide. *Am J Clin Nutr* **85**:1457–1464.

Brossard N, Croset M, Pachiaudi C, Riou JP, Tayot JL, and Lagarde M. 1996. Retroconversion and metabolism of [13C]22:6n-3 in humans and rats after intake of a single dose of [13C]22:6n-3-triacylglycerols. *Am J Clin Nutr* **64**:577–586.

Burdge GC, Jones AE, and Wootton SA. 2002. Eicosapentaenoic and docosapentaenoic acids are the principal products of alpha-linolenic acid metabolism in young men*. *Br J Nutr* **88**:355–363.

Calderon F and Kim HY. 2007. Role of RXR in neurite outgrowth induced by docosahexaenoic acid. *Prostaglandins Leukot Essent Fatty Acids* **77**:227–232.

Calon F. 2011. Omega-3 polyunsaturated fatty acids in Alzheimer's disease: Key questions and partial answers. *Curr Alzheimer Res* **8**:470–478.

Calon F and Cole G. 2007. Neuroprotective action of omega-3 polyunsaturated fatty acids against neurodegenerative diseases: Evidence from animal studies. *Prostaglandins Leukot Essent Fatty Acids* **77**:287–293.

Calon F, Lim GP, Morihara T, Yang F, Ubeda O, Salem N Jr., Frautschy SA, and Cole GM. 2005. Dietary n-3 polyunsaturated fatty acid depletion activates caspases and decreases NMDA receptors in the brain of a transgenic mouse model of Alzheimer's disease. *Eur J Neurosci* **22**:617–626.

Calon F, Lim GP, Yang F, Morihara T, Teter B, Ubeda O, Rostaing P, Triller A, Salem N Jr., Ashe KH et al. 2004. Docosahexaenoic acid protects from dendritic pathology in an Alzheimer's disease mouse model. *Neuron* **43**:633–645.

Cao D, Kevala K, Kim J, Moon HS, Jun SB, Lovinger D, and Kim HY. 2009. Docosahexaenoic acid promotes hippocampal neuronal development and synaptic function. *J Neurochem* **111**:510–521.

Carlson SE. 2009. Docosahexaenoic acid supplementation in pregnancy and lactation. *Am J Clin Nutr* **89**:678S–684S.

Chan CP, Wan TS, Watkins KL, Pelsers MM, Van der Voort D, Tang FP, Lam KH, Mill J, Yuan Y, Lehmann M et al. 2005. Rapid analysis of fatty acid-binding proteins with immunosensors and immunotests for early monitoring of tissue injury. *Biosens Bioelectron* **20**:2566–2580.

Chen N and Napoli JL. 2008. All-trans-retinoic acid stimulates translation and induces spine formation in hippocampal neurons through a membrane-associated RARalpha. *FASEB J* **22**:236–245.

Chen S and Subbaiah PV. 2013. Regioisomers of phosphatidylcholine containing DHA and their potential to deliver DHA to the brain: Role of phospholipase specificities. *Lipids* **48**:675–686.

Chen W, Jump DB, Esselman WJ, and Busik JV. 2007. Inhibition of cytokine signaling in human retinal endothelial cells through modification of caveolae/lipid rafts by docosahexaenoic acid. *Invest Ophthalmol Vis Sci* **48**:18–26.

Chiu SL and Cline HT. 2010. Insulin receptor signaling in the development of neuronal structure and function. *Neural Dev* **5**:7.

Connor JR and Menzies SL. 1996. Relationship of iron to oligodendrocytes and myelination. *Glia* **17**:83–93.

Courtes S, Vernerey J, Pujadas L, Magalon K, Cremer H, Soriano E, Durbec P, and Cayre M. 2011. Reelin controls progenitor cell migration in the healthy and pathological adult mouse brain. *PLoS One* **6**:e20430.

Debski EA and Cline HT. 2002. Activity-dependent mapping in the retinotectal projection. *Curr Opin Neurobiol* **12**:93–99.

Doretto S, Malerba M, Ramos M, Ikrar T, Kinoshita C, De Mei C, Tirotta E, Xu X, and Borrelli E. 2011. Oligodendrocytes as regulators of neuronal networks during early postnatal development. *PLoS One* **6**:e19849.

Duraisamy Y, Lambert D, O'Neill CA, and Padfield PJ. 2007. Differential incorporation of docosahexaenoic acid into distinct cholesterol-rich membrane raft domains. *Biochem Biophys Res Commun* **360**:885–890.

EFSA Panel on Dietetic Products, Nutrition and Allergies (NDA). 2012. Scientific opinion related to the tolerable upper intake level of eicosapentaenoic acid (EPA), docosahexaenoic acid (DHA) and docosapentaenoic acid (DPA). *EFSA Journal* **10**:2815[48pp.].

Emken EA, Adlof RO, and Gulley RM. 1994. Dietary linoleic acid influences desaturation and acylation of deuterium-labeled linoleic and linolenic acids in young adult males. *Biochim Biophys Acta* **1213**:277–288.

Farkas O, Lifshitz J, and Povlishock JT. 2006. Mechanoporation induced by diffuse traumatic brain injury: An irreversible or reversible response to injury? *J Neurosci* **26**:3130–3140.

Farooqui AA, Horrocks LA, and Farooqui T. 2007. Modulation of inflammation in brain: A matter of fat. *J Neurochem* **101**:577–599.

Farooqui AA, Ong WY, and Horrocks LA. 2004. Biochemical aspects of neurodegeneration in human brain: Involvement of neural membrane phospholipids and phospholipases A2. *Neurochem Res* **29**:1961–1977.

Fedorova I, Hussein N, Baumann MH, Di Martino C, and Salem N Jr. 2009. An n-3 fatty acid deficiency impairs rat spatial learning in the Barnes maze. *Behav Neurosci* **123**:196–205.

Fedorova-Dahms I, Thorsrud BA, Bailey E, and Salem N Jr. 2014. A 3-week dietary bioequivalence study in preweaning farm piglets of two sources of docosahexaenoic acid produced from two different organisms. *Food Chem Toxicol* **65**:43–51.

Florent S, Malaplate-Armand C, Youssef I, Kriem B, Koziel V, Escanye MC, Fifre A, Sponne I, Leininger-Muller B, Olivier JL et al. 2006. Docosahexaenoic acid prevents neuronal apoptosis induced by soluble amyloid-beta oligomers. *J Neurochem* **96**:385–395.

Flores AI, Narayanan SP, Morse EN, Shick HE, Yin X, Kidd G, Avila RL, Kirschner DA, and Macklin WB. 2008. Constitutively active Akt induces enhanced myelination in the CNS. *J Neurosci* **28**:7174–7183.

Folsom TD and Fatemi SH. 2013. The involvement of Reelin in neurodevelopmental disorders. *Neuropharmacology* **68**:122–135.

Freund Levi Y, Vedin I, Cederholm T, Basun H, Faxen Irving G, Eriksdotter M, Hjorth E, Schultzberg M, Vessby B, Wahlund LO et al. 2014. Transfer of omega-3 fatty acids across the blood-brain barrier after dietary supplementation with a docosahexaenoic acid-rich omega-3 fatty acid preparation in patients with Alzheimer's disease: The OmegAD study. *J Intern Med* **275**:428–436.

Futerman AH and Banker GA. 1996. The economics of neurite outgrowth—the addition of new membrane to growing axons. *Trends Neurosci* **19**:144–149.

Garcia ML, Lobsiger CS, Shah SB, Deerinck TJ, Crum J, Young D, Ward CM, Crawford TO, Gotow T, Uchiyama Y et al. 2003. NF-M is an essential target for the myelin-directed "outside-in" signaling cascade that mediates radial axonal growth. *J Cell Biol* **163**:1011–1020.

Gawrisch K, Soubias O, and Mihailescu M. 2008. Insights from biophysical studies on the role of polyunsaturated fatty acids for function of G-protein coupled membrane receptors. *Prostaglandins Leukot Essent Fatty Acids* **79**:131–134.

Gebauer SK, Psota TL, Harris WS, and Kris-Etherton PM. 2006. n-3 fatty acid dietary recommendations and food sources to achieve essentiality and cardiovascular benefits. *Am J Clin Nutr* **83**:1526S–1535S.

Ghiani CA, Mattan NS, Nobuta H, Malvar JS, Boles J, Ross MG, Waschek JA, Carpenter EM, Fisher RS, and de Vellis J. 2011. Early effects of lipopolysaccharide-induced inflammation on foetal brain development in rat. *ASN Neuro* **3**:233–245.

Giza CC and Hovda DA. 2001. The neurometabolic cascade of concussion. *J Athl Train* **36**:228–235.

Gladman SJ, Huang W, Lim SN, Dyall SC, Boddy S, Kang JX, Knight MM, Priestley JV, and Michael-Titus AT. 2012. Improved outcome after peripheral nerve injury in mice with increased levels of endogenous omega-3 polyunsaturated fatty acids. *J Neurosci* **32**:563–571.

Goodenowe DB, Cook LL, Liu J, Lu Y, Jayasinghe DA, Ahiahonu PW, Heath D, Yamazaki Y, Flax J, Krenitsky KF et al. 2007. Peripheral ethanolamine plasmalogen deficiency: A logical causative factor in Alzheimer's disease and dementia. *J Lipid Res* **48**:2485–2498.

Goti D, Balazs Z, Panzenboeck U, Hrzenjak A, Reicher H, Wagner E, Zechner R, Malle E, and Sattler W. 2002. Effects of lipoprotein lipase on uptake and transcytosis of low density lipoprotein (LDL) and LDL-associated alpha-tocopherol in a porcine in vitro blood-brain barrier model. *J Biol Chem* **277**:28537–28544.

Green KN, Martinez-Coria H, Khashwji H, Hall EB, Yurko-Mauro KA, Ellis L, and LaFerla FM. 2007. Dietary docosahexaenoic acid and docosapentaenoic acid ameliorate amyloid-beta and tau pathology via a mechanism involving presenilin 1 levels. *J Neurosci* **27**:4385–4395.

Gururajan A and van den Buuse M. 2014. Is the mTOR-signalling cascade disrupted in Schizophrenia? *J Neurochem* **129**:377–387.

Hack I, Hellwig S, Junghans D, Brunne B, Bock HH, Zhao S, and Frotscher M. 2007. Divergent roles of ApoER2 and Vldlr in the migration of cortical neurons. *Development* **134**:3883–3891.

Hall JC, Priestley JV, Perry VH, and Michael-Titus AT. 2012. Docosahexaenoic acid, but not eicosapentaenoic acid, reduces the early inflammatory response following compression spinal cord injury in the rat. *J Neurochem* **121**:738–750.

He F, Lupu DS, and Niculescu MD. 2014. Perinatal alpha-linolenic acid availability alters the expression of genes related to memory and to epigenetic machinery, and the Mecp2 DNA methylation in the whole brain of mouse offspring. *Int J Dev Neurosci* **36**:38–44.

He K, Rimm EB, Merchant A, Rosner BA, Stampfer MJ, Willett WC, and Ascherio A. 2002. Fish consumption and risk of stroke in men. *JAMA* **288**:3130–3136.

Head BP, Patel HH, and Insel PA. 2014. Interaction of membrane/lipid rafts with the cytoskeleton: Impact on signaling and function: Membrane/lipid rafts, mediators of cytoskeletal arrangement and cell signaling. *Biochim Biophys Acta* **1838**:532–545.

Henderson ST. 2008. Ketone bodies as a therapeutic for Alzheimer's disease. *Neurotherapeutics* **5**:470–480.

Herz J and Chen Y. 2006. Reelin, lipoprotein receptors and synaptic plasticity. *Nat Rev Neurosci* **7**:850–859.

Hicks DA, Nalivaeva NN, and Turner AJ. 2012. Lipid rafts and Alzheimer's disease: Protein-lipid interactions and perturbation of signaling. *Front Physiol* **3**:189.

Hippenmeyer S. 2014. Molecular pathways controlling the sequential steps of cortical projection neuron migration. *Adv Exp Med Biol* **800**:1–24.

Hoffman DR, Boettcher JA, and Diersen-Schade DA. 2009. Toward optimizing vision and cognition in term infants by dietary docosahexaenoic and arachidonic acid supplementation: A review of randomized controlled trials. *Prostaglandins Leukot Essent Fatty Acids* **81**:151–158.

Huang TT, Zou Y, and Corniola R. 2012. Oxidative stress and adult neurogenesis—effects of radiation and superoxide dismutase deficiency. *Semin Cell Dev Biol* **23**:738–744.

Igarashi M, Ma K, Gao F, Kim HW, Rapoport SI, and Rao JS. 2011. Disturbed choline plasmalogen and phospholipid fatty acid concentrations in Alzheimer's disease prefrontal cortex. *J Alzheimers Dis* **24**:507–517.

Innis SM. 2008. Dietary omega 3 fatty acids and the developing brain. *Brain Res* **1237**:35–43.

Insitute of Medicine. 2011. *Nutrition and Traumatic Brain Injury. Improving Acute and Subacute Health Outcomes in Military Personnel.* The National Academy Press, Washington DC.

Ishii A, Fyffe-Maricich SL, Furusho M, Miller RH, and Bansal R. 2012. ERK1/ERK2 MAPK signaling is required to increase myelin thickness independent of oligodendrocyte differentiation and initiation of myelination. *J Neurosci* **32**:8855–8864.

Janssen CI and Kiliaan AJ. 2014. Long-chain polyunsaturated fatty acids (LCPUFA) from genesis to senescence: The influence of LCPUFA on neural development, aging, and neurodegeneration. *Prog Lipid Res* **53**:1–17.

Jaworski J, Spangler S, Seeburg DP, Hoogenraad CC, and Sheng M. 2005. Control of dendritic arborization by the phosphoinositide-3'-kinase-Akt-mammalian target of rapamycin pathway. *J Neurosci* **25**:11300–11312.

Jeffrey BG, Weisinger HS, Neuringer M, and Mitchell DC. 2001. The role of docosahexaenoic acid in retinal function. *Lipids* **36**:859–871.

Katz LC and Shatz CJ. 1996. Synaptic activity and the construction of cortical circuits. *Science* **274**:1133–1138.

Kim HY and Spector AA. 2013. Synaptamide, endocannabinoid-like derivative of docosahexaenoic acid with cannabinoid-independent function. *Prostaglandins Leukot Essent Fatty Acids* **88**:121–125.

Koletzko B, Lien E, Agostoni C, Bohles H, Campoy C, Cetin I, Decsi T, Dudenhausen JW, Dupont C, Forsyth S et al. 2008. The roles of long-chain polyunsaturated fatty acids in pregnancy, lactation and infancy: Review of current knowledge and consensus recommendations. *J Perinat Med* **36**:5–14.

Krstic D, Pfister S, Notter T, and Knuesel I. 2013. Decisive role of Reelin signaling during early stages of Alzheimer's disease. *Neuroscience* **246**:108–116.

Kumar V, Zhang MX, Swank MW, Kunz J, and Wu GY. 2005. Regulation of dendritic morphogenesis by Ras-PI3K-Akt-mTOR and Ras-MAPK signaling pathways. *J Neurosci* **25**:11288–11299.

Larsson SC and Orsini N. 2011. Fish consumption and the risk of stroke: A dose–response meta-analysis. *Stroke* **42**:3621–3623.

Learoyd AE and Lifshitz J. 2012. Comparison of rat sensory behavioral tasks to detect somatosensory morbidity after diffuse brain-injury. *Behav Brain Res* **226**:197–204.

Lee CW, Shih YH, Wu SY, Yang T, Lin C, and Kuo YM. 2013. Hypoglycemia induces tau hyperphosphorylation. *Curr Alzheimer Res* **10**:298–308.

Lee PR and Fields RD. 2009. Regulation of myelin genes implicated in psychiatric disorders by functional activity in axons. *Front Neuroanat* **3**:4.

Lemaitre-Delaunay D, Pachiaudi C, Laville M, Pousin J, Armstrong M, and Lagarde M. 1999. Blood compartmental metabolism of docosahexaenoic acid (DHA) in humans after ingestion of a single dose of [13.C]DHA in phosphatidylcholine. *J Lipid Res* **40**:1867–1874.

Lengqvist J, Mata De Urquiza A, Bergman AC, Willson TM, Sjovall J, Perlmann T, and Griffiths WJ. 2004. Polyunsaturated fatty acids including docosahexaenoic and arachidonic acid bind to the retinoid X receptor alpha ligand-binding domain. *Mol Cell Proteomics* **3**:692–703.

Lewis M, Ghassemi P, and Hibbeln J. 2013. Therapeutic use of omega-3 fatty acids in severe head trauma. *Am J Emerg Med* **31**:273 e275–278.

Lewis MD and Bailes J. 2011. Neuroprotection for the warrior: Dietary supplementation with omega-3 fatty acids. *Mil Med* **176**:1120–1127.

Lidvall HF, Linderoth B, and Norlin B. 1974. Causes of the post-concussional syndrome. *Acta Neurol Scand Suppl* **56**:3–144.

Lin YH, Llanos A, Mena P, Uauy R, Salem N Jr. and Pawlosky RJ. 2010. Compartmental analyses of 2H5-alpha-linolenic acid and C-U-eicosapentaenoic acid toward synthesis of plasma labeled 22:6n-3 in newborn term infants. *Am J Clin Nutr* **92**:284–293.

Lin YH and Salem N Jr. 2007. Whole body distribution of deuterated linoleic and alpha-linolenic acids and their metabolites in the rat. *J Lipid Res* **48**:2709–2724.

Lingwood D, Ries J, Schwille P, and Simons K. 2008. Plasma membranes are poised for activation of raft phase coalescence at physiological temperature. *Proc Natl Acad Sci U S A* **105**:10005–10010.
Liu K, Lu Y, Lee JK, Samara R, Willenberg R, Sears-Kraxberger I, Tedeschi A, Park KK, Jin D, Cai B et al. 2010. PTEN deletion enhances the regenerative ability of adult corticospinal neurons. *Nat Neurosci* **13**:1075–1081.
Liu RZ, Mita R, Beaulieu M, Gao Z, and Godbout R. 2010. Fatty acid binding proteins in brain development and disease. *Int J Dev Biol* **54**:1229–1239.
Lizard G, Rouaud O, Demarquoy J, Cherkaoui-Malki M, and Iuliano L. 2012. Potential roles of peroxisomes in Alzheimer's disease and in dementia of the Alzheimer's type. *J Alzheimers Dis* **29**:241–254.
Llorens-Maritin M, Jurado J, Hernandez F, and Avila J. 2014. GSK-3beta, a pivotal kinase in Alzheimer disease. *Front Mol Neurosci* **7**:46.
Lorenzetto E, Panteri R, Marino R, Keller F, and Buffelli M. 2008. Impaired nerve regeneration in reeler mice after peripheral nerve injury. *Eur J Neurosci* **27**:12–19.
Mahley RW and Huang Y. 2012. Apolipoprotein e sets the stage: Response to injury triggers neuropathology. *Neuron* **76**:871–885.
Makrides M, Gibson RA, McPhee AJ, Collins CT, Davis PG, Doyle LW, Simmer K, Colditz PB, Morris S, Smithers LG et al. 2009. Neurodevelopmental outcomes of preterm infants fed high-dose docosahexaenoic acid: A randomized controlled trial. *JAMA* **301**:175–182.
Martinez M and Vazquez E. 1998. MRI evidence that docosahexaenoic acid ethyl ester improves myelination in generalized peroxisomal disorders. *Neurology* **51**:26–32.
Massalini S, Pellegatta S, Pisati F, Finocchiaro G, Farace MG, and Ciafre SA. 2009. Reelin affects chain-migration and differentiation of neural precursor cells. *Mol Cell Neurosci* **42**:341–349.
Matsuki T, Zaka M, Guerreiro R, van der Brug MP, Cooper JA, Cookson MR, Hardy JA, and Howell BW. 2012. Identification of Stk25 as a genetic modifier of Tau phosphorylation in Dab1-mutant mice. *PLoS One* **7**:e31152.
McAllister TW. 1992. Neuropsychiatric sequelae of head injuries. *Psychiatr Clin North Am* **15**:395–413.
McNamara RK and Carlson SE. 2006. Role of omega-3 fatty acids in brain development and function: Potential implications for the pathogenesis and prevention of psychopathology. *Prostaglandins Leukot Essent Fatty Acids* **75**:329–349.
Medhi B and Chakrabarty M. 2013. Insulin resistance: An emerging link in Alzheimer's disease. *Neurol Sci* **34**:1719–1725.
Melamed O, Levav-Rabkin T, Zukerman C, Clarke G, Cryan JF, Dinan TG, Grossman Y, and Golan HM. 2014. Long-lasting glutamatergic modulation induced by neonatal GABA enhancement in mice. *Neuropharmacology* **79**:616–625.
Meyer U, Nyffeler M, Yee BK, Knuesel I, and Feldon J. 2008. Adult brain and behavioral pathological markers of prenatal immune challenge during early/middle and late fetal development in mice. *Brain Behav Immun* **22**:469–486.
Michael-Titus AT and Priestley JV. 2014. Omega-3 fatty acids and traumatic neurological injury: From neuroprotection to neuroplasticity? *Trends Neurosci* **37**:30–38.
Mills JD, Hadley K, and Bailes JE. 2011. Dietary supplementation with the omega-3 fatty acid docosahexaenoic acid in traumatic brain injury. *Neurosurgery* **68**:474–481; discussion 481.
Mitchell DC, Niu SL, and Litman BJ. 2012. Quantifying the differential effects of DHA and DPA on the early events in visual signal transduction. *Chem Phys Lipids* **165**:393–400.
Mitchell LS, Gillespie SC, McAllister F, Fanarraga ML, Kirkham D, Kelly B, Brophy PJ, Griffiths IR, Montague P and Kennedy PG. 1992. Developmental expression of major myelin protein genes in the CNS of X-linked hypomyelinating mutant rumpshaker. *J Neurosci Res* **33**:205–217.

Moriguchi T and Salem N Jr. 2003. Recovery of brain docosahexaenoate leads to recovery of spatial task performance. *J Neurochem* **87**:297–309.

Morse NL. 2012. Benefits of docosahexaenoic acid, folic acid, vitamin D and iodine on foetal and infant brain development and function following maternal supplementation during pregnancy and lactation. *Nutrients* **4**:799–840.

Mukherjee PK, Chawla A, Loayza MS, and Bazan NG. 2007. Docosanoids are multifunctional regulators of neural cell integrity and fate: Significance in aging and disease. *Prostaglandins Leukot Essent Fatty Acids* **77**:233–238.

Muller C, Bauer NM, Schafer I, and White R. 2013. Making myelin basic protein from mRNA transport to localized translation. *Front Cell Neurosci* **7**:169.

Narayanan SP, Flores AI, Wang F, and Macklin WB. 2009. Akt signals through the mammalian target of rapamycin pathway to regulate CNS myelination. *J Neurosci* **29**:6860–6870.

Nishikawa M, Kimura S, and Akaike N. 1994. Facilitatory effect of docosahexaenoic acid on N-methyl-D-aspartate response in pyramidal neurones of rat cerebral cortex. *J Physiol* **475**:83–93.

Niu SL, Mitchell DC, Lim SY, Wen ZM, Kim HY, Salem N Jr. and Litman BJ. 2004. Reduced G protein-coupled signaling efficiency in retinal rod outer segments in response to n-3 fatty acid deficiency. *J Biol Chem* **279**:31098–31104.

Ojo JO, Mouzon B, Greenberg MB, Bachmeier C, Mullan M, and Crawford F. 2013. Repetitive mild traumatic brain injury augments tau pathology and glial activation in aged hTau mice. *J Neuropathol Exp Neurol* **72**:137–151.

Orr SK, Palumbo S, Bosetti F, Mount HT, Kang JX, Greenwood CE, Ma DW, Serhan CN, and Bazinet RP. 2013. Unesterified docosahexaenoic acid is protective in neuroinflammation. *J Neurochem* **127**:378–393.

Ouellet M, Emond V, Chen CT, Julien C, Bourasset F, Oddo S, LaFerla F, Bazinet RP, and Calon F. 2009. Diffusion of docosahexaenoic and eicosapentaenoic acids through the blood–brain barrier: An in situ cerebral perfusion study. *Neurochem Int* **55**:476–482.

Pan HC, Kao TK, Ou YC, Yang DY, Yen YJ, Wang CC, Chuang YH, Liao SL, Raung SL, Wu CW et al. 2009. Protective effect of docosahexaenoic acid against brain injury in ischemic rats. *J Nutr Biochem* **20**:715–725.

Panteri R, Mey J, Zhelyaznik N, D'Altocolle A, Del Fa A, Gangitano C, Marino R, Lorenzetto E, Buffelli M, and Keller F. 2006. Reelin is transiently expressed in the peripheral nerve during development and is upregulated following nerve crush. *Mol Cell Neurosci* **32**:133–142.

Paterniti I, Impellizzeri D, Di Paola R, Esposito E, Gladman S, Yip P, Priestley JV, Michael-Titus AT, and Cuzzocrea S. 2014. Docosahexaenoic acid attenuates the early inflammatory response following spinal cord injury in mice: In-vivo and in-vitro studies. *J Neuroinflammation* **11**:6.

Pawlosky RJ, Hibbeln JR, Lin Y, Goodson S, Riggs P, Sebring N, Brown GL, and Salem N Jr. 2003. Effects of beef- and fish-based diets on the kinetics of n-3 fatty acid metabolism in human subjects. *Am J Clin Nutr* **77**:565–572.

Pawlosky RJ and Salem N Jr. 2004. Perspectives on alcohol consumption: Liver polyunsaturated fatty acids and essential fatty acid metabolism. *Alcohol* **34**:27–33.

Perederiy JV and Westbrook GL. 2013. Structural plasticity in the dentate gyrus—revisiting a classic injury model. *Front Neural Circuits* **7**:17.

Peterson BS, Vohr B, Staib LH, Cannistraci CJ, Dolberg A, Schneider KC, Katz KH, Westerveld M, Sparrow S, Anderson AW et al. 2000. Regional brain volume abnormalities and long-term cognitive outcome in preterm infants. *JAMA* **284**:1939–1947.

Plourde M and Cunnane SC. 2007. Extremely limited synthesis of long chain polyunsaturates in adults: Implications for their dietary essentiality and use as supplements. *Appl Physiol Nutr Metab* **32**:619–634.

Pluta R, Jolkkonen J, Cuzzocrea S, Pedata F, Cechetto D, and Popa-Wagner A. 2011. Cognitive impairment with vascular impairment and degeneration. *Curr Neurovasc Res* **8**:342–350.

Polozova A and Litman BJ. 2000. Cholesterol dependent recruitment of di22:6-PC by a G protein-coupled receptor into lateral domains. *Biophys J* **79**:2632–2643.
Polozova A and Salem N Jr. 2007. Role of liver and plasma lipoproteins in selective transport of n-3 fatty acids to tissues: A comparative study of 14C-DHA and 3H-oleic acid tracers. *J Mol Neurosci* **33**:56–66.
Quinn JF, Raman R, Thomas RG, Yurko-Mauro K, Nelson EB, Van Dyck C, Galvin JE, Emond J, Jack CR Jr., Weiner M et al. 2010. Docosahexaenoic acid supplementation and cognitive decline in Alzheimer disease: A randomized trial. *JAMA* **304**:1903–1911.
Rakic P. 2006. A century of progress in corticoneurogenesis: From silver impregnation to genetic engineering. *Cereb Cortex* **16 Suppl 1**:i3–17.
Risdall JE and Menon DK. 2011. Traumatic brain injury. *Philos Trans R Soc Lond B Biol Sci* **366**:241–250.
Robson LG, Dyall S, Sidloff D, and Michael-Titus AT. 2010. Omega-3 polyunsaturated fatty acids increase the neurite outgrowth of rat sensory neurones throughout development and in aged animals. *Neurobiol Aging* **31**:678–687.
Romanelli RJ and Wood TL. 2008. Directing traffic in neural cells: Determinants of receptor tyrosine kinase localization and cellular responses. *J Neurochem* **105**:2055–2068.
Rossel M, Loulier K, Feuillet C, Alonso S, and Carroll P. 2005. Reelin signaling is necessary for a specific step in the migration of hindbrain efferent neurons. *Development* **132**:1175–1185.
Rusca A, Di Stefano AF, Doig MV, Scarsi C, and Perucca E. 2009. Relative bioavailability and pharmacokinetics of two oral formulations of docosahexaenoic acid/eicosapentaenoic acid after multiple-dose administration in healthy volunteers. *Eur J Clin Pharmacol* **65**:503–510.
Rutherford WH, Merrett JD, and McDonald JR. 1979. Symptoms at one year following concussion from minor head injuries. *Injury* **10**:225–230.
Ryan AS, Astwood JD, Gautier S, Kuratko CN, Nelson EB, and Salem N Jr. 2010. Effects of long-chain polyunsaturated fatty acid supplementation on neurodevelopment in childhood: A review of human studies. *Prostaglandins Leukot Essent Fatty Acids* **82**:305–314.
Ryan AS, Keske MA, Hoffman JP, and Nelson EB. 2009. Clinical overview of algal-docosahexaenoic acid: Effects on triglyceride levels and other cardiovascular risk factors. *Am J Ther* **16**:183–192.
Saha N, Kolev M, and Nikolov DB. 2014. Structural features of the Nogo receptor signaling complexes at the neuron/myelin interface. *Neurosci Res* **87C**:1–7.
Salem N Jr., Litman B, Kim HY, and Gawrisch K. 2001. Mechanisms of action of docosahexaenoic acid in the nervous system. *Lipids* **36**:945–959.
Sarkadi-Nagy E, Wijendran V, Diau GY, Chao AC, Hsieh AT, Turpeinen A, Nathanielsz PW, and Brenna JT. 2003. The influence of prematurity and long chain polyunsaturate supplementation in 4-week adjusted age baboon neonate brain and related tissues. *Pediatr Res* **54**:244–252.
Schulz A, Kyselyova A, Baader SL, Jung MJ, Zoch A, Mautner VF, Hagel C, and Morrison H. 2014. Neuronal merlin influences ERBB2 receptor expression on Schwann cells through neuregulin 1 type III signalling. *Brain* **137**:420–432.
Shaikh SR, Dumaual AC, Castillo A, LoCascio D, Siddiqui RA, Stillwell W, and Wassall SR. 2004. Oleic and docosahexaenoic acid differentially phase separate from lipid raft molecules: A comparative NMR, DSC, AFM, and detergent extraction study. *Biophys J* **87**:1752–1766.
Shirai N, Suzuki H, Tokairin S, Ehara H, and Wada S. 2002. Dietary and seasonal effects on the dorsal meat lipid composition of Japanese (Silurus asotus) and Thai catfish (Clarias macrocephalus and hybrid Clarias macrocephalus and Clarias galipinus). *Comp Biochem Physiol A Mol Integr Physiol* **132**:609–619.
Shirai N, Terayama M, and Takeda H. 2002. Effect of season on the fatty acid composition and free amino acid content of the sardine Sardinops melanostictus. *Comp Biochem Physiol B Biochem Mol Biol* **131**:387–393.

Snigdha S, Smith ED, Prieto GA, and Cotman CW. 2012. Caspase-3 activation as a bifurcation point between plasticity and cell death. *Neurosci Bull* **28**:14–24.

Spielman LJ, Little JP, and Klegeris A. 2014. Inflammation and insulin/IGF-1 resistance as the possible link between obesity and neurodegeneration. *J Neuroimmunol* **273**:8–21.

Stein DG. 2013. A clinical/translational perspective: Can a developmental hormone play a role in the treatment of traumatic brain injury? *Horm Behav* **63**:291–300.

Stillwell W, Shaikh SR, Zerouga M, Siddiqui R, and Wassall SR. 2005. Docosahexaenoic acid affects cell signaling by altering lipid rafts. *Reprod Nutr Dev* **45**:559–579.

Sutherland C, Leighton IA, and Cohen P. 1993. Inactivation of glycogen synthase kinase-3 beta by phosphorylation: New kinase connections in insulin and growth-factor signalling. *Biochem J* **296** (Pt 1):15–19.

Tavazoie SF, Alvarez VA, Ridenour DA, Kwiatkowski DJ, and Sabatini BL. 2005. Regulation of neuronal morphology and function by the tumor suppressors Tsc1 and Tsc2. *Nat Neurosci* **8**:1727–1734.

Teague H, Ross R, Harris M, Mitchell DC, and Shaikh SR. 2013. DHA-fluorescent probe is sensitive to membrane order and reveals molecular adaptation of DHA in ordered lipid microdomains. *J Nutr Biochem* **24**:188–195.

Tuszynski MH, Steeves JD, Fawcett JW, Lammertse D, Kalichman M, Rask C, Curt A, Ditunno JF, Fehlings MG, Guest JD et al. 2007. Guidelines for the conduct of clinical trials for spinal cord injury as developed by the ICCP Panel: Clinical trial inclusion/exclusion criteria and ethics. *Spinal Cord* **45**:222–231.

Umhau JC, Zhou W, Carson RE, Rapoport SI, Polozova A, Demar J, Hussein N, Bhattacharjee AK, Ma K et al. 2009. Imaging incorporation of circulating docosahexaenoic acid into the human brain using positron emission tomography. *J Lipid Res* **50**:1259–1268.

Umhau JC, Zhou W, Thada S, Demar J, Hussein N, Bhattacharjee AK, Ma K, Majchrzak-Hong S, Herscovitch P, Salem N Jr. et al. 2013. Brain docosahexaenoic acid [DHA] incorporation and blood flow are increased in chronic alcoholics: A positron emission tomography study corrected for cerebral atrophy. *PLoS One* **8**:e75333.

van Neerven S, Kampmann E, and Mey J. 2008. RAR/RXR and PPAR/RXR signaling in neurological and psychiatric diseases. *Prog Neurobiol* **85**:433–451.

Vandal M, Alata W, Tremblay C, Rioux-Perreault C, Salem N Jr., Calon F, and Plourde M. 2014. Reduction in DHA transport to the brain of mice expressing human APOE4 compared to APOE2. *J Neurochem* **129**:516–526.

Veerkamp JH, Van M, Ht, and Zimmerman AW. 2000. Effect of fatty acid-binding proteins on intermembrane fatty acid transport studies on different types and mutant proteins. *Eur J Biochem* **267**:5959–5966.

Virtanen JK, Siscovick DS, Longstreth WT Jr., Kuller LH, and Mozaffarian D. 2008. Fish consumption and risk of subclinical brain abnormalities on MRI in older adults. *Neurology* **71**:439–446.

Wang C, Harris WS, Chung M, Lichtenstein AH, Balk EM, Kupelnick B, Jordan HS, and Lau J. 2006. n-3 Fatty acids from fish or fish-oil supplements, but not alpha-linolenic acid, benefit cardiovascular disease outcomes in primary- and secondary-prevention studies: A systematic review. *Am J Clin Nutr* **84**:5–17.

Weisinger HS, Vingrys AJ, Bui BV, and Sinclair AJ. 1999. Effects of dietary n-3 fatty acid deficiency and repletion in the guinea pig retina. *Invest Ophthalmol Vis Sci* **40**:327–338.

Wellhauser L and Belsham DD. 2014. Activation of the omega-3 fatty acid receptor GPR120 mediates anti-inflammatory actions in immortalized hypothalamic neurons. *J Neuroinflammation* **11**:60.

White R and Kramer-Albers EM. 2014. Axon-glia interaction and membrane traffic in myelin formation. *Front Cell Neurosci* **7**:284.

Won SJ, Kim SH, Xie L, Wang Y, Mao XO, Jin K, and Greenberg DA. 2006. Reelin-deficient mice show impaired neurogenesis and increased stroke size. *Exp Neurol* **198**:250–259.

Wu A, Ying Z, and Gomez-Pinilla F. 2004. Dietary omega-3 fatty acids normalize BDNF levels, reduce oxidative damage, and counteract learning disability after traumatic brain injury in rats. *J Neurotrauma* **21**:1457–1467.

Wu A, Ying Z, and Gomez-Pinilla F. 2011. The salutary effects of DHA dietary supplementation on cognition, neuroplasticity, and membrane homeostasis after brain trauma. *J Neurotrauma* **28**:2113–2122.

Wu A, Ying Z, and Gomez-Pinilla F. 2014. Dietary strategy to repair plasma membrane after brain trauma: Implications for plasticity and cognition. *Neurorehabil Neural Repair* **28**:75–84.

Xiong M, Li J, Ma SM, Yang Y, and Zhou WH. 2013. Effects of hypothermia on oligodendrocyte precursor cell proliferation, differentiation and maturation following hypoxia ischemia in vivo and in vitro. *Exp Neurol* **247**:720–729.

Yamashima T. 2012. 'PUFA-GPR40-CREB signaling' hypothesis for the adult primate neurogenesis. *Prog Lipid Res* **51**:221–231.

Yang XL, Xiong WC, and Mei L. 2004. Lipid rafts in neuregulin signaling at synapses. *Life Sci* **75**:2495–2504.

Yaqoob P. 2009. The nutritional significance of lipid rafts. *Annu Rev Nutr* **29**:257–282.

Yavin E, Himovichi E, and Eilam R. 2009. Delayed cell migration in the developing rat brain following maternal omega 3 alpha linolenic acid dietary deficiency. *Neuroscience* **162**:1011–1022.

Young SG and Zechner R. 2013. Biochemistry and pathophysiology of intravascular and intracellular lipolysis. *Genes Dev* **27**:459–484.

Yurko-Mauro K, McCarthy D, Rom D, Nelson EB, Ryan AS, Blackwell A, Salem N Jr., and Stedman M. 2010. Beneficial effects of docosahexaenoic acid on cognition in age-related cognitive decline. *Alzheimers Dement* **6**:456–464.

Zamarbide M, Etayo-Labiano I, Ricobaraza A, Martinez-Pinilla E, Aymerich MS, Luis Lanciego J, Perez-Mediavilla A and Franco R. 2014. GPR40 activation leads to CREB and ERK phosphorylation in primary cultures of neurons from the mouse CNS and in human neuroblastoma cells. *Hippocampus* **24**:733–739.

Zhou W, Xu D, Peng X, Zhang Q, Jia J, and Crutcher KA. 2008. Meta-analysis of APOE4 allele and outcome after traumatic brain injury. *J Neurotrauma* **25**:279–290.

10 Vitamin E
Defining Status for Optimal Health

Michael I. McBurney

CONTENTS

10.1 INTRODUCTION

Vitamin E, discovered in 1922, consists of eight structurally related antioxidant molecules (α-, β-, γ-, and δ-tocopherols and α-, β-, γ-, and δ-tocotrienols) produced by plants or synthetically (Niki and Traber 2012). Of the eight stereoisomeric forms, it is the four 2R α-tocopherol forms (α- and γ-tocopherol) maintained in human plasma that are considered biologically important (Traber 2013). Because of the specificity of α-tocopherol transfer protein (α-TPP) in the liver (Reboul et al. 2009), the major form in circulation across all forms of lipoprotein fractions is α-tocopherol despite the predominance of γ-tocopherol as a US dietary source (Ford et al. 2006). Thus, α-tocopherol is the most abundant form in tissues and the only form retained at high levels in humans (Cohn 1997). Unlike other fat-soluble vitamins, for example, vitamins A and D, α-tocopherol does not accumulate in the liver or extra-hepatic tissues (IOM 2000). Using isotopically labeled α-tocopherol, blood sampling and complete urinary and fecal collections in six men and six women, (Chuang et al. 2011) measured apparent absorption of 79% with feces being the major route of elimination (23%) followed by urine (4%). The half-life of ^{14}C-tracer, measured over 70 days (d), was 7.5 days and 15.2 days for plasma and red blood cells (RBC), respectively. Other non-α-tocopherol forms of vitamin E are metabolized and excreted. Tocotrienols are detected in high-density lipoprotein (HDL) cholesterol, peaking between 4 and 8 h, before being cleared from circulation (Fairus et al. 2006).

In the cells of plants and animals, vitamin E protects polyunsaturated fatty acids (PUFA) from oxidation by reacting with peroxyl radicals (Valk and Hornstra 2000, Traber 2013). The amount of tocopherol required to protect fatty acids from peroxidation increases as the proportion of unsaturated fatty acids increases (Valk and Hornstra 2000). Vitamin E does this by reacting 1000 times faster with fat-soluble radicals than these molecules can react with other double bonds within PUFAs (Traber 2013).

10.2 DEFICIENCY REQUIREMENTS

Approximately 25 years ago, a risk assessment model was adopted to establish estimated average requirements (EAR) and tolerable upper intake levels (UL) (IOM 1998). The EAR is the daily intake of a nutrient estimated to meet the nutrient requirement of half the healthy individuals in a life stage and gender group. Using specific criterion for adequacy, the recommended dietary allowance (RDA) is the average daily dietary intake level to meet the nutrient intake of nearly all (97%–98%) healthy individuals in a particular gender and life stage group.

Unlike the current recommendations for calcium and vitamin D (IOM 2011) which consider nutrient requirements based on indicators of adequacy as well as to prevent deficiency (i.e., rickets), a plasma α-tocopherol concentration corresponding to <12% hydrogen peroxide-induced in vitro erythrocyte (RBC) lysis in vitamin E-deficient subjects was chosen as a criterion of adequacy (IOM 2000). Intake levels required to prevent RBC hemolysis do not necessarily reflect the optimal vitamin E status required to maintain healthy function of all cell types. Moreover, the EAR for vitamin E is based exclusively on the 2R-steroisomeric forms of α-tocopherol whereas the UL was determined using all forms of supplemental α-tocopherol. Vitamin E deficiency, is not described until the 1980s, usually caused by a genetic defect in the α-tocopherol transfer protein (Niki and Traber 2012). However, with respect to the general healthy population, it is timely to reconsider vitamin E intake recommendations based on the vitamin E status needed to maintain optimal antioxidant status to support normal cellular function and human health (Peter et al. 2013).

10.3 STATUS ASSESSMENT

Ford et al. (2006) analyzed serum α-tocopherol concentrations in 4087 adults participating in the National Health and Nutrition Examination Survey (1999–2000). In adults ≥20 years, α-tocopherol concentrations range between 12 and 46 μmol/L (Ford et al. 2006). Serum α-tocopherol levels are affected by age (positively), ethnicity, and smoking (Schleicher et al. 2013). Approximately 40% of Americans ≥60 years have α-tocopherol concentrations <30 μmol/L (Ford et al. 2006). In all men and women, the proportion is ≈66% and 61%, respectively. Generally, serum α-tocopherol concentrations rank as follows: Whites > Mexican Americans > African Americans. Because many US children consume inadequate amounts of vitamin E daily (Kim et al. 2006), they are likely to have plasma concentrations near deficient levels (<11 μmol/L).

These results correlate with other surveys. Wang et al. (2013) reported serum α-tocopherol concentrations in 2912 participants from the 2005–2006 National Health and Nutrition Examination Survey, age ≥40 years, who self-reported a presence or absence of glaucoma. The five quintiles for serum α-tocopherol concentrations were ≤22.4, >22.4, >27.0, >31.6, and >40.0 μmol/L. In other words, 60% were <27.0 μmol/L and 80% were <31.6 μmol/L. In 1997, Winklhofer-Roob, van't Hof, and Shmerling (1997) reported that most Swiss persons had plasma α-tocopherol levels below 30 μmol/L and these values were intermediate when compared to other nations. Illison et al. (2011) randomly selected individuals with diabetes from a database in Brazil. They reported that 36% were vitamin E-deficient with plasma α-tocopherol concentrations ≤12 μmol/L, while the remainder were <30.8 μmol/L.

Because blood α-tocopherol concentrations do not correlate well with dietary intake and lipid peroxidation markers are not specific to vitamin E status (Ford et al. 2006, Lebold et al. 2012), other markers of oxidative status would be beneficial. F2-isoprostanes are formed non-enzymatically by free radical-mediated peroxidation of arachidonic acid (Morrow et al. 1990). Plasma concentrations of F2-isoprostanes are often used to assess oxidative stress in vivo because they reflect dietary patterns (Meyer et al. 2013), and a linear relationship exists between vitamin E dosage and percent reduction in plasma F_2-isoprostane concentrations (Roberts et al. 2007). However, maximum suppression of plasma concentrations of F_2-isoprostanes does not occur until 16 weeks of supplementation (Roberts et al. 2007). Urinary metabolites of vitamin E, α-carboxyethyl hydroxychroman (α-CECH), and α-carboxymethylbutyl hydroxychroman (α-CMBHC) appear to be more reliable markers of vitamin E status (Lebold et al. 2012). Because 3–5 times more α-CECH is produced from *all-rac*-α-tocopherol than RRR-α-tocopherol (Bruno et al. 2005), it is important to separate subjects who use dietary supplements or fortified foods from those who do not (Lebold et al. 2012). More research is needed to measure vitamin E intake, concentrations of α-tocopherol, and its metabolites in biological samples and functional outcomes.

10.4 GENETIC FACTORS

Genetics may also affect α-tocopherol status (Girona et al. 2008, Sundl et al. 2007, Borel et al. 2007, Di Donato et al. 2010). A single-nucleotide polymorphism close to the apolipoprotein A5 gene (rs12272004) has been associated with higher plasma α-tocopherol concentrations (Ferrucci et al. 2009). Using a genome-wide association study approach with over 5000 men of European descent, Major et al. (2011) identified three loci associated with α-tocopherol levels (rs2108622, rs11057830, and rs964184). Susceptibility to respiratory infections among the elderly may be influenced by genetic polymorphisms that interact with vitamin E needs (Belisle et al. 2010). Asleh and Levy (2010) demonstrated that impaired HDL function in HP 2-2 individuals (but not those with HP 1-1 or HP 1-2 genotypes) with diabetes could be mitigated with vitamin E (400 IU daily), but not vitamin C.

10.5 OPTIMAL VITAMIN E STATUS

Observational studies assessing only the relationship between dietary intakes of antioxidant nutrients, for example, vitamin E and cancer prevention, have reported inconsistent results (Lin et al. 2009, Gaziano et al. 2009). It should not be surprising that yes/no responses to questionnaires do not provide a reasonable assessment of nutrient status and disease risk (Dietrich et al. 2009, Neuhouser et al. 2009, Song et al. 2009, Del Rio et al. 2011, Larsson et al. 2010, Roberts et al. 2010, Christen et al. 2010, Gaziano et al. 2012).

During the last quarter of the twentieth century, a number of randomized, placebo-controlled intervention trials (RCTs) were conducted using vitamin E at pharmacologic doses. See meta-analyses by Miller et al. (2005) and Biesalski et al. (2010). The results were analyzed as a pharmaceutical drug vs. placebo with some consideration of dose, compliance, and duration of the intervention (Miller et al. 2005, Biesalski et al. 2010). In the majority, the RCTs were flawed because the investigators failed to assess α-tocopherol status or relevant biomarkers (Blumberg and Frei 2007). They also lacked markers to evaluate the effect of any given antioxidant interventions (Steinberg and Witztum 2002).

Levels ≥30 μmol/L have been proposed for primary prevention of cardiovascular disease and cancer (Gey and Puska 1989). In their review, Traber, Frei, and Beckman (2008) note that the Alpha-Tocopherol, Beta-Carotene Cancer Prevention (ATBC) Study found that those in the lowest serum α-tocopherol quintile had significantly higher risk of total and cause-specific mortality than those in the highest quintile (ATBC 1994). The median baseline α-tocopherol level was 26.7 μmol/L with 20th and 80th percentiles of 21.6 and 33 μmol/L, respectively. Basically, three quarters of these volunteers had lower α-tocopherol concentrations than the starting point for the RCTS reviewed by Miller et al. (2005) and Biesalski et al. (2010). The optimum reduction in mortality measured in ATBC (1994) occurred at 30 μmol/L, below the starting point for most of the subsequent vitamin E intervention trials. A close analysis of Figure 10.1 shows that the greatest positive impact on relative risk for total mortality is achieved by increasing serum α-tocopherol levels from 16 to 30 μmol/L (Wright et al. 2006). While a modest increased risk in mortality was observed with serum α-tocopherol concentrations that had increased beyond 30 μmol/L, most Americans have circulating concentrations of α-tocopherol below 30 μmol/L (Ford et al. 2006, Schleicher et al. 2013, Wang et al. 2013), in a range where they could benefit from increased vitamin E intake. A level of 30 μmol/L is consistent with a daily recommended dietary intake of 13 mg α-tocopherol (Traber and Stevens 2011).

RCTs conducted in individuals with optimal vitamin E concentrations are unlikely to benefit from increased intake. Moreover, nutrient intervention trials need to be designed differently than drug studies because everyone has some level of nutrient intake. It is impossible to have a true placebo group with zero intake. Single-agent nutrition intervention studies must be designed to ensure the study subpopulation is representative of the general population in terms of disease risk and nutritional status (Gann 2009). This is not always the case. For example, the physicians responding to the letters of invitation for the Physicians' Health Study were 19 and 16% lower total

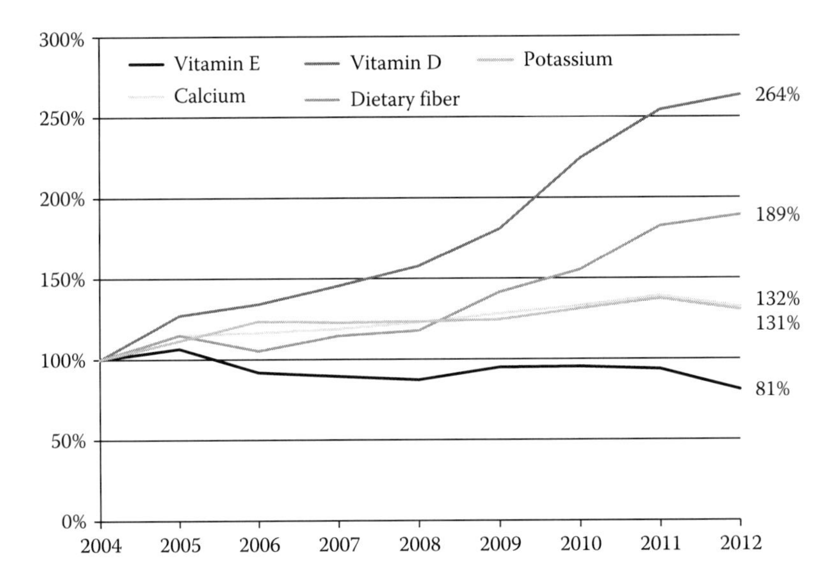

FIGURE 10.1 Percent change in annual number of scientific citations by nutrient in PubMed between 2004 and 2012. PubMed searches were conducted on October 17, 2013 using "clinical trials, classical articles, comparative study, controlled clinical trial, randomized controlled trial, and humans."

and cardiovascular mortality rates than unwilling respondents (Sesso et al. 2002). While data may not support pharmacologic doses of vitamin E (Gann 2009), nutrition science should not turn a blind eye to the need to defining optimal vitamin E status. More research is needed to assess vitamin E intake, vitamin E status, and functional outcomes in the general population.

10.6 VITAMIN E STATUS AND NON-COMMUNICABLE DISEASES

10.6.1 Cancer

Lippman et al. (2009) reported that vitamin E supplementation, alone or in combination, did not prevent prostate cancer in healthy men. Once again, the males included in this study had baseline α-tocopherol levels averaging more than 28 μmol/L. Although they did not report plasma α-tocopherol concentrations in the Somen's Antioxidant Cardiovascular Study (WACS), Lin et al. (2009) concluded that supplementation with vitamin E offered no overall benefit. However, blood α-tocopherol levels were taken to evaluate compliance in 30 local participants; average placebo levels were >28 μmol/L (Cook et al. 2007). Men with pre-diagnostic (baseline) serum α-tocopherol levels averaging 30 μmol/L had a 10% lower risk of developing prostate cancer compared to those at 18.6 μmol/L (Weinstein et al. 2007).

Men who smoke have a reduced risk of pancreatic risk as serum α-tocopherol concentrations increase from ≈18 μmol/L (Stolzenberg-Solomon et al. 2009).

In reporting the Health Professionals Follow-up Study results, Maserejian et al. (2007) concluded that increased vitamin E intake was correlated with increased risk of oral pre-malignant lesions in men without assessing blood vitamin E levels. The assertion was based on correlations of total dietary vitamin E intakes with plasma α-tocopherol levels ranging between 19 and 35 μmol/L (Ascherio et al. 1992). The crude correlation coefficients between food frequency questionnaire (FFQ) and plasma concentrations were 0.24 and 0.27 in women, and these correlations decreased significantly when participants who reported using dietary supplements containing vitamin E were excluded (Ascherio et al. 1992). More research is needed to elucidate the relationship between suboptimal vitamin E status and cancer.

10.6.2 Brain Health, Cognition, and Depression

The brain, especially rich in the long-chain polyunsaturated omega-3 fatty acid docosahexaenoic acid (DHA) has high levels of α-tocopherol, which are preserved during periods of inadequate vitamin E intake (Vatassery et al. 1984). Bowman et al. (2012) examined the cross-sectional relationship of plasma α-tocopherol concentrations in 104 elderly (average age 87 years) individuals participating in the Oregon Brain Aging Study cohort. Higher plasma profiles of vitamins C, E, B, and D and marine omega-3 fatty acids were positively associated with brain volume and cognitive function. In conjunction with automated structural magnetic resonance imaging (MRI), plasma α-tocopherol levels can help differentiate individuals with Alzheimer's disease from those with mild cognitive impairment from cognitively intact control subjects (Mangialasche et al. 2013). Controls had α-tocopherol levels >30 μmol/L whereas those with Alzheimer's had an average <30 μmol/L (Mangialasche et al. 2013). Among patients with mild to moderate Alzheimer's, 2000 IU vitamin E daily slowed functional decline by 19% compared to placebo over 6 months (Dysken et al. 2014). This finding is especially relevant as there is no drug in the market for individuals with Alzheimer's disease.

Beydoun et al. (2013) examined the relationship of antioxidant status with depressive symptoms in US adults aged 20–85 years. Women with elevated depressive symptoms had lower serum levels of vitamins E (26 vs. 30 μmol/L) and C (43 vs. 60 μmol/L) as well as all carotenoids compared with their non-depressed counterparts. Maes et al. (2000) reported lower vitamin E concentrations (≈23 μmol/L) in American individuals with major depression vs. normal volunteers (≈32 μmol/L), as did Owen et al. (2005) in Australians. Tiemeir and colleagues (2002) did not find a statistically significant relationship between vitamin E status and depression symptoms in the Rotterdam study, but both controls and subjects had average vitamin E concentrations close to 30 μmol/L. More research is needed to understand the interaction between dietary intakes of vitamin E and DHA, markers of nutrient status, and brain function.

10.6.3 Liver Function

Severe thermal injury rapidly depletes plasma vitamin E levels in children (Traber et al. 2010). In a pilot trial, vitamin E supplementation normalized liver enzyme levels in obese children with non-alcoholic steatohepatitis (NASH) (Lavine 2000).

Supplementation with antioxidant vitamins, C and E, have also been effective in improving fibrosis scores in NASH patients (Harrison et al. 2003). Vitamin E supplementation (800 IU/day) has been used to help treat NASH in adults, but α-tocopherol status was not reported (Sanyal et al. 2010). Because of the high prevalence of overweight and obesity globally, more research is needed to understand the relationship between vitamin E status and the prevalence of NASH in overweight or obese individuals.

10.6.4 Metabolic Syndrome, Diabetes, and Cardiovascular Health

Metabolic syndrome is a constellation of risk factors contributing to diabetes, cardiovascular disease, and other non-communicable diseases. Czernichow et al. (2009) retrospectively analyzed the effect of antioxidant supplementation on the risk of metabolic syndrome in adults participating in the Supplementation en VItamines et Mineraux AntioXydants (SU.VI.MAX) primary prevention trial. Like the original SU.VI.MAX report (Zureik et al. 2004), vitamin E supplementation did not change disease risk in individuals with baseline serum α-tocopherol levels of >31 μmol/L. However, the relationship is less clear in individuals with suboptimal vitamin E status.

The release of hemoglobin into plasma during the normal turnover of RBCs or into extravascular spaces following hemorrhage is being recognized to mediate oxidative reactions and disease risk (Melamed-Frank et al. 2001, Rother et al. 2005). Haptoglobin is an antioxidant protein which helps prevent hemoglobin-induced tissue oxidation (Melamed-Frank et al. 2001). In the early 1990s, before knowledge of genetic polymorphisms, Fuller et al. (1996) reported that vitamin E supplementation (1200 IU/day) in patients with diabetes and baseline plasma α-tocopherol ≈22–24 μmol/L, significantly increased plasma α-tocopherol levels and reduced LDL oxidative susceptibility. Since then, three polymorphisms of the haptoglobin (HP) gene have been characterized: HP 1-1, HP 2-1, and HP 2-2 (Asleh et al. 2003). Differences in antioxidant activity against hemoglobin between HP 1-1 and HP 2-2 are exaggerated when hemoglobin is glycosylated (Asleh et al. 2005). In five independent longitudinal studies, the HP 2-2 genotype has been predictive of a three- to five-fold increased risk of cardiovascular disease compared to individuals with diabetes without the HP 2-2 genotype (Costacou et al. 2008, Levy et al. 2002, Milman et al. 2008, Roguin et al. 2003, Suleiman et al. 2005). The HDL particle seems to be an important target for HP 2-hemoglobin-mediated oxidation (Asleh et al. 2008). Asleh and Levy (2010) demonstrated that impaired HDL function in HP 2-2 individuals with diabetes could be mitigated with vitamin E but not vitamin C. Although serum vitamin C levels are also dependent upon haptoglobin type, it appears to be vitamin E that is more protective (Levy et al. 2004). Vitamin E appears to inhibit oxidative modifications of HDL structure and lipid oxidation in persons with the HP 2-2 genotype (Farbstein et al. 2011). In human plaques taken from individuals with the HP 2-2 genotype (vs. HP 1-1/2-1), iron content and expression of oxidized phospholipids have increased (Purushothaman et al. 2012). Based on the prevalence of the HP 1-1 genotype (16%), the HP 2-2 genotype (36%), and the HP 2-1 genotype (48%) in western populations, over a third of individuals with diabetes may benefit from vitamin E treatment (Vardi et al. 2012, Langlois and Delanghe 1996). Although there is evidence that vitamin E supplementation may reduce the risk of cardiovascular death in persons with the HP 2-2 genotype, little is known about the vitamin E status of these individuals.

10.6.5 Urinary and Reproductive Health

According to global statistics, approximately 20%–25% of couples have fertility problems (Menezo et al. 2014). Oxidative stress is recognized as a cause of male infertility because sperm plasma membranes are rich in the polyunsaturated fatty acid, DHA. Benedetti et al. (2012) showed that infertile men had lower sperm (1.48 vs. 1.68 μmol/L) and serum α-tocopherol (17.8 vs. 22.0 μmol/L) concentrations than fertile males. In women with unexplained infertility, vitamin E supplementation (400 IU/day) improved the endometrial response during controlled ovarian stimulation (Cicek et al. 2012). Serum vitamin E status has been suggested as a predictor of pre-eclampsia (Siddiqui et al. 2013). Pre-eclampsia is associated with significantly lower vitamin E levels, yet we still do not understand the effect of vitamin E status on male and female fertility.

10.7 FUTURE DIRECTIONS

Dietary supplementation has shifted from preventing deficiency to promoting wellness and preventing diseases (Bjelakovic and Gluud 2011). As suggested by Zingg et al. (2008), increasingly there is a strong scientific basis to establish guidelines for recommending personalized antioxidant vitamin supplementation (i.e., vitamin E) based on individual polymorphisms. Since 2004, there has been a significant decline in vitamin E research compared to other "nutrients of concern" (Figure 10.1). The field should adopt the nutrient specific physiological recommendations of Heaney (2014) to further define the role of vitamin E in protecting lipid-rich membranes and cells from oxidative damage. It is time to seek consensus on markers of vitamin E status and optimal levels for health (Peter et al. 2013). Studies are needed to assess the vitamin E status in persons representative of the general population.

REFERENCES

Ascherio, A., M. J. Stampfer, G. A. Colditz, E. B. Rimm, L. Litin, and W. C. Willett. 1992. Correlations of vitamin A and E intakes with the plasma concentrations of carotenoids and tocopherols among American men and women. *J Nutr* 122 (9):1792–801.

Asleh, R., S. Blum, S. Kalet-Litman, J. Alshiek, R. Miller-Lotan, R. Asaf, W. Rock, M. Aviram, U. Milman, C. Shapira, et al. 2008. Correction of HDL dysfunction in individuals with diabetes and the haptoglobin 2-2 genotype. *Diabetes* 57 (10):2794–800. doi: 10.2337/db08-0450 db08-0450 [pii].

Asleh, R., J. Guetta, S. Kalet-Litman, R. Miller-Lotan, and A. P. Levy. 2005. Haptoglobin genotype- and diabetes-dependent differences in iron-mediated oxidative stress in vitro and in vivo. *Circ Res* 96 (4):435–41. doi: 01.RES.0000156653.05853.b9 [pii] 10.1161/01.RES.0000156653.05853.b9.

Asleh, R. and A. P. Levy. 2010. Divergent effects of alpha-tocopherol and vitamin C on the generation of dysfunctional HDL associated with diabetes and the Hp 2-2 genotype. *Antioxid Redox Signal* 12 (2):209–17. doi: 10.1089/ars.2009.2829.

Asleh, R., S. Marsh, M. Shilkrut, O. Binah, J. Guetta, F. Lejbkowicz, B. Enav, N. Shehadeh, Y. Kanter, O. Lache, et al. 2003. Genetically determined heterogeneity in hemoglobin scavenging and susceptibility to diabetic cardiovascular disease. *Circ Res* 92 (11):1193–200. doi: 10.1161/01.RES.0000076889.23082.F1 01.RES.0000076889.23082.F1 [pii].

ATBC. 1994. The effect of vitamin E and beta carotene on the incidence of lung cancer and other cancers in male smokers. *New Engl J Med* 330 (15):1029–35. doi:10.1056/NEJM199404143301501.

Belisle, S. E., D. H. Hamer, L. S. Leka, G. E. Dallal, J. Delgado-Lista, B. C. Fine, P. F. Jacques, J. M. Ordovas, and S. N. Meydani. 2010. IL-2 and IL-10 gene polymorphisms are associated with respiratory tract infection and may modulate the effect of vitamin E on lower respiratory tract infections in elderly nursing home residents. *Am J Clin Nutr* 92 (1):106–14. doi: 10.3945/ajcn.2010.29207 ajcn.2010.29207 [pii].

Benedetti, S., M. C. Tagliamonte, S. Catalani, M. Primiterra, F. Canestrari, S. De Stefani, S. Palini, and C. Bulletti. 2012. Differences in blood and semen oxidative status in fertile and infertile men, and their relationship with sperm quality. *Reprod BioMed Online* 25 (3):300–6. doi: http://dx.doi.org/10.1016/j.rbmo.2012.05.011.

Beydoun, M. A., H. A. Beydoun, A. Boueiz, M. R. Shroff, and A. B. Zonderman. 2013. Antioxidant status and its association with elevated depressive symptoms among US adults: National Health and Nutrition Examination Surveys 2005-6. *Br J Nutr* 109 (9):1714–29. doi: 10.1017/S0007114512003467.

Biesalski, H. K., T. Grune, J. Tinz, I. Zollner, and J. B. Blumberg. 2010. Reexamination of a meta-analysis of the effect of antioxidant supplementation on mortality and health in randomized trials. *Nutrients* 2 (9):929–49. doi: 10.3390/nu2090929.

Bjelakovic, G. and C. Gluud. 2011. Vitamin and mineral supplement use in relation to all-cause mortality in the Iowa Women's Health Study. *Arch Intern Med* 171 (18):1633–4. doi: 10.1001/archinternmed.2011.459171/18/1633 [pii].

Blumberg, J. B. and B. Frei. 2007. Why clinical trials of vitamin E and cardiovascular diseases may be fatally flawed. Commentary on The relationship between dose of vitamin E and suppression of oxidative stress in humans. *Free Radic Biol Med* 43 (10):1374–6. doi: S0891-5849(07)00588-6 [pii]10.1016/j.freeradbiomed.2007.08.017.

Borel, P., M. Moussa, E. Reboul, B. Lyan, C. Defoort, S. Vincent-Baudry, M. Maillot, M. Gastaldi, M. Darmon, H. Portugal, et al. 2007. Human plasma levels of vitamin E and carotenoids are associated with genetic polymorphisms in genes involved in lipid metabolism. *J Nutr* 137 (12):2653–9. doi: 137/12/2653 [pii].

Bowman, G. L., L. C. Silbert, D. Howieson, H. H. Dodge, M. G. Traber, B. Frei, J. A. Kaye, J. Shannon, and J. F. Quinn. 2012. Nutrient biomarker patterns, cognitive function, and MRI measures of brain aging. *Neurology* 78 (4):241–9. doi: 10.1212/WNL.0b013e3182436598WNL.0b013e3182436598 [pii].

Bruno, R. S., S. W. Leonard, J. Li, T. M. Bray, and M. G. Traber. 2005. Lower plasma alpha-carboxyethyl-hydroxychroman after deuterium-labeled alpha-tocopherol supplementation suggests decreased vitamin E metabolism in smokers. *Am J Clin Nutr* 81 (5):1052–9. doi: 81/5/1052 [pii].

Christen, W. G., R. J. Glynn, H. D. Sesso, T. Kurth, J. MacFadyen, V. Bubes, J. E. Buring, J. E. Manson, and J. M. Gaziano. 2010. Age-related cataract in a randomized trial of vitamins E and C in men. *Arch Ophthalmol* 128 (11):1397–405. doi: 10.1001/archophthalmol.2010.266128/11/1397 [pii].

Chuang, J. C., H. D. Matel, K. P. Nambiar, S. H. Kim, J. G. Fadel, D. M. Holstege, and A. J. Clifford. 2011. Quantitation of [5-14CH3]-(2R, 4'R, 8'R)-alpha-tocopherol in humans. *J Nutr* 141 (8):1482–8. doi: 10.3945/jn.111.138925jn.111.138925 [pii].

Cicek, N., O. G. Eryilmaz, E. Sarikaya, C. Gulerman, and Y. Genc. 2012. Vitamin E effect on controlled ovarian stimulation of unexplained infertile women. *J Assist Reprod Genet* 29 (4):325–8. doi: 10.1007/s10815-012-9714-1.

Cohn, W. 1997. Bioavailability of vitamin E. *Eur J Clin Nutr* 51 Suppl 1:S80–5.

Cook, N. R., C. M. Albert, J. M. Gaziano, E. Zaharris, J. MacFadyen, E. Danielson, J. E. Buring, and J. E. Manson. 2007. A randomized factorial trial of vitamins C and E and beta carotene in the secondary prevention of cardiovascular events in women: Results from the Women's Antioxidant Cardiovascular Study. *Arch Intern Med* 167 (15):1610–8. doi: 167/15/1610 [pii]10.1001/archinte.167.15.1610.

Costacou, T., R. E. Ferrell, and T. J. Orchard. 2008. Haptoglobin genotype: A determinant of cardiovascular complication risk in type 1 diabetes. *Diabetes* 57 (6):1702–6. doi: 10.2337/db08-0095db08-0095 [pii].

Czernichow, S., A. C. Vergnaud, P. Galan, J. Arnaud, A. Favier, H. Faure, R. Huxley, S. Hercberg, and N. Ahluwalia. 2009. Effects of long-term antioxidant supplementation and association of serum antioxidant concentrations with risk of metabolic syndrome in adults. *Am J Clin Nutr* 90 (2):329–35. doi: 10.3945/ajcn.2009.27635ajcn.2009.27635 [pii].

Del Rio, D., C. Agnoli, N. Pellegrini, V. Krogh, F. Brighenti, T. Mazzeo, G. Masala, B. Bendinelli, F. Berrino, S. Sieri, et al. 2011. Total antioxidant capacity of the diet is associated with lower risk of ischemic stroke in a large Italian cohort. *J Nutr* 141 (1):118–23. doi: 10.3945/jn.110.125120 jn.110.125120 [pii].

Di Donato, I., S. Bianchi, and A. Federico. 2010. Ataxia with vitamin E deficiency: Update of molecular diagnosis. *Neurol Sci* 31 (4):511–5. doi: 10.1007/s10072-010-0261-1.

Dietrich, M., P. F. Jacques, M. J. Pencina, K. Lanier, M. J. Keyes, G. Kaur, P. A. Wolf, R. B. D'Agostino, and R. S. Vasan. 2009. Vitamin E supplement use and the incidence of cardiovascular disease and all-cause mortality in the Framingham Heart Study: Does the underlying health status play a role? *Atherosclerosis* 205 (2):549–53. doi: 10.1016/j.atherosclerosis.2008.12.019 S0021-9150(08)00900-3 [pii].

Dysken, M. W., M. Sano, S. Asthana, J. E. Vertrees, M. Pallaki, M. Llorente, S. Love, G. D. Schellenberg, J. R. McCarten, J. Malphurs, et al. 2014. Effect of vitamin E and memantine on functional decline in Alzheimer disease: The TEAM-AD VA cooperative randomized trial. *JAMA* 311 (1):33–44. doi: 10.1001/jama.2013.282834.

Fairus, S., R. M. Nor, H. M. Cheng, and K. Sundram. 2006. Postprandial metabolic fate of tocotrienol-rich vitamin E differs significantly from that of alpha-tocopherol. *Am J Clin Nutr* 84 (4):835–42.

Farbstein, D., S. Blum, M. Pollak, R. Asaf, H. L. Viener, O. Lache, R. Asleh, R. Miller-Lotan, I. Barkay, M. Star, et al. 2011. Vitamin E therapy results in a reduction in HDL function in individuals with diabetes and the haptoglobin 2-1 genotype. *Atherosclerosis* 219 (1):240–4. doi: 10.1016/j.atherosclerosis.2011.06.005 S0021-9150(11)00482-5 [pii].

Ferrucci, L., J. R. Perry, A. Matteini, M. Perola, T. Tanaka, K. Silander, N. Rice, D. Melzer, A. Murray, C. Cluett, et al. 2009. Common variation in the beta-carotene 15,15'-monooxygenase 1 gene affects circulating levels of carotenoids: A genome-wide association study. *Am J Hum Genet* 84 (2):123–33. doi: 10.1016/j.ajhg.2008.12.019 S0002-9297(09)00010-X [pii].

Ford, E. S., R. L. Schleicher, A. H. Mokdad, U. A. Ajani, and S. Liu. 2006. Distribution of serum tocs in US. *Am J Clin Nutr* 84:375–83.

Fuller, C. J., M. Chandalia, A. Garg, S. M. Grundy, and I. Jialal. 1996. RRR-alpha-tocopheryl acetate supplementation at pharmacologic doses decreases low-density-lipoprotein oxidative susceptibility but not protein glycation in patients with diabetes mellitus. *Am J Clin Nutr* 63 (5):753–9.

Gann, P. H. 2009. Randomized trials of antioxidant supplementation for cancer prevention: First bias, now chance—Next, cause. *JAMA* 301 (1):102–3. doi: 10.1001/jama.2008.863 2008.863 [pii].

Gaziano, J. M., R. J. Glynn, W. G. Christen, T. Kurth, C. Belanger, J. MacFadyen, V. Bubes, J. E. Manson, H. D. Sesso, and J. E. Buring. 2009. Vitamins E and C in the prevention of prostate and total cancer in men: The Physicians' Health Study II randomized controlled trial. *JAMA* 301 (1):52–62. doi: 10.1001/jama.2008.862 2008.862 [pii].

Gaziano, J. M., H. D. Sesso, W. G. Christen, V. Bubes, J. P. Smith, J. Mac Fadyen, M. Schvartz, J. E. Manson, R. J. Glynn, and J. E. Buring. 2012. Multivitamins in the prevention of cancer in men: The Physicians' Health Study II randomized controlled trial. *JAMA* 308 (18):1871–80.

Gey, K. F. and P. Puska. 1989. Plasma vitamins E and A inversely correlated to mortality from ischemic heart disease in cross-cultural epidemiology. *Ann N Y Acad Sci* 570:268–82.

Girona, J., M. Guardiola, A. Cabre, J. M. Manzanares, M. Heras, J. Ribalta, and L. Masana. 2008. The apolipoprotein A5 gene-1131T—>C polymorphism affects vitamin E plasma concentrations in type 2 diabetic patients. *Clin Chem Lab Med* 46 (4):453–7. doi: 10.1515/CCLM.2008.110.

Harrison, S. A., S. Torgerson, P. Hayashi, J. Ward, and S. Schenker. 2003. Vitamin E and vitamin C treatment improves fibrosis in patients with nonalcoholic steatohepatitis. *Am J Gastroenterol* 98 (11):2485 90. doi: 10.1111/j.1572-0241.2003.08699.x.

Heaney, R. P. 2014. Guidelines for optimizing design and analysis of clinical studies of nutrient effects. *Nutr Rev* 72 (1):48–54. doi: 10.1111/nure.12090.

Illison, V. K., P. H. C. Rondó, A. M. de Oliveira, F. H. D'Abronzo, and K. F. Campos. 2011. The relationship between plasma alpha-tocopherol concentration and vitamin E intake in patients with type 2 diabetes mellitus. *Int J Vitam Nutr Res* 81 (1):12–20. doi: 10.1024/0300-9831/a000046.

IOM. 1998. *Dietary Reference Intakes: A Risk Assessment Model for Establishing Upper Intake Levels for Nutrients*. doi: NBK45189 [bookaccession].

IOM. 2000. *Dietary Reference Intakes for Vitamin C, Vitamin E, Selenium, and Carotenoids*.

IOM. 2011. *Dietary Reference Intakes for Calcium and Vitamin D*. doi: NBK56070 [bookaccession].

Kim, Y. N., K. R. Lora, D. W. Giraud, and J. A. Driskell. 2006. Nonsupplemented children of Latino immigrants have low vitamin E intakes and plasma concentrations and normal vitamin C, selenium, and carotenoid intakes and plasma concentrations. *J Am Diet Assoc* 106 (3):385–91. doi: S0002-8223(05)02083-3 [pii] 10.1016/j.jada.2005.12.010.

Langlois, M. R. and J. R. Delanghe. 1996. Biological and clinical significance of haptoglobin polymorphism in humans. *Clin Chem* 42 (10):1589–600.

Larsson, S. C., A. Akesson, L. Bergkvist, and A. Wolk. 2010. Multivitamin use and breast cancer incidence in a prospective cohort of Swedish women. *Am J Clin Nutr* 91 (5):1268–72. doi: 10.3945/ajcn.2009.28837 ajcn.2009.28837 [pii].

Lavine, J. E. 2000. Vitamin E treatment of nonalcoholic steatohepatitis in children: A pilot study. *J Pediatr* 136 (6):734–8.

Lebold, K. M., A. Ang, M. G. Traber, and L. Arab. 2012. Urinary-carboxyethyl hydroxychroman can be used as a predictor of -tocopherol adequacy, as demonstrated in the Energetics Study. *Am J Clin Nutr* 96 (4):801–9. doi: 10.3945/ajcn.112.038620.

Levy, A. P., P. Friedenberg, R. Lotan, P. Ouyang, M. Tripputi, L. Higginson, F. R. Cobb, J. C. Tardif, V. Bittner, and B. V. Howard. 2004. The effect of vitamin therapy on the progression of coronary artery atherosclerosis varies by haptoglobin type in postmenopausal women. *Diabetes Care* 27 (4):925–30.

Levy, A. P., I. Hochberg, K. Jablonski, H. E. Resnick, E. T. Lee, L. Best, and B. V. Howard. 2002. Haptoglobin phenotype is an independent risk factor for cardiovascular disease in individuals with diabetes: The Strong Heart Study. *J Am Coll Cardiol* 40 (11):1984–90. doi: S0735109702025342 [pii].

Lin, J., N. R. Cook, C. Albert, E. Zaharris, J. M. Gaziano, M. Van Denburgh, J. E. Buring, and J. E. Manson. 2009. Vitamins C and E and beta carotene supplementation and cancer risk: A randomized controlled trial. *J Natl Cancer Inst* 101 (1):14–23. doi: 10.1093/jnci/djn438 djn438 [pii].

Lippman, S. M., E. A. Klein, P. J. Goodman, M. S. Lucia, I. M. Thompson, L. G. Ford, H. L. Parnes, L. M. Minasian, J. M. Gaziano, J. A. Hartline, et al. 2009. Effect of selenium and vitamin E on risk of prostate cancer and other cancers: The Selenium and Vitamin E Cancer Prevention Trial (SELECT). *JAMA* 301 (1):39–51. doi: 10.1001/jama.2008.864 2008.864 [pii].

Maes, M., N. De Vos, R. Pioli, P. Demedts, A. Wauters, H. Neels, and A. Christophe. 2000. Lower serum vitamin E concentrations in major depression. Another marker of lowered antioxidant defenses in that illness. *J Affect Disord* 58 (3):241–6.

Major, J. M., K. Yu, W. Wheeler, H. Zhang, M. C. Cornelis, M. E. Wright, M. Yeager, K. Snyder, S. J. Weinstein, A. Mondul, et al. 2011. Genome-wide association study identifies common variants associated with circulating vitamin E levels. *Hum Mol Genet* 20 (19):3876–83. doi: 10.1093/hmg/ddr296 ddr296 [pii].

Mangialasche, F., E. Westman, M. Kivipelto, J. S. Muehlboeck, R. Cecchetti, M. Baglioni, R. Tarducci, G. Gobbi, P. Floridi, H. Soininen, et al. 2013. Classification and prediction of clinical diagnosis of Alzheimer's disease based on MRI and plasma measures of alpha-/gamma-tocotrienols and gamma-tocopherol. *J Intern Med* 273 (6):602–21. doi: 10.1111/joim.12037.

Maserejian, N. N., E. Giovannucci, B. Rosner, and K. Joshipura. 2007. Prospective study of vitamins C, E, and A and carotenoids and risk of oral premalignant lesions in men. *Int J Cancer* 120 (5):970–7. doi: 10.1002/ijc.22448.

Melamed-Frank, M., O. Lache, B. I. Enav, T. Szafranek, N. S. Levy, R. M. Ricklis, and A. P. Levy. 2001. Structure-function analysis of the antioxidant properties of haptoglobin. *Blood* 98 (13):3693–8.

Menezo, Y., D. Evenson, M. Cohen, and B. Dale. 2014. Effect of antioxidants on sperm genetic damage. *Adv Exp Med Biol* 791:173–89. doi: 10.1007/978-1-4614-7783-9_11.

Meyer, K. A., F. P. Sijtsma, J. A. Nettleton, L. M. Steffen, L. Van Horn, J. M. Shikany, M. D. Gross, J. Mursu, M. G. Traber, and D. R. Jacobs, Jr. 2013. Dietary patterns are associated with plasma F(2)-isoprostanes in an observational cohort study of adults. *Free Radic Biol Med* 57:201–9. doi: 10.1016/j.freeradbiomed.2012.08.574 S0891-5849(12)01081-7 [pii].

Miller III, E. R., R. Pastor-Barriuso, D. Dalal, R. A. Riemersma, L. J. Appel, and E. Guallar. 2005. Meta-analysis: High-dosage vitamin e supplementation may increase all-cause mortality. *Ann Intern Med* 142 (1):37–46. doi: 10.7326/0003-4819-142-1-200501040-00110.

Milman, U., S. Blum, C. Shapira, D. Aronson, R. Miller-Lotan, Y. Anbinder, J. Alshiek, L. Bennett, M. Kostenko, M. Landau, et al. 2008. Vitamin E supplementation reduces cardiovascular events in a subgroup of middle-aged individuals with both type 2 diabetes mellitus and the haptoglobin 2-2 genotype: A prospective double-blinded clinical trial. *Arterioscler Thromb Vasc Biol* 28 (2):341–7. doi: ATVBAHA.107.153965 [pii] 10.1161/ATVBAHA.107.153965.

Morrow, J. D., K. E. Hill, R. F. Burk, T. M. Nammour, K. F. Badr, and L. J. Roberts, 2nd. 1990. A series of prostaglandin F2-like compounds are produced in vivo in humans by a non-cyclooxygenase, free radical-catalyzed mechanism. *Proc Natl Acad Sci U S A* 87 (23):9383–7.

Neuhouser, M. L., S. Wassertheil-Smoller, C. Thomson, A. Aragaki, G. L. Anderson, J. E. Manson, R. E. Patterson, T. E. Rohan, L. van Horn, J. M. Shikany, et al. 2009. Multivitamin use and risk of cancer and cardiovascular disease in the Women's Health Initiative cohorts. *Arch Intern Med* 169 (3):294–304. doi: 10.1001/archinternmed.2008.540 169/3/294 [pii].

Niki, E. and M. G. Traber. 2012. A history of vitamin E. *Ann Nutr Metab* 61 (3):207–12. doi: 10.1159/000343106.

Owen, A. J., M. J. Batterham, Y. C. Probst, B. F. Grenyer, and L. C. Tapsell. 2005. Low plasma vitamin E levels in major depression: Diet or disease? *Eur J Clin Nutr* 59 (2):304–6. doi: 10.1038/sj.ejcn.1602072.

Peter, S., U. Moser, S. Pilz, M. Eggersdorfer, and P. Weber. 2013. The challenge of setting appropriate intake recommendations for vitamin E: Considerations of status and functionality to define nutrient requirements. *Int J Vitam Nutr Res* 83 (2):129–136. doi: 10.1024/0300-9831/a000153.

Purushothaman, K. R., M. Purushothaman, A. P. Levy, P. A. Lento, S. Evrard, J. C. Kovacic, K. C. Briley-Saebo, S. Tsimikas, J. L. Witztum, P. Krishnan, et al. 2012. Increased expression of oxidation-specific epitopes and apoptosis are associated with haptoglobin genotype: Possible implications for plaque progression in human atherosclerosis. *J Am Coll Cardiol* 60 (2):112–9. doi: 10.1016/j.jacc.2012.04.011 S0735-1097(12) 01424-6 [pii].

Reboul, E., D. Trompier, M. Moussa, A. Klein, J. F. Landrier, G. Chimini, and P. Borel. 2009. ATP-binding cassette transporter A1 is significantly involved in the intestinal absorption of alpha- and gamma-tocopherol but not in that of retinyl palmitate in mice. *Am J Clin Nutr* 89 (1):177–84. doi: 10.3945/ajcn.2008.26559 ajcn.2008.26559 [pii].

Roberts, J. M., L. Myatt, C. Y. Spong, E. A. Thom, J. C. Hauth, K. J. Leveno, G. D. Pearson, R. J. Wapner, M. W. Varner, J. M. Thorp, Jr., et al. 2010. Vitamins C and E to prevent complications of pregnancy-associated hypertension. *N Engl J Med* 362 (14):1282–91. doi: 10.1056/NEJMoa0908056362/14/1282 [pii].

Roberts, L. J., 2nd, J. A. Oates, M. F. Linton, S. Fazio, B. P. Meador, M. D. Gross, Y. Shyr, and J. D. Morrow. 2007. The relationship between dose of vitamin E and suppression of oxidative stress in humans. *Free Radic Biol Med* 43 (10):1388–93. doi: S0891-5849(07)00455-8 [pii]10.1016/j.freeradbiomed.2007.06.019.

Roguin, A., W. Koch, A. Kastrati, D. Aronson, A. Schomig, and A. P. Levy. 2003. Haptoglobin genotype is predictive of major adverse cardiac events in the 1-year period after percutaneous transluminal coronary angioplasty in individuals with diabetes. *Diabetes Care* 26 (9):2628–31.

Rother, R. P., L. Bell, P. Hillmen, and M. T. Gladwin. 2005. The clinical sequelae of intravascular hemolysis and extracellular plasma hemoglobin: A novel mechanism of human disease. *JAMA* 293 (13):1653–62. doi: 293/13/1653 [pii] 10.1001/jama.293.13.1653.

Sanyal, A. J., N. Chalasani, K. V. Kowdley, A. McCullough, A. M. Diehl, N. M. Bass, B. A. Neuschwander-Tetri, J. E. Lavine, J. Tonascia, A. Unalp, et al. 2010. Pioglitazone, vitamin E, or placebo for nonalcoholic steatohepatitis. *N Engl J Med* 362 (18):1675–85. doi: 10.1056/NEJMoa0907929 NEJMoa0907929 [pii].

Schleicher, R. L., M. R. Sternberg, and C. M. Pfeiffer. 2013. Race-ethnicity is a strong correlate of circulating fat-soluble nutrient concentrations in a representative sample of the U.S. population. *J Nutr* 143 (6):966S–76S. doi: 10.3945/jn.112.172965.

Sesso, H. D., J. M. Gaziano, M. Van Denburgh, C. H. Hennekens, R. J. Glynn, and J. E. Buring. 2002. Comparison of baseline characteristics and mortality experience of participants and nonparticipants in a randomized clinical trial: The Physicians' Health Study. *Control Clin Trials* 23 (6):686–702. doi: S0197245602002350 [pii].

Siddiqui, I. A., A. Jaleel, H. M. Al'Kadri, S. Akram, and W. Tamimi. 2013. Biomarkers of oxidative stress in women with pre-eclampsia. *Biomark Med* 7 (2):229–34. doi: 10.2217/bmm.12.109.

Song, Y., N. R. Cook, C. M. Albert, M. Van Denburgh, and J. E. Manson. 2009. Effects of vitamins C and E and beta-carotene on the risk of type 2 diabetes in women at high risk of cardiovascular disease: A randomized controlled trial. *Am J Clin Nutr* 90 (2):429–37. doi: 10.3945/ajcn.2009.27491 ajcn.2009.27491 [pii].

Steinberg, D. and J. L. Witztum. 2002. Is the oxidative modification hypothesis relevant to human atherosclerosis?: Do the antioxidant trials conducted to date refute the hypothesis? *Circulation* 105 (17):2107–2111. doi: 10.1161/01.cir.0000014762.06201.06.

Stolzenberg-Solomon, R. Z., S. Sheffler-Collins, S. Weinstein, D. H. Garabrant, S. Mannisto, P. Taylor, J. Virtamo, and D. Albanes. 2009. Vitamin E intake, alpha-tocopherol status, and pancreatic cancer in a cohort of male smokers. *Am J Clin Nutr* 89 (2):584–91. doi: 10.3945/ajcn.2008.26423 ajcn.2008.26423 [pii].

Suleiman, M., D. Aronson, R. Asleh, M. R. Kapeliovich, A. Roguin, S. R. Meisel, M. Shochat, A. Sulieman, S. A. Reisner, W. Markiewicz, et al. 2005. Haptoglobin polymorphism predicts 30-day mortality and heart failure in patients with diabetes and acute myocardial infarction. *Diabetes* 54 (9):2802–6. doi: 54/9/2802 [pii].

Sundl, I., M. Guardiola, G. Khoschsorur, R. Sola, J. C. Vallve, G. Godas, L. Masana, M. Maritschnegg, A. Meinitzer, N. Cardinault, et al. 2007. Increased concentrations of circulating vitamin E in carriers of the apolipoprotein A5 gene - 1131T > C variant and associations with plasma lipids and lipid peroxidation. *J Lipid Res* 48 (11):2506–13. doi: M700285-JLR200 [pii] 10.1194/jlr.M700285-JLR200.

Traber, M. G. 2013. Mechanisms for the prevention of vitamin E excess. *J Lipid Res* 54 (9):2295–306. doi: 10.1194/jlr.R032946 jlr.R032946 [pii].

Traber, M. G., B. Frei, and J. S. Beckman. 2008. Vitamin E revisited: Do new data validate benefits for chronic disease prevention? *Curr Opin Lipidol* 19 (1):30–8. doi: 10.1097/MOL.0b013e3282f2dab6 00041433-200802000-00007 [pii].

Traber, M. G., S. W. Leonard, D. L. Traber, L. D. Traber, J. Gallagher, G. Bobe, M. G. Jeschke, C. C. Finnerty, and D. Herndon. 2010. alpha-Tocopherol adipose tissue stores are depleted after burn injury in pediatric patients. *Am J Clin Nutr* 92 (6):1378–84. doi: 10.3945/ajcn.2010.30017 ajcn.2010.30017 [pii].

Traber, M. G. and J. F. Stevens. 2011. Vitamins C and E: Beneficial effects from a mechanistic perspective. *Free Radic Biol Med* 51 (5):1000–13. doi: 10.1016/j.freeradbiomed.2011.05.017 S0891-5849(11)00319-4 [pii].

Valk, E. E. and G. Hornstra. 2000. Relationship between vitamin E requirement and polyunsaturated fatty acid intake in man: A review. *Int J Vitam Nutr Res* 70 (2):31–42.

Vardi, M., S. Blum, and A. P. Levy. 2012. Haptoglobin genotype and cardiovascular outcomes in diabetes mellitus - natural history of the disease and the effect of vitamin E treatment. Meta-analysis of the medical literature. *Eur J Intern Med* 23 (7):628–32. doi: 10.1016/j.ejim.2012.04.009 S0953-6205(12)00096-9 [pii].

Vatassery, G. T., C. K. Angerhofer, and F. J. Peterson. 1984. Vitamin E concentrations in the brains and some selected peripheral tissues of selenium-deficient and vitamin E-deficient mice. *J Neurochem* 42 (2):554–8.

Wang, S. Y., K. Singh, and S. C. Lin. 2013. Glaucoma and vitamins A, C, and E supplement intake and serum levels in a population-based sample of the United States. *Eye* 27 (4):487–94. doi: 10.1038/eye.2013.10.

Weinstein, S. J., M. E. Wright, K. A. Lawson, K. Snyder, S. Mannisto, P. R. Taylor, J. Virtamo, and D. Albanes. 2007. Serum and dietary vitamin E in relation to prostate cancer risk. *Cancer Epidemiol Biomarkers Prev* 16 (6):1253–9. doi: 16/6/1253 [pii] 10.1158/1055-9965.EPI-06-1084.

Winklhofer-Roob, B. M., M. A. van't Hof, and D. H. Shmerling. 1997. Reference values for plasma concentrations of vitamin E and A and carotenoids in a Swiss population from infancy to adulthood, adjusted for seasonal influences. *Clin Chem* 43 (1):146–53.

Wright, M. E., K. A. Lawson, S. J. Weinstein, P. Pietinen, P. R. Taylor, J. Virtamo, and D. Albanes. 2006. Higher baseline serum concentrations of vitamin E are associated with lower total and cause-specific mortality in the Alpha-Tocopherol, Beta-Carotene Cancer Prevention Study. *Am J Clin Nutr* 84 (5):1200–7. doi: 84/5/1200 [pii].

Zingg, J. M., A. Azzi, and M. Meydani. 2008. Genetic polymorphisms as determinants for disease-preventive effects of vitamin E. *Nutr Rev* 66 (7):406–14. doi: 10.1111/j.1753-4887.2008.00050.x NURE050 [pii].

Zureik, M., P. Galan, S. Bertrais, L. Mennen, S. Czernichow, J. Blacher, P. Ducimetière, and S. Hercberg. 2004. Effects of long-term daily low-dose supplementation with antioxidant vitamins and minerals on structure and function of large arteries. *Arterioscler Thromb Vasc Biol* 24 (8):1485–1491. doi: 10.1161/01.ATV.0000136648.62973.c8.

11 Iodine Nutrition Is Required for Thyroid Function and Neurodevelopment

Iodine Supplementation in Pregnancy

Swetha L. Kommareddy and Elizabeth N. Pearce

CONTENTS

11.1 INTRODUCTION

Iodine is a trace element that is essential for thyroid hormone synthesis. Thyroid hormones affect the function of virtually every organ system and are critical for fetal and infant neurodevelopment in utero and in early life. Iodine deficiency disorders (IDD) have multiple adverse effects on growth and development, including endemic goiter, cretinism, intellectual impairments, growth retardation, and neonatal hypothyroidism.[1] Low maternal thyroid hormones due to iodine deficiency can cause irreversible fetal brain damage.[2]

More than 90% of dietary iodine is absorbed by the stomach and duodenum.[3] Depending on whether iodine intake is sufficient, the proportion of iodine taken up by the thyroid ranges from 10%–80% of the absorbed iodine.[3] Active transport of iodide into the thyroid gland is regulated by iodine levels in blood and by thyroid stimulating hormone (TSH) from the pituitary.[5] This active transport of iodide is mediated by sodium iodide symporter (NIS) present on the basolateral surface of thyroid epithelial cells. Iodine that is not actively transported into the thyroid gland is primarily excreted in the urine, and a small percentage is excreted in feces and saliva.[3]

There are two forms of thyroid hormone: Thyroxine (T4) and Triiodothyronine (T3). T4 is the primary hormone produced by the thyroid gland and T3 is the biologically active hormone. Some T3 is produced by the thyroid gland, but most of the T3 is produced in other tissues by deiodination of T4. The majority of circulating thyroid hormone (>99%) is bound to proteins, especially to thyroxine binding globulin (TBG). Therefore, changes in serum TBG levels can lead to changes in measured levels of total thyroid hormones. Only free (unbound) thyroid hormones (fT4 and fT3) are biologically available. TSH produced from anterior pituitary gland regulates thyroid hormone production. There is a regulatory feedback system so that the secretion of TSH is inhibited by fT4 and fT3.

A highly effective strategy for the elimination of IDD in most regions worldwide has been fortification of salt with iodine. It is simple and cost-effective. The annual cost of salt iodization is estimated at only $0.02–$0.05 per person.[4] Approximately 70% of all households worldwide, currently have access to adequately iodized salt.[1] The main sources of dietary iodine in the United States are iodized salt (due to fortification), dairy foods (due to iodine in cattle feeds and iodophor cleansers), and bread dough (due to use of iodate as a dough conditioner).[5]

11.2 ASSESSMENT OF IODINE STATUS IN POPULATIONS

Iodine status assessment is essential for public health planning. There are several accepted methods for monitoring the iodine sufficiency of populations, including use of median urinary iodine concentrations (UICs), total goiter rates (TGR), and serum thyroglobulin levels (Tg).[1,11] Assessment of thyroid size may be used to assess iodine status, either by palpation or by thyroid ultrasound. The World Health Organization (WHO) has described a grading system based on the prevalence of thyroid enlargement by palpation.[11] IDD severity in populations (assessed in school-aged children) is defined as TGR <5%—iodine sufficiency, TGR 5%–19%—mild deficiency, TGR 20%–29%—moderate deficiency, and TGR >30%—severe deficiency.[11] However, use of the goiter rate alone may cause over-estimation of the prevalence of iodine deficiency following iodine fortification of foods, since goiter regression may take a long time, especially in adults and older children, after iodine deficiency is corrected.[6,7] In addition, in areas of mild to moderate iodine deficiency, goiter estimation by palpation alone has poor sensitivity and specificity and thyroid ultrasound is preferable. International standards for age-specific and body surface area-specific thyroid volumes in school-aged children have been described.[8]

As more than 90% of iodine is renally excreted,[9,10] median spot UICs can be used as a measure of recent iodine intake in populations. Population iodine sufficiency is defined by a median UIC of 100–299 μg/L in school-aged children, and 150–249 μg/L in pregnant women.[11] UIC cannot be used to determine the iodine status of individuals, due to substantial day-to-day variation in dietary iodine intake.[12] Due to these variations, it has been shown that in order to estimate individual iodine status, at least ten repeat spot urine collections are needed.[13,14] UICs are most frequently sampled in school-aged children. However, recent studies have demonstrated that median UIC in this group may not be the representative of the iodine status of the whole population, including pregnant women.[15,16]

Dried blood spot thyroglobulin levels can also be used to monitor population iodine status. Thyroglobulin is synthesized only in the thyroid. When iodine intake is sufficient, the serum thyroglobulin level is usually <10 μg/L.[17] However, in iodine deficient areas, higher serum TSH levels stimulate the thyroid gland, causing an increase in thyroid size, and thereby leading to higher serum thyroglobulin levels.[18] A median thyroglobulin value of <13 μg/L and/or <3% of thyroglobulin values >40 μg/L in school-aged children is consistent with iodine sufficiency.[11,71]

11.3 EPIDEMIOLOGY

In 1993, WHO estimated that 110 countries were affected by IDD. The United Nations Children's Fund (UNICEF), the WHO, and Iodine Global Network (formerly the International Council for the control of Iodine Deficiency Disorders, or ICCIDD) have made a concerted effort since then to eliminate IDD worldwide.[19] In 2011, 32 countries remained iodine deficient,[20] of which 9 countries were moderately deficient and 23 were mildly deficient. No country is currently considered severely iodine deficient.[20] Globally, 1.88 billion people have inadequate iodine intake, a decrease of 6.4% compared to 2007.[20] Overall, there has been progress in many regions of the world. However, a decrease in UICs has been noted in the last two decades in several industrialized countries, including the USA, Australia, and the UK.

According to recent National Health and Nutrition Examination Surveys (NHANES), the median UIC for US adults decreased by more than 50% between the early 1970s and the 1990s.[21] The median UIC in the United States is currently 144 μg/L, consistent with iodine sufficiency.[22] However, between the 1970s and the 1990s, the prevalence of low UIC (<50 μg/L) in women of childbearing age increased from 4% to 15%. This is of particular concern since women of childbearing age are most vulnerable to the harmful effects of iodine deficiency. Most recently, in 2005–2010, median UIC in pregnant women consistently dropped below 150 μg/L, indicating that US pregnant women are mildly iodine deficient.[23,22]

11.4 IODINE REQUIREMENT IN PREGNANCY AND LACTATION

Iodine requirements increase in pregnancy for several reasons. Maternal thyroid hormone production increases by approximately 50% in early pregnancy. In early gestation, human chorionic gonadotropin (hCG) stimulates the thyroid gland, as hCG and TSH share a common alpha subunit structure.[24] High levels of estrogen during pregnancy decrease the catabolism of TBG, which leads to increased levels of bound and total thyroid hormones (T4 and T3). This, in turn, leads to an increased requirement for thyroid hormone production in order to maintain free hormone levels.[25] The placenta acts as a site for thyroid hormone metabolism due to the presence of the enzyme type 3 deiodinase.[26] Some iodine crosses the placenta to be used by the fetus. Finally, an increase in maternal glomerular filtration rate (GFR) leads to an increased renal iodine clearance.[27]

Women who maintain adequate iodine intake before conception and during pregnancy, have adequate intrathyroidal iodine stores and are hence able to meet increased iodine requirements during gestation. However, women with inadequate iodine intake may be unable to meet the increased demand. Fetal thyroid function is absent in the first trimester and the fetus is dependent on maternal thyroid hormone which crosses the placenta in small amounts. The fetal thyroid becomes functional at approximately 20 weeks of gestation. Once functional, the fetal thyroid gland is dependent on maternal iodine intake, and maternal iodine deficiency during pregnancy may lead to both maternal and fetal hypothyroidism.[2]

Iodine is concentrated in breast milk due to expression of NIS on lactating breast cells.[28] Iodine in breast milk is the only source of iodine for exclusively breastfed infants. Therefore, adequate iodine intake during lactation is important for both maternal and child health.

The US Institute of Medicine recommends that women ingest 220 μg of iodine daily in pregnancy and 290 μg daily during lactation.[29] The WHO, similarly, recommends 250 μg daily iodine intake during pregnancy and lactation, higher than the 150 μg daily required by non-pregnant adults.[11]

11.5 EFFECTS OF IODINE DEFICIENCY IN PREGNANCY

11.5.1 Severe Iodine Deficiency: Maternal Effects

Severe IDD is associated with poor maternal outcomes including spontaneous abortion, prematurity, and stillbirth.[11] Iodine deficiency can also lead to maternal hypothyroidism and development of goiter. The risk for goiter increases with parity and smoking.[30,31]

11.5.2 Severe Iodine Deficiency: Fetal Effects

Severe iodine deficiency during pregnancy has adverse fetal effects, including low birth weight and decreased head circumference; increased infant mortality; impaired intellectual development; and, in severe cases, cretinism. Cretinism is characterized by severe mental retardation, squint, deaf mutism, and motor spasticity.[3] Iodine deficiency remains the leading cause of preventable mental retardation worldwide. A Chinese metanalysis by Quan et al. showed that children born in iodine-sufficient areas had 12 points higher IQ, on average, than those born in iodine deficient regions.[32] Another metanalysis, by Bleichrodt et al., demonstrated that the average IQ of children from iodine-sufficient areas was 13.5 points higher than that of children from areas of moderate to severe deficiency.[33]

11.5.3 Mild to Moderate Iodine Deficiency: Fetal Effects

Several observational studies have shown that maternal hypothyroxinemia (low fT4) and mild hypothyroidism during pregnancy are associated with adverse effects on child neurocognitive development. In the 1990s, Haddow et al. demonstrated that the IQ scores of 7–9 year old children of women with mild TSH elevations in the second trimester were 7 points lower than those of children born to women who were euthyroid during pregnancy.[34] These children also had delays in motor skills, language, and attention. Pop et al. evaluated 10-month-old infants born to women who had fT4 levels below the 10th percentile in early pregnancy, and showed that these infants had lower psychomotor scores when compared to those born to women with normal fT4 during early pregnancy.[35] In the Generation R study in the Netherlands, Heinrichs et al. reported that lower maternal fT4 was associated with increased risk of expressive language delay.[36] It is important to note that all these studies were done in iodine-sufficient regions.

More recently, studies have specifically examined the effects of mild to moderate iodine deficiency during pregnancy on child development. A study in the UK demonstrated that mild to moderate maternal iodine deficiency in early pregnancy was associated with increased risk of suboptimal verbal IQ scores in children at eight years of age. These children also had decreased reading and comprehension scores at age nine.[37] In a study conducted in Tasmania, children whose mothers had iodine deficiency during pregnancy showed decreased performance in spelling, grammar, and general English literacy on standardized testing, when compared to children born to iodine-sufficient mothers.[38] In a study done in the Netherlands in 2012, Van Mil et al. showed that low urinary iodine during pregnancy is associated with impaired executive functioning in children.[39] The prevalence of attention deficit and hyperactivity disorders (ADHD) is higher in children born to women living in iodine deficient areas than those in iodine-replete areas.[40]

11.6 EFFECTS OF IODINE EXCESS IN PREGNANCY

Most individuals tolerate high iodine doses well. When there is an excess iodine load, the acute Wolff-Chaikoff effect, a homeostatic mechanism, normally leads to transient inhibition of thyroid hormone synthesis.[41] The mechanism responsible is thought to be the formation of intrathyroidal iodolactones, which lead to inhibition of thyroid peroxidase activity.[42] With continued exposure, the thyroid "escapes" from the acute Wolff-Chaikoff effect by downregulating the NIS and decreasing the active transport of iodine into the thyroid.[43] In susceptible individuals, there may be a failure of either the acute Wolff-Chaikoff effect or the escape, resulting in thyroid dysfunction. The fetal thyroid gland cannot fully escape from the acute Wolff-Chaikoff effect until approximately 36 weeks of gestation.[44] Therefore, iodine excess during pregnancy can selectively cause fetal hypothyroidism, even when the mother remains euthyroid.[45] The Institute of Medicine recommends an upper limit of 1100 μg of dietary iodine daily in pregnancy and lactation, while the WHO, more conservatively, recommends a threshold of 500 μg/day.[29,11]

11.7 SAFETY AND EFFICACY OF IODINE SUPPLEMENTATION DURING PREGNANCY

11.7.1 Effects on Maternal Thyroid Function

Several clinical trials of iodine supplementation for mildly to moderately iodine deficient pregnant women have been conducted in Europe. Pederson et al. treated 28 mildly iodine deficient Danish women with 200 μg daily iodine starting at 17–18 weeks gestation. When compared to controls, the treated group had lower TSH, T4, Tg levels, and thyroid volumes.[46] Similarly, in a Belgian study by Glinoer et al., women were randomized to potassium iodide (KI) 100 μg/day, KI with 100 μg of levothyroxine per day, or placebo starting at 14 weeks gestation. Women in the placebo group had higher serum TSH at the time of delivery when compared to those in KI group. Serum Tg was higher in the controls and they had greater thyroid volumes.[47]

Nohr et al. randomized 49 women to 150 μg/day of iodine in a multivitamin vs. no supplements starting in the first trimester. Maternal TSH and Tg were lower in the supplemented group.[48] Romano et al. randomized 35 pregnant women to two groups: 17 women received 120–180 μg/day of iodine in the form of iodized salt starting in the first trimester and 18 women served as controls. No differences in serum TSH were noted between the groups. Thyroid volumes were greater in the control group.[49] In Germany, Leisenkotter et al. treated women with 300 μg of KI starting at 10–12 weeks gestation. When compared to untreated controls, no differences in serum TSH, T4, Tg, or thyroid volume were noted.[50]

In an Italian study by Antonangeli et al., 86 women were randomized to receive either 50 or 200 μg iodide daily starting at 10–16 weeks of gestation. No differences in serum TSH, T4, Tg, or thyroid volume were noted between the groups.[51] Most recently, in Spain, Santiago et al. randomized 131 pregnant women to three groups: iodine fortification of cooking salt; 200 μg of KI daily; or 300 μg of KI daily, all starting in the first trimester. No differences were found in TSH, free T4, free T3, or thyroid volume between the three groups,[52] suggesting that all forms of iodine intake were equally effective.

In an observational study by Moleti et al., consumption of iodized salt for 2 years preconception (long-term) was associated with lower TSH and lower rates of maternal hypothyroidism when compared to women who started iodine supplementation during pregnancy (short-term), indicating that long-term iodine supplementation might be more beneficial.[53] Rebagliato et al. reported higher serum TSH levels in women who took >200 μg iodine daily when compared to those who took <200 μg/day.[54]

All these studies were done in women living in areas of mild to moderate iodine deficiency. Overall, they demonstrated that women with adequate iodine intake in the form of supplementation/fortification during pregnancy and preconception have smaller thyroid volumes and, in most studies, have lower serum TSH than women who were not treated. No adverse effects were noted in supplemented women, except in the study by Rebagliato et al. which reported higher TSH in women who took more than 200 μg of iodine. Long-term iodine supplementation before pregnancy appears to be more effective than initiation during pregnancy or late in gestation.

11.7.2 Neonatal Effects of Iodine Supplementation during Pregnancy: Neonatal Thyroid Function

To date, four randomized trials have examined the effect of iodine supplementation on neonatal thyroid function.[46,47,50,52] No differences in TSH were noted in supplemented versus control groups. Thyroid volume was higher in offspring of mothers who were not supplemented in two of the studies,[47,50] but no difference in neonatal thyroid volumes was noted in another study.[52]

11.7.3 Fetal Neurodevelopment

11.7.3.1 Severe Iodine Deficiency

The evidence supporting iodine supplementation for severely iodine deficient pregnant women is clear. In a landmark study in Papua New Guinea by Pharoah et al., preconception supplementation with iodized oil caused a significant reduction in the prevalence of cretinism at 4 and 10 years follow-up.[55] In a study in Zaire, children of pregnant women treated with iodized oil at 28 weeks of pregnancy showed higher psychomotor development scores at 72 months of age when compared to children of untreated mothers.[56] Similar results have subsequently been noted in other studies conducted in areas of severe iodine deficiency.[57]

Iodine supplementation in severely iodine deficient regions also has positive effects on birth weight, head circumference, and infant mortality rates. Iodine supplementation of pregnant women in each trimester of pregnancy and children from birth to 3 years of age, in a severely iodine deficient region in China reduced the prevalence of microcephaly to 11% compared to 27% in untreated children.[58] The prevalence of neurological abnormalities was lower in children born to mothers supplemented in early pregnancy.[58] In an Asian study, use of iodized salt was associated with increased birth weights.[59] In a study conducted in China by Delong et al., the addition of potassium iodate to drinking water resulted in a reduction in infant mortality.[60]

11.7.3.2 Mild to Moderate Iodine Insufficiency

Limited evidence suggests that iodine supplementation for women with mild to moderate iodine deficiency improves neurological development of the offspring. In an uncontrolled prospective study by Velasco et al., pregnant women were supplemented with 300 μg of iodine daily during the first trimester. Children of iodine-supplemented women had higher psychomotor scores at 3 to 18 months than those of women who did not receive any iodine supplements during pregnancy.[61] A study by Berbel et al. showed that neurocognitive scores at 18 months of age were higher in children of women who started 200 μg daily iodine supplementation at 4–6 weeks of gestation when compared to those who started supplementation only at week 12–14 or at delivery. This suggests that timing of iodine supplementation is critical.[62] However, in a study by Murcia et al. iodine supplementation of ≥150 μg/day was associated with lower psychomotor development scores (PDI) in infants when compared to infants of mothers who took <100 μg/day.[63] In a study by Santiago et al.[52] no differences in neurocognitive function were seen between infants of women who were randomized to receive either iodized salt or KI (200 or 300 μg daily).

Current data suggests that iodine supplementation for mildly to moderately iodine deficient females during pregnancy may be beneficial for child development. However, definitive high-quality studies have not been performed to date. It is unclear why results from the study by Murcia et al. are discrepant with those of other studies. Randomized, placebo-controlled trials of iodine supplementation in early pregnancy in regions of mild to moderate iodine deficiency are needed. Such trials are currently underway in India and Thailand.[64]

11.8 CURRENT RECOMMENDATIONS FOR IODINE SUPPLEMENTATION IN PREGNANCY

In a 2007 consensus statement, the WHO recommended that in countries or regions where the proportion of households consuming iodized salt is <90%, pregnant and lactating women should take iodine supplements in order to ensure daily iodine intake of 250 μg per day.[65] This can be done in the form of daily iodine supplement or, in resource-poor regions where daily supplementation is not feasible. An annual oral dose of 400 mg of iodized oil supplement can be used.[65] Due to concerns that pregnant women in the United States are mildly iodine deficient, the American Thyroid Association (ATA) and Endocrine Society have recommended 150 μg/day of iodine supplementation for the US women who are in the preconception period or pregnant or breastfeeding.[66,67] This recommendation is also supported by the Society of Neurobehavioral Teratology and the American Academy of Pediatrics.[68,72]

11.9 ADOPTION OF RECOMMENDATIONS

According to NHANES data from 2001 to 2006, only 20% of pregnant US women reported taking iodine containing supplements.[69] In part, this may be due to a lack of availability. In 2009, of the 223 different prenatal vitamin types marketed in the United States (both prescription and non-prescription), only 114 (51%) contained iodine. Those with kelp as the iodine source had more variable iodine content than those which contained potassium iodide.[70] Therefore, the ATA and Endocrine Society recommend oral iodine supplements delivered in the form of potassium iodide.

11.10 CONCLUSIONS

Pregnant and lactating women have increased iodine requirements. Iodine deficiency can lead to adverse effects on maternal and fetal thyroid function. Iodine deficiency has significant and irreversible effects on neurological development of the fetus.

Iodine supplementation of severely iodine deficient women clearly improves obstetric and developmental outcomes. Large-scale, prospective, randomized studies are needed to further evaluate the effects of iodine supplementation in early pregnancy on the neurological development of the fetus in areas of mild to moderate iodine deficiency. However, in light of present data, it is recommended that all US women who are in the preconception period or pregnant or lactating should take 150 μg/day iodine supplements. Recommended strategies for ensuring adequate iodine nutrition vary elsewhere around the world, depending on the availability of supplements and dietary iodine intake in pregnancy.

REFERENCES

1. Zimmermann, M.B. 2009. Iodine deficiency. *Endocr Rev* 30:376–408.
2. de Escobar, G.M., Obregon, M.J., del Rey, F.E. 2007. Iodine deficiency and brain development in the first half of pregnancy. *Public Health Nutr* 10:1554–70.
3. Zimmermann, M.B., Jooste, P.L., Pandav, C.S. 2008. Iodine-deficiency disorders. *Lancet* 372:1251–62.
4. Caulfield, L.E., Richard, S.A., Rivera, J.A., Musgrove, P., Black, R.E. 2006. Stunting, wasting, and micronutrient deficiency disorders. In: *Disease Control Priorities in Developing Countries*, Eds. D.T. Jamison, J.G. Breman, A.R. Measham et al., Chapter 28, 2nd edition. Washington (DC): World Bank.
5. Pearce, E.N., Pino, S., He, X., Bazrafshan, H.R., Lee, S.L., Braverman, L.E. et al. 2004. Sources of dietary iodine: Bread, cows' milk, and infant formula in the Boston area. *J Clin Endocrinol Metab* 89:3421–4.
6. Aghini-Lombardi, F., Antonangeli, L., Pinchera, A. et al. 1997. Effect of iodized salt on thyroid volume of children living in an area previously characterized by moderate iodine deficiency. *J Clin Endocrinol Metab* 82:1136–39.
7. Zimmermann, M.B., Hess, S.Y., Adou, P. et al. 2003. Thyroid size and goiter prevalence after introduction of iodized salt: A 5-y prospective study in schoolchildren in Cote d'Ivoire. *Am J Clin Nutr* 77:663–67.
8. Zimmermann, M.B., Hess, S.Y., Molinari, L. et al. 2004. New reference values for thyroid volume by ultrasound in iodine-sufficient schoolchildren: A World Health Organization/Nutrition for Health and Development Iodine Deficiency Study Group Report. *Am J Clin Nutr* 79:231–7.
9. Nath, S.K., Moinier, B., Thuillier, F., Rongier, M., Desjeux, J.F. 1992. Urinary excretion of iodide and fluoride from supplemented food grade salt. *Int J Vitam Nutr Res* 62:66–72.
10. Jahreis, G., Hausmann, W., Kiessling, G., Franke, K., Leiterer, M. 2001. Bioavailability of iodine from normal diets rich in dairy products–results of balance studies in women. *Exp Clin Endocrinol Diabetes* 109:163–7.
11. World Health Organization. 2007. Assessment of Iodine Deficiency Disorders and Monitoring their Elimination. 3rd edition. Geneva, Switzerland.
12. Rasmussen, L.B., Ovesen, L., Christiansen, E. 1999. Day-to-day and within-day variation in urinary iodine excretion. *Eur J Clin Nutr* 53:401–7.
13. König, F., Andersson, M., Hotz, K., Aeberli, I., Zimmermann, M.B. 2011. Ten repeat collections for urinary iodine from spot samples or 24-hour samples are needed to reliably estimate individual iodine status in women. *J Nutr* 141:2049–54.
14. Andersen, S., Karmisholt, J., Pedersen, K.M., Laurberg, P. 2008. Reliability of studies of iodine intake and recommendations for number of samples in groups and in individuals. *Br J Nutr* 99:813–8.

15. Wong, E.M., Sullivan, K.M., Perrine, C.G., Rogers, L.M., Peña-Rosas, J.P. 2011. Comparison of median urinary iodine concentration as an indicator of iodine status among pregnant women, school-age children, and nonpregnant women. *Food Nutr Bull* 32:206–12.
16. Gowachirapant, S., Winichagoon, P., Wyss, L. et al. 2009. Urinary iodine concentrations indicate iodine deficiency in pregnant Thai women but iodine sufficiency in their school-aged children. *J Nutr* 139:1169–72.
17. Spencer, C.A., Wang, C.C.1995. Thyroglobulin measurement. Techniques, clinical benefits, and pitfalls. *Endocrinol Metab Clin North Am* 24:841–63.
18. Knudsen, N., Bulow, I., Jorgensen, T., Perrild, H., Ovesen, L., Laurberg, P. 2001. Serum Tg – a sensitive marker of thyroid abnormalities and iodine deficiency in epidemiological studies. *J Clin Endocrinol Metab* 86:3599–603.
19. World Health Organization, United Nations Children's Fund, International Council for Control of Iodine Deficiency Disorders. 1993. Global prevalence of iodine deficiency disorders. Micronutrient Deficiency Information System working paper 1.
20. Andersson, M., Karumbunathan, V., Zimmermann, M.B. 2012. Global iodine status in 2011 and trends over the past decade. *J Nutr* 142:744–50.
21. Hollowell, J.G., Staehling, N.W., Hannon, W.H. et al. 1998. Iodine nutrition in the United States. Trends and public health implications: Iodine excretion data from National Health and Nutrition Examination Surveys I and III (1971–1974 and 1988–1994). *J Clin Endocrinol Metab* 83:3401–08.
22. Caldwell, K.L., Pan, Y., Mortinsen, M.E., Makhmudov, A., Merrill, L., Moye, J. 2013. Iodine status in pregnant women in the National Children's Study and in U.S. women (15–44 years), NHANES 2005–2010. *Thyroid* 23:927–37.
23. Sullivan, K.M., Perrine, C., Pearce, E.N., Caldwell, K.L. 2013. Monitoring the iodine status of pregnant women in the United States. *Thyroid* 23:520–21.
24. Hershman, J.M. 2004. Physiological and pathological aspects of the effect of human chorionic gonadotropin on the thyroid. *Best Pract Res Clin Endocrinol Metab* 18:249–65.
25. Glinoer, D. 2001. Pregnancy and iodine. *Thyroid* 11:471–81.
26. Roti, E., Fang, S.L., Emerson, C.H., Braverman, L.E. 1981. Placental inner ring iodothyronine deiodination: A mechanism for decreased passage of T4 and T3 from mother to fetus. *Trans Assoc Am Physicians* 94:183–89.
27. Dafnis, E., Sabatini, S. 1992. The effect of pregnancy on renal function: Physiology and pathophysiology. *Am J Med Sci* 303:184–205.
28. Pearce, E.N., Leung, A.M., Blount, B.C. et al. 2007. Breast milk iodine and perchlorate concentrations in lactating Boston-area women. *J Clin Endocrinol Metab* 92:1673–77.
29. Institute of Medicine. 2001. Dietary reference in takes for vitamin a, vitamin k, arsenic, boron, chromium, copper, iodine, iron, manganese, molybdenum, nickel, silicon, vanadium, and zinc. National Academy Press.
30. Rotondi, M., Amato, G., Biondi, B. et al. 2000. Parity as a thyroid size-determining factor in areas with moderate iodine deficiency. *J Clin Endocrinol Metab* 85:4534–7.
31. Knudsen, N., Bülow, I., Laurberg, P., Ovesen, L., Perrild, H., Jørgensen, T. 2002. Parity is associated with increased thyroid volume solely among smokers in an area with moderate to mild iodine deficiency. *Eur J Endocrinol* 146:39–43.
32. Qian, M., Wang, D., Watkins, W.E. 2005. The effects of iodine on intelligence in children: A meta-analysis of studies conducted in China. *Asia Pac J Clin Nutr* 14:32–42.
33. Bleichrodt, N., Born, M.P. 1994. A metaanalysis of research on iodine and its relationship to cognitive development. In: *The Damaged Brain of Iodine Deficiency*, Ed. J.B. Stanbury, 195–200. New York: Cognizant Communication Corporation.
34. Haddow, J.E., Palomaki, G.E., Allan, W.C. et al. 1999. Maternal thyroid deficiency during pregnancy and subsequent neuropsychological development of the child. *N Engl J Med* 341:549–55.

35. Pop, V.J., Kuijpens, J.L., van Baar, A.L. et al. 1999. Low maternal free thyroxine concentrations during early pregnancy are associated with impaired psychomotor development in infancy *Clin Endocrinol (Oxf)* 50:149–55.
36. Henrichs, J., Bongers-Schokking, J.J., Schenk, J.J. et al. 2010. Maternal thyroid function during early pregnancy and cognitive functioning in early childhood: The generation R study. *J Clin Endocrinol Metab* 95:4227–34.
37. Bath, S.C., Steer, C.D., Golding, J., Emmett, P., Rayman, M.P. 2013. Effect of inadequate iodine status in UK pregnant women on cognitive outcomes in their children: Results from the Avon Longitudinal Study of Parents and Children (ALSPAC) *Lancet* 382:331–7.
38. Hynes, K.L., Otahal, P., Hay, I., Burgess, J.R. 2013. Mild iodine deficiency during pregnancy is associated with reduced educational outcomes in the offspring: 9-year follow-up of the gestational iodine cohort. *J Clin Endocrinol Metab* 98:1954–62.
39. Van Mil, N.H., Tiemeier, H., Bongers-Schokking, J.J. et al. 2012. Low urinary iodine excretion during early pregnancy is associated with alterations in executive functioning in children. *J Nutr* 142:2167–74.
40. Vermiglio, F., Lo Presti, V.P., Moleti, M. et al. 2004. Attention deficit and hyperactivity disorders in the offspring of mothers exposed to mild-moderate iodine deficiency: A possible novel iodine deficiency disorder in developed countries. *J Clin Endocrinol Metab* 89:6054–60.
41. Wolf, J., Chaikoff, I.L. 1949. The temporary nature of the inhibitory action of excess iodine on organic iodine synthesis in the normal thyroid. *Endocrinology* 45:504–13.
42. Markou, K., Georgopoulos, N., Kyriazopoulou, V., Vagenakis, A.G. 2001. Iodine-induced hypothyroidism. *Thyroid* 11:501–10.
43. Braverman, L.E., Ingvar, S.H. 1963. Changes in thyroidal function during adaptation to large doses of iodide. *J Clin Invest* 42:1216–31.
44. Bartalena, L., Bogazzi, F., Braverman, L.E., Martino, E. 2001. Effects of amiodarone administration during pregnancy on neonatal thyroid function and subsequent neurodevelopment. *J Endocrinol Invest* 24:116–30.
45. Connelly, K.J., Boston, B.A., Pearce, E.N. et al. 2012. Congenital hypothyroidism caused by excess prenatal maternal iodine ingestion. *J Pediatr* 161:760–2.
46. Pedersen, K.M., Laurberg, P., Iversen, E. 1993. Amelioration of some pregnancy-associated variations in thyroid function by iodine supplementation. *J Clin Endocrinol Metab* 77:1078–83.
47. Glinoer, D., De Nayer, P., Delange et al. 1995. A randomized trial for the treatment of mild iodine deficiency during pregnancy: Maternal and neonatal effects. *J Clin Endocrinol Metab* 80:258–69.
48. Nøhr, S.B., Laurberg, P. 2000. Opposite variations in maternal and neonatal thyroid function induced by iodine supplementation during pregnancy. *J Clin Endocrinol Metab* 85:623–7.
49. Romano, R., Jannini, E.A., Pepe, M. et al. 1991. The effects of iodoprophylaxis on thyroid size during pregnancy. *Am J Obstet Gynecol* 164:482–485.
50. Liesenkötter, K.P., Göpel, W., Bogner, U., Stach, B., Grüters, A. 1996. Earliest prevention of endemic goiter by iodine supplementation during pregnancy. *Eur J Endocrinol* 134:443–448.
51. Antonangeli, L., Maccherini, D., Cavaliere, R. et al. 2002. Comparison of two different doses of iodide in the prevention of gestational goiter in marginal iodine deficiency: A longitudinal study. *Eur J Endocrinol* 147:29–34.
52. Santiago, P., Velasco, I., Muela, J.A. 2013. Infant neurocognitive development is independent of the use of iodised salt or iodine supplements given during pregnancy. *Br J Nutr* 110:831–9.
53. Moleti, M., Lo Presti, V.P., Campolo, M.C. et al. 2008. Iodine prophylaxis using iodized salt and risk of maternal thyroid failure in conditions of mild iodine deficiency. *J Clin Endocrinol Metab* 93:2616–21.

54. Rebagliato, M., Murcia, M., Espada, M. et al. 2010. Iodine intake and maternal thyroid function during pregnancy. *Epidemiology* 21:62–9
55. Pharoah, P.O., Connolly, K.J. 1987. A controlled trial of iodinated oil for the prevention of endemic cretinism: A long-term follow-up. *Int J Epidemiol* 16:68–73.
56. Thilly, C.H., Delange, F., Lagasse, R. et al. 1978. Fetal hypothyroidism and maternal thyroid status in severe endemic goiter. *J Clin Endocrinol Metab* 47:354–60.
57. Zimmermann, M.B. 2012. The effects of iodine deficiency in pregnancy and infancy. *Paediatr Perinat Epidemiol* 26 Suppl 1:108–17.
58. Cao, X.Y., Jiang, X.M., Dou, Z.H. 1994. Timing of vulnerability of the brain to iodine deficiency in endemic cretinism. *N Engl J Med* 331:1739–44.
59. Mason, J.B., Deitchler, M., Gilman, A. et al. 2002. Iodine fortification is related to increased weight-for-age and birthweight in children in Asia. *Food Nutr Bull* 23:292–308.
60. DeLong, G.R., Leslie, P.W., Wang, S.H. et al. 1997. Effect on infant mortality of iodination of irrigation water in a severely iodine-deficient area of China. *Lancet* 350:771–3.
61. Velasco, I., Carreira, M., Santiago, P. et al. 2009. Effect of iodine prophylaxis during pregnancy on neurocognitive development of children during the first two years of life. *J Clin Endocrinol Metab* 94:3234–41.
62. Berbel, P., Mestre, J.L., Santamaria, A. et al. 2009. Delayed neurobehavioral development in children born to pregnant women with mild hypothyroxinemia during the first month of gestation: The importance of early iodine supplementation. *Thyroid* 19:511–9.
63. Murcia, M., Rebagliato, M., Iniguez, C. et al. 2011. Effect of iodine supplementation during pregnancy on infant neurodevelopment at 1 year of age. *Am J Epidemiol* 173:804–12.
64. Melse-Boonstra, A., Gowachirapant, S., Jaiswal, N., Winichagoon, P., Srinivasan, K., Zimmermann, M.B. 2012. Iodine supplementation in pregnancy and its effect on child cognition. *J Trace Elem Med Biol* 26:134–6.
65. Andersson, M., de Benoist, B., Delange, F., Zupan, J. 2007. Prevention and control of iodine deficiency in pregnant and lactating women and in children less than 2-years-old: Conclusions and recommendations of the Technical Consultation. *Public Health Nutr* 10:1606–11.
66. Stagnaro-Green, A., Abalovich, M., Alexander, E. 2011. Guidelines of the American Thyroid Association for the diagnosis and management of thyroid disease during pregnancy and postpartum, American Thyroid Association Taskforce on Thyroid Disease During Pregnancy and Postpartum. *Thyroid* 21:1081–125.
67. De Groot, L., Abalovich, M., Alexander, E.K. et al. 2012. Management of thyroid dysfunction during pregnancy and postpartum: An Endocrine Society clinical practice guideline. *J Clin Endocrinol Metab* 97:2543–65.
68. Obican, S.G., Jahnke, G.D., Soldin, O.P., Scialli, A.R. 2012. Teratology public affairs committee position paper: Iodine deficiency in pregnancy. *Birth Defects Res A Clin Mol Teratol* 94:677–682.
69. Gregory, C.O., Serdula, M.K., Sullivan, K.M. 2009. Use of supplements with and without iodine in women of childbearing age in the United States. *Thyroid* 19:1019–20.
70. Leung, A.M., Pearce, E.N., Braverman, L.E. 2009. Iodine content of prenatal multivitamins in the United States. *N Engl J Med* 360:939–40.
71. Zimmermann, M.B., Aeberli, I., Andersson, M. et al. 2013. Thyroglobulin is a sensitive measure of both deficient and excess iodine intakes in children and indicates no adverse effects on thyroid function in the UIC range of 100–299 μg/L: A UNICEF/ICCIDD study group report. *J Clin Endocrinol Metab* 98:1271–80.
72. Council on Environmental Health, Rogan, W.J., Paulson, J.A. et al. 2014. Iodine deficiency, pollutant chemicals, and the thyroid: New information on an old problem. *Pediatrics* 133:1163–6.

12 Possible Benefits of Lutein and Zeaxanthin for Visual Symptoms of Mild Traumatic Brain Injury

Emily R. Bovier and Billy R. Hammond, Jr.

CONTENTS

12.1 OVERVIEW

Most of the reported cases of traumatic brain injury (TBI) in the United States are classified as a concussion or a mild traumatic brain injury (MTBI). This approximation (75% of the annual 1.7 million cases; Faul et al., 2010) is likely underestimated since epidemiological reports do not include cases assessed outside of hospital settings, such as data from the military, or incidents that go untreated. MTBI is becoming a major public health problem, not only with respect to the general population, but also for specific groups of individuals such as athletes and military personnel. The growing concern regarding consequences of MTBI is evident in the recent media attention given to athletes and soldiers suffering from deficits associated with concussive events. According to U.S. Military Casualty Statistics from the 2010 Congressional Research Service Report for Congress, the incidence of MTBI between 2000 and 2010 was 137,328 cases (out of 178,876 total TBI cases).

Typically, when the quality of life of patients with TBI is considered, attention is given to patients with more severe forms of TBI or to secondary symptoms related to depression and anxiety. Although MTBI is less severe than the other forms of brain injury (i.e., cases that result in extensive structural damage or coma), the outcome of MTBI may still have a lasting impact, since patients are likely to experience permanent secondary deficits, for example, visual disturbances, such as increased sensitivity to light, are common and long lasting side effects of MTBI. Furthermore, individuals with a history of MTBI may experience visual symptoms despite preserved ocular health and normal CT scans.

Lasting problems with visual function are an example of "late symptoms" (Ryan and Warden, 2003) since they often occur days or even weeks after the injury. Late-symptom clusters are referred to as post-concussion syndrome (PCS) if symptomatology persists for longer than a few months. A specific set of criteria for "post-concussional syndrome (PCS)" is outlined in The ICD-10 Classification of Mental and Behavioural Disorders (World Health Organization, 1992), and the Diagnostic and Statistical Manual of Mental Disorders (DSM-IV-TR; American Psychiatric Association, 2000) has criteria for "post-concussional disorder (PCD)."

Consistent with classification systems for behavioral disorders, a diagnosis of PCS/PCD is based on the presence of a combination of symptoms from a larger checklist. For example, the DSM-IV-TR lists eight symptoms, and a diagnosis of PCD requires the presence of at least three symptoms for three months. The symptoms include the following: becoming easily fatigued, disordered sleep, headache, vertigo or dizziness, irritability or aggression with little or no provocation, anxiety, depression, or affective lability, changes in personality (e.g., social or sexual inappropriateness), and apathy or lack of spontaneity (adapted from DSM-IV-TR; American Psychiatric Association, 2000). The symptom list for the ICD-10 is quite similar, although it includes additional symptoms related to memory and concentration. Despite overlapping symptoms, these two classification systems can result in differential diagnoses. Indeed, Boake et al. (2005) demonstrated a higher prevalence of PCS when using the ICD-10 checklist compared to the DSM-IV checklist. In general, assessment of injury severity and monitoring of symptomatology following MTBI includes a major focus on cognitive domains such as concentration and memory, whereas sensory components tend to lack specificity. However, sensory dysfunction, particularly visual disturbances, can be detrimental to daily functioning and may also contribute to other subjective complaints, such as headaches and vertigo.

Often the subjective experiences of visual disruption after an MTBI take the form of changes in visual function. The mechanisms related to disruptions in visual processing after brain injury are not well understood (e.g., Stern, 2011). Manifestations of the disturbance could vary from a subjective intolerance to bright light, reduced visibility in dim lighting, difficulty reading, etc. Disruptions to visual function have been reported in light-sensitive patients, such as changes in adaptation (e.g., photopic and scotoptic thresholds; Zihl and Kerkhoff, 1990) and changes in temporal vision (e.g., critical flicker fusion (CFF) thresholds; Chang et al., 2007). Early detection of impairments in visual function can be paired with rehabilitative methods to alleviate symptoms and improve quality of life. The use of tinted lenses, for example, is one palliative approach to alleviating light sensitivity (e.g., Jackowski et al., 1996). Perhaps one of the more promising approaches with respect to visual disturbances, however, and the subject of this review, is treatment, simultaneously preventive and palliative, using specific components of the diet. The plant pigments known as carotenoids have been the most studied, specifically the xanthophylls lutein and zeaxanthin.

Dietary lutein and zeaxanthin may be particularly beneficial for visual symptoms associated with MTBI since they are concentrated in very high proportions in the retina (1000 times the levels in the serum) and throughout the rest of the central nervous system. There is a striking parallel between some of the known functions of lutein and zeaxanthin and deficits associated with MTBI. Patients with MTBI experience visual discomfort and disability, such as sensitivity to bright light and visual disability in glare. Temporal vision may be impaired after MTBI (e.g., disruptions to flicker sensitivity and processing speed). Higher levels of lutein and zeaxanthin in the retina have been associated with reduced photophobia, reduced glare disability, and improvements in temporal processing speed.

Lutein and zeaxanthin are known to function as optical filters, enhancers of cellular communication, and protective antioxidants and anti-inflammatories. When deposited in the retina, lutein and zeaxanthin filter short-wave light that contributes to visual discomfort and disability. Throughout the cortex, lutein and zeaxanthin may mediate neural efficiency, for example, by enhancing gap junction communication. Patients with MTBI may have slowed processing and disruptions in attention that may be accounted for by deficits in neural communication. The protective effects of lutein and zeaxanthin are the result of the nutrient's ability to reduce oxidative stress and inflammation. Individuals with a history of brain injury are likely to have elevated levels of oxidative stress and be particularly vulnerable to subsequent injury.

To summarize, MTBI is a public health concern due to the increasing incidence, financial costs, and negative impact on the patients' quality of life. One likely innocuous strategy for enhancing resilience and reducing the sequelae of symptoms following injury would be to increase central levels of protective agents like lutein and zeaxanthin. This review summarizes the existing evidence for this approach. Although the focus is on lutein and the zeaxanthins, this can be considered a specific example of a general principle: The nervous system is composed and maintained by elements of the diet, an optimal diet will lead to maximal hardiness and resistance to injuries that were likely common throughout our evolutionary past (like MTBI). Indeed, humans, similar to other animals, likely evolved synergies with many plants and micro-organisms and these synergies were often beneficial to the host (e.g., aiding recovery). Modern lifestyles (e.g., with excess calories but deficient in micronutrients) represent a mismatch with our evolutionary biology and this results in decreased ability to handle stressors such as concussive injury. Xanthophyllic carotenoids, widely available in green leafy vegetables, seem uniquely suited to diminishing damage and symptoms caused by physical trauma to the brain. The American diet is deficient in these specific food components which may increase our susceptibility to central nervous system damage and degeneration with age.

12.2 DEFINING MILD TRAUMATIC BRAIN INJURY

TBI is caused by the head impacting an object and/or forceful movements of the brain due to acceleration or deceleration forces. Physical trauma from an external source can result in focal and/or diffuse damage, depending on the nature of the injury. For example, direct contact with an object, or a skull-penetrating injury in more extreme cases, results in focal damage that is identifiable with structural scans and is often associated with functional deficits related to the area of injury. Acceleration forces on the other hand usually lead to diffuse injury. This wide-spread damage, common to mild forms of TBI, is often characterized by the presence of axonal swelling.

MTBI, or concussion, is defined based on the loss of consciousness and memory loss. Compared to more severe TBI, MTBI occurs with a loss of consciousness that lasts 30 min or less, and post-traumatic amnesia that is present for no longer than 24 h. These specific criteria are a part of the definition of MTBI put forth by the Mild Traumatic Brain Injury Committee (1993), a special interest group of the American Congress of Rehabilitative Medicine, and have been maintained in a definition established by the World Health Organization Collaborative Center Task Force on Mild Traumatic Brain Injury (Carroll et al., 2004). The Glasgow Coma Scale is used to score the extent of the injury based on motor (e.g., flexion and extension), verbal (e.g., alertness, coherence of speech), and eye-opening responses (e.g., whether eyes open spontaneously, to speech or pain, or not at all). Comparatively, other definitions of MTBI, such as that provided by the American Congress of Rehabilitation Medicine, include a wider range of physical symptoms (e.g., headaches, lethargy, sensory loss, etc.) along with cognitive (e.g., executive functions, concentration, language, etc.), and emotional responsiveness.

Separate scales have been established for both athletes and military personnel. The American Academy of Neurology (1997) established criteria for classifying the severity of an injury and for sideline evaluation of athletes. A concussion can be labeled as Grade 1, 2, or 3. Grade 3 involves loss of consciousness, whereas Grade 1 and 2 classifications are determined by the time course of symptom resolution (e.g., less than 15 min for Grade 1). Criteria for sideline evaluation include mental status testing (e.g., orientation, concentration, and memory), exertion (e.g., the completion of physical tasks such as sprints, pushups, etc. and monitoring of any symptoms such as dizziness), and neurological tests (e.g., pupillary reactivity/symmetry, coordination, and proprioception/vestibular functioning). The Defense and Veterans Brain Injury Center has its own definition of MTBI for military situations, although it is relatively consistent with that of the CDC and WHO. Diagnosis of MTBI in military personnel is facilitated by the Military Acute Concussion Evaluation, which includes four cognitive domains: orientation, immediate memory, concentration, and memory recall (French et al., 2008). The tasks used to assess each domain of functioning are similar to those used for athletes (e.g., digit backward task for concentration, immediate and delayed recall of objects for memory functioning).

12.3 VISUAL SYMPTOMS OF MILD TRAUMATIC BRAIN INJURY

Patients with MTBI may have a complex presentation of visual dysfunction. For example, Kapoor and Ciuffreda (2002) categorized symptoms based on dysfunction related to accommodation, version, vergence, visual field deficits, and photosensitivity. Specific ocular deficits, however, are often absent despite the presence of subjective visual side effects. Symptoms frequently manifest as increased sensitivity to light. Patients who report elevated light sensitivity after injury typically have deficits in visual performance that are not evident in patients without a subjective experience of light sensitivity.

Lane (1963) hypothesized that disruptions to central vision (e.g., as a result of brain injury) leads to an increased dependence on peripheral vision, the effectiveness of which is reduced by bright light, leading to visual distress. Based on this mechanistic theory (i.e., light disrupting the peripheral retinal input), Lane described the visual distress as cortical in nature and a consequence of adaptation problems. Zihl and Kerkhoff (1990) speculated that brain damage has a global effect on visual function, as opposed to deficits with a specific injury-related origin. Finally, Stern (2011) classified the etiology of light sensitivity in brain-injury patients into mechanisms related to magnocellular deficits, deficits of inhibition related to an imbalance of neurotransmitters, binocular vision disorders, and side-effects of post-trauma vision syndrome related to primary visual pathway deficits.

12.4 VISUAL DISABILITY AND DISCOMFORT

Bright headlights, or walking outside on a bright day after being in a dark room, may be perceived as painful or aversive (glare discomfort). Light entering the eye can be scattered by the anterior media and when this light is sufficiently intense (i.e., greater than one's current adaptive state), it leads to glare disability. Scattering effects (both intra- and extra ocular) can reduce visual function even at low light levels. For example, luminance differences (e.g., contrast between objects) ultimately enable visibility of objects in the environment, therefore any reduction in contrast can degrade the integrity of the visual stimulus and interfere with detection. If the intensity of a light source is sufficient to bleach the photoreceptors responsible for transducing the light stimulus to a neural signal, then visibility is reduced until photoreceptors regenerate visual pigment.

Individuals with disruptions to the visual system as a result of disease or injury (such as MTBI) are more susceptible to experiencing visual disability or discomfort. In a "normal" visual system, light that is ultimately transduced into a neural signal by retinal receptors is first focused by the optical components of the eye. Light incident on the surface of the eye is refracted by the cornea before passing through the pupil, the size of which is altered by the dilator and sphincter muscles of the iris in order to regulate the amount of incoming light. The lens then accommodates to bring light to a focus on the retina, which is comprised of photopigment-containing receptors that capture quanta of light and transduce the energy to a neural signal. A network of vertical and lateral connections (which serve to enhance luminance differences via lateral inhibition) among photoreceptors, bipolar cells, horizontal cells, and amacrine cells ultimately results in the activation of ganglion cells, which carry the signal to the brain via the optic nerve. Luminance information is carried by the fibers in the rod-driven magnocellular pathway en route to the visual cortex, whereas detailed information is mediated by the cone-driven parvocellular pathway. Although this is a simplistic overview of a highly complex sensory system, it highlights the various stages of processing that, if disrupted, could result in visual disability or discomfort.

Visibility can be degraded as a result of forward light scatter (incident light scattering toward the retina), which reduces the contrast between a target and its background. Changes in the optics of the eye or the progression of aberrations as a result of certain conditions (e.g., those that affect the lens, intraocular pressure, or pupillary function) can cause intraocular light scatter. For example, the lens becomes more opaque with age as a result of yellowing and the formation of clumps from proteins in the lens. Consequently, light passing through the lens is disrupted: Patients with age-related cataracts, for instance, have significantly more forward light-scatter (e.g., de Waard et al., 1992).

Increased intraocular pressure, characteristic of glaucoma as a result of disruption to the flow of aqueous humor from the anterior chamber, has also been associated with a change in light tolerance. This can disrupt the visual experience to a point where it interferes with quality of life. For example, in a sample of patients with glaucoma, 70% reported difficulties with glare and high ambient lighting, which was a specific factor established by Nelson et al. (1999) in a questionnaire for visual difficulties experienced by individuals with glaucoma. Specific items depicting daily activities that were related to this factor included glare in general and adaptation to different levels of lighting.

Changes in pupil size, such as those that characterize MTBI, can result in spherical aberrations that degrade visibility. For example, a larger pupil size in low light conditions can cause increased scatter since the refractive index of the lens, along with numerous aberrations, is greater along the edge relative to the center of the lens. The size of the pupil is regulated by the pupillary light reflex, which begins with signals sent from light-sensitive ganglion cells (e.g., melanopsin-containing, or intrinsically photosensitive, retinal ganglion cells) that travel to the optic nerve and pretectal nucleus of the upper midbrain, and then project to the Edinger-Wetsphal nucleus (part of the oculomotor nerve). Parasympathetic projections from the oculomotor nerve synapse with cililary ganglion neurons, which innervate the constrictor muscle of the iris. Damage to these projections, or alterations as a result of drug use, could result in the failure of the pupil to constrict when exposed to bright light.

Visual discomfort refers to light exposure that does not necessarily influence visibility but is perceived as discomforting to the viewer (Vos, 2003). Physiological responses to glare, such as pupil restriction, are accompanied by behavioral responses such as shielding the eyes or averting the gaze from the source. Visual discomfort is often associated with the term photophobia, which literally means "fear of light," however, specific definitions of photophobia have varied. The term has been used interchangeably with "light sensitivity" and at other times more specific operational definitions for quantifying a photophobic response have been proposed (e.g., Stringham et al.'s (2003) definition of a photophobia threshold based on squinting responses). Generally, though, photophobia is used to depict the experience of pain or discomfort from bright light (Lebensohn, 1934). This is a common symptom of migraines, for example, and could be the result of deficits along the magnocellular and parvocellular pathways (e.g., Coleston et al., 1994).

12.4.1 Light Sensitivity in Mild Traumatic Brain Injury

Empirical evidence suggests that patients with brain injuries experience changes in their tolerance to various lighting conditions (e.g., outdoor lighting, fluorescent lighting, etc.) and changes in visual performance as evidenced by certain behavioral tasks (e.g., reading rate, Jackowski et al., 1996). Entering a bright room after being in dim lighting, exposure to bright sunlight, or exposure to vehicle headlights at night are common causes of visual disability and discomfort. For patients with MTBI, however, even standard room lighting may be intolerable. For example, in a study by Bohnen et al. (1991), patients with PCS tolerated light intensities of 500, 600, 1000, and 1500 lux significantly less well than non-PCS and healthy controls (a 500 lux stimulus is typical for offices with fluorescent lighting, for example, and a 1000 lux stimulus is equivalent to an overcast day). Zihl and Kerkhoff (1990) identified TBI patients with photopic adaptation deficits, 85% of which had complaints of "blinding" vision, and found significantly lower reading lamp levels rated as "too bright" compared to individuals without subjective complaints of light sensitivity.

Military personnel are especially vulnerable to MTBI-induced light sensitivity, particularly if they have experienced a blast-related injury. Capo-Aponte et al. (2012) found that 50% of the blast-induced MTBI patients reported light sensitivity and 30% reported glare sensitivity, whereas only 10% of non-MTBI subjects reported light and glare sensitivity. Goodrich et al. (2013) found statistically significant differences in the frequency of light sensitivity between blast related and non-blast related TBI patients. This wide array of visual problems in MTBI is significant. A good majority of the information processing done by the brain is based on visual input. Sensory loss is well known to proceed and predict later cognitive problems (sensory loss is often described at the "gateway" to cognitive loss) such as those eventually experienced in patients with MTBI. By correcting early visual issues, later problems might be averted.

A good example is provided by Jackowski et al. (1996). This group tested whether filtering lenses could improve visual function (specifically contrast sensitivity and reading rate) for TBI patients who indicated "photophobia" as a visual complaint. Reading rates for TBI patients significantly improved with the use of a Corning Photogchromic Filter 450 (154.03 words/min compared to 123.91 words/min, mean improvement of 26%, $p < 0.05$). The CPF 450 filter also significantly improved contrast sensitivity ($p < 0.01$) in five out of the six TBI patients. Subjective reports of improved reading ability from TBI patients included comments related to print clarity, reduction in the "crowding" of print, and reduced reading effort. Patients from this study continued to wear the CPF lenses over the next year for multiple tasks aside from reading, such as driving and all indoor tasks. Subject reports were consistent with the laboratory findings, and symptoms reappeared when the patients did not use the filters.

12.4.2 Optical Filtering by Lutein and Zeaxanthin

Although extrinsic spectacle lenses might be a useful adjuvant, the eye contains natural dietary-based filters that could even be more effective. Lutein and zeaxanthin (and the lutein conversion product, meso-zeaxanthin) function as an intraocular filter by accumulating in the central retina (here, termed macular pigment; MP) and absorbing short-wave light. The effects of lutein and zeaxanthin on visual function have been detailed in several empirical reports. MP has been shown to absorb light scattered by the ocular media, thereby reducing the veil of obscuration, and improving visual performance in glare (Stringham and Hammond, 2007; 2008, Stringham et al., 2011). The positive effect of increased MP level has been shown not only in cross-sectional studies (Stringham and Hammond, 2007), but also in a within-subject lutein and zeaxanthin supplementation study (Stringham and Hammond, 2008). Exposure to relatively intense light can also cause bleaching of photopigments. Photostress recovery refers to the physiological process necessary for regeneration of photopigments. Perceptually, photostress often manifests as a ghostly afterimage that gradually fades away. Until the recovery process has sufficiently progressed, objects are "hidden" beneath the afterimage, resulting in severely compromised visual performance. TBI patients often exhibit slowed or abnormal photostress recovery times (Du et al., 2005). In normal subjects, Stringham and Hammond (2007) showed that higher levels of MP were associated with faster photostress recovery times. A subsequent lutein and zeaxanthin supplementation study showed that increases in MP within subjects resulted in commensurate decreases in photostress recovery time (Stringham and Hammond, 2008). The average decrease in photostress recovery time after 6 months of lutein and zeaxanthin supplementation was 5 s. In practical terms, this translates into visual recovery, a full 440 ft earlier if driving at a speed of 60 mph.

Stringham et al. (2003) showed that photophobia was reduced significantly as a function of MP, in subjects with a wide range of MP levels. In other words, a person with a higher level of MP can tolerate substantially more light before experiencing visual discomfort. This effect is not trivial—the optical density of MP appears to be linearly related to the logarithm of the intensity of the light source. This means that if someone's MP level could be doubled (an increase that has been experimentally demonstrated), s(he) would be able to withstand twice as much light energy before experiencing discomfort. As lutein and zeaxanthin, and hence MP, are obtained solely via the diet (e.g., from leafy green vegetables), there is high variability among people in MP level—some have very low or no MP, whereas measures as high as 1.5 log optical density have been reported (Hammond, 1997). Dietary modification or supplementation with lutein and zeaxanthin has been shown to reliably increase MP levels (Hammond, 1997; Bone and Landrum, 1997; Stringham et al., 2008). Therefore, an effective, benign strategy for reducing photophobia would appear to be dietary modification to include higher dietary levels of lutein and zeaxanthin, or lutein and zeaxanthin supplementation. Although this type of study has not yet been conducted, cross-sectional data suggest that increases in MP will lead to decreases in photophobia and could represent a meaningful improvement in the photophobia symptoms commonly found in TBI patients.

12.5 TEMPORAL PROCESSING SPEED

The most comprehensive way to quantify temporal vision is to measure the complete temporal contrast sensitivity function (Wooten et al., 2010). This function is defined as contrast sensitivity (the inverse of contrast threshold) for sinusoidally modulated light over a wide range of temporal frequencies. Measuring the entire function is useful because it is thought to be the envelope of multiple temporal filters tuned to different frequencies. In other words, changes in the function could in principle be due to changes at multiple levels of the visual system. For example, CFF thresholds and the high frequency cut-off of the temporal contrast sensitivity function, are thought to reflect cortical activity and provide a means of defining the upper limit of an individual's processing capacity. CFF thresholds have also been associated with cognitive performance, which suggests a common mechanism related to neural processing speed (Bovier et al., 2013). Behavioral indices related to speed of processing in the visual domain may reflect the efficiency of the neural system.

One central tenet of the concept of neural efficiency is inherent in the name; the efficiency of neural communication, whether it be related to speed of communication or signal strength. Efficiency of the neural system could be influenced by several factors:

1. The speed of conduction that leads to neural activation. Slowed neural conduction could be accounted for by the degradation of myelin, for example. This has been a proposed model of cognitive decline in Alzheimer's disease (e.g., Bartzokis, 2004).
2. The number of connections, such as the number of gap junctions or the number of dendritic spines on a neuron, for example, both of which influence signal conduction.
3. Lateral connections, such as gap junctions, which can enhance communication between neurons and influence the neural signal in a way to optimize behavior. For example, lateral connections in the retina serve to enhance contrast differences in the environment via lateral inhibition, thereby improving visibility.
4. The amount of a neural network needed to complete a task. Indeed, elderly individuals have been posited to compensate for age related degradation of the brain via activation of more neural circuits (e.g., the scaffolding theory of aging and cognition, Park and Reuter-Lorenz, 2009), which results in slowed processing.

12.5.1 Disrupted Temporal Processing in Mild Traumatic Brain Injury

Kurylo et al. (2006) noted that impairments for patients with acquired brain injury were the most significant for tasks involving temporal information. They suggest that this reflects a reduction of processing speed specific to the processing of stimuli, which may be due to increased demand on neurons responsible for information integration. Deficits could be accounted for by disruptions in perceptual organization, since information processing can be considered a hierarchy in which perceptual organization occurs at an earlier level. Kurylo et al. describe perceptual organization of visual information as the integration of spatial properties of the scene (e.g., proximal relationships and luminance or chromatic contrast) and temporal relationships (e.g., motion coherence and luminance modulation). If the structural integrity of the neural fibers connecting processing modules is compromised, then perceptual organization will be disrupted. In their study, patients with acquired brain injury exhibited higher grouping thresholds (i.e., required a greater amount of target proximity or similarity for perceptual organization) and extended processing time (i.e., needed greater target exposure time prior to the presentation of a masking stimulus in order to perceptually organize the target) compared to healthy controls.

Chang et al. (2007) assessed critical flicker frequency and subjective reports of light and motion sensitivity for MTBI patients ($N = 18$) and healthy controls ($N = 56$). CFF was not significantly different between patients and controls; however, within the patient sample, CFF was significantly higher for patients who were light sensitive ($t = 2.698$, $p = 0.016$) and motion sensitive ($t = -2.813$, $p = 0.013$) compared to patients with no reported sensitivity or symptoms. The authors suggest that patients with subjective experiences of light and motion sensitivity may have reduced inhibition of temporal processing as a result of their injury, thereby resulting in increased sensitivity (i.e., increased sensitivity to bright flicker is in part affected by efferent pathways that influence sensory awareness).

Using the same method described by Chang et al. (2007), Schrupp et al. (2009) measured CFF in the parafovea in order to determine if temporal processing outside of the retina was disrupted in patients with MTBI. This was predicated on the notion that motion and flicker perception is processed in the magnocellular pathway, which receives more input from the parafoveal retina compared to the foveal retina. Consistent with Chang et al.'s findings, CFF in the fovea was not significantly different between patients and controls; however, mean variability was 45% greater for the MTBI group. No significant differences in parafoveal CFF (assessed in either the right or left hemifield) were found, but MTBI patient variability was 9 and 4% higher, respectively. When comparing CFF in the fovea and parafovea for both groups, foveal CFF was significantly higher than CFF assessed in the right or left hemifield. Subjective reports of light and motion sensitivity were not significantly related to any measure of CFF.

Based on the studies by Chang et al. and Schrupp et al., it appears as though MTBI patients who experience light sensitivity may have disrupted temporal processing, although the results from the two studies are not consistent. Inconsistency could be attributed to the subjective rating scale used to quantify light sensitivity (i.e., a scale of 1–4, with one depicting "never" experiencing light sensitivity and four depicting "marked" sensitivity) paired with a small sample size of patients (18 in Chang et al.'s study and 14 in Schrupp et al.'s study).

12.5.2 Lutein and Zeaxanthin and Temporal Processing Speed

Hammond and Wooten (2005) first tested the influence of lutein and zeaxanthin on temporal vision and formally proposed the neural efficiency hypothesis. They assessed the relationship between macular pigment and CFF thresholds with stimuli expressly chosen to reflect post-receptoral processing presumably localized within the visual cortex (e.g., Powell, 1983). Macular pigment was significantly related to CFF in a sample of 134 subjects aged 17–92 years ($r = 0.30$; $p < 0.001$). This relationship was still significant after statistical adjustment for age and also maintained for stratified age groups (younger: $r = 0.33$, $p < 0.013$; middle: $r = 0.32$, $p < 0.015$; older: $r = 0.27$, $p = 0.04$). Based on these results, the authors suggested that lutein and zeaxanthin could improve the efficiency of neural signals throughout the visual system. Indeed, individuals with higher macular pigment have higher sensitivity according to assessments of the full temporal contrast sensitivity function (Renzi and Hammond, 2010).

Hammond and Wooten's hypothesis is consistent with evidence from cellular models showing that carotenoids improve gap junction communication between somatosensory cells (Stahl et al., 1997) and reversed declines of neuronal transduction in rat models as a result of dietary supplementation with spinach (Joseph et al., 1998). Indeed, specific cortical concentrations of lutein and zeaxanthin have been identified by tissue analyses of the brains of elderly humans (Craft et al., 2004; Johnson et al., 2013), infants (Vishwanathan et al., 2011), and primates (Vishwanathan et al., 2013). These studies support the neural efficiency hypothesis since they provide evidence that lutein and zeaxanthin accumulate throughout cortical tissue and are therefore in place to influence neural function.

Mechanisms that may account for the ability of lutein and zeaxanthin to promote neural efficiency are also based on tubulin as a binding site for lutein and zeaxanthin (e.g., Bernstein et al., 1997). Potential outcomes of the xanthophyll's association with tubulin (which forms microtubules) could be related to the cytoskeleton of dendrites and axonal tracks. Microtubules have been identified in dendritic spines (e.g., Gu et al., 2008) and implicated in their formation and plasticity. An increase in the length of dendritic spines and total number of spines is one mechanism that could account for enhanced neural efficiency. Microtubules are also present in the cytoskeleton of axonal tracts. As lutein and zeaxanthin bind to tubulin and have a horizontal orientation in lipid bilayers (e.g., Pasenkiewicz-Gierula et al., 2012), this may improve the structural integrity of myelin, resulting in preserved or increased axonal conduction speed. One final mechanism by which lutein and zeaxanthin could promote neural efficiency is through increased gap junction communication (e.g., Stahl et al., 1997), which has been demonstrated in somatic tissue. The underlying biology of how exactly this occurs is unknown; however, it has been shown that carotenoids stimulate the production of connexin proteins (e.g., Bertram, 1999), which form gap junctions. It may be that lutein and zeaxanthin's ability to bind to tubulin influences the association between microtubules and ribosomes, resulting in an increased production of connexin proteins. Although reasonable, direct functional studies on neurons themselves are needed in order to adequately evaluate the potential of these carotenoids to promote direct change within nervous tissue.

12.6 GENERAL CONCLUSIONS

Lutein and zeaxanthin are found throughout the retina and brain and, in addition to filtering and neural effects, may be uniquely suited to affecting the long-term diseases processes known to be initiated by concussive events (such as inflammatory stress). Previous research has shown that a wave of secondary injury begins immediately after impact in patients suffering closed head injuries and that this is likely a major contribution to delayed neuron dysfunction and loss. Inflammation is both an acute and chronic response to concussive head injury that has been studied extensively (for a review, see Cederberg et al., 2010). Lutein has been shown to decrease the expression of COX-2, which is a pro-inflammatory protein, and reduce the production of nNOS (neuronal Nitric Oxide Synthsase) in a dose-dependent manner in rat retinas after induced ischemia via high intraocular pressure (Choi et al., 2005). Another common cellular characteristic of TBI is damage to plasma membranes (e.g, Koob et al., 2008). Such damage can have numerous effects such as disrupting interneuronal signaling and energy transfer. Lutein and zeaxanthinco localize with n-3 fatty membrane acids and are also known to stabilize membranes (sometimes described as transmembrane rivets between lipid bilayers) and bind to microtubules (Bernstein et al., 1997) in the cytoskeleton. Finally, increased free radical oxygen species (ROS) production plays a key role in neuronal loss following MTBI (e.g., Dash et al., 2008). As antioxidants, lutein and zeaxanthin protect long-chain polyunsaturated fatty acids (PUFAs) in neural membranes (Sommerburg, 1999; Rapp, 2000).

Taken together, existing evidence supports the use of lutein and zeaxanthin as both a means of increasing resiliency and ameliorating concussive damage once it has occurred. This conclusion, however, awaits careful clinical study. Since MP optical density can easily be measured in neural tissue (retina), this permits an in vivo assessment of an individual's lutein/zeaxanthin status. This allows prospective study of at risk groups (e.g., football players at the beginning of a season). Similarly, the existence of purified lutein and zeaxanthin supplements allows for classic double-blind placebo-controlled evaluations of palliative effects. Dietary interventions of this sort provide hope for an innocuous and possibly clinically significant approach to this common and debilitating condition.

REFERENCES

ACRM; Mild Traumatic Brain Injury Committee. 1993. Definition of mild traumatic brain injury. *J Head Trauma Rehabil* 8:86–87.

American Academy of Neurology. 1997. Practice parameter: The management of concussion in sports (summary statement). Report of the Quality Standards Subcommittee. *Neurology* 48:581–585.

American Psychiatric Association. 2000. Diagnostic and statistical manual of mental disorders: DSM-IV-TR. Washington, DC.

Bartzokis, G. 2004. Age-related myelin breakdown: A developmental model of cognitive decline and Alzheimer's disease. *Neurobiol of Aging* 25:5–18.

Bernstein, P.S., Balashov, N.A., Tsong, E.D., and Rando, R.R. 1997. Retinal tubulin binds retinal carotenoids. *Invest Ophthalmol Vis Sci* 38:167–175.

Bertram, J.S. 1999. Carotenoids and gene regulation. *Nutr Rev* 57:182–191.

Boake, C., McCauley, S.R., Levin, H.S. et al. 2005. Diagnostic criteria for postconcussional syndrome after mild to moderate traumatic brain injury. *J Neuropsychiatry Clin Neurosci* 17:350–356.

Bohnen, N., Twijnstra, A., Wijnen, G., and Jolles, J. 1991. Tolerance for light and sound of patients with persistent post-concussional symptoms 6 months after mild head injury. *J Neurol* 238:443–446.

Bovier, E.R., Fletcher, L.M., Thorne, S.A., Hammond, B.R., and Renzi, L.M. 2013. Critical flicker fusion thresholds: Relations to neurocognitive function. *Eur J Ophthalmol* 23:610.

Carroll, L.J., Cassidy, J.D., Holm, L., Kraus, J., and Coronado, V.G. 2004. Methodological issues and research recommendations for mild traumatic brain injury: The WHO Collaborating Centre Task Force on Mild Traumatic Brain Injury. *J Rehabil Med* Suppl. 43:113–125.

Cederberg, D. and Siesio, P. 2010. What has inflammation to do with traumatic brain injury? *Childs Nerv Syst* 26:221–226.

Chang, T.T., Ciuffreda, K.J., and Kapoor, N. 2007. Critical flicker frequency and related symptoms in mild traumatic brain injury. *Brain Inj* 21:1055–1062.

Choi, J., Kim, D., Hong, Y., Mizuno, S., and Joo, C. 2005. Inhibition of nNOS and COX-2 expression by lutein in acute retinal ischemia. *Nutrition* 22: 668–671.

Coleston, D.M., Chronicle, E., Ruddock, K.H., and Kennard, C. 1994. Precortical dysfunction of spatial and temporal visual processing in migraine, *J Neurol Neurosurg Psychiatry* 57:1208–1211.

Du, T., Ciuffreda, J., and Kapoor, N. 2005. Elevated dark adaptation thresholds in traumatic brain injury. *Brain Inj* 19:1125–1138.

de Waard, P.W.T., IJspeert, J.K., van den Berg, T.J.T.P., and de Jong, P.T.V.M. 1992. Intraocular light scattering in age-related cataracts. *Invest Ophthalmol Vis Sci* 33:618–625.

Faul, M., Xu, L., Wald, M.M., and Coronado, V.G. 2010. Traumatic brain injury in the United States: Emergency department visits, hospitalizations, and deaths. Centers for Disease Control and Prevention, National Center for Injury Prevention and Control, Atlanta, GA.

French, L., McCrea, M., and Baggett, M. 2008. The military acute concussion evaluation (MACE). *J Spec Oper Med* 8:68–77.

Joseph, J.A., Shukitt-Hale, B., Denisova, N.A. et al. 1998. Long-term dietary strawberry, spinach, or vitamin-E supplementation retards the onset of age-related neuronal signal-transduction and cognitive behavioral deficits. *J Neurosci* 18:8047–8055.

Gu, J., Firestein, B.L., and Zheng, J.Q. 2008. Microtubules in dendritic spine development. *J Neurosci* 28:12120–12124.

Hammond, BR., Johnson, E.J., Russell, R.M. et al. 1997. Dietary modification of human macular pigment density. *Invest Ophthalmol Vis Sci* 38:1795–1801.

Hammond, B.R. and Wooten, B.R. 2005. CFF thresholds: Relation to macular pigment optical density. *Ophthalmic Physiol Opt* 25:315–319.

Jackowski, M.M., Sturr, J.F., Taub, H.A., and Turk, M.A. 1996. Photophobia in patients with traumatic brain injury: Uses of light-filtering lenses to enhance contrast sensitivity and reading rate. *Neuro Rehabilitation* 6:193–201.

Joseph, J.A., Shukitt-Hale, B., Denisova, N.A., Prior, R.L., Cao, G., Martin, A., Taglialatela, G., and Bickford, P.C. 1998. Long-term dietary strawberry, spinach, or vitamin-E supplementation retards the onset of age-related neuronal signal-transduction and cognitive behavioral deficits. *J Neurosci* 18:8047–8055.

Kapoor, N. and Ciuffreda, K.J. 2002. Vision disturbances following traumatic brain injury. *Curr Treat Options in Neurol* 4:271–280.

Koob, A., Colby, J.M., and Borgens, R.B. 2008. Behavioral recovery from traumatic brain injury after membrane reconstruction using polyethylene glycol. *J Biol Eng* 2:9 doi:10.1186/1754-1611-2-9.

Kurylo, D.D., Waxman, R., and Kezin, O. 2006. Spatial-temporal characteristics of perceptual organization following acquired brain injury. *Brain Inj* 20:237–244.

Lane, B.C. 1963. Functional photophobia: Preliminary observations from optometric analysis of 100 cases. *Eastern Seaboard Conference on Visual Training* 8:32–51.

Lebenshon, J.E. 1934. The nature of photophobia. *Arch of Ophthalmol* 12:380–390.

Nelson, P., Aspinall, P., and O'Brien, C. 1999. Patients' perception of visual impairment in glaucoma: A pilot study. *Br J Ophthalmol* 83:546–552.

Park, D.C. and Reuter-Lorenz, P. 2009. The adaptive brain: Aging and neurocognitive scaffolding. *Annu Rev Psychol* 60:173–196.

Pasenkiewics-Gierula, M., Krzysztof, B., Murzyn, K., and Markiewicz, M. 2012. Orientation of lutein in a lipid bilayer – revisited. *Acta Biochim Pol* 59:115–118.

Rapp, L.M., Maple, S.S., and Choi, J.H. 2000. Lutein and zeaxanthin concentrations in rod outer segment membranes from perifoveal and peripheral human retina. *Invest Ophthalmol Vis Sci* 41:1200–1209.

Ryan, L.M. and Warden, D.L. 2003. Post concussion syndrome. *Int Rev of Psychiatry* 15:310–316.

Salthouse, T.A. 2004. What and when of cognitive aging. *Curr Dir in Psychol Sci* 13:140–144.

Schrupp, L.E., Ciuffreda, K.J., and Kapoor, N. 2009. Foveal versus eccentric retinal critical flicker frequency in mild traumatic brain injury. *Optometry* 80:642–650.

Sommerberg, O., Siems, W.G., Hurst, J.S., Lewis, J.W., Kliger, D.S., and Frederik, J.G.M. 1999. Lutein and zeaxanthin are associated with photoreceptors in the human retina. *Curr Eye Res* 19:491–495.

Stahl, W., Nicolai, S., Briviba, K. et al. 1997. Biological activities of natural and synthetic carotenoids: Induction of gap junctional communication and singlet oxygen quenching. *Carcinogenesis* 18:89–92.

Stern, C.D. 2011. Photophobia, light, and color in acquired brain injury. In *Vision Rehabilitation: Multidisciplinary Care of the Patient Following Brain Injury*, Eds. P.S. Suter and L.H. Harvey, 283–300. Boca Raton, FL: CRC Press.

Stringham, J.M., Fuld, K., and Wenzel, A.J. 2003. Action spectrum for photophobia. *J Opt Soc Am A Opt Image Sci Vis* 20:1852–1858.

Stringham, J.M. and Hammond, B.R. 2007. The glare hypothesis of macular pigment function. *Optom Vis Sci* 84:859–864.

Stringham, J.M. and Hammond, B.R. 2008. Macular pigment and visual performance under glare conditions. *Optometry and Vision Science* 85:82–88.

Vishwanathan, R., Kuchan, M.J., and Johnson, E.J. 2011. Lutein is the predominant carotenoid in infant brain. *Acta Biologica Cracoviensia* 53:Suppl. 1, 1.23.

Vishwanathan, R., Neuringer, M., Snodderly, D.M., Schalch, W., and Johnson, E.J. 2013. Macular lutein and zeaxanthin are related to brain lutein and zeaxanthin in primates. *Nutr Neurosci* 16:21–29.

Vos, J.J. 2003. Reflections on glare. *Light Res and Technol* 35:163–176.

Wooten, B.R., Renzi, L.R., Moore, R., and Hammond, B.R. 2010. A practical method of measuring the human temporal contrast sensitivity function. *Biomed Opt Express* 1:47–58.

World Health Organization. 1992. The ICD-10 classification of mental and behavioural disorders: Clinical descriptions and diagnostic guidelines. World Health Organization, Geneva.

Zihl, J. and Kerkhoff, G. 1990. Foveal photopic and scotopic adaptation in patients with brain damage. *Clin Vis Sci* 5:185–195.

13 Flavonoid Supplementation and Cardiovascular Disease

Weston Bussler, Joseph Hildebrand, Catherine Mixon, Ty Wagoner, Slavko Komarnytsky, and Gabriel Keith Harris

CONTENTS

13.1 FLAVONOID SUPPLEMENTATION AND CARDIOVASCULAR DISEASE

The connection between flavonoids and cardiovascular health was observed as early as the 1930s, when the Hungarian scientist Albert Szent-Györgyi observed the effects of the flavone hesperidin on changes on the permeability of the vascular epithelium (Pearson 1957). Over the past 80 years, there has been a continued rise in cardiovascular diseases (CVD), reaching an annual \$108.9 billion in healthcare costs (Heidenreich et al. 2011). CVD is a blanket term that refers to a number of diseases and conditions that affect the circulatory system. Within this classification are two of the leading causes of death in humans—heart attack and stroke. Researchers are studying treatments that may reduce the impact of risk factors, which are leading to these death-causing events. Growing interest has been placed on the relationship of plant-derived secondary metabolites and health, particularly the group of plant polyphenols known as flavonoids. Research on flavonoids has increased significantly over the past two decades (Figure 13.1).

This chapter will explore the prevalence and risk of CVD, the different types of flavonoids, the metabolic functions of flavonoids, the outcomes of flavonoid supplementation on CVD, the potential complications of high-dose supplementation, and the mechanisms of flavonoid–CVD interaction. In addition, this chapter will clarify

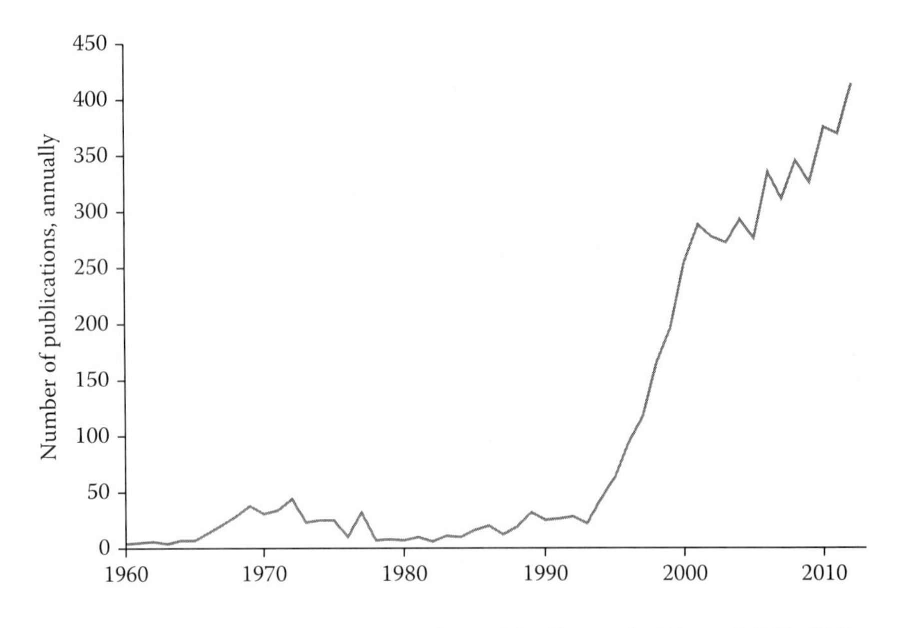

FIGURE 13.1 PubMed Search of "Flavonoids and Cardiovascular Disease" 1960–2012.

some of the gaps and confusing aspects of flavonoid actions as they relate to CVD, including location of bioactivity, acute and chronic intake levels, flavonoids as a treatment or preventative agent, as well as age-appropriate interventions and relevant doses for desired metabolic effects. Finally, the future course for flavonoid research and investigational efforts will be provided.

13.2 IMPACT OF HEART AND VASCULAR DISEASES

As diagnosis of various vascular and heart diseases rises, so do the overall healthcare costs. In the United States, CVD costs roughly $272.5 billion annually (Heidenreich et al. 2011). This amount includes the direct costs of healthcare services, medications, which does not include the indirect costs associated with losses in productivity. To put this into perspective, approximately $1 of every $6 spent on healthcare in the United States is spent on CVD treatments and services. The direct healthcare costs of four types of CVD are shown in Table 13.1.

According to the CDC, in 2009–2010, 35.7% of American adults and 16.9% of adolescents and children were considered overweight or obese. Also, 67 million, or roughly 1 in 3 Americans, have been diagnosed with hypertension. Another 25.8 million people, about 30%, have been diagnosed with Type II Diabetes. Obesity, hypertension, and Type II Diabetes are major risk factors for CVD. Today, 49% of the population has one or more of these risk factors, increasing their risk of being diagnosed with CVD.

The numbers shown in Table 13.2 reflect the massive number of people who suffer from CVD and the differences in the types of CVD—outlined in Table 13.3—that

TABLE 13.1
Direct US Healthcare Costs of Major Cardiovascular Diseases 2010

Cardiovascular Disease	Cost ($B)
Coronary heart disease	$108.9
Hypertensive disease	$93.5
Stroke	$53.9
Heart failure	$34.4

TABLE 13.2
Total Deaths in 2008 Due to Cardiovascular Diseases Globally (AHA 2011)

Region	Ischemic	Cerebrovascular	Rheumatic	Overall CVD
Americas (North/South)	881,000	437,000	10,000	1,944,000
Europe	2,195,000	1,278,000	25,000	4,584,000
East Mediterranean	587,000	292,000	22,000	1,195,000
Africa	374,000	449,000	11,000	1,254,000
South-East Asia	1,834,000	1,192,000	56,000	3,616,000
Western-Pacific	1,383,000	2,504,000	96,000	4,735,000
Total deaths	7,254,000	6,152,000	220,000	17,327,000

TABLE 13.3
Cardiovascular Events and Conditions that Contribute to Mortality

Condition	Symptoms
	Chronic CVD (Contributes to CVD Mortality Events)
Atherosclerosis	Plaque builds up inside arteries. Plaque can be made up of fat, cholesterol, calcium, and/or any other compounds found in blood. Atherosclerosis is a precursor to heart attack and stroke.
Hypercholes-terolemia	Hypercholesterolemia is a disorder characterized by high levels of blood cholesterol. Cholesterol is manufactured primarily in the liver and then carried to the cells throughout the body by LDL. As cholesterol and other fats do not dissolve in water, they cannot travel through the body unaided. Lipoproteins are particles formed in the liver to transport cholesterol and other fats through the bloodstream. For CVD, high cholesterol constitutes high levels of LDL cholesterol or low HDL cholesterol. Having either of these, increases the CVD mortality risk by allowing more LDL to be oxidized and congest the arteries.
Congenital heart disease	Birth defect that can cause a narrowing of the aorta or holes in the wall that separates the left and right ventricle (Krikler 1992).
Rheumatic heart disease	Chronic condition that is characterized by the development of fibrosis in the heart valves following Rheumatic fever. Bacterial infection (Rhumatic fever) that causes fibrosis of heart valves, living in areas without access to antibiotics. A total of 15.6 million people are currently affected worldwide. About 1% of all school children in Africa, Asia, the Eastern Mediterranean region, and Latin America show signs of the disease.
Peripheral arterial disease	Atherosclerosis that usually affects the arteries and legs.
Peripheral vascular disease	Circulation problems that inhibit proper circulation primarily in the legs. People that have this disease will have pain in their calves, especially when they are walking.
Oxidative stress	An imbalance of prooxidants and antioxidants. The excessive formation of reactive species leads to atherosclerosis.
Chronic inflammation	Typically associated with prolonged OS. A low level chronic immune response leads to vascular damage and atherosclerosis.
Hypertension	A systolic blood pressure at or above 140 mmHg and/or a diastolic blood pressure at or above 90 mmHg. Systolic BP = the maximum pressure in the arteries when the heart contracts. Diastolic BP = the minimum pressure in the arteries between the hearts contractions.
	Acute CVD (Death Causing Events)
Ischemic heart disease	Problems circulating blood to the heart muscle. A lack of enough oxygenated blood (ischemia) causing angina (chest pain) and dyspnea (shortness of breath) and myocardial infarction, commonly known as a heart attack.
Cerebrovascular disease (Stroke)	Occurs when there are problems circulating blood through the blood vessels of the brain. A blockage with effects lasting less than 24 h is referred to as a transient ischemic attack. A complete blockage with long-term effects is referred to as a cerebrovascular thrombosis (clot) or a stroke. Sometimes, a blood vessel in the brain can burst, resulting in a long-term brain damage.

(*Continued*)

TABLE 13.3 (*Continued*)
Cardiovascular Events and Conditions that Contribute to Mortality

Condition	Symptoms
1. Ischemic stroke	Complete blockage of blood flow to the brain
2. Hemorrhagic stroke	Obstruction within a blood vessel supplying blood to the brain
3. Heart failure	The pumping action of the heart can no longer provide enough blood to the rest of the body to serve required functions. Symptoms include, shortness of breath from congested lungs, swelling of legs from water retention due to little blood reaching the kidneys, increased need for urination, stomach bloating/loss of appetite, dizziness/fatigue/weakness from less blood reaching the brain, and finally a rapid or irregular heartbeat.

are afflicting people from different areas. Ischemic heart disease deaths predominate Europe, both America and the Eastern Mediterranean; Cerebrovascular deaths are much more prominent in comparison to Africa, Southeast Asia, and the Western-Pacific. Lifestyle differences have been attributed to these different rates, with diet representing a major portion. Research over the past two decades has shown that flavonoid supplementation may have an effect on decreasing the risk factors of CVD and many other chronic diseases. Local consumption of flavonoids also might explain why there are different rates of CVD in different regions of the world.

13.3 FLAVONOID OVERVIEW

Plants synthesize a number of polyphenolic compounds with many biological purposes such as biochemical defense and pigmentation. These compounds are classified by their chemical structure into ten different classes, one of which is the flavonoids. Recent evaluations state that more than 5500 different naturally occurring flavonoids have been discovered (Yamane and Kato 2012). They are characterized by an aromatic ring structure with one or more hydroxyl groups. The characteristic ring structures of flavonoid compounds and their subsequent functional groups contain a large amount of electron density, thereby creating partial negative charges. These partial negative charges become targets for chemical reactions such as functional group modification, metal chelation, redox reactions, or protein/enzyme interactions (Pourcel et al. 2007). They also provide plants with antimicrobial properties, protection from ultraviolet rays, and limit the ability of herbivore digestive enzymes. These features are able to help the plants survive and thrive (Pourcel et al. 2007). Flavonoids are categorized into six subclasses based on oxidation state or the connection between aromatic rings. The subclasses are listed in Table 13.4.

The majority of flavonoids are derived from a flavone backbone, namely, 2-phenyl-1,4-benzopyrene, shown in Figure 13.2, which gives them their characteristic structure. Isoflavones are derived from a slightly different 3-phenyl-1,4-benzopyrene backbone. Flavonoids generally exist in two forms: Flavonoid glycosides, which are

TABLE 13.4
Classification of Flavonoids with Common Examples and Associated Foods

Flavonoid Class	Examples	Associated Foods[a,b]
Flavanols	Catechin, epicatechin, gallocatechin	Tea, cocoa, wine
Flavonones	hesperetin, naringenin	Citrus, grapefruit, lemon
Isoflavones	Genistein, glycitein	Soybean, chickpea
Flavonols	Quercetin, myricetin, kaempferol	Onion, wine, most fruits
Flavones	Luteolin, apigenin	Thyme, oregano, celery, and parsley
Anthocyanidins	Cyanidin, malvidin, delphinidin	Red, blue, and purple berries

[a] Arts and Hollman (2005).
[b] de Pascual-Teresa, Moreno, and García-Viguera (2010).

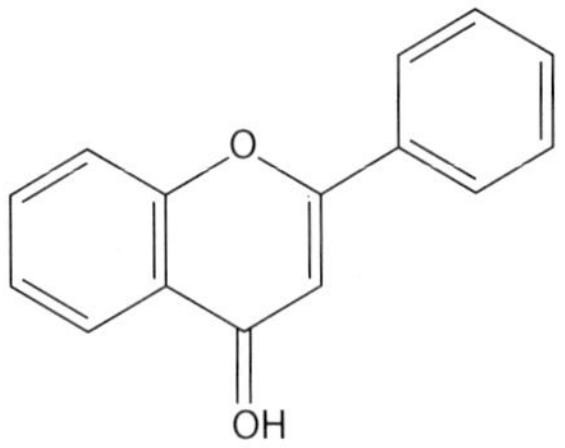

FIGURE 13.2 Basic structural backbone of flavonoids.

attached to sugars, and aglycones, which are not. Glycosides are the more dominant form of most flavonoids with the exception of flavanols (Williamson 2003). Attachment to sugars plays an important role in bioavailability by altering absorption routes. The general structure of the flavonoid classifications is shown in Figure 13.3. Most features of the 2-phenyl-1,4-benzopyrene structure are shown below, while isoflavones are derived from 3-phenyl-1,4-benzopyrene.

13.3.1 Flavonols

Flavonols are the most commonly consumed flavonoids because they are found in a variety of common fruits and vegetables. The most abundant flavonols in food are quercetin, myricetin, and kaempferol. These compounds are commonly associated with onions, apples, and wine, although they are present in most fruits and vegetables. Quercetin is the main dietary source of flavonols, with an estimated daily intake of 25–30 mg making up roughly 65% of the global daily flavonoid consumption (Ross and Kasum 2002; Perez-Vizcaino and Duarte 2010). Due to its abundance in food supply, quercetin is the most studied flavonoid to date (Perez-Vizcaino and Duarte 2010).

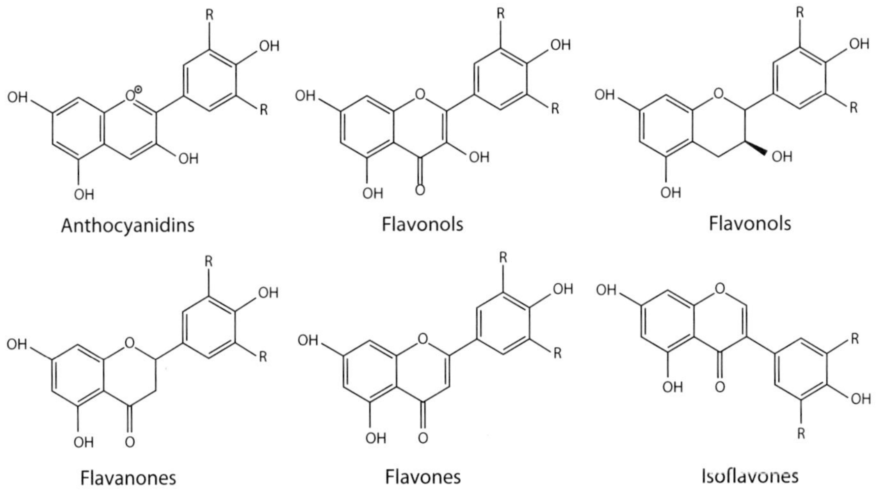

FIGURE 13.3 Basic structure of the six flavonoid classes.

13.3.2 Flavanols

Flavanols, often referred to as flavan-3-ols, have also been studied extensively because they are commonly found in two highly consumed foods: tea and chocolate. Other sources of flavan-3-ols are grape products and some legumes. The common flavanols catechin, epicatechin, and gallocatechin exist as monomers, mainly in the aglycone form (de Pascual-Teresa, Moreno, and García-Viguera 2010). Flavanols also commonly exist in a polymerized form as proanthocyanidins.

13.3.3 Anthocyanidins

Anthocyanidins are the aglycone derivative of anthocyanins, which are attached to sugars for solubility and stability. These compounds are extremely sensitive to pH, light, and oxidative conditions. They exhibit a well-characterized color change from red to blue with increasing pH. Anthocyanins are water-soluble pigments. Six types of anthocyanidins are commonly found in red and purple berries: pelargonidin, cyanidin, delphinidin, petunidin, peonidin, and malvidin. Other foods that contain anthocyanidins are red wines, cereals, and some leafy/root vegetables. Cyanidin is the most common anthocyanidin in foods; black grapes contain up to 600 mg/100 g and berries can contain up to 500 mg/100 g (Erdman et al. 2007).

13.3.4 Flavonones

Flavonones are present in highest concentrations in citrus fruits. These compounds are generally found in a glycosylated form. Flavonones such as narigenin—which are commonly found in citrus fruits such as grapefruit—feature an attached neohesperidose that imparts a bitter flavor (Manach et al. 2004). Research is limited on flavanones because natural sources are limited in human diets.

13.3.5 Isoflavones

While all of the flavonoid classes have been tested individually in vivo, isoflavones are the most widely tested in humans due to their abundance in food supply. There are conflicting scientific reports on the potential health benefits, but they are marketed online as cures to heart disease and inflammation (Espín, García-Conesa, and Tomás-Barberán 2007). They are unique flavonoids in that they belong to the phytoestrogen class. The two most common isoflavones are genistein and glycitein, which are commonly found in soybeans, chickpeas, and other legumes. Although they do not participate in hormonal signaling, they feature similar conformations of hydroxyl groups to estradiol giving them pseudo-hormonal properties (Manach et al. 2004).

13.3.6 Flavones

Flavones are the least common flavonoid found in fruits and vegetables (Manach et al. 2004). Apigenin and luteolin are the most common flavone glycosides, and are mainly found in celery and parsley (Erdman et al. 2007).

13.3.7 Absorption and Bioavailability

Like all nutrients, flavonoids pass through the digestive system and interact with many of the nutrient uptake mechanisms. Note that the ingestion of flavonoid-rich foods does not directly lead to increased levels in the body. Factors such as absorption efficiency, metabolism, protein interactions, and excretion of these compounds impact the bioavailability of flavonoids.

When consumed by humans, limited levels of flavonoid glycosides are absorbed through the SGLUT-1 transporters in enterocytes. Other methods of flavonoid absorption come when the glycoside is hydrolyzed to the aglycone form after reactions in either the oral cavity or via microbial metabolism in the large intestine (Walle 2004). The glycoside forms have a greater ability for absorption (Hollman and Katan 1997).

More recent research has examined the synergistic effects of diet on absorption of flavonoids. Low-fat diets are recommended as a way to curb cardiovascular risk factors, but dietary fat may improve the absorption of potentially beneficial flavonoids. Plasma concentration of flavonoids taken with a high fat diet improved by 45% when compared to a fat-free meal (Guo et al. 2013). Studies with green tea catechins have shown that flavonoids can complex with lipoproteins and alter the lipid usability of fatty acids within lipoproteins, increasing the excretion of lipids (Koo and Noh 2007). Flavonoid derivatives have a high affinity for proteins, and flavonoids commonly interact with human serum albumin (HSA) in the blood. This affinity is amplified by increased dietary oleic acid, the type of fatty acid found in olive and peanut oils (Bolli et al. 2010).

The number of clinical trials investigating flavonoid bioavailability and absorption has gradually increased over the past two decades. These studies commonly measure flavonoid levels in blood plasma or urine to determine the extent at which these compounds are absorbed by the body. The methods used to determine flavonoid bioavailability are the post-prandial test, oral–intravenous balance, oral–fecal balance, and observation of effects of chronic consumption. Post-prandial tests look at the area under the curve in the blood after a single dose and are considered the most suitable test to measure flavonoid bioavailability (Erdman et al. 2007).

Flavonoids are a diverse group of molecules with many possible modifications, so it is not surprising that some are more efficiently absorbed than others. The conjugated form of flavonoids has an impact on the location of absorption, and the level of glucosylation has a direct impact on absorption (Arts and Hollman 2005). Early research suggested that the glycone conjugates of quercetin, which are naturally found in onions, have higher absorption than aglycone or rutinoside conjugates that may be present in supplements (Hollman et al. 1995). Manach also found onion sources of quercetin to be more bioavailable than quercetin commonly found in apples or green tea (Manach et al. 2005).

As flavonoids are metabolized, they undergo a variety of conformational modifications during the passage from the small intestine to the blood stream (Crozier, Jaganath, and Clifford 2009). These may include deglycosylation, glucuronidation, sulfation, and methylation. The resulting metabolic byproducts are different from the glycone and aglycone conjugates that are almost exclusively found in plants (Williams, Spencer, and Rice-Evans 2004). Typical flavonoid concentrations in plasma are less than 1 μmol/L (Manach et al. 2004). Isoflavones are known to be particularly well absorbed in humans, as are quercetin glucosides. The least well-absorbed flavonoids are proanthocyanidins and flavan-3-ols, but this could be a result of the instability of these compounds in the body rather than poor absorption. For example, a 50 mg dose of epicatechin translates in to a maximum plasma concentration between 0.4 and 2.5 μM (Erdman et al. 2007).

Modification of flavonoids may make them more available to absorption by humans. One such example is a solid dispersion of quercetin with polyvinylpyrrolidone, Kollidon 25®. This modified version increased solubility 436 times over quercetin (Costa et al. 2011). Moving forward, to properly assess flavonoids and their ability to alter the prognosis of CVD, the safety and effectiveness of the increased bioavailable forms must be proven. Flavonoid supplementation has the potential to provide a number of health benefits, but the possible negatives must be understood.

Without a specific uptake mechanism in humans, these alternate routes of absorption present many possible routes of flavonoid entry into the bloodstream. Further research in absorption and bioavailability of flavonoids is still needed. An important concept that has been lacking in the literature is the relationship between absorption efficiency and age. Not only are there inherent regulators of absorption, as mentioned above, age-related complications add another dimension to the puzzle. The body's efficiency in all processes declines with age, which will have a direct impact on the metabolism and processing of nutrients, and may later affect flavonoid dose recommendations. Once absorbed, flavonoids impact a variety of metabolic pathways.

13.4 FUNCTIONS OF FLAVONOIDS IN METABOLISM

Flavonoids have the ability to induce many different biochemical responses in humans. The main functions that are applicable to CVD include antioxidant potential by scavenging and preventing the formation of free radicals, reduction of chronic inflammation, phase II enzyme detoxification, and interactions with microflora metabolism. This section also identifies potential negative metabolic effects (García-Lafuente et al. 2009; Lu, Xiao, and Zhang 2013). Each of these activities is unique, but they are also closely related to one another.

13.4.1 Flavonoids as Antioxidants

Free radicals are extremely reactive molecules because they contain unbound electrons. Free radicals are constantly created in biological systems either intentionally or unintentionally, and they are involved in a number of required physiological functions, such as NADPH oxidase activity (Actis-Goretta et al. 2003). Unintended radical compounds can interfere with cellular functions, leading to oxidative stress (OS) (Aruoma, Kaur, and Halliwell 1991). OS results from an imbalance in the ratio of prooxidant and antioxidant compounds in humans (Jones 2006). Examples of damaging effects of OS in organisms include peroxidation of membrane lipids, oxidative damage to nucleic acids, and the oxidation of sulfhydryl groups in proteins. Chronic OS has been identified as an inducing risk factor for a number of fatal diseases in humans, including CVD. The primary free radicals of concern in humans are reactive oxygen and nitrogen species (ROS and RNS) (Wang et al. 2006).

13.4.2 Nitric Oxide Production

Nitric oxide (NO) is a compound produced from the amino acid arginine and nitric oxide synthase (NOS). Multiple genes are used to make the NOS family of enzymes; each is regulated differently and produces NO for a different biological purpose. The functions and biological locations of the different NOS types are described in Table 13.5. Production of NO is often used as a marker of CVD treatment efficacy because epithelial NO is a key regulator of vascular health. The scientific literature offers confusing explanations of the positive and negative effects of NO. Ultimately,

TABLE 13.5
Types of Nitric Oxide Synthase and Their Biological Functions

Nitric Oxide Synthase Type	Biological Location	Function
Neuronal nitric oxide synthase (nNOS)	Nervous tissue and skeletal muscle	Cell signaling and communication
Endothelial nitric oxide synthase (eNOS)	Endothelium	Vasodilation
Inducible nitric oxide synthase (iNOS)	Immune and cardiovascular systems	Immune response to pathogens and foreign materials

increasing concentrations of NO can either protect from or lead to CVD depending on where it is produced in the body.

NO alone can be cytotoxic by reacting with a superoxide anion, forming a damaging RNS called peroxynitrite. The development of RNS in humans focuses mainly on iNOS-derived NO rather than eNOS, in which production of NO can be viewed as a positive for preventing CVD mortality by increasing blood flow. The triggers for iNOS activity and NO release are lipopolysaccharides (LPS), bacteria, viruses, and proinflammatory cytokines. Excess NO production leads to more RNS and ROS, causing more OS. Antioxidants are molecules that have the ability to absorb the free radicals of oxidative compounds, negating the negative health impacts (García-Lafuente et al. 2009). Many flavonoids show great antioxidant potential in vitro by scavenging and negating radical compounds (Wang et al. 2006); however, the actual impact of flavonoids as antioxidants may not be as great because the concentration of flavonoids circulating in the blood is much lower than that of other free-radical scavenging molecules in humans (Williams, Spencer, and Rice-Evans 2004). This suggests that the antioxidant potential of flavonoids is not their only CVD related bioactivity.

In addition to decreasing the damaging effects of iNOS derived NO, flavonoids have the ability to increase the eNOS in vascular endothelial cells to promote the formation of NO. An increase in NO production promotes vasodilation that limits hypertension (Duffy and Vita 2003). By activating eNOS, flavonoids can reduce blood pressure. This is a primary reason why the effects of flavonoids are being investigated in patients with blood circulation issues, specifically those with hypertension and improper blood flow.

13.4.3 Inflammation Reduction

NO biosynthesis—along with prostaglandins—is involved in a variety of inflammatory reactions. The proper regulation of this pathway is crucial to management of cardiovascular health (González-Gallego, Sánchez-Campos, and Tuñón 2007). Inflammation is a biological process where the immune system responds to triggers of infection or injury by quickly creating a specifically targeted destructive environment to resolve the infection, repair any damage to the cell, and restore the original equilibrium. The ideal inflammation process is short, self-limiting, and specific to the intended spot. When inflammation functions properly there are no dangers; when left unchecked, overactive immune responses can lead to the development of debilitating chronic diseases (García-Lafuente et al. 2009). Cyclooxygenase-2 (COX-2) is responsible for the conversion of arachidonic acid to prostaglandins. COX-2 is needed for normal body function even though excess levels signal chronic inflammation (González-Gallego, Sánchez-Campos, and Tuñón 2007).

Flavonoids inhibit enzyme activity by acting on the protein kinases involved in signal transduction. This limits the ability of transcription factors, nuclear factor-κB (NF-κB), and activator protein-1 (AP-1), along with increasing antioxidant defenses through activation of nuclear factor erythroid-derived-2 (NF-E2). NFκB is a protein complex responsible for controlling DNA transcription in animal cells; it is involved in cellular responses to stress, cytokines, free radicals, oxidized low-density lipoprotein (LDL), ultraviolet radiation, and bacterial/viral antigens. AP-1 is a group of leucine zipper transcription factors that bind to DNA and promote cellular differentiation, proliferation, and apoptosis (Fujioka et al. 2004). NF-E2 has shown to be a primary cellular defense mechanism against cytotoxic effects of OS (Linker et al. 2011; Gilmore 2006; González-Gallego, Sánchez-Campos, and Tuñón 2007). These anti-inflammatory mechanisms work together to reduce reactive species that may lead to the oxidation of LDL and eventually atherosclerotic plaques.

13.4.4 Phase II Enzyme Detoxification

Phase II enzymes play a role in the elimination and excretion of toxic substances from the body, including ROS and other electrophilic compounds. Increasing the activity of these enzymes leads to an increased resistance to oxidative damage that may lead to atherosclerosis (Li, Cao, and Zhu 2006). Green tea catechins have been shown to increase activity of these elements in HepG2 cells (Chen et al. 2000). Similar results were seen in rats when fed green tea leaves, which contain high levels of catechins, by increasing the activity of the glutathione-S-transferase (GST) family of Phase II enzymes in the liver (Lin et al. 1998).

13.4.5 Microflora Interactions

More recent research proposes that the health related benefits of flavonoids might be due to their effects on intestinal microbiota as opposed to a direct benefit on human epithelial cells. Flavonoids have a flexible structure that allows for interactions with a wide variety of enzymes, suggesting that they may have an innate ability to regulate microbial metabolic enzymes. Recent studies have identified more than 900 metabolic targets of flavonoids that have homologues in the genomes of human intestinal bacteria. These pathways benefit the intestinal bacteria by inducing changes in metabolism that indirectly benefit humans (Lu, Xiao, and Zhang 2013). Future research should expand on the recent developments of the microbiome flavonoid interactions in humans.

13.4.6 Potential Complications from Flavonoid Supplementation

As consumers look for a "magic bullet" to alleviate health problems, flavonoid supplements have gained attention. Supplements have limited regulation by the FDA, so claims and dosage information are not strictly monitored. There has been an increase in evidence showing specific drug interactions between flavonoids and conventional medications that can present detrimental health effects. One proposed mechanism for this interaction is the presence of flavonoids altering the bioavailability of drugs in the body.

Despite evidence suggesting health benefits from flavonoid consumption, dosage plays an enormous role; there are potential risks associated with high dose supplementation of flavonoids. The risks of consuming high levels of these compounds are not well understood due to the vast number of compounds in the flavonoid family, the lack of adequate dietary intake information evaluating exact amounts that are consumed by people, and limited studies investigating the risk factors of flavonoid compounds. Many foods that have been long consumed by humans are rich in these compounds, giving them the Generally Recognized as Safe (GRAS) moniker. However, some hazards have been identified including anti-nutritional effects, thyroid toxicity, drug interactions, genotoxicity/carcinogenicity, and developmental effects. Human clinical studies supplementing quercetin show adverse effects after a single dose over 4 g; however, a treatment under 500 mg twice daily for a month did not show adverse effects (Russo et al. 2012).

The anti-nutritional effect of flavonoids can come from a number of mechanisms. There is a potential for inhibition of proteolysis within the gut, reduced glucose uptake, impaired food utilization, and impaired mineral absorption. Flavones can inhibit the activity of catechol-O-methyl-transferase, resulting in an increase of norepinephrine concentration and activation of fat oxidation (Dulloo et al. 1999). Epigallocatechin (EGC) and epigallocatechin gallate (EGCG) from green tea have the potential to inhibit glucose uptake by competing for sodium-glucose-cotransporter-1 (Kobayashi et al. 2000). While some researchers cite this action as a negative impact of consuming flavonoids, others conclude that this may be beneficial because it slows glucose uptake, protecting from diabetes mellitus and metabolic syndrome (Johnston et al. 2005). Dietary non-heme iron absorption was reduced by 50%–70% when consumed in tandem with 20–50 mg of polyphenols. This inhibition was increased to 60%–90% when the polyphenol consumption was increased to 100–400 mg (Hurrell, Reddy, and Cook 1999).

High levels of quercetin supplementation have been of some concern because of the potential toxicity of their oxidized product quercetin-quinone (QQ). QQ is a semiquinone radical that has the ability to arylate protein thiols, creating electrophilic compounds that can damage cells. Despite potential concerns, this theory has not yet been proved in any human-based models (Russo et al. 2012).

Plants produce some flavonoids as toxins to deter other animals from eating the plants, so it is reasonable to assume potential toxicity in humans as well. Although some of the beneficial health effects of flavonoids are related to their antioxidative properties, flavonoids at high concentrations can act as prooxidants in the presence of redox-active heavy metals (Galati and O'Brien 2004). This oxidative capacity can lead to the formation of ROS that can damage biological compounds. In the presence of Cu^{2+} and oxygen in vitro, flavonoids can produce radicals that damage DNA (Sakihama et al. 2002).

Potentially harmful effects on the liver have been seen in vivo mice models with EGCG and polymeric tannins (Li et al. 2002; Gali-Muhtasib, Yamout, and Sidani 2000). Both of these compounds can be found in herbal supplements, so there are potential safety implications with very large doses of these compounds. However, it is important to note that toxic doses of flavonoids are much greater than the levels found in dietary sources, so toxicity would more likely be associated with large dose supplements (Galati and O'Brien 2004). Moreover, the prooxidant effect of flavonoids is catalyzed by free copper, ascorbate, and peroxidase activity in vitro. When scaling up to a human some discrepancies occur, most notably the in vivo copper is not usually in the free form that is most damaging, and peroxidase is compartmentalized making these in vitro effects not directly translatable to humans (Erdman et al. 2007).

One example that has been identified is the flavonoid naringenin—present in grapefruits—inhibiting cytochrome P450 3A4 activity (Veronese et al. 2003). These drug interactions need to be considered by persons attempting to consume excessive flavonoid concentrations in their diets (Morris and Zhang 2006). With these possible negative effects identified, the latent therapeutic potential of flavonoids on CVD and its risk factors can be explored in experiment models. The full range of flavonoid effects on metabolism are crucial to developing proper recommendations for them as supplements to treat CVD.

13.5 CARDIOVASCULAR DISEASE

CVD is not just a single disease; it is a complex collection of diseases and risk factors that take different forms in different individuals. These risk factors are better understood if classified into two categories: diseases that can directly lead to death (such as ischemia, heart failure, and stroke), and chronic diseases that contribute to these events (such as atherosclerosis, hypertension, and peripheral heart disease). Explanations of these events are presented in Tables 13.3. Other risk factors to consider for prevention of CVD are insulin resistance, obesity, smoking, lack of exercise, age, gender, family history, alcohol consumption, and race.

Studies use in vitro and animal models to understand some of the factors that can lead to chronic CVD. The complex mechanisms for altering risk factors such as atherosclerosis and inflammation are used to understand flavonoid CVD activity more than the acute events. Acute events such as MI and stroke are more easily recorded, so large-scale epidemiological and meta-analyses are used to correlate flavonoids with CVD risk reduction. Table 13.3 refers to both the chronic and acute forms of heart disease.

13.5.1 Risk Factors for CVD

The development of CVD cannot be isolated to one specific risk. Rather, a cascade of possible factors contributes to the development of CVD. Figure 13.4 attempts to outline some of the major modifiable risk factors that lead to CVD in individuals. The relationship is very complex and specific answers are hard to come by; however, any action that might reduce a risk factor should be investigated. The remainder of this chapter will review studies that observe the relationship between supplementing flavonoids and the impact they have on CVD and risk factors.

13.6 FLAVONOID SUPPLEMENTATION EFFECT ON CHRONIC CVD

13.6.1 Blood Lipid Profile

Blood lipid modifications are recommended by both the American Heart Association and National Cholesterol Education to prevent CVD (Kim et al. 2011). Specifically, they recognize the association of high levels of total cholesterol, LDL cholesterol, and blood triglycerides, and as well as the low levels of HDL cholesterol and

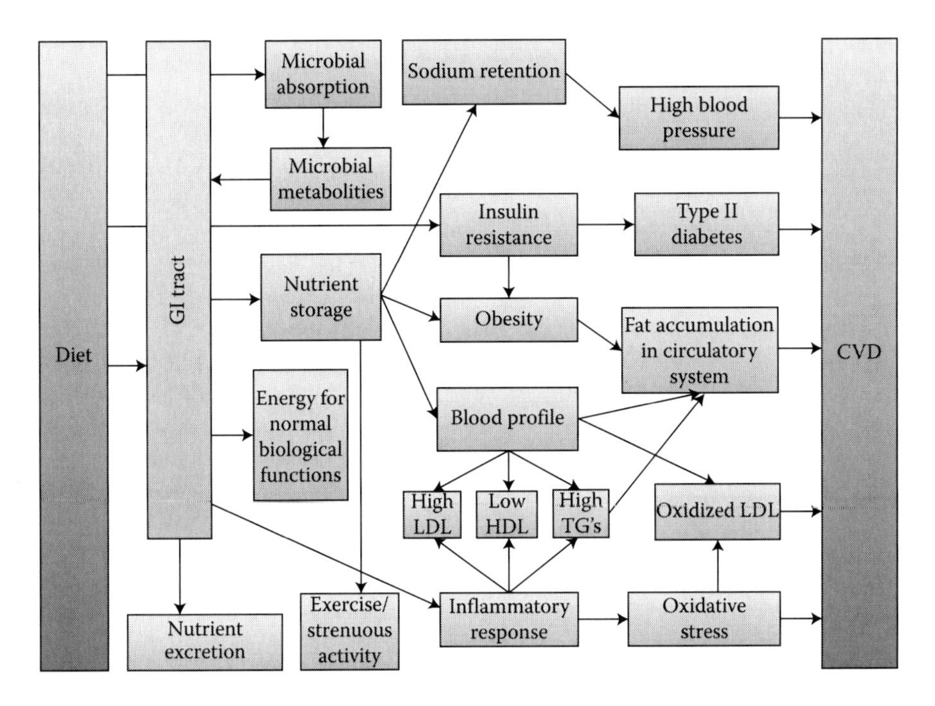

FIGURE 13.4 Illustration of the complex relationship between diet and CVD development.

their relationship to cardiovascular morbidity and mortality (Kim et al. 2011). Hypercholesterolemia is a condition characterized by high cholesterol concentrations throughout the blood of an individual. High total cholesterol, high LDL cholesterol, high blood triglycerides, and low HDL cholesterol are risk factors predicting development of other more damaging CVD. Drug- and diet-formulated treatment plans are recommended to improve blood lipid profiles.

The oxidation of lipids in LDLs that become trapped in the extracellular matrix of the subendothelial space causes events that induce inflammation, which can eventually damage blood lipid profiles, leading to atherosclerosis and other forms of CVD (Berliner et al. 1995). Transcription factors are activated by the oxidized lipids, leading to the production of proteins and an inflammatory response that ultimately causes a fatty streak in arteries. This progression inhibits the mechanical abilities of the artery wall, while also allowing predisposition to plaque ruptures at sites of monocytic infiltration. This eventually induces thrombosis, or other obstructions, making blood flow less efficient (Berliner et al. 1995).

Long-term supplementation of flavonoids may be effective in improving blood lipid profiles by decreasing serum concentrations of inflammation markers. Anthocyanins have been shown to reduce chronic inflammatory markers and cytokines in hypercholesterolemic adults (Zhu et al. 2012). Twice daily doses of 320 mg anthocyanins for 24 weeks resulted in a 21.6% decrease in serum levels of high sensitivity C-reactive protein (hsCRP), a 12.3% reduction in soluble vascular cell adhesion molecule-1 (sVCAM-1), and a 12.8% decrease in Interleukin-1 beta (IL-1beta).

Serum LDL cholesterol was also reduced by 10.4%, and HDL was increased by 14% (Zhu et al. 2012).

In vitro models have demonstrated that flavonoids have the ability to sequester chronic inflammation. When tested on primary human adipocytes, flavonoids were shown to reduce inflammation (Chuang et al. 2010). The anti-inflammatory action of flavonoids has been attributed to the inhibition of inflammatory enzymes. Flavonoids can reduce the expression of iNOS, cyclooxygenase (COX-2), lipooxygenase, prostanoids, leukotrienes, chemokines, adhesion molecules, and cytokines (García-Lafuente et al. 2009). Prostaglandins and NO biosynthesis are involved in the pathway for inflammatory response to stimuli. The isoforms of iNOS and COX-2 are responsible for producing the majority of these pathway mediators. Flavonoids have the capability to inhibit both of these enzymes, as well as other enzymes in the inflammatory process such as adhesion molecules and C-reactive protein. Overexpression of these molecules in the inflammation pathway is attributed to the development of chronic diseases (Tuñón et al. 2009).

Cocoa flavanols (catechin and epicatechin) have shown the ability to inhibit proinflammatory cytokine and leukotriene production, while also inducing vessel relaxation. These improvements on the blood lipid profile may reduce damage from oxidation and inflammation, which are leading risk factors for CVD (Mathur et al. 2002).

13.6.2 Hypercholesterolemia

Between 1988 and 2008, high total cholesterol rates have decreased for men and women, aged 45–75 years or older. The CDC reports that roughly one in four Americans in this demographic (about 32 million) take statins, cholesterol lowering drugs (CDC 2013). The high cholesterol rates for men and women aged 20–44 have increased over the same time period. This data trend in older adults has shown that interventions with statins have decreased cholesterol rates (CDC 2013). The data also show that cholesterol levels are on the rise for younger adults, increasing their need for early cholesterol-lowering interventions. One of the major problems with starting a statin regimen in younger individuals is adherence. Data have shown that only 57% of patients continue their treatment (Grundy 2013).

Reasons for stopping statin treatment include observed side effects (10%–20% of patients experience muscle problems), fear of some side effects reported by patients but not confirmed by FDA (some patients claim to experience memory loss, a fuzzy feeling, or lack of focusing ability), medication costs, lack of insurance coverage, not understanding the treatment benefits, and an overall lack of commitment to the treatment (Grundy 2013). Supplementation of flavonoids may provide a safer and more manageable alternative to the current prescribed statin treatment. Adequate flavonoid supplementation alone, or in addition to statins has shown an active ability to improve blood lipid profiles.

Flavonoids are thought to act on uptake mechanisms for cholesterol by the small intestine effectively reducing circulating cholesterol (Ikeda et al. 1992). Investigating the changes brought on by consuming a metabolite on blood lipid profile is an easy way to determine if it may present a health benefit. One such study examined the protective effect of quercetin in hypercholesterolemic rats. The results showed that quercetin supplementation in combination with a high cholesterol diet was able to decrease liver triglycerides by 24%, reduce total cholesterol by 22%, and reduce serum cholesterol by 20% (Mariee, Abd-Allah, and El-Beshbishy 2012).

These protective effects seem to translate to humans as well. One study assessed the effect of dietary flavonoid supplementation on CVD in post-menopausal women taking statins to treat Type II Diabetes. The dosage was set at 27 g/day of chocolate with 850 mg flavan-3-ols and 100 mg isoflavones, or a placebo, for one year. The results showed that the treatment group had a significant reduction in total cholesterol, LDL/HDL ratio, and total LDL cholesterol. They concluded that high flavonoid diets can work well with drug treatments to reduce lipid profile risk factors (Curtis et al. 2012).

A cohort study based in Finland examined the food intake of 2748 men and 2385 women, 30–69 years of age and free of any known heart disease. After a 26-year period, five major flavonoid intakes—quercetin, kaempferol, myricetin, luteolin, and apigenin—were estimated based on dietary data. Median flavonoid intake was found to be 3–4 mg/day with approximately 95% of the total intake coming from quercetin. The incidence of coronary mortality was found to be higher in populations with low dietary flavonoid intake. The protective effect of flavonoids was associated with a diet high in apple and onion intake. The proposed mechanism for the effect was the prevention of oxidation of LDL particles, however, other mechanisms could have also contributed. The beneficial effect of high fruit and vegetable diets correlated to their flavonoid content (Knekt et al. 2002).

Other blood lipid profile studies found that cocoa powder flavonoids reduced oxidative susceptibility of LDL cholesterol while keeping prostaglandin concentrations stable (Wan et al. 2001). Ingestion of green tea catechins may alter blood lipid profile by moderately reducing the intestinal absorption and delivery of cholesterol (Koo and Noh 2007).

13.6.3 Hypertension and Blood Circulation

Proper blood circulation is necessary to life, and any impediments to blood circulation can be very damaging. One important CVD risk factor is atherosclerosis, which is the medical condition in which fat, cholesterol, and other substances build up on the walls of arteries and form hard structures called plaques. Plaques are created when these materials are oxidized, causing them to adhere to the walls of arteries. This can eventually lead to partial or full occlusion as well as creation of thrombogenic material potentially leading to stroke.

Atherosclerosis is a chronic condition; it progresses slowly and is asymptomatic until abnormal narrowing of a blood vessel occurs. This narrowing can become so severe that blood supply to tissues becomes insufficient or plaques break off and become thrombogenic material, leading to ischemia. Flavonoids interact with this narrowing mechanism by increasing the vasodilation of blood vessels. Specifically, a 2013 study showed high berry anthocyanin consumption was able to increase flow mediated dilation at two intervals, 1 and 6 h (Rodriguez-Mateos et al. 2013). In a meta-analysis published by the European Society of Cardiology, chronic and acute intakes of flavan-3-ol rich foods, such as chocolate or cocoa, reduced diastolic blood pressure and improved flow-mediated dilation. Additionally, the improvements were found at all dose levels (Wright et al. 2012).

When treating hypertensive patients with quercetin supplements, an observed reduction in markers for OS—ferric reducing ability of plasma (FRAP) and poly ADP ribose polymerase (PARP)—was observed. However, this effect was only seen in patients with Stage I Hypertension; prehypertension patients were not significantly affected (Edwards et al. 2007).

The Kuopio Ischemic Heart Disease Risk Factor Study (KIHD) consisted of 1380 middle-aged eastern Finnish men in which the mean common carotid artery intima-media thickness (CCA-IMT) was studied. The study identified a trend for an inverse association between intake of flavonols and mean CCA-IMT (Mursu et al. 2008). A different double-blinded randomized study found the flavonoid intervention did not significantly change CCA-IMT, augmentation index, or blood pressure, but pulse pressure variability improved. In a subgroup with pulse wave velocity data, a 10% CV risk reduction over control patients was observed in high risk patients already using cholesterol lowering drugs (Curtis et al. 2013). These findings suggest that a high flavonoid diet would prevent further circulatory damage.

13.6.4 Atherosclerosis

Atherosclerosis is often the underlying pathological condition of CVD. The condition involves the initiation and perpetuation of atherosclerotic lesions, which erode or rupture, resulting in acute CVD events, such as poor blood flow, myocardial infarction, or cerebrovascular attack. Atherosclerosis is a risk factor for many CVD, and is caused by oxidation of cholesterol, lipids, and other products resulting in narrower passageways for blood circulation. It can be thought of as a combination of poor blood lipid status, constricted blood vessels, and blood circulation issues. Atherosclerosis can lead to any of the acute CVD death events, so prevention and treatment can reduce its impact on CVD. Flavonoids are often studied specifically for their therapeutic potential on atherosclerosis.

OS results from an imbalance between excessive formation of reactive oxygen or nitrogen species and limited antioxidant defenses. Endothelium and NO are key regulators of vascular health. NO bioavailability is modulated by ROS that degrade NO, uncouple NO synthase, and inhibit synthesis. These processes lead to the development of endothelial dysfunction, which has been identified as an initial step to atherosclerosis. Flavonoids have shown to improve vascular function through increased endothelial nitric oxide (eNOS) production in animals and humans, but many of these studies have lacked placebo controls and large sample sizes (Rimbach et al. 2009). Red wine has been evaluated as a way of reducing LDL oxidation and lowering atherosclerosis risk. The results indicate that cells treated with red wine showed a reduced amount of copper-induced LDL (Kerry and Abbey 1997).

Licorice root has been used in traditional Chinese medicine to treat a number of ailments; when examined for flavonoid content, licorice root extract yielded five flavonoids: liquiritin, liquiritigenin, isoliquiritigenin, and 7,4′-dihydroxyflavone (Jayaprakasam et al. 2009). Supplementation of licorice root extract to hypercholesterolemic patients for a period of 1 month, followed by an additional 1 month of placebo consumption was examined. Licorice consumption resulted in a moderate reduction in the patients' plasma susceptibility to lipid peroxidation (by 19%), and a marked reduction in the susceptibility of plasma LDL oxidation. LDL oxidation slowed by 55%, in comparison to the lag time of LDL isolated from plasma derived before licorice extract consumption (Aviram 2004).

A study by Kapetivadze examined the effect of flavonoid supplementation in combination with the anti-hypertension drug indapamide in diabetic patients. After 10 weeks, results showed an observed reduction of total cholesterol by 7%, LDL cholesterol was reduced by 10%, total glucose was reduced by 9.4%, and HDL cholesterol concentration increased by 8%. These results suggest a benefit for flavonoid supplementation in combination with drug treatment for atherosclerosis (Kapetivadze et al. 2010).

Various medications are recommended to assist in treating this condition including ACE inhibitors, antiplatelet drugs, and many others. Recent studies have found that flavonoids function in many of the same ways as ACE inhibitors and antiplatelet drugs. Individuals with high intakes of flavonoids show effective dilation of blood vessels. Flavonoids also have been shown to inhibit the formation of clots in the blood (Wright et al. 2012).

13.7 FLAVONOID SUPPLEMENTATION AND ACUTE CVD/CVD MORTALITY

13.7.1 Congestive Heart Failure

Congestive heart failure is a diagnosis of various issues that pertain to the efficiency at which the heart pumps blood through the body and the declining strength of the heart muscle. Congestive heart failure can be caused by many other conditions, including coronary artery disease (CAD), peripheral arterial disease (PAD), atherosclerosis, heart attack, cardiomyopathy, and conditions that overwork the heart, such as hypertension (AHA 2011).

There are different types of heart failure, affecting different areas in the heart and inhibiting the amount of blood filling the heart. This limits the amount of oxygen-rich blood pumped throughout the body. Systolic dysfunction occurs when the heart muscle does not contract with enough force; therefore, decreased amounts of oxygenated blood will be pumped throughout the body (AHA 2011). Diastolic dysfunction mainly affects the ventricles of the heart. The heart muscles contract normally; however, the ventricles cannot properly relax or become stiff, inhibiting the heart's normal filling capacity, meaning less blood will exit the heart; this inhibits major organs and tissues from receiving the required amounts of blood in order to normally function (AHA 2011). Angioplasty and stents are medical procedures that attempt to unblock heart arteries. In cases where the two above methods do not succeed, heart bypass surgery is necessary to unblock coronary arteries (AHA 2011). These are costly interventions, and they may not be able to be administered in time to prolong life. Flavonoid consumption has been investigated as a way to avoid the development of congestive heart failure (Wright et al. 2012).

According to various studies, many experts have recommended increased intakes of flavonoid-rich diets for heart failure preventative purposes (Peterson et al. 2012).

In the Dutch Zutphen Elderly Study cohort, flavonoids in the diet were analyzed for 805 men, aged 65–84. Their diet consisted of: tea (61%), onions (13%), and apples (10%). Their total flavonoid intake was 25.9 mg per day. At both 5 and 10-year follow-ups, flavones and flavonols were associated with reduced coronary heart disease (CHD) mortality. Also, higher intake of flavan-3-ols, specifically, catechins and epicatechins, showed a reduced risk of CHD after a 10-year follow-up. Similarly, in Finnish populations, quercetin and kaempferol were associated with lower CHD mortality; quercetin showed a significant decrease in mortality, while kaempferol showed a small effect on mortality (Knekt et al. 2002).

13.7.2 Ischemic Heart Disease and Myocardial Infarction

Ischemic heart disease is characterized by a blockage in the coronary arteries that reduces the flow of blood as it returns to the heart. Myocardial infarction (MI) is the most common diagnosis when referring to these types of blockages. MI is the irreversible death of heart muscle tissue due to the loss of oxygen via insufficient blood flow to a section of the heart. Many studies have analyzed the effect that various flavonoids have on the prevention of MI in select populations. Despite some disagreement, the results are promising, suggesting that flavonoid consumption may have a positive effect on the prevention of MI.

A cohort study that was conducted over an 18-year time span yielded promising information correlating anthocyanin intake with a lower risk of developing MI. When 93,600 women were examined over an 18-year period, 405 cases of MI were reported. When analyzing the diets of patients the biggest inverse association correlated with women who consumed 58–643 mg of flavonoids per day (2–35 mg were anthocyanins). The 15 mg increase in anthocyanins decreased risk of MI by 17%. Interestingly, the authors also concluded that combined intakes of blueberries and strawberries decreased risk of MI compared to participants who consumed less than three servings per week of those fruits (Cassidy et al. 2013).

Many cohort studies estimate dietary consumption of flavonoids and relate it to the observed incidence of CVD. Table 13.6 summarizes a portion of these results. The Rotterdam Study released by the American Journal of Clinical Nutrition compared MI incidence in black tea-drinkers and nondrinkers. A longitudinal study of 4807 individuals with no previous MI history reported that the relative risk of MI was lower for subjects consuming >375 mL tea per day compared with non-tea drinkers (RR = 0.57; 033–0.98). Drinking tea even more strongly lowered the risk of fatal MI (RR = 0.35; 0.13–0.98) when the highest and lowest tertiles of tea consumption were compared (Geleijnse et al. 2002).

The Finnish Mobile Clinic Health Examination Survey also found an inverse correlation between quercetin intake and ischemic heart disease. Comparing the highest and lowest levels of quercetin intake as determined from surveys shows RR = 0.79; 0.63–0.99, with statistically significant results ($p < 0.02$) (Knekt et al. 2002).

Two of the largest health studies in the United States did not find a significant inverse correlation between flavonoids and ischemia. The Women's Health Study observed 38,445 women for 6.9 years for CVD risks and events. The highest level of flavonoid consumption had an age-adjusted RR = 0.88 (0.63–1.24), but the results

TABLE 13.6
Table Summarizing Several Flavonoid Studies on Acute CVD and Their Outcomes

Location	Population	Mean Follow-Up	Outcome	Diet	Results (Relative Risk, 95% Confidence Interval)	Source
Zutphen elderly study (Netherlands)	804 M	10 years	CHD mortality and MI outcome	Flavonol	RR of CHD mortality for the highest tertile of daily flavonol consumption (more than 29 mg) compared to the lowest (less than 19 mg) was 0.47 (0.27–0.82) $p = 0.006$. RR for MI incidence for highest tertile compared to lowest was 0.62 (0.24–1.05) $p = 0.078$.	Hertog et al. (1997)
Caerphilly Study (UK)	1900 M	14 years	IHD mortality	Black tea	Flavonol intake, highest compared to lowest quartile, was weakly positively corellated to IHD mortality RR = 1.6 (0.9–2.9) $p = 0.119$.	Hertog et al. (1997)
Rotterdam study (Netherlands)	4807 M and W	5.6 years	MI incidence and MI fatality	Flavonoids, tea	The RR of MI incidence for highest tertile (>375 mL/daily) compared to non-drinkers was 0.57 (0.33–0.98). The intake of dietary flavonoids was significantly inversely associated with fatal MI (RR: 0.35 (0.13–0.98)) in upper compared with lower tertiles of intake.	Geleijnse et al. (2002)
Finnish Mobile clinic health examination survey	10,054 M and W	28 years	IHD mortality	Quercetin	The highest quartile of quercetin intake was correlated with lower mortality from IHD compared to lowest quartile, RR: 0.79 (0.63–0.99) $p = 0.02$.	Knekt et al. (2002)
Womens health study (USA)	38,445 W	6.9 years	CVD risk and events	Flavonoids, tea	For both CVD and important vascular events, age and treatment adjusted RR was 0.88 (0.63, 1.24) $p = 0.16$. A small proportion of women consuming >4 cups tea/d had a non-significant ($p = 0.07$) reduction in event risk. Flavonoid intakes were non-significantly inversely correllated with CVD risks and events.	Sesso et al. (2003)

(Continued)

TABLE 13.6 (*Continued*)
Table Summarizing Several Flavonoid Studies on Acute CVD and Their Outcomes

Location	Population	Mean Follow-Up	Outcome	Diet	Results (Relative Risk, 95% Confidence Interval)	Source
Nurses health study (USA)	66,360 W	12 years	MI and CHD fatality	Flavonol, flavone	Women in the highest quintile of flavonol and flavone intake had RR for nonfatal MI (RR: 1.05, 0.85, 1.29; $p = 0.55$) and CHD death (RR: 0.81, 0.57–1.16; $p = 0.29$) compared to lowest quintile. Both results were non-significant.	Lin et al. (2007)
Iowa womens study (USA)	34,489 W	16 years	CHD, CVD and total mortality	Anthocyanidins, flavanones, flavones	Adjusted RR between highest and lowest consumption quintiles for anthocyanidins and CHD (0.88 (0.78, 0.99)) and CVD (0.91 (0.83, 0.99)); between flavanones and CHD (RR: 0.78 (0.65, 0.94)); and between flavones and total mortality (RR: 0.88 (0.82, 0.96)). These results were all significant ($p < 0.05$).	Mink et al. (2007)

weren't significant ($p < 0.07$). Consumption of more than four cups tea per day also non-significantly correlated with the risk of cardiovascular events (Sesso et al. 2003). The Nurses Health Study also found non-significant relationships between total flavonol and flavone intake and non-fatal MI (RR = 1.05; 0.85–1.29; $p < 0.55$) and fatal CHD event (RR = 0.81; 0.57–1.16; $p < 0.29$) (J. Lin et al. 2007). The Iowa Women's Study analyzed intake of anthocyanins, flavanones, and flavones separately, finding significant differences. Comparing the highest and lowest quintiles of consumption, anthocyanidins were associated with reduced risk of CHD (RR = 0.88; 0.78–0.99) and CVD (RR = 0.91; 0.83–0.99), while flavanones were associated with reduced risk of CHD (RR = 0.78; 0.82–0.96) and flavones with total mortality (RR = 0.88; 0.82–0.96)(Mink et al. 2007).

Several animal studies have also shown individual flavonoids to have a protective effect against ischemia. One study used rats to look at the modulation of vascular ion channels stemming from NO release after flavonoid consumption as a way to reduce ischemic disease. Pre-treatment with flavonoids with these substitutions decreased the time required to reach half-maximal contracture and the maximum ischemic contracture, while the non-substituted flavonoids (4'-hydroxyflavanone, 6-hydroxyflavanone, and 7-hydroxyflavanone) did not improve post-ischemia functional parameters (Testai et al. 2013). Also, these flavonoids improved post-ischemia recovery.

The preventative effects of epicatechin on lysosomal alterations—a marker that accompanies ischemic myocellular damage—showed that when the lysosomal membrane is compromised there could be an elevation of undesirable enzymes in intra- and extracellular space. The ability to maintain normal levels of lysosomal enzymes in body fluids/tissues would also be compromised in this state. When there is localization of acid hydrolases in the cardiac myocytes of the lysosomes, enzyme release into the cytosol will follow, leading to myocardial injury or cellular death. Alterations in the activity of lysosomal enzymes have been connected to patients that experience MI. Epicatechin reduced myocardial damage in MI-induced rats (Stanely and Prince 2013). This suggests that certain flavonoids provide a specific benefit to treating and preventing ischemic heart disease (Testai et al. 2013).

13.7.3 Stroke

Stroke is the second leading cause of death both in developed and developing countries (WHO 2013), and there are a growing number of studies examining the relationship between flavonoids and stroke incidence. Some earlier studies examined total stroke occurrence, rather than separating into categories based on the nature of the cardiovascular event. These two main categories are ischemic and hemorrhagic stroke.

Ischemic stroke occurs when blood flow is restricted to the brain. This most often results due to narrowing of the blood vessels in the brain caused by atherosclerosis. Hypertension is the greatest controllable risk factor for ischemic stroke (Roger et al. 2012). In terms of both mortality and frequency of occurrence, ischemic stroke is more dominant than hemorrhagic stroke in the United States.

Hemorrhagic strokes occur after vascular rupture in the brain (intracerebral), or just outside the brain (subarachnoid), forces blood into the surrounding area causing compression on the brain tissue. The most important diet-related risk factor for hemorrhagic stroke is hypertension, which strains the blood vessels, although the causes of hemorrhagic stroke are less known than ischemic stroke. Due to the different mechanisms of action, ischemic and hemorrhagic stroke should be analyzed separately in future cohort studies. Due to the difficulty of directly measuring the effects of flavonoids on stroke, especially in small, clinical trials, many studies assess a number of risk factors for stroke instead. These risk factors may include atherosclerosis, hypertension, HDL, and LDL cholesterol levels, and flow-mediated dilation. Table 13.7 describes the large, population-based studies that have been conducted to date examining the effects of flavonoid intake on stroke risk.

The potential health effects of dietary flavonoids have been studied extensively, but the relationship between flavonoids and stroke have been inconsistent. The Zutphen study (Keli et al. 1996) was an early prospective cohort study that examined total dietary intake of flavonoids based on participant evaluations. The relative risk (RR) of stroke incidence for flavonoid consumption of 28.6 mg/day or greater was 0.27 (0.11–0.70) compared to consumption of less than 18.3 mg/day. They also examined tea intake, showing a RR of 0.31 (0.12–0.84) for daily consumption of more than 4.7 cups of tea compared to less than 2.6 cups. While this study brought early attention to flavonoids as having possible benefits on stroke incidence, the small sample (n = 552) only examined men.

More recent studies have focused on tea as a primary source of flavonoids. Excluding water, tea is the most commonly consumed beverage in the world (Cheng 2006). Black tea is the most commonly produced variety, with an estimated 76%–78% of total production. In the USA, 80% of tea consumption is black tea (Basu and Lucas 2007). Tea varieties have been studied independently, including green tea (Tanabe et al. 2008) or black tea (Gans et al. 2010). More recent studies have looked at total tea intake (Lopez-Garcia et al. 2009; Larsson, Virtamo, and Wolk 2013; Leurs et al. 2010). The Tokamachi–Nakasato study focused specifically on several levels of green tea intake in Japan (n = 6,358) (Tanabe et al. 2008). Both middle (several times per week: RR = 0.43, 0.25–0.74; $p < 0.002$) and high (several cups daily: RR = 0.41, 0.24–0.70; $p < 0.001$) tea intakes were associated with a considerably lower risk of total stroke incidence. Even after separation of cerebral infarction and cerebral hemorrhage, the results were consistently statistically significant. Similar results were found when looking primarily at black tea consumption (Gans et al. 2010). After adjusting for age and sex, high tea consumption (4.1–6 cups a day) was associated with a reduced risk of total stroke (RR = 0.69, 0.50–0.95, $p < 0.07$). However, the trend was non-significant when adjusted for additional lifestyle variables such as physical activity, waist circumference and alcohol consumption (RR = 0.92, 0.66–1.28; $p < 0.63$). Despite the large sample size (n = 37,514), only 70 incidences of stroke-related mortality were observed. Additional studies are needed to evaluate this relationship.

A more recent Finnish study with a great number of stroke occurrences also found an inverse correlation between tea intake and total stroke(Larsson, Virtamo, and Wolk 2013). Consumption of more than four cups of tea per day showed had a statistically significant impact (RR = 0.77, 0.61–0.98) on all strokes, split up by the type of event.

European studies have also embraced the potential protective power of the flavonoids in chocolate. Early research on the subject suggested that chocolate

TABLE 13.7
Table Summarizing Several Flavonoid Studies on Stroke Risk and Their Outcomes

Location	Population	Mean Follow-Up	Diet	Results	Source
Finland	34,670 W 40,291 M	10.2 years	Tea	More than four cups of tea a day showed statistically significant decrease in stroke risk. RR = 0.77 (95% CI, 0.61–0.98)	Larsson et al. (2013)
Swedish mammography	33,372 W	10.4 years	Cocoa	The adjusted RR for a 50 g/week increase of chocolate consumption were 0.89 (95% CI: 0.73–1.09) for women with a history of hypertension and 0.85 (95% CI, 0.74–0.97) for women without hypertension.	Larsson et al. (2011)
Swedish cohort of men	37,103 M	10.2 years	Cocoa	The multivariate relative risk of stroke comparing the highest quartile of chocolate consumption (median 62.9 g/week) with the lowest quartile (median 0 g/week) was 0.83 (95% CI, 0.70–0.99).	Larson et al. (2012)
Nurses Health study (US)	69,622 W	14.0 years	Dietary flavonoids	Women in the highest compared to lowest quintile of flavanone intake had a relative risk (RR) of ischemic stroke of 0.81 and 95% CI = 0.66–0.99, $p = 0.04$. Citrus fruits/juices, the main dietary source of flavanones, tended to be associated with a reduced risk for ischemic stroke (RR = 0.90 and 95% CI = 0.77–1.05).	Cassidy et al. (2012)
Zutphen study	552 M	15.0 years	Dietary flavonoids	The relative risk (RR) of the highest vs the lowest quartile of flavonoid intake (> or = 28.6 mg/d vs <18.3 mg/d) was 0.27 (95% confidence interval [CI], 0.11–0.70). Black tea contributed about 70% to flavonoid intake. The RR for a daily tea consumption of 4.7 cups or more vs less than 2.6 cups was 0.31 (95% CI, 0.12–0.84).	Keli et al. (1996)

(*Continued*)

TABLE 13.7 (*Continued*)

Table Summarizing Several Flavonoid Studies on Stroke Risk and Their Outcomes

Germany	10,904 M 16,644 W	8 years	Cocoa	The adjusted RR for comparing top vs. bottom quartiles was 0.52 (0.30–0.89) for stroke.	Buijsse et al. (2010)
Tokamachi-Nakasato (Japan)	2087 M 4271 W	5 years	Tea	A lower risk was observed for total stroke incidence in both the middle (multivariable HR, 0.43; 95% CI, 0.25–0.74; $p = 0.002$) and the high (multivariable HR, 0.41; 95% CI, 0.24–0.70; $p = 0.001$) categories of green tea consumption.	Tanabe et al. (2008)
Nurses health study (US)	83,076 W	24 years	Tea	RR = 0.79 (0.49–1.29) 0.19	Lopez-Garcia et al. (2010)
Netherlands cohort study	120,852 M and W	10 years	Tea	For tea, moderate (1–2 cups/d) and high tea consumption (3 cups/d) were inversely related to IHD mortality in men (HR: 0–75; 95% CI 0–61, 0–93 and HR: 0–71, 95% CI 0–57, 0–88, respectively ($p = 0.007$)) compared with 0–1 cup/d of tea consumption	Leurs et al. (2010)
Epic-NL cohort (Dutch)	37,514 M and W	13 years	Tea	Tea consumption tended to be associated ($p = 0.07$) with a reduced risk of stroke with the lowest HR for 4.1 to 6.0 cups per day (0.69; 95% CI, 0.50–0.95). This relation attenuated to nonsignificant after multivariate adjustment (HR, 0.92; 95% CI, 0.66–1.28; Ptrend = 0.63).	de Koning Gans et al. (2010)

consumption may reduce blood pressure by increasing NO production. A review of the dietary intake of chocolate in Germany found that increased chocolate intake was associated with a lower total risk of stroke (RR = 0.52, 0.30–0.89). The authors of the study proposed that the beneficial effects of chocolate intake were due to reductions in blood pressure, a risk factor for stroke (Buijsse et al. 2010).

More recent studies have built on this framework by examining the effects of chocolate on both ischemic and hemorrhagic stroke, separately. The Swedish Mammography study evaluated women (n = 33,372) over 10.4 years, and found that a 50 g/week increase in chocolate consumption was associated with a decreased risk for total stroke (RR = 0.86, 0.77–0.96), cerebral infarction (RR = 0.88, 0.77–0.99), and hemorrhagic stroke (RR = 0.73, 0.54–0.99). However, the results were only significant for women in the highest quartile of chocolate consumption, suggesting higher doses are necessary for a protective effects (Larsson, Virtamo, and Wolk 2011). The Swedish cohort of Men (n = 37,103) found similar results after 10.2 years, but even higher chocolate consumption was necessary for a protective effect. Men in the highest quartile of consumption (62.9 g/week) had a relative risk for total stroke of 0.83 (0.70–0.99) compared to the lowest quartile (Larsson, Virtamo, and Wolk 2012).

These results of these three studies are promising, however, the caloric density of chocolate is a concern. Daily doses of 100 g dark chocolate have been shown to decrease systolic blood pressure, but the increased daily caloric intake (nearly 480 kcal) may counteract the cardiovascular benefits (Taubert D et al. 2003). An extract of flavonoids from cocoa, if effective, may provide the protective benefits in a less calorie-dense form.

Not all prospective cohort studies have found flavonoids to be protective against stroke. The Nurses Health Study in the United States (n = 69,622) found no evidence for an inverse association between flavonoid intake (flavonols and flavanones) and total, ischemic, or hemorrhagic stroke (Cassidy et al. 2012). However, there were only 253 cases of hemorrhagic stroke, so additional studies are needed. The same study also compared stroke risk with green and black tea consumption. High consumption levels (more than 4 cups/day) tended to be associated with a reduced risk of total stroke (RR = 0.79, 0.49–1.29), but the results were not significant ($p < 0.19$) (Lopez-Garcia et al. 2009).

There is a growing amount of evidence suggesting flavonoids may provide protective benefits from stroke, but additional studies are warranted before clear recommendations can be made. Individual flavonoids need to be evaluated in randomized studies to determine if the protective effects are due to the flavonoids, their metabolites, or synergistic effects between flavonoids and their food source.

13.8 PROPOSED MECHANISMS OF FLAVONOID-INDUCED CVD PREVENTION AND TREATMENT

The complexity of biological systems makes it difficult to understand the mechanisms flavonoids use to prevent and treat CVD. The flavonoid mechanisms in metabolism outlined in Section 3 present many possibilities for CVD interactions. The many forms of CVD outlined in Table 13.3 provide different symptoms and risk factors. Over 5000 flavonoids have been characterized that provide different cellular impacts. The following focuses on the mechanisms of flavonoid CVD prevention and treatment.

Ingestion of green tea catechins may prevent CVD by reducing the intestinal absorption of cholesterol and other dietary lipids. It appears that EGCG interferes with the emulsification of fats by limiting digestion through inhibition of phospholipase A2 and micellar solubilization of lipids; thus, limiting fat absorption efficiency (Koo and Noh 2007).

In vitro studies of red wine flavonoids found an association with CVD prevention, which was attributed to the prevention of LDL oxidation through flavonoids antioxidant potential (Kerry and Abbey 1997). Flavonoids are efficient free-radical scavengers in vitro, but serum concentrations are typically much lower than other dietary antioxidants (Chun, Kim, and Lee 2003).

In animal models, flavonoids have the potential to reduce inflammation and protect against hypertension and atherosclerosis. Chronic quercetin supplementation in mice reduces LPS-induced inflammation (Patil et al. 2003). Green tea consumption protects against hypertension by reportedly decreasing OS and inflammation (Bhardwaj and Khanna 2013). Nuclear factor (erythroid-derived 2)-like 2 (Nrf2) is a transcriptional regulator of phase II antioxidant enzymes, and activation of Nrf2 has been suggested to be an important step in reducing OS associated with CVD (Reuland et al. 2013).

In vivo work has found that the epicatechins present in green tea inhibit the formation of oxidized serum cholesterol, which prevents progression toward atherosclerosis (Basu and Lucas 2007). Flavonoids can improve cerebral blood flow and prevent platelet aggregation (Perez-Vizcaino and Duarte 2010). Flavonoids also promote activation of eNOS, which increases the bioavailability of NO in the system by reducing formation of RNS and leads to dilatory effects (Sudano et al. 2012). Hypertension is considered the most important risk factor for cerebral infarction (Tanabe et al. 2008; Ikeda et al. 2007). Green tea also led to a reduction in atherosclerosis in rabbits by decreasing vascular endothelial growth factors expressed in atherosclerotic plaque (Kavantzas et al. 2006).

Flavan-3-ols, flavonols and proanthocyanidins have shown an effect on ACE activity by inhibiting the conversion of angiotensin, thus preventing blood pressure increases (Actis-Goretta et al. 2003; Balasuriya and Rupasinghe 2012). This suggests that the in vivo reduction in blood pressure is related to the ACE inhibition of flavonols. Flavonoids may also inhibit PDI reductase, an enzyme that participates in thrombus formation, which can lead to stroke. The flavonol rutin was shown to inhibit PDI reductase in vitro (Jasuja et al. 2012).

Modulation of vascular ion channels stemming from NO release is a major way flavonoids reduce ischemia mortality, likely due to flavonoids' antioxidant capabilities (Testai et al. 2013). Previous studies conducted by these researchers have found that the flavones, apigenin, kaempferol, naringenin, and the isoflavone, daidzein, have demonstrated vasodilatory properties. There has also been recent evidence that flavonoids, vitexin, proanthocyanidin, orientin, and luteolin, exhibit cardioprotective effects in experimental models of myocardial I/R injury (Testai et al. 2013).

Compared to the hearts from the vehicle-treated rats, the rats pre-treated with the flavonoids that had the hydroxy or methoxy substitution exhibited higher rate pressure product and coronary flow values throughout the entire reperfusion time.

In addition to the prevention of stroke, several studies have proposed flavonoid supplementation as a means of reducing the severity of acute stroke damage (Chen et al. 2011; Perez-Vizcaino and Duarte 2010). Epicatechin doses administered to mice showed a neuroprotective effect during the 6-h window from stroke onset to irreversible neuron death (Shah et al. 2010). Reducing stroke severity may increase the likelihood of surviving the stroke. High anthocyanin consumption was found to impact neutrophil NADPH oxidase activity ultimately increasing blood flow (Rodriguez-Mateos et al. 2013). Inhibiting NADPH oxidase limited the ROS in the brain, reducing the damage after a stroke (Actis-Goretta et al. 2003).

Researchers have found that only the 5-hydroxy-substituted derivatives (5-hydroxy flavone, apigenin, chrysin, naringenin) improved post-ischemia functional recovery and a decrease in tissue injuries (Testai et al. 2013); 5-methoxy-flavone showed similar effects as well. Therefore, the capabilities of flavonoids were attributed to the 5-hydroxy-substituted derivatives (Testai et al. 2013). Further research is needed both in CVD development and flavonoid activity to pinpoint the exact way that flavonoid supplementation works to prevent CVD.

13.9 CONCLUSION

In this chapter, evidence was collected in order to better understand the mechanisms by which flavonoids prevent CVD and other risk factors. The powerful connection between flavonoid consumption and heart health has been identified through various studies. It should also be noted that there is a potential concern with over supplementation of flavonoid extracts, specifically those that have high absorption capabilities. The doses found in dietary sources of flavonoids appear to be safe.

In many previous studies, antioxidant and anti-inflammatory activity are separated; however, they work together. For example, antioxidants quench reactive reactions but regulation of iNOS prevents the formation of those radicals in the first place. The main functions of flavonoids in human metabolism include: antioxidant potential and formation prevention, reduction of chronic inflammation, phase II enzyme detoxification, microflora metabolism/interactions, and potential negative metabolic effects. The interactions between intestinal microbiota and flavonoids have not been characterized, which is a new frontier of possible research.

Many epidemiological studies use specific events such as heart attack and stroke to evaluate the protective benefits of flavonoids. The complexity of biological systems makes it difficult to understand exactly how flavonoids impact CVD. There are many possible effects of flavonoid supplementation: flavonoids lower LDL/blood lipid profiles by reducing absorption and decreasing delivery; they reduce chronic inflammation by preventing radical formation; they reduce COX enzyme activity and decrease iNOS production and flavonoids work as antioxidants to prevent LDL oxidation/foam cell development. The vasodilatory impact on hypertension, increasing eNOS (dilatory effects), preventing platelet aggregation, and performing phase II enzymatic detoxification; however, these correlations ignore the possible protection that flavonoids may provide earlier in life. Age plays an important role in metabolism and absorption, and additional research on younger subjects may help evaluate the role of flavonoids before the onset and progression of CVD.

Moving forward, there will be foods that are developed specifically with higher or more bioavailable flavonoid contents. For example, genetically engineered tomatoes have been produced that have increased levels of rutin and kaempferol (Le Gall et al. 2003). Innovations in increasing bioavailability and creating isolated supplements need to be tested thoroughly before being distributed. Randomized trials are needed to establish the bioavailability of individual flavonoids and their metabolites, and to determine if the beneficial effects are actually due to the individual compounds or to synergistic effects between flavonoids and their food source. The importance of flavonoid dosage is absent from much of the literature. The preventative effects appear to be dose dependent, and high dose supplementation may lead to adverse health effects.

When investigating CVD and the impact of flavonoids, it is beneficial to understand that CVD is a collection of diseases and risk factors that affect individuals differently. The two categories of risk factors are better understood as diseases that can directly lead to death (such as ischemia, heart failure and stroke) and chronic diseases (such as atherosclerosis, hypertension, and peripheral heart disease). Therefore, the various flavonoids mentioned have different mechanisms and effects on these conditions. Separating the different types of CVD and specific causes can allow for cross-referencing flavonoid types, and the mechanisms of prevention they may exhibit.

For every $6 spent on health care, $1 goes toward treatment for CVD, and this trend is projected to increase over the next several decades. This is an exponential amount of resources that includes health care services, medications, and losses in productivity. Looking at the different types of CVD diagnoses on a global scale, ischemic heart disease predominates Europe, North and South America, and the Eastern Mediterranean. Cerebrovascular CVD deaths are more prominent in Africa, Southeast Asia, and the Western-Pacific. These regional differences are linked with lifestyle differences, mainly diet. Looking at these statistics and the different dietary habits of different populations, the data exhibits the effect that food has on heart health.

It can be concluded that flavonoid consumption has strong potential to improve heart and vascular health by inhibiting various risk factors that lead to CVD diagnoses in individuals all over the world.

REFERENCES

Actis-Goretta, Lucas, Javier I. Ottaviani, Carl L. Keen, and Cesar G. Fraga. 2003. Inhibition of angiotensin converting enzyme (ACE) activity by flavan-3-ols and procyanidins. *FEBS Letters* 555 (3) (December 18): 597–600.

Arts, Ilja C. W. and Peter C. H. Hollman. 2005. Polyphenols and disease risk in epidemiologic studies. *The American Journal of Clinical Nutrition* 81 (1) (January 1): 317S–325S.

Aruoma, Okezie I., Harparkash Kaur, and Barry Halliwell. 1991. Oxygen free radicals and human diseases. *The Journal of the Royal Society for the Promotion of Health* 111 (5) (October 1): 172–177.

Aviram, Michael. 2004. Flavonoids-rich nutrients with potent antioxidant activity prevent atherosclerosis development: The licorice example. *International Congress Series* 1262 (May): 320–327.

Balasuriya, Nileeka, and H. P. Vasantha Rupasinghe. 2012. Antihypertensive properties of flavonoid-rich apple peel extract. *Food Chemistry* 135 (4) (December 15): 2320–2325.

Basu, Arpita, and Edralin A. Lucas. 2007. Mechanisms and effects of green tea on cardiovascular health. *Nutrition Reviews* 65 (8): 361–375.

Berliner, J. A., Mohamad Navab, Alan M. Fogelman, Joy S. Frank, Linda L. Demer, Peter A. Edwards, Andrew D. Watson, and Aldons J. Lusis. 1995. Atherosclerosis: Basic mechanisms. oxidation, inflammation, and genetics. *Circulation* 91 (9) (May 1): 2488–2496.

Bhardwaj, Pooja, and Deepa Khanna. 2013. Green tea catechins: Defensive role in cardiovascular disorders. *Chinese Journal of Natural Medicines* 11 (4) (July): 345–353.

Bolli, Alessandro, Maria Marino, Gerald Rimbach, Gabriella Fanali, Mauro Fasano, and Paolo Ascenzi. 2010. Flavonoid binding to human serum albumin. *Biochemical and Biophysical Research Communications* 398 (3) (July 30): 444–449.

Buijsse, Brian, Cornelia Weikert, Dagmar Drogan, Manuela Bergmann, and Heiner Boeing. 2010. Chocolate consumption in relation to blood pressure and risk of cardiovascular disease in german adults. *European Heart Journal* 31 (13) (July 1): 1616–1623.

Cassidy, Aedín, Kenneth J. Mukamal, Lydia Liu, Mary Franz, A. Heather Eliassen, and Eric B. Rimm. 2013. High anthocyanin intake is associated with a reduced risk of myocardial infarction in young and middle-aged women. *Circulation* 127 (2) (January 14): 188–196.

Cassidy, Aedín, Eric B. Rimm, Éilis J. O'Reilly, Giancarlo Logroscino, Colin Kay, Stephanie E. Chiuve, and Kathryn M. Rexrode. 2012. Dietary flavonoids and risk of stroke in women. *Stroke* 43 (4) (April 1): 946–951.

CDC–DHDSP. 2013. High cholesterol prevention: What you can do. Accessed December 1. http://www.cdc.gov/cholesterol/what_you_can_do.htm.

Chen, Chi, Rong Yu, Edward D. Owuor, and A. N. Tony Kong. 2000. Activation of antioxidant-response element (ARE), mitogen-activated protein kinases (MAPKs) and caspases by major green tea polyphenol components during cell survival and death. *Archives of Pharmacological Research* 23 (6) (December): 605–612.

Chen, Lei, Xiao-ying Bi, Li-xun Zhu, Yi-qing Qiu, Su-ju Ding, and Ben-qiang Deng. 2011. Flavonoids of puerarin versus tanshinone II A for ischemic stroke: A randomized controlled trial. *Journal of Chinese Integrative Medicine* 9 (11) (November): 1215–1220.

Cheng, Tsung O. 2006. All teas are not created equal: The chinese green tea and cardiovascular health. *International Journal of Cardiology* 108 (3) (April 14): 301–308.

Chuang, Chia-Chi, Kristina Martinez, Guoxiang Xie, Arion Kennedy, Akkarach Bumrungpert, Angel Overman, Wei Jia, and Michael K McIntosh. 2010. Quercetin is equally or more effective than resveratrol in attenuating tumor necrosis factor-α-mediated inflammation and insulin resistance in primary human adipocytes. *The American Journal of Clinical Nutrition* 92 (6) (December): 1511–1521.

Chun, Ock Kyoung, Dae-Ok Kim, and Chang Yong Lee. 2003. Superoxide radical scavenging activity of the major polyphenols in fresh plums. *Journal of Agricultural and Food Chemistry* 51 (27) (December 31): 8067–8072.

Costa, Ana Rita de Mello, Flávia Silva Marquiafável, Mirela Mara de Oliveira Lima Leite Vaz, Bruno Alves Rocha, Paula Carolina Pires Bueno, Pedro Luiz M. Amaral, Hernane da Silva Barud, and Andresa Ap Berreta-Silva. 2011. Quercetin-PVP K25 solid dispersions. *Journal of Thermal Analysis and Calorimetry* 104 (1) (April 1): 273–278.

Crozier, Alan, Indu B. Jaganath, and Michael N. Clifford. 2009. Dietary phenolics: Chemistry, bioavailability and effects on health. *Natural Product Reports* 26 (8) (July 22): 1001–1043.

Curtis, Peter J., John Potter, Paul A. Kroon, Paddy Wilson, Ketan Dhatariya, Mike Sampson, and Aedín Cassidy. 2013. Vascular function and atherosclerosis progression after 1 y of flavonoid intake in statin-treated postmenopausal women with type 2 diabetes: A double-blind randomized controlled trial. *American Journal of Clinical Nutrition* 97 (5) (April 3): 936–942.

Curtis, Peter J., Mike Sampson, John Potter, Ketan Dhatariya, Paul A. Kroon, and Aedín Cassidy. 2012. Chronic ingestion of flavan-3-ols and isoflavones improves insulin sensitivity and lipoprotein status and attenuates estimated 10-year CVD risk in medicated postmenopausal women with type 2 diabetes a 1-year, double-blind, randomized, controlled trial. *Diabetes Care* 35 (2) (February 1): 226–232.

de Pascual-Teresa, Sonia, Diego A. Moreno, and Cristina García-Viguera. 2010. Flavanols and anthocyanins in cardiovascular health: A review of current evidence. *International Journal of Molecular Sciences* 11 (4) (April 13): 1679–1703.

Duffy, Stephen J, and Joseph A Vita. 2003. Effects of phenolics on vascular endothelial function. *Current Opinion in Lipidology* 14 (1) (February): 21–27.

Dulloo, Abdul G., Claudette Duret, Dorothee Rohrer, Lucien Girardier, Nouri Mensi, Marc Fathi, Philippe Chantre, and Jacques Vandermander. 1999. Efficacy of a green tea extract rich in catechin polyphenols and caffeine in increasing 24-h energy expenditure and fat oxidation in humans. *The American Journal of Clinical Nutrition* 70 (6) (December): 1040–1045.

Edwards, Randi L., Tiffany Lyon, Sheldon E. Litwin, Alexander Rabovsky, J. David Symons, and Thunder Jalili. 2007. Quercetin reduces blood pressure in hypertensive subjects. *The Journal of Nutrition* 137 (11) (November 1): 2405–2411.

Erdman, John W., Douglas Balentine, Lenore Arab, Gary Beecher, Johanna T. Dwyer, John Folts, James Harnly et al. 2007. Flavonoids and heart health: Proceedings of the ILSI north america flavonoids workshop, May 31–June 1, 2005, Washington, DC. *The Journal of Nutrition* 137 (3) (March 1): 718S–737S.

Espín, Juan Carlos, María Teresa García-Conesa, and Francisco A. Tomás-Barberán. 2007. Nutraceuticals: Facts and fiction. *Phytochemistry* 68 (22–24) (November): 2986–3008.

Fujioka, Shuichi, Jiangong Niu, Christian Schmidt, Guido M. Sclabas, Bailu Peng, Tadashi Uwagawa, Zhongkui Li, Douglas B. Evans, James L. Abbruzzese, and Paul J. Chiao. 2004. NF-κB and AP-1 Connection: Mechanism of NF-κB-dependent regulation of AP-1 activity. *Molecular and Cellular Biology* 24 (17) (September 1): 7806–7819.

Galati, Giuseppe, and Peter J. O'Brien. 2004. Potential toxicity of flavonoids and other dietary phenolics: Significance for their chemopreventive and anticancer properties. *Free Radical Biology and Medicine* 37 (3) (August 1): 287–303.

Gali-Muhtasib, Hala U., Sawsan Z. Yamout, and Mazen M. Sidani. 2000. Tannins protect against skin tumor promotion induced by ultraviolet-B radiation in hairless mice. *Nutrition and Cancer* 37 (1): 73–77.

Gans, J. Margot de Koning, Cuno S. P. M. Uiterwaal, Yvonne T. van der Schouw, Jolanda M. A. Boer, Diederick E. Grobbee, W. M. Monique Verschuren, and Joline W. J. Beulens. 2010. Tea and coffee consumption and cardiovascular morbidity and mortality. *Arteriosclerosis, Thrombosis, and Vascular Biology* 30 (8) (August 1): 1665–1671.

García-Lafuente, Ana, Eva Guillamón, Ana Villares, Mauricio A. Rostagno, and José Alfredo Martínez. 2009. Flavonoids as anti-inflammatory agents: Implications in cancer and cardiovascular disease. *Inflammation Research* 58 (9) (September 1): 537–552.

Geleijnse, Johanna M., Lenore J. Launer, Deirdre A. M. van der Kuip, Albert Hofman, and Jacqueline C. M. Witteman. 2002. Inverse association of tea and flavonoid intakes with incident myocardial infarction: The rotterdam study. *The American Journal of Clinical Nutrition* 75 (5) (May 1): 880–886.

Gilmore, T. D. 2006. Introduction to NF-κB: Players, pathways, perspectives. *Oncogene* 25 (51): 6680–6684.

González-Gallego, J, S. Sánchez-Campos, and M. J. Tuñón. 2007. Anti-inflammatory properties of dietary flavonoids. *Nutrición Hospitalaria* 22 (3) (June): 287–293.

Grundy, Scott M. 2013. Statin discontinuation and intolerance: The challenge of lifelong therapy. *Annals of Internal Medicine* 158 (7) (April 2): 562–563.

Guo, Yi, Eunice Mah, Catherine G. Davis, Thunder Jalili, Mario G. Ferruzzi, Ock K. Chun, and Richard S. Bruno. 2013. Dietary fat increases quercetin bioavailability in overweight adults. *Molecular Nutrition and Food Research* 57 (5): 896–905.

Heidenreich, Paul A., Justin G. Trogdon, Olga A. Khavjou, Javed Butler, Kathleen Dracup, Michael D. Ezekowitz, Eric Andrew Finkelstein et al. 2011. Forecasting the future of cardiovascular disease in the united states a policy statement from the american heart association. *Circulation* (January 24).

Hertog, Michaël G. L., Edith J. M. Feskens, and Daan Kromhout. 1997. Antioxidant flavonols and coronary heart disease risk. *The Lancet* 349 (9053) (March 8): 699.

Hollman, P. C. and M. B. Katan. 1997. Absorption, metabolism and health effects of dietary flavonoids in man. *Biomedicine and Pharmacotherapy = Biomédecine and Pharmacothérapie* 51 (8): 305–310.

Hollman, P. C., J. H. de Vries, S. D. van Leeuwen, M. J. Mengelers, and M. B. Katan. 1995. Absorption of dietary quercetin glycosides and quercetin in healthy ileostomy volunteers. *The American Journal of Clinical Nutrition* 62 (6) (December 1): 1276–1282.

Hurrell, Richard F., Manju Reddy, and James D. Cook. 1999. Inhibition of non-haem iron absorption in man by polyphenolic-containing beverages. *British Journal of Nutrition* 81: 289–295.

Ikeda, Ikuo, Youji Imasato, Eiji Sasaki, Mioko Nakayama, Hirosi Nagao, Tadakazu Takeo, Fumihisa Yayabe, and Michihiro Sugano. 1992. Tea catechins decrease micellar solubility and intestinal absorption of cholesterol in rats. *Biochimica et Biophysica Acta (BBA)–Lipids and Lipid Metabolism* 1127 (2) (July 29): 141–146.

Ikeda, Masahiko, Chinatsu Suzuki, Keizo Umegaki, Kieko Saito, Masaki Tabuchi, and Takako Tomita. 2007. Preventive effects of green tea catechins on spontaneous stroke in rats. *Medical Science Monitor: International Medical Journal of Experimental and Clinical Research* 13 (2) (February): BR40–45.

Jasuja, Reema, Freda H. Passam, Daniel R. Kennedy, Sarah H. Kim, Lotte van Hessem, Lin Lin, Sheryl R. Bowley et al. 2012. Protein disulfide isomerase inhibitors constitute a new class of antithrombotic agents. *The Journal of Clinical Investigation* 122 (6) (June 1): 2104–2113.

Jayaprakasam, Bolleddula, Srinivasulu Doddaga, Rong Wang, Daniel Holmes, Joseph Goldfarb, and Xiu-Min Li. 2009. Licorice flavonoids inhibit eotaxin-1 secretion by human fetal lung fibroblasts in vitro. *Journal of Agricultural and Food Chemistry* 57 (3) (February 11): 820–825.

Johnston, Kelly, Paul Sharp, Michael Clifford, and Linda Morgan. 2005. Dietary polyphenols decrease glucose uptake by human intestinal caco-2 cells. *FEBS Letters* 579 (7) (March): 1653–1657.

Jones, Dean P. 2006. Redefining oxidative stress. *Antioxidants and Redox Signaling* 8 (9–10) (October): 1865–1879.

Kapetivadze, V., R. Tabukashvili, K. Tchaava, N. Gegeshidze, Z. Grigorashvili, and I. Kapetivadze. 2010. Ms423 treatment of atherosclerosis patients with type 2 diabetes by soybean flavonoid supplements and indapamide. *Atherosclerosis Supplements* 11 (2) (June): 195.

Kavantzas, N., A. Chatziioannou, A. E. Yanni, D. Tsakayannis, D. Balafoutas, G. Agrogiannis, and D. Perrea. 2006. Effect of green tea on angiogenesis and severity of atherosclerosis in cholesterol-fed rabbit. *Vascular Pharmacology* 44 (6) (June): 461–463.

Keli, Sirving O., Michael G. L. Hertog, Edith J. M. Feskens, and Daan Kromhout. 1996. Dietary flavonoids, antioxidant vitamins, and incidence of stroke: The zutphen study. *Archives of Internal Medicine* 156 (6) (March 25): 637–642.

Kerry, Nicole L, and Mavis Abbey. 1997. Red wine and fractionated phenolic compounds prepared from red wine inhibit low density lipoprotein oxidation in vitro. *Atherosclerosis* 135 (1) (November): 93–102.

Kim, Amie, Andrew Chiu, Meredith K. Barone, Diane Avino, Fei Wang, Craig I. Coleman, and Olivia J. Phung. 2011. Green tea catechins decrease total and low-density lipoprotein cholesterol: A systematic review and meta-analysis. *Journal of the American Dietetic Association* 111 (11) (November): 1720–1729.

Knekt, Paul, Jorma Kumpulainen, Ritva Järvinen, Harri Rissanen, Markku Heliövaara, Antti Reunanen, Timo Hakulinen, and Arpo Aromaa. 2002. Flavonoid intake and risk of chronic diseases. *The American Journal of Clinical Nutrition* 76 (3) (September 1): 560–568.

Kobayashi, Yoko, Miho Suzuki, Hideo Satsu, Soichi Arai, Yukihiko Hara, Koichi Suzuki, Yusei Miyamoto, and Makoto Shimizu. 2000. Green tea polyphenols inhibit the sodium-dependent glucose transporter of intestinal epithelial cells by a competitive mechanism. *Journal of Agricultural and Food Chemistry* 48 (11) (November): 5618–5623.

Koo, Sung I, and Sang K Noh. 2007. Green tea as inhibitor of the intestinal absorption of lipids: Potential mechanism for its lipid-lowering effect. *The Journal of Nutritional Biochemistry* 18 (3) (March): 179–183.

Larsson, Susanna C, Jarmo Virtamo, and Alicja Wolk. 2012. Chocolate consumption and risk of stroke: A prospective cohort of men and meta-analysis. *Neurology* 79 (12) (September 18): 1223–1229.

Larsson, Susanna C., Jarmo Virtamo, and Alicja Wolk. 2011. Chocolate consumption and risk of stroke in women. *Journal of the American College of Cardiology* 58 (17) (October 18): 1828–1829.

Larsson, Susanna C., Jarmo Virtamo, and Alicja Wolk. 2013. Black tea consumption and risk of stroke in women and men. *Annals of Epidemiology* 23 (3) (March): 157–160.

Le Gall, Gwénaëlle, M. Susan DuPont, Fred A. Mellon, Adrienne L. Davis, Geoff J. Collins, Martine E. Verhoeyen, and Ian J. Colquhoun. 2003. Characterization and content of flavonoid glycosides in genetically modified tomato (lycopersicon esculentum) fruits. *Journal of Agricultural and Food Chemistry* 51 (9) (April): 2438–2446.

Leurs, Lina J, Leo J Schouten, R Alexandra Goldbohm, and Piet A van den Brandt. 2010. Total fluid and specific beverage intake and mortality due to IHD and stroke in the netherlands cohort study. *The British Journal of Nutrition* 104 (8) (October): 1212–1221. doi:10.1017/S0007114510001923.

Li, Yunbo, Zhuoxiao Cao, and Hong Zhu. 2006. Upregulation of endogenous antioxidants and phase 2 enzymes by the red wine polyphenol, resveratrol in cultured aortic smooth muscle cells leads to cytoprotection against oxidative and electrophilic stress. *Pharmacological Research* 53 (1) (January): 6–15.

Li, Zhi Gang, Yutaka Shimada, Fumiaki Sato, Masato Maeda, Atsushi Itami, Junichi Kaganoi, Izumi Komoto, Atsushi Kawabe, and Masayuki Imamura. 2002. Inhibitory effects of epigallocatechin-3-gallate on N-nitrosomethylbenzylamine-induced esophageal tumorigenesis in F344 rats. *International Journal of Oncology* 21 (6) (December 1): 1275–1283.

Lin, Jennifer, Kathy M. Rexrode, Frank Hu, Christine M. Albert, Claudia U. Chae, Eric B. Rimm, Meir J. Stampfer, and JoAnn E. Manson. 2007. Dietary intakes of flavonols and flavones and coronary heart disease in US women. *American Journal of Epidemiology* 165 (11) (June 1): 1305–1313.

Lin, Yu-Li, Chong-Yurn Cheng, Ya-Ping Lin, Yong-Wei Lau, I-Ming Juan, and Jen-Kun Lin. 1998. Hypolipidemic effect of green tea leaves through induction of antioxidant and phase II enzymes including superoxide dismutase, catalase, and glutathione S-transferase in rats. *Journal of Agricultural and Food Chemistry* 46 (5) (May 1): 1893–1899.

Linker, Ralf A., De-Hyung Lee, Sarah Ryan, Anne M. van Dam, Rebecca Conrad, Pradeep Bista, Weike Zeng et al. 2011. Fumaric acid esters exert neuroprotective effects in neuroinflammation via activation of the Nrf2 antioxidant pathway. *Brain* 134 (3) (March 1): 678–692.

Lopez-Garcia, Esther, Fernando Rodriguez-Artalejo, Kathryn M. Rexrode, Giancarlo Logroscino, Frank B. Hu, and Rob M. van Dam. 2009. Coffee consumption and risk of stroke in women. *Circulation* 119 (8) (March 3): 1116–1123.

Lu, Ming-Feng, Zheng-Tao Xiao, and Hong-Yu Zhang. 2013. Where do health benefits of flavonoids come from? Insights from flavonoid targets and their evolutionary history. *Biochemical and Biophysical Research Communications* 434 (4) (May 17): 701–704.

Manach, Claudine, Augustin Scalbert, Christine Morand, Christian Rémésy, and Liliana Jiménez. 2004. Polyphenols: Food sources and bioavailability. *The American Journal of Clinical Nutrition* 79 (5) (May 1): 727–747.

Manach, Claudine, Gary Williamson, Christine Morand, Augustin Scalbert, and Christian Rémésy. 2005. Bioavailability and bioefficacy of polyphenols in humans. I. Review of 97 bioavailability studies. *The American Journal of Clinical Nutrition* 81 (1) (January 1): 230S–242S.

Mariee, Amr D., Gamil M. Abd-Allah, and Hesham A. El-Beshbishy. 2012. Protective effect of dietary flavonoid quercetin against lipemic-oxidative hepatic injury in hypercholesterolemic rats. *Pharmaceutical Biology* 50 (8) (August): 1019–1025.

Mathur, Surekha, Sridevi Devaraj, Scott M. Grundy, and Ishwarlal Jialal. 2002. Cocoa products decrease low density lipoprotein oxidative susceptibility but do not affect biomarkers of inflammation in humans. *The Journal of Nutrition* 132 (12) (December 1): 3663–3667.

Mink, Pamela J., Carolyn G. Scrafford, Leila M. Barraj, Lisa Harnack, Ching-Ping Hong, Jennifer A. Nettleton, and David R. Jacobs. 2007. Flavonoid intake and cardiovascular disease mortality: A prospective study in postmenopausal women. *The American Journal of Clinical Nutrition* 85 (3) (March 1): 895–909.

Morris, Marilyn E., and Shuzhong Zhang. 2006. Flavonoid–drug interactions: Effects of flavonoids on ABC transporters. *Life Sciences* 78 (18) (March 27): 2116–2130.

Mursu, Jaakko, Sari Voutilainen, Tarja Nurmi, Tomi-Pekka Tuomainen, Sudhir Kurl, and Jukka T. Salonen. 2008. Flavonoid intake and the risk of ischaemic stroke and CVD mortality in middle-aged finnish men: The kuopio ischaemic heart disease risk factor study. *British Journal of Nutrition* 100 (4) (October): 890–895.

Patil, Chandrashekhar S., Vijay Pal Singh, P. S. V. Satyanarayan, Naveen K. Jain, Amarjit Singh, and Shrinivas K. Kulkarni. 2003. Protective effect of flavonoids against aging- and lipopolysaccharide-induced cognitive impairment in mice. *Pharmacology* 69 (2): 59–67.

Pearson W. N. 1957. FLavonoids in human nutrition and medicine. *Journal of the American Medical Association* 164 (15) (August 10): 1675–1678.

Perez-Vizcaino, Francisco, and Juan Duarte. 2010. Flavonols and cardiovascular disease. *Molecular Aspects of Medicine* 31 (6) (December): 478–494.

Peterson, Julia J, Johanna T Dwyer, Paul F Jacques, and Marjorie L McCullough. 2012. Associations between flavonoids and cardiovascular disease incidence or mortality in european and US populations. *Nutrition Reviews* 70 (9) (September): 491–508.

Pourcel, Lucille, Jean-Marc Routaboul, Véronique Cheynier, Loïc Lepiniec, and Isabelle Debeaujon. 2007. Flavonoid oxidation in plants: From biochemical properties to physiological functions. *Trends in Plant Science* 12 (1) (January): 29–36.

Reuland, Danielle J., Shadi Khademi, Christopher J. Castle, David C. Irwin, Joe M. McCord, Benjamin F. Miller, and Karyn L. Hamilton. 2013. Upregulation of phase II enzymes through phytochemical activation of Nrf2 protects cardiomyocytes against oxidant stress. *Free Radical Biology and Medicine* 56 (March): 102–111.

Rimbach, Gerald, Mona Melchin, Jennifer Moehring, and Anika E. Wagner. 2009. Polyphenols from cocoa and vascular health—A critical review. *International Journal of Molecular Sciences* 10 (10) (September 30): 4290–4309.

Rodriguez-Mateos, Ana, Catarina Rendeiro, Triana Bergillos-Meca, Setareh Tabatabaee, Trevor W. George, Christian Heiss, and Jeremy PE Spencer. 2013. Intake and time dependence of blueberry flavonoid–induced improvements in vascular function: A randomized, controlled, double-blind, crossover intervention study with mechanistic insights into biological activity. *The American Journal of Clinical Nutrition* 98 (5) (November 1): 1179–1191.

Roger, Véronique L, Alan S Go, Donald M Lloyd-Jones, Emelia J Benjamin, Jarett D Berry, William B Borden, Dawn M Bravata et al. 2012. Executive summary: Heart disease and stroke statistics—2012 update: A report from the american heart association. *Circulation* 125 (1) (January 3): 188–197.

Ross, Julie A., and Christine M. Kasum. 2002. Dietary flavonoids: Bioavailability, metabolic effects, and safety. *Annual Review of Nutrition* 22 (1) (July): 19–34.

Russo, Maria, Carmela Spagnuolo, Idolo Tedesco, Stefania Bilotto, and Gian Luigi Russo. 2012. The flavonoid quercetin in disease prevention and therapy: Facts and fancies. *Biochemical Pharmacology* 83 (1) (January 1): 6–15.

Sakihama, Yasuko, Michael F Cohen, Stephen C Grace, and Hideo Yamasaki. 2002. Plant phenolic antioxidant and prooxidant activities: Phenolics-induced oxidative damage mediated by metals in plants. *Toxicology* 177 (1) (August 1): 67–80.

Sesso, Howard D., J. Michael Gaziano, Simin Liu, and Julie E. Buring. 2003. Flavonoid intake and the risk of cardiovascular disease in women. *The American Journal of Clinical Nutrition* 77 (6) (June 1): 1400–1408.

Shah, Zahoor A., Rung-chi Li, Abdullah S. Ahmad, Thomas W. Kensler, Masayuki Yamamoto, Shyam Biswal, and Sylvain Doré. 2010. The flavanol (-)-epicatechin prevents stroke damage through the Nrf2/HO1 pathway. *Journal of Cerebral Blood Flow and Metabolism* 30 (12): 1951–1961.

Stanely, Ponnian, and Mainzen Prince. 2013. Epicatechin prevents alterations in lysosomal glycohydrolases, catepsins and reduces myocardial infact size in isoproterenol-induced myocardial infarcted rats. *Elsevier European Journal of Pharmacology* 706 (February 27): 63–69.

Sudano, Isabella, Andreas J. Flammer, Susanne Roas, Frank Enseleit, Frank Ruschitzka, Roberto Corti, and Georg Noll. 2012. Cocoa, blood pressure, and vascular function. *Current Hypertension Reports* 14 (4) (June 9): 279–284.

Tanabe, Naohito, Hiroshi Suzuki, Yoshifusa Aizawa, and Nao Seki. 2008. Consumption of green and roasted teas and the risk of stroke incidence: Results from the tokamachi–nakasato cohort study in japan. *International Journal of Epidemiology* 37 (5) (October 1): 1030–1040.

Taubert, Dirk, Reinhard Berkels, Renate Roesen, and Wolfgang Klaus. 2003. Chocolate and blood pressure in elderly individuals with isolated systolic hypertension. *JAMA* 290 (8) (August 27): 1029–1030.

Testai, Lara, Alma Martelli, Mario Cristofaro, Maria C. Breschi, and Vincenzo Calderone. 2013. Cardioprotective effects of different flavonoids against myocardial ischaemia/reperfusion injury in langendorff-perfused rat hearts. *Journal of Pharmacy and Pharmacology* 65 (5) (May 26): 750–756.

Tuñón, M J, M V García-Mediavilla, S Sánchez-Campos, and J González-Gallego. 2009. Potential of flavonoids as anti-inflammatory agents: Modulation of pro-inflammatory gene expression and signal transduction pathways. *Current Drug Metabolism* 10 (3) (March): 256–271.

Veronese, Maria L., Lisa P. Gillen, Joanne P. Burke, Ellen P. Dorval, Walter W. Hauck, E. Pequignot, Scott A. Waldman, and Howard E. Greenberg. 2003. Exposure-dependent inhibition of intestinal and hepatic CYP3A4 in vivo by grapefruit juice. *The Journal of Clinical Pharmacology* 43 (8): 831–839.

Walle, Thomas. 2004. Absorption and metabolism of flavonoids. *Free Radical Biology and Medicine* 36 (7) (April 1): 829–837.

Wan, Y, J. A. Vinson, T. D. Etherton, J. Proch, S. A. Lazarus, and P. M. Kris-Etherton. 2001. Effects of cocoa powder and dark chocolate on LDL oxidative susceptibility and prostaglandin concentrations in humans. *The American Journal of Clinical Nutrition* 74 (5) (November): 596–602.

Wang, Lisu, Yi-Chen Tu, Tzi-Wei Lian, Jing-Ting Hung, Jui-Hung Yen, and Ming-Jiuan Wu. 2006. Distinctive antioxidant and antiinflammatory effects of flavonols. *Journal of Agricultural and Food Chemistry* 54 (26) (December 1): 9798–9804.

WHO. 2013. The top 10 causes of death, WHO. Accessed October 18. http://who.int/mediacentre/factsheets/fs310/en/.

Williams, Robert J, Jeremy P. E. Spencer, and Catherine Rice-Evans. 2004. Flavonoids: Antioxidants or signalling molecules? *Free Radical Biology and Medicine* 36 (7) (April 1): 838–849.

Williamson, Gary. 2003. Common features in the pathways of absorption and metabolism of flavonoids. In *Phytochemicals*, edited by Mark Meskin, Wayne Bidlack, Audra Davies, Douglas Lewis, and R Keith Randolph. CRC Press.

Wright, Bernice, Jeremy P. E. Spencer, Julia A. Lovegrove, and Jonathan M. Gibbins. 2012. Insights into dietary flavonoids as molecular templates for the design of anti-platelet drugs. *European Society of Cardiology* (September 27): 13–22.

Yamane, Kazuya, and Yuudai Kato. 2012. *Handbook on Flavonoids: Dietary Sources, Properties, and Health Benefits*. Nova Science Publishers, Inc.

Zhu, Y., W. Ling, H. Guo, F. Song, Q. Ye, T. Zou, D. Li et al. 2012. Anti-inflammatory effect of purified dietary anthocyanin in adults with hypercholesterolemia: A randomized controlled trial. *Metabolism and Cardiovascular Diseases* (August).

14 Butterbur and Beyond *Dietary Supplements for Migraine Prevention*

Margaret Slavin

CONTENTS

14.1 INTRODUCTION

Migraine is a recurring, debilitating primary headache condition affecting approximately 17% of women and 6% of men annually in the United States (Diamond et al. 2007), though the recent Global Burden of Disease study recorded slightly higher worldwide rates at 18.8% in women and 10.7% in men (Vos et al. 2012). There are two major subtypes; migraine with and without aura. Migraine without aura is classified in individuals who have had at least five headache attacks lasting 4–72 h, with pain characteristics that fulfill two or more of the following: moderate to severe intensity; unilateral location; pulsating quality; or aggravation upon routine physical activity or avoidance thereof, and is accompanied by nausea, vomiting, photophobia or phonophobia (Headache Classification Committee of the IHS 2013). Migraine with aura occurs when an individual experiences reversible sensory disturbances (most frequently in the form of visual aura) with headache, which may or may not meet the criteria of migraine without aura.

When episodic migraines increase in frequency above 15 headache days/month, the patient's condition is said to have "transformed" to chronic migraine (Silberstein et al. 1996). Chronic migraine cases represent 7.7% of all migraineurs, or about 1% of the overall US population (Buse et al. 2012). Not surprisingly then, an individual migraineur and society carry a heavy burden because of the disease. In the 2010 Global Burden of Disease study, migraine ranked as the eighth most disabling disorder, measured in global years lived with disability (YLD), accounting for half of all the neurological disease-induced disabilities in the world and responsible for more disability worldwide than diabetes and ostheoarthritis (Vos et al. 2012). Beyond individual suffering, migraine poses a significant cost burden. The projected national direct monetary burden of migraine in 2004 was $11.07 billion annually, including $5.21 billion for outpatient care, and $4.61 billion for prescriptions (Hawkins et al. 2007). The cost to treat individuals has recently been assessed at an annual cost of $4144 for individual chronic migraine and $1533 for individuals with episodic migraine in the USA, with 72% and 68% of those costs going toward medications, respectively (Stokes et al. 2011).

Pharmaceutical medications are available to alleviate migraine attacks acutely and to prevent migraine in those with more significant symptoms. These treatments are well reviewed elsewhere, and are not discussed in depth here (Silberstein et al. 2012; Goadsby and Sprenger 2010). Beyond the drawback of the significant cost, migraine medications are notably inefficient at times. A prophylactic medication is considered effective when a 50% reduction in headache days is achieved (Shapiro 2012). Thus, many dietary supplement trials discussed below report "responder rate" as the number of patients who respond to the treatment with greater than 50% reduction migraine symptoms. Also, when considering acute medications taken to abort a migraine which has already started, symptoms return in 25% of the patients after taking the most common class of headache abortive medications, the triptans (Bolay and Ertas 2011). Additional concerns of pharmaceutical treatments include prohibitive side effects, incomplete childhood and pregnancy safety data, and the potential for inducing medication-overuse headaches with certain acute treatments. Beyond this, a significant population of candidates for acute and preventative pharmaceutical migraine therapy do not receive it (Diamond et al. 2007; Lipton et al. 2007). The use of preventive medication(s) decreased with household income (Diamond et al. 2007), suggesting that the cost of obtaining the prescriptions may be prohibitive for lower income migraineurs.

Meanwhile, evidence is building to suggest that a number of dietary supplements may have beneficial effects in the prevention of migraine. Reports regarding the strength of the evidence, as assessed by various organizations, are presented in Table 14.1. However, there are no widely accepted guidelines as to criteria for when to initiate prophylactic treatment with supplements, and even so with pharmaceuticals. A US Headache Consortium report in 2000 loosely described characteristics deserving attention when considering pharmacological strategies to prevent migraine, including "recurring migraines that, in the patients' opinion, significantly interfere with their daily routines; contraindication to, failure of, or overuse of acute therapies; and the cost of both acute and preventive therapies," among others (Ramadan et al.). The American Migraine Prevalence and Prevention study later assembled a panel of 12 experts to operationally define which patients need preventive treatment for research purposes based on the subject's level of impairment, though these are not explicit recommendations for use in clinical management (Lipton et al. 2007):

1. Prevention should be *offered* in patients who report 6+ headache days/month, 4+ headache days/month with some impairment, or 3+ headache days/month with severe impairment.

TABLE 14.1
Comparison of Evidence Quality Assignments for Dietary Supplements by Major Migraine Prevention Guidelines

	AHS/AAN Guidelines[a]	Canadian Guidelines[b]	EFNS Guidelines[c]
Butterbur (*Petasites hybridus*)	A	Strong, moderate-quality evidence	B
Magnesium	B	Strong, low-quality evidence	C
Riboflavin	B	Strong, low-quality evidence	C
CoEnzyme Q10	C	Strong, low-quality evidence	C
Feverfew (*Tanacetum parthenium*)	B	Do not use	C

Source: Adapted from Loder E, Burch R, and Rizzoli P. 2012. *Headache*. 52: 930–945.
Note: Here Level A = high-quality evidence, first-line treatment; Level B = moderate-quality evidence, second-line treatment; Level C = low-quality evidence, third-line treatments.
AAN = American Academy of Neurology; AHS = American Headache Society; EFNS = European Federation of Neurological Societies.
[a] Holland et al. (2012).
[b] Pringsheim et al. (2012).
[c] Evers et al. (2009).

2. Prevention should be *considered* when patients experience 4 or 5 migraine days/month with normal functioning, 3 migraine days with some impairment, or 2 migraine days with severe impairment.
3. Prevention is *not indicated* in migraineurs with less than 4 headache days/month with no impairment of function, or in people with only 1 headache day/month of any level of impairment.

It remains to the judgment of the medical care provider to assemble the entirety of the migraineur's symptoms, rule out other potential causes, and weigh the risks and benefits of treatment, before recommending a preventive therapy or not. It is generally accepted that a trial period of 2–3 months is necessary to determine if a migraine preventive treatment is working, as evidenced by the typical study length of 3 months. Because of their low cost and generally positive safety profiles, dietary supplements offer an evidence-based alternative to pharmaceuticals in reducing the burden of migraine and have the potential to save significant disability time and health-care costs. The dietary supplements with the most promising clinical evidence for efficacy in migraine prevention are presented here for consideration.

14.2 DIETARY SUPPLEMENTS WITH CLINICAL EVIDENCE

14.2.1 Butterbur (*Petasites hybridus*)

Butterbur is a botanical supplement prepared as an extract of the root of the perennial flowering shrub native to parts of Europe. In its native state, the plant components contain hepatotoxic and carcinogenic pyrrolizidine alkaloids, and thus, must be consumed as purified extracts to reap the purported anti-inflammatory and antispasmodic benefits. The most widely studied commercial extract is Petadolex, which is produced in Germany and standardized to contain a minimum of 15% petasins (*Eremophilane sesquiterpenoids*; www.petadolex.com), the suspected active components (Sutherland and Sweet 2010), and no detectable levels (<0.08 ppm) of pyrrolizidine alkaloids (Danesch and Rittinghausen 2003).

Two double-blind, placebo-controlled, randomized controlled trials demonstrating butterbur's preventive effects against migraine are available in the literature (Diener et al. 2004; Lipton et al. 2004). Both trials used Petadolex and showed a decrease in migraine attack frequency in subjects treated with Petasites as compared to the placebo, though the Diener study detected a difference in control at a lower dose (50 mg twice daily) than the Lipton study, where a dose of 75 mg twice daily was necessary to reach statistical difference from the placebo. The latter study included two doses: 50 mg and 75 mg twice daily. Interestingly, though the 50 mg dose did not reach statistical significance from the control, it did achieve an intermediate effect between the control and high dose, appearing to suggest a dose-dependent relationship. Notably, both studies showed a large proportion of patients who experienced reductions of migraine frequency by 50% or greater; 48% of those receiving 50 mg twice daily (Diener et al. 2004) and 69% of those receiving 75 mg twice daily (Lipton et al. 2004). As common in migraine research, both studies experienced high-placebo response rates.

The quality of these study designs, combined with their consistent results, resulted in *Petasites* being the only dietary supplement labeled as having "established efficacy," with recommendations as a first-line treatment in a recent systematic review conducted jointly by the Quality Standards Subcommittee of the American Academy of Neurology and the American Headache Society (Holland et al. 2012). Alternate but older systematic reviews are not quite as generous, pegging the results of these studies as "moderate evidence of effectiveness" for the 150 mg daily dose (Agosti et al. 2006). The European Federation of Neurological Sciences guidelines named *Petasites* (2×75 mg daily dose) as a Level B migraine prophylactic drug, meaning it is a "second choice" behind numerous pharmaceuticals, but it was the highly recommended of the dietary supplements (by US regulatory definitions) and nonprescription treatments (Evers et al. 2009). The Canadian Headache Society guidelines interpret the data to make a strong recommendation to offer 75 mg butterbur twice daily, with moderate quality evidence (Pringsheim et al. 2012). A comparison of recommendations from the various headache organizations is available in Table 14.1.

Additionally, an open study with children was published shortly after the two randomized controlled trials (Pothmann and Danesch 2005). The open trial without a control group was selected due to ethical controls in research with children. Nonetheless, with limited options for migraine prevention in children, the results are still enlightening. The study provided children and adolescents (6–18 years old) with 50–150 mg butterbur daily (depending on age), and followed them for 4 months. Results identified a very high portion of the treated children (86%) and adolescents (74%) who experienced reductions of migraine attack frequency of greater than 50% (Pothmann and Danesch 2005).

Long-term safety data (beyond 4 months) regarding *Petasites* are lacking. Safety during pregnancy and breastfeeding has also not been established (Sutherland and Sweet 2010), and further evidence in children is desired. Foremost for safety, consumers should not consume unprocessed *Petasites* products, and instead should look for purified extracts which have verified the removal of the hepatotoxic pyrrolizidine alkaloids (i.e., "certified PA-free"). Common side effects of administration of these purified extracts are generally reported to be mild and include belching and gastrointestinal upset (Sutherland and Sweet 2010). Notably, butterbur has the potential to cause allergic reactions in those who are allergic to other plants in the Asteraceae family (Sutherland and Sweet 2010).

14.2.2 Magnesium

Magnesium is an essential mineral, acting as a cofactor in at least 300 enzyme systems in the body. Low levels of magnesium have been detected in migraineurs, both during attacks and interictally. Assays have included blood serum, saliva, cerebrospinal fluid, red blood cells, and in vivo in the brain using ^{31}P magnetic resonance imaging (Sun-Edelstein and Mauskop 2009). Longstanding speculation suggests that magnesium loss may be enhanced during migraine (Sun-Edelstein and Mauskop 2009; Rybica et al. 2012), but it remains to be studied whether migraineurs have outright higher magnesium demands than the general population. Nonetheless, a number of magnesium supplementation trials have been performed, suggesting its potential effectiveness in the prevention of migraine.

Several systematic reviews have weighed the evidence for magnesium supplementation, and conclude (with varying language) that there appears to be credence to the migraine preventive hypothesis. A comparison of the recommendations made by major migraine prevention guidelines is shown in Table 14.1. The American Academy of Neurology and the American Headache Society report concluded that magnesium supplementation is "probably effective" (Level B) for migraine prevention based on multiple Class II trials, and is worthy of consideration for migraine prevention, though no specific dose was cited (Holland et al. 2012). Canadian Headache Society guidelines make a "strong recommendation" with "low quality evidence" that clinicians "offer magnesium to eligible patients for migraine prophylaxis" (Pringsheim et al. 2012). The recommended dose is 600 mg of elemental magnesium in the form of magnesium citrate. Sun-Edelstein and Mauskop (2009) provided a review of migraine research, speculations on its role in pathogenesis, and a recommended dose of 400 mg magnesium in one of several forms (chelated magnesium, magnesium oxide or slow-release magnesium) to migraineurs.

The debate continues in the migraine community, with some positing that daily 400 mg magnesium supplements should be given to "all migraine patients" (Mauskop and Varughese 2012) based on their low cost, low-risk profile, and their estimation that it could benefit half of all the migraineurs. Meanwhile, the counterargument gives the negative and mixed study results more weight and suggests that pharmacological agents are available with better evidence (Pardutz and Vecsei 2012).

Double-blind, placebo-controlled trials showing a beneficial impact of magnesium supplementation have used various forms and doses of magnesium;

magnesium pyrrolidone carboxylic acid salt (360 mg elemental Mg [eMg]—Facchinetti et al. 1991), trimagnesium citrate (600 mg eMg—Peikert et al. 1996; 600 mg eMg—Koseoglu et al. 2008; 300 mg eMg—Dermirkaya et al. 2000), and magnesium oxide (300 mg eMg—Efsanjani et al. 2012). Dosing differed across administration times and frequencies, but each of these showed a decrease in attack frequency, with the exception of Facchinetti et al.'s work, which did not measure frequency but rather showed a decrease in pain total index. A widely reviewed study using the magnesium-L-aspartate-hydrochloride-trihydrate (243 mg eMg) in a double-blind, placebo-controlled clinical trial did not show benefit of supplementing Mg as compared to placebo (Pfaffenrath et al. 1996). However, the results are jeopardized by the significant side effects of this alternate form of Mg. Nearly half of the patients in the treatment group reported adverse effects, primarily related to gastrointestinal upset in the form of soft stools or diarrhea, which raises into question the bioavailability of Mg using this aspartate-salt form and the applicability of the results. Lastly, a double-blind, placebo-controlled trial in children aged 3–17 showed a statistically significant decrease in headache frequency in children taking the magnesium oxide (9 mg/kg/day), as well as lower headache severity (Wang et al. 2003).

When approaching the subject of safety and adverse effects, it is worthy of mention that the UL value (the tolerable upper intake limit) for magnesium is fairly low, 350 mg/day of magnesium from "pharmacological agents" for adult men and women (Dietary Reference Intakes Report 2006). The UL value was set primarily because of the common endpoint of diarrhea in multiple non-food high-magnesium studies (Dietary Reference Intakes Report 2006), and this outcome does appear in the adverse effects of high-dose magnesium supplementation for migraine prophylaxis trials. Though the adverse effects of magnesium supplementation beyond diarrhea appear rare (as increasing consumption results in less efficient absorption), the proximity of doses recommended for migraine to the UL makes it prudent to discuss magnesium toxicity symptoms beyond diarrhea, including loss of tendon reflexes and muscle weakness, metabolic alkalosis, cardiorespiratory arrest, and death.

14.2.3 Riboflavin

Riboflavin (vitamin B_2) is an essential water-soluble vitamin with numerous known functions, including as a coenzyme in various steps of energy metabolism, which has been suggested as a potential link to migraine. Its effectiveness in migraine was suggested as early as in 1946, with a report of improvement of ophthalmic and simple migraine cases when 10–15 mg riboflavin/day were administered (Smith 1946).

In systematic reviews of migraine prophylaxis, the work of Schoenen et al. (1994, 1998) remains the primary driver of recommendations in favor of riboflavin as an effective agent in the prevention of migraines. An initial open study of 49 patients supplemented 400 mg riboflavin daily (with or without 75 mg aspirin) and showed a dramatic 67% decrease in migraine days/month after 3 months of treatment (Schoenen et al. 1994). Soon thereafter, a well-designed randomized double-blind placebo-controlled trial with 55 patients echoed the results: patients treated with 400 mg riboflavin daily reported a statistically significant reduction in migraine frequency, total migraine days, headache severity after 3 months of treatment, as compared to placebo (Schoenen et al. 1998). Beyond this, those treated with riboflavin were significantly more likely to be a "responder", by experiencing a greater than 50% reduction in headache symptoms, seen in 56% of those treated with riboflavin versus 19% of the placebo group.

Since these original trials ($n = 23$), another small, open study, reported a significant decrease in migraine frequency by about half with 400 mg riboflavin supplementation daily by 3 months, with stable symptoms at 6 months, though differences in migraine duration and severity were not detected (Boehnke et al. 2004). Furthermore, a randomized supplement-drug comparison trial of 100 migraine patients compared the effectiveness of 100 mg riboflavin to 80 mg of propranolol, the well-regarded pharmaceutical migraine prophylactic (Nambiar et al. 2011). The trial was not blinded, but both treatments showed similar decreases in frequency (42%–43%), duration (26%–32%), and severity (26%–27%) of migraine headaches after 3 months of treatment. Furthermore, the riboflavin group reported significantly fewer adverse effects than propranolol. The authors therefore concluded riboflavin may be a preferable migraine prophylactic treatment because of its agreeable safety and tolerability while exhibiting comparable reductions in migraine indicators as the drug propranolol.

The strength of this evidence, in combination with riboflavin's well-regarded safety (there is no UL value), is interpreted and presented in Table 14.1 in the recommendations for migraine prevention by the major neurological and headache societies. The American guidelines consider riboflavin to be "probably effective" on the basis of Schoenen work alone (Holland et al. 2012). Similarly, the Canadian guidelines recommend the daily use of 400 mg riboflavin strongly, partly because of the good safety profile, though they consider the evidence to be low (Pringsheim et al. 2012). European guidelines rate riboflavin as Level C, having only "probable evidence" at 400 mg (Evers et al. 2009). Notably, none of these recommendations has taken into account the 2011 randomized comparison trial of riboflavin versus propranolol (Nambiar et al. 2011).

The well-regarded safety of riboflavin as a supplement has also drawn interest in the community of pediatric and adolescent migraine research, for obvious reasons. However, two randomized, double-blind, placebo-controlled trials in children and adolescents showed no reduction in migraine frequency (MacLennan et al. 2008; Bruijn et al. 2010). Notably, both studies were fairly small (48 and 42 patients, respectively) and plagued by high-placebo responder rates, as is common in migraine research with young patients (Lewis et al. 2005). Meanwhile, a similarly sized ($n = 41$) retrospective study of patients with resistant migraine, aged 8–18 showed a decrease in migraine frequency with doses of both 200 and 400 mg riboflavin/day (Condo et al. 2009).

14.2.4 Coenzyme Q10

Coenzyme Q10 (CoQ10), like riboflavin, is intimately involved with energy metabolism via the electron transport chain, as well as possessing antioxidant properties. Although its most recognized clinical application is in the area of cardiac health promotion (Littarru and Tiano 2010), CoQ10 has also been studied in relation to migraine prevention on the hypothesis that mitochondrial dysfunction is to blame in some migraineurs.

Migraine prevention guidelines across the international organizations are in unusual agreement with regard to CoQ10 (see Table 14.1), likely because only one true randomized controlled trial was available in adults for interpretation (Sandor et al. 2005), though with promising results. In the trial with 42 enrolled adults, the treatment group received 100 mg CoQ10 three times per day, and showed a decrease in frequency, headache days, and days with nausea after 3 months. The responder rate of adults who experienced at least a 50% decrease in symptoms was 47.6%, as compared to 14.4% of those receiving placebo (Sandor et al. 2005). From the results of this one study, the American and European guidelines classify CoQ10 as a Level C treatment, as drugs which may be considered as a third choice because of "only probable efficacy," while the Canadian Headache Society guidelines make a strong recommendation with low-quality evidence in support of its use at 100 mg, three times daily, indicative that they believe the potential benefits outweigh the minimal risks associated with CoQ10 at this dose (Holland et al. 2012; Evers et al. 2009; Pringsheim et al. 2012).

Other research with CoQ10 includes a preceding open-label trial, published in 2002, where 32 patients receiving 150 mg CoQ10 daily showed an average decrease in migraine frequency by 55.3%, with an overall responder rate of 61.3% (Rozen et al. 2002). CoQ10 has also been assessed in children, with one prospective, but uncontrolled study using serum levels of CoQ10 below 0.7 μg/mL as an indicator triggering treatment with oral doses of 1–3 mg/kg/day in children aged 3–22. Of those who reported taking the CoQ10 treatment for an average follow-up of 97 days, 46.3% reported a reduction of symptoms by at least 50% (Hershey et al. 2007). The only placebo-controlled, double-blind, randomized crossover control trial in children that has been conducted did not detect a difference between the placebo and CoQ10 treatment group outcomes (Slater et al. 2011). However, the trial was plagued by high dropout rates (out of 120 initial patients, only 50 completed the endpoint data collection at 224 days) and a very high-placebo response rate.

The investigations of CoQ10 for its cardiac benefits have produced a body of supplementation research that allows for a broad evaluation of adverse effects. Hidaka et al. (2008) reviewed these preclinical, clinical, and pharmacokinetic data and found CoQ10 to be "highly safe for use as a dietary supplement." Adverse effects are generally recognized to be minimal and transient. An acceptable daily intake was calculated as 12 mg/kg/day using standard methods and a 100-fold safety factor (equivalent to approximately 720 mg/day for a 60 kg adult, well above the levels used in migraine prophylactic studies; Hidaka et al. 2008).

14.2.5 Feverfew

Feverfew (*Tanacetum parthemium* L.) is a flowering perennial shrub whose common name arises from the Latin *febrifugia*, or "fever reducer", an allusion to its traditional use that traces back millennia (Pareek et al. 2011). The most recognized bioactive chemical is parthenolide, a sesquiterpene lactone, found in the leaves of the plant (Pareek et al. 2011); although its role in migraine prevention has been questioned due to a lack of definitive evidence linking it to clinical results (Pittler and Ernst 2009). Feverfew dietary supplements are available for purchase in various forms: powdered leaves, extracts, and extracts standardized for parthenolide content.

Results of clinical trials with feverfew in migraine prophylaxis have yielded mixed results. Differences in protocols are evident in the form of feverfew administered (ground leaves and extracts of various solvents), dose and dosing protocols, as well as selection criteria of patients. Earlier studies which used ground feverfew leaves showed significant decreases in frequency (Murphy et al. 1988) and intensity/severity (Palevitch 1997) of migraines in crossover trials. An ethanolic extract of feverfew, standardized to contain 0.5 mg of parthenolide did not display a prophylactic effect in a crossover trial (De Weerdt et al. 1996). Later, a stable, standardized supercritical CO_2 extract of feverfew (MIG-99) was developed and tested in a parallel-group trial, showing that doses of 6.25 mg MIG-99 (0.5 mg parthenolid equivalent) administered three times/day could decrease frequency of migraine in a subgroup of high-frequency migraineurs, but not those with lower-frequency migraine (Pfaffenrath et al. 2002). The study was followed by a larger trial, which detected a statistically significant reduction in migraine frequency of 1.9/month in a broader population of migraineurs, as compared to a reduction of 1.3 in the placebo group (Diener et al. 2005). Also, rates of patients who saw 50% or greater decreases in migraine frequency were used to calculate an odds ratio, showing a 3.4 times greater likelihood of experiencing a response while taking MIG-99, as compared to placebo.

Still, inconsistencies in research protocols across the studies have made the results difficult to compile, leading to various interpretations of these feverfew results. Table 14.1 shows the disagreement regarding feverfew amongst major migraine prevention guidelines. Although the American agencies rate the supporting evidence as Level B ("probably effective"), justifying its presence as a second-line treatment, the EFNS considers the same evidence to justify a Level C recommendation (Holland et al. 2012; Evers et al. 2009). Meanwhile, the Canadian guidelines make a strong recommendation with moderate quality evidence *against* the use of feverfew as a migraine prophylactic agent, stating that evidence shows feverfew is no better than placebo (Pringhseim et al. 2012). Lastly, a Cochrane review of publications through 2003 found "insufficient evidence…to suggest an effect of feverfew over placebo" (Pittler and Ernst 2009).

As with many other botanical supplements, long-term safety data is unavailable. In clinical trials, feverfew is generally well tolerated. However, a common adverse event in earlier trials using ground leaves included ulceration or inflammation of the mouth (Murphy et al. 1988; Johnson et al. 1985). More recent studies with extracts did not detect a difference in adverse events reported by treatment and placebo groups (Pfaffenrath et al. 2002; Diener et al. 2005). Notably, two studies have reported a "post-feverfew syndrome" when patients stop using feverfew, including "augmentation" of headache symptoms (Palevitch et al. 1997) and joint pain/stiffness, anxiety and poor sleep (Johnson et al. 1985), which may be a factor when deciding on a preventive strategy.

14.3 CONCLUSIONS

Till date, evidence supporting the use of dietary supplements in migraine prevention is promising, but remains in need of significantly more high-quality clinical studies to provide more definitive answers. As yet, butterbur has the highest level of evidence with two high-quality randomized controlled trials in support of its efficacy in reducing migraine occurrences. The general difficulty of assessing migraine outcomes, high-placebo response rates, and at times a lack of standardized methods continue to complicate clinical migraine prevention research. Potential mechanisms of action of these supplements are discussed in detail elsewhere (Taylor 2011), though without a definitive understanding of the true pathophysiology of migraine, much remains to be learned in this regard, which could also inform future clinical research.

As with any existing migraine preventive treatment, expectations of efficacy of dietary supplements for the individual patient must be tempered because there is no available treatment that will eliminate migraine. A 50% reduction in migraine frequency or headache days is considered successful. That said, individuals with headaches are not recommended to self-medicate, as migraine preventative treatments—including dietary supplements—are best prescribed by a qualified medical professional who has ruled out other potentially more serious diagnoses with similar symptoms and determined that a preventive measure is appropriate.

Still, current recommendations do not explicitly exist regarding when practitioners should consider preventive agents in patients with episodic migraine. (Considerations on the matter are discussed in the introduction.) As with any medical treatment, the decision is made by weighing risks and benefits. Though not without risk, dietary supplements discussed here have limited reported adverse effects, and may provide similar preventive abilities as pharmaceuticals with greater potential for adverse effects. Also, as initial reports suggest that poorly optimized treatment of episodic migraines may lead to a greater risk of transformation to chronic migraine (Lipton et al. 2013), the amount of potential "benefit" to be reaped by these supplements may be seen beyond the immediate prevention of headache—there may also be long-term implications to preventing migraines in patients who wouldn't otherwise justify the "risk" of pharmaceutical preventive treatments. Additionally, advances in our understanding of biological mechanisms underpinning clinical efficacy may allow for combination therapies to be developed (dietary supplements, drugs, or a mix thereof) with additive, or even synergistic, results.

REFERENCES

Agosti R, Duke RK, Chrubasik JE, and Chrubasik S. 2006. Effectiveness of *Petasites hybridus* preparations in the prophylaxis of migraine: A systematic review. *Phytomedicine.* 13: 743–746.

Boehnke C, Reuter U, Flach U, Schuh-Hofer S, Einhaupl KM, and Arnold G. 2004. High-dose riboflavin treatment is efficacious in migraine prophylaxis: An open study in a tertiary care centre. *European Journal of Neurology.* 11: 475–477.

Bolay H and Ertas M. 2011. Advances in migraine treatment. *CML—Neurology.* 27(4): 101–113.

Bruijn J, Duivenvoorden H, Passchier J, Locher H, Dijkstra N, and Arts W-F. 2010. Medium-dose riboflavin as a prophylactic agent in children with migraine: A preliminary placebo-controlled, randomized, double-blind, cross-over trial. *Cephalagia.* 30(12): 1426–1434.

Buse DC, Manack AN, Fanning KM, Serrano D, Reed ML Turkel CC, and Lipton RB. 2012. Chronic migraine prevalence, disability, and sociodemographic factors: Results from the American migraine prevalence and prevention study. *Headache.* 52: 1456–1470.

Condo M, Posar A, Arbizzani A, and Parmeggiani A. 2009. Riboflavin prophylaxis in pediatric and adolescent migraine. *Journal Headache Pain*. 10: 361–365.

Danesch U and Rittinghausen R. 2003. Safety of a patented special butterbur root extract for migraine prevention. *Headache*. 43: 76–78.

De Weerdt CJ, Bootsma HPR, and Hendriks H. 1996. Herbal medicines in migraine prevention. *Phytomedicine*. 3(3): 225–230.

Dermirkaya S, Dora B, Topcuoglu MA, Ulas UH, and Vural O. 2000. A comparative study of magnesium, flunarizine and amitriptyline in the prophylaxis of migraine. *Journal Headache Pain*. 1: 179–186.

Diamond S, Bigal ME, Silberstein S, Loder E, Reed M, Lipton RB. 2007. Patterns of diagnosis and acute and preventive treatment for migraine in the United States: Results from the American migraine prevalence and prevention study. *Headache*. 47: 355–363.

Diener HC, Rahlfs VW, and Danesch U. 2004. The first placebo-controlled trial of a special butterbur root extract for the prevention of migraine: Reanalysis of efficacy criteria. *European Neurology*. 51: 89–97.

Diener HC, Pfaffenrath V, Schnitker J, Friede, and Henneicke-von Zepelin HH. 2005. Efficacy and safety of 6.25 mg t.i.d. feverfew CO_2-extract (MIG-99) in migraine prevention—a randomized, double-blind, multicenter, placebo-controlled study. *Cephalagia*. 25: 1031–1041.

Dietary reference intakes—the essential guide to nutrient requirements. 2006. Eds. Otten JJ, Hellwig JP, and Meyers LD. The National Academies Press: Washington, DC.

Efsanjani AT, Mahdavi R, Mameghani ME, Talebi M, Nikniaz Z, and Safaiyan A. 2012. The effects of magnesium, L-carnitine, and concurrent magnesium-L-carnitine supplementation in migraine prophylaxis. *Biological Trace Element Research*. 150: 42–48.

Evers S, Afra J, Frese A, Goadsby PJ, Linde M, May A, and Sandor PS. 2009. EFNS guideline on the drug treatment of migraine—revised report of an EFNS task force. *European Journal of Neurology*. 16: 968–981.

Facchinetti F, Sances G, Borella P, Genazzani AR, and Nappi G. 1991. Magnesium prophylaxis of menstrual migraine: Effects on intracellular magnesium. *Headache*. 31: 298–301.

Goadsby PJ and Sprenger T. 2010. Current practice and future directions in the prevention and acute management of migraine. *Lancet Neurology*. 9: 285–298.

Hawkins K, Wang S, and Rupnow M. 2007. Direct cost burden among insured U.S. employees with migraine. *Headache*. 48: 553–563.

Headache Classification Committee of The International Headache Society. 2013. The international classification of headache disorders, 3rd edition (beta version). *Cephalagia*. 33(9): 629–808.

Hershey AD, Powers SW, Vockell A-LB, LeCates SL, Ellinor PL, Segers A, Burdine D, Manning P, and Kabbouche MA. 2007. Coenzyme Q10 deficiency and response to supplementation in pediatric and adolescent migraine. *Headache*. 47: 73–80.

Hidaka T, Fujii K, Funahashi I, Fukutomi N, and Hosoe K. 2008. Safety assessment of coenzyme Q_{10} (CoQ_{10}). *BioFactors*. 32: 199–208.

Holland S, Silberstein SD, Freitag F, Dodick DW, Argoff C, and Ashman E. 2012. Evidence-based guideline update: NSAIDs and other complementary treatments for episodic migraine prevention in adults. *Neurology*. 78: 1346–1353.

Johnson ES, Kadam NP, Hylands DM, and Hylands PJ. 1985. Efficacy of feverfew as prophylactic treatment of migraine. *British Medical Journal*. 291: 569–573.

Koseoglu E, Talashoglu A, Gonul AS, and Kula M. 2008. The effects of magnesium prophylaxis in migraine without aura. *Magnesium Research*. 21(2): 101–108.

Lewis DW, Winner P, and Wasiewski W. 2005. The placebo responder rate in children and adolescents. *Headache*. 45: 232–239.

Lipton RB, Gobel H, Einhaupl KM, Wilks K, and Mauskop A. 2004. *Petasites hybridus* (butterbur) is an effective preventive treatment for migraine. *Neurology*. 63: 2240–2244.

Lipton RB, Bigal ME, Diamond M, Freitag F, Reed ML, and Stewart WF. 2007. Migraine prevalence, disease burden, and the need for preventive therapy. *Neurology*. 68: 343–349.

Lipton RB, Buse DC, Fanning KM, Serrano D, and Reed ML. 2013. Suboptimal acute treatment of episodic migraine (EM) is associated with an increased risk of progression to chronic migraine (CM): Results of the American migraine prevalance and prevention (AMPP) study [Abstract]. *Cephalagia*. 33(11): 954–955.

Littarru GP and Tiano L. 2010. Clinical aspects of coenzyme Q_{10}: An update. *Nutrition*. 26: 250–254.

Loder E, Burch R, and Rizzoli P. 2012. The 2012 AHS/AAN guidelines for prevention of episodic migraine: A summary and comparison with other recent clinical practice guidelines. *Headache*. 52: 930–945.

MacLennan SC, Wade FN, Forrest KML, Ratanayake PD, Fagan E, and Antony J. 2008. High-dose riboflavin for migraine prophylaxis in children: A double-blind, randomized, placebo-controlled trial. *Journal of Child Neurology*. 23(11): 1300–1304.

Mauskop A and Varughese J. 2012. Why all migraine patients should be treated with magnesium. *J Neural Transmission*. 119: 575–579.

Murphy JJ, Heptinstall S, and Mitchell JRA. 1988. Randomised double-blind placebo-controlled trial of feverfew in migraine prevention. *The Lancet*. 332(8604): 189–192.

Nambiar NJ, Aiyappa C, and Srinivasa R. 2011. Oral riboflavin versus oral propranolol in migraine prophylaxis: An open label randomized controlled trial. *Neurology Asia*. 16(3): 223–229.

Palevitch D, Earon G, and Carasso R. 1997. Feverfew (*Tanacetum parthenium*) as a prophylactic treatment for migraine: A double-blind placebo-controlled study. *Phytotherapy Research*. 11: 508–511.

Pardutz A and Vecsei L. 2012. Should magnesium be given to every migraineur? No. *Journal Neural Transmission*. 119: 581–585.

Pareek A, Suthar M, Rathore GS, and Bansal V. 2011. Feverfew (*Tanacetum parthenium* L.): A systematic review. *Pharmacognosy Reviews*. 5(9): 103–110.

Peikert A, Wilimzig C, and Kohne-Volland R. 1996. Prophylaxis of migraine with oral magnesium: Results from a prospective, multi-center, placebo-controlled and double-blind randomized study. *Cephalagia*. 16: 257–263.

Petadolex. Available at: www.petadolex.com. Last accessed January 31, 2014.

Pfaffenrath V, Wessely P, Meyer C, Isler HR, Evers S, Grotemeyer KH, Taneri Z, Soyka D, Gobel H, and Fischer M. 1996. Magnesium in the prophylaxis of migraine—a double-blind, placebo-controlled study. *Cephalagia*. 16: 436–440.

Pfaffenrath V, Diener HC, Fischer M, Friede M, and Henneicke-von Zepelin HH. 2002. The efficacy and safety of *Tanacetum parthenium* (feverfew) in migraine prophylaxis—a double-blind, multicenter, randomized placebo-controlled dose-response study. *Cephalagia*. 22: 523–532.

Pittler MH and Ernst E. 2009. Feverfew for preventing migraine (review). *Cochrane Database of Systematic Reviews*, Issue 1. Art. No.: CD002286. DOI: 10.1002/14651858.CD002286.pub2.

Pothmann R and Danesch U. 2005. Migraine prevention in children and adolescents: Results of an open study with a special butterbur root extract. *Headache*. 45: 196–203.

Pfaffenrath V, Wessely P, Meyer C, Isler HR, Evers S, Grotemeyer KH, Taneri Z, Soyka D, Gobel H, and Fischer M. 1996. Magnesium in the prophylaxis of migraine—a double-blind, placebo-controlled study. *Cephalagia*. 16: 436–440.

Pringsheim T, Davenport WJ, Mackie G, Worthington I, Aube M, Christie SN, Gladstone J, and Becker WJ. 2012. Systematic review: Medications for migraine prophylaxis—Section II. *Canadian Journal Neurology Science*. 39(Suppl 2): S8–S28.

Ramadan NM, Silberstein SD, Freitag FG et al. Evidence-based guidelines for migraine headache in the primary care setting: Pharmacological management for prevention of migraine. U.S. Headache Consortium. Available at: http://tools.aan.com/professionals/practice/pdfs/gl0090.pdf. Last accessed March 12, 2015.

Rozen TD, Oshinsky ML, Gebeline CA, Bradley KC, Young WB, Shechter AL, and Silberstein SD. 2002. Open label trial of coenzyme Q10 as a migraine preventive. *Cephalagia*. 22: 137–141.

Rybica M, Baranowska-Bosiacka I, Zyluk B, Nowacki P, and Chlubek D. 2012. The role of magnesium in migraine pathogenesis. Potential use of magnesium compounds in prevention and treatment of migraine headaches. *Journal Elementary*. 17(2): 345–356.

Sandor PS, Di Clemente L, Coppola G, Saenger U, Fumal A, Magis D, Seidel L, Agosti RM, and Schoenen J. 2005. Efficacy of coenzyme Q10 in migraine prophylaxis: A randomized controlled trial. *Neurology*. 64: 713–715.

Schoenen J, Lenaerts M, and Bastings E. 1994. High-dose riboflavin as a prophylactic treatment of migraine: Results of an open pilot study. *Cephalagia*. 14: 328–329.

Schoenen J, Jacquy J, and Lenaerts M. 1998. Effectiveness of high-dose riboflavin in migraine prophylaxis. *Neurology*. 50: 466–470.

Shapiro RE. 2012. Preventive treatment of migraine. *Headache*. 52(Suppl. 2): 65–69.

Silverstein SD, Lipton RB, and Sliwinski M. 1996. Classification of daily and near-daily headaches: Field trial of revised HIS criteria. *Neurology*. 47: 871–875.

Silberstein SD, Holland S, Freitan F, Dodick DW, Argoff C, and Ashman E. 2012. Evidence-based guideline update: Pharmacologic treatment for episodic migraine prevention in adults. *Neurology*. 78: 1337–1345.

Slater SK, Nelson TD, Kabbouche MA, LeCates SL, Horn P, Segers A, Manning P, Powers SW, and Hershey AD. A randomized, double-blinded, placebo-controlled, crossover, add-on study of CoEnzyme Q10 in the prevention of pediatric and adolescent migraine. *Cephalagia*. 31(8): 897–905.

Smith CB. 1946. The role of riboflavin in migraine. *Canadian Medical Association Journal*. 54: 589–591.

Stokes M, Becker WJ, Lipton RB, Sullivan SD, Wilcox TK, Wells L, Manack A, Proskorovsky I, Gladstone J, Buse DC, Varon SF, Goadsby PJ, and Blumenfeld AM. 2011. Cost of health care among patients with chronic and episodic migraine in Canada and the USA: Results from the international burden of migraine study (IBMS). *Headache*. 51: 1058–1077.

Sun-Edelstein C and Mauskop A. 2009. Role of magnesium in the pathogenesis and treatment of migraine. *Expert Review Neurotherapeutics*. 9(3): 369–379.

Sutherland A and Sweet BV. 2010. Butterbur: An alternative therapy for migraine prevention. *American Journal Health-System Pharmacology*. 67: 705–711.

Taylor FR. 2011. Nutraceuticals and headache: The biological basis. *Headache*. 51: 484–501.

Vos T et al. 2012. Years lived with disability (YLDs) for 1160 sequelae of 289 diseases and injuries 1990–2010: A systematic analysis for the global burden of disease study 2010. *Lancet*. 380: 2163–2196.

Wang F, Van Den Eeden SK, Ackerson LM, Salk SE, Reince RH, and Elin RJ. 2003. Oral magnesium oxide prophylaxis of frequent migrainous headache in children: A randomized, double-blind, placebo-controlled trial. *Headache*. 43: 601–610.

15 Probiotics—From Gut to Cognition

Virginia Robles-Alonso, Claudia Herrera, and Francisco Guarner

CONTENTS

15.1 SUMMARY

A large and diverse community of commensal microbes is harbored in the human gut, in a synbiotic arrangement that influences both physiology and pathology in the host. First, the gut microbes conduct a multitude of biochemical reactions and they can be collectively conceived as a "metabolic organ." Second, they provide an important barrier for defense against invasion by pathogens, and finally, host–microbes interactions in the gut play a role in the development and regulation of local and distant host structures and organs, like mucosal and systemic immunity, liver, heart, and brain. Microbial ecology in the gut can be modulated by pharmacological, and nutritional intervention with probiotics and prebiotics, and a balanced microbial environment would likely help to boost the synbiotic functions of bacteria on host's health. In controlled human studies, probiotics and prebiotics have been used, safely and successfully, for improving certain metabolic functions of the microbiota (lactose digestion, calcium absorption, stimulation of bowel transit, and prevention of hepatic encephalopathy (HE)), for protection against infections (prevention and treatment of acute diarrhea, prevention of bacterial translocation) and for modulation of the immuno-inflammatory disorders (prevention and treatment of atopic diseases, necrotizing enterocolitis, chronic pouchitis). Current experimental and clinical research aims at establishing a potential role of probiotics and prebiotics in the prevention and control of obesity, metabolic syndrome, colon cancer, and even psychological disorders.

15.2 GUT MICROBIOTA

15.2.1 Host–Microbes Relationships

The term "microbiota" refers to the community of living micro-organisms assembled in a particular ecological niche of a host individual. Chronic microbial colonization that inflicts no evident harm on the host, only attracted minor scientific attention during the past century (Moran 2006). However, vertebrate and invertebrate animals are in permanent association with such microbial communities maternally inherited at birth or acquired from the environment during the first stages of life (Moran 2006). Associations that benefit the host as well as the microbe are grouped under the term "symbiosis" and the microbial partners are called "symbionts." The prevalence of symbiosis has long been recognized on the basis of observations from microscopy, but most aspects of symbiont origins and functions have remained unexplored, before the age of molecular techniques, because of the difficulties to cultivate and isolate a large majority of these microbial species. The development of novel gene sequencing technologies as well as availability of powerful bioinformatic analysis tools have allowed a dramatic proliferation of research studies over the past few years.

Although all epithelial surfaces of mammalians are colonized by microorganisms, the gastrointestinal tract has the largest microbial burden. In humans, the gastrointestinal tract houses over 10^{14} microbial cells with over 1000 microbial species, most of them belonging to the domain bacteria (Qin et al. 2010). The human gut is the natural habitat for a complex ecosystem of microbial communities that have adapted to live on the mucosal surfaces or in the lumen (Guarner and Malagelada 2003, Dethlefsen et al. 2007). Gut bacteria include native species that colonize the tract permanently and a variable set of living micro-organisms that transit through the tract temporarily. Native bacteria are mainly acquired at birth and during the first years of life, whereas transient bacteria are continuously being ingested from the environment (food, drinks, etc.).

The mucosa of the gastrointestinal tract constitutes a major interface with the external environment, and is the body's principal site for interaction with the microbial world. The gastrointestinal mucosa exhibits a very large surface (considering the villus-crypt structure in an unfolded disposition, a flat extension of up to 4000 ft^2 is estimated), and contains adapted structures and functions for bi-directional communication with microorganisms, including a number of preformed receptors, microbial recognition mechanisms, host–microbe cross-talk pathways, and microbe-specific adaptive responses (Cummings et al. 2004, MacDonald et al. 2011). The stomach and the duodenum harbor a very low number of microorganisms adhering to the mucosal surface or in transit, typically less than 10^3 bacteria cells (colony forming units (CFU)) per gram of contents. Acid, bile, and pancreatic secretions kill most ingested microbes, and the phasic propulsive motor activity impedes stable colonization of the lumen. There is a progressive increase in the number of bacteria along the jejunum and ileum, from approximately 10^4 in the jejunum to 10^7 CFU/g of contents at the ileal end. The large intestine is heavily populated by anaerobes with numbers in the region of 10^{12} CFU/g of luminal contents. In the upper gut, transit is rapid and bacterial density is low, but the impact on immune function is thought to be important by interactions of bacteria with the organized lymphoid structures of the small intestinal mucosa. In the colon, however, transit time is slow and microorganisms have the opportunity to proliferate by fermenting available substrates derived from either the diet or endogenous secretions. By far, the colon harbors the largest population of human microbial symbionts, which contribute to 60% of the solid colonic contents (O'Hara and Shanahan 2006). Several 100 g of bacteria living within the colonic lumen certainly affect the host homoeostasis.

Some resident bacteria in the human gut are associated with toxin formation and pathogenicity when they become dominant, e.g., *Clostridium difficile.* Some other resident species are potential pathogens when the integrity of the mucosal barrier is functionally breached. However, the normal interaction between gut bacteria and their host is a symbiotic relationship, defined as mutually beneficial for both partners. The host provides a nutrient-rich habitat, and the intestinal bacteria confer important benefits on the host's health (Hooper et al. 2002). Several beneficial features of gut bacteria are widely recognized, including production of short-chain fatty acids, vitamin synthesis, secretion of defensins or bacteriocins, and inhibition of pathogens through a multiplicity of mechanisms (Guarner and Malagelada 2003, O'Hara and Shanahan 2006). Our current knowledge on the benefits derived from microbial colonization is mainly supported by observations using germ-free animal models.

15.2.2 Primary Functions of the Microbiota

Comparison of animals bred under germ-free conditions with their conventionally raised counterparts (conventional microflora) has revealed a series of anatomic characteristics and physiological functions that are associated with the presence of the microbiota (Wostmann 1981) (Figure 15.1). Organ weights (heart, lung, and liver), cardiac output, intestinal wall thickness, intestinal motor activity, serum gamma-globulin levels, lymph nodes, among other characteristics, are all reduced or atrophic in germ-free animals, suggesting that gut bacteria have important and specific functions on the host. These functions are ascribed into three categories, i.e., metabolic, protective, and trophic functions (Guarner and Malagelada 2003, O'Hara and Shanahan 2006).

Germ-free vs. Colonized mice

Reduced
- Organ weight (heart, liver, lungs)
- Cardiac output
- Oxygen consumption

Increased
- Food intake

Reduced
- Mesenteric and systemic lymph nodes
- Mucosa-associated lymphoid tissue
- Serum immunoglobulin levels

Increased
- Susceptibility to infection

FIGURE 15.1 Germ-free animals have increased nutritional requirements in order to sustain body weight, are highly susceptible to infections, and show structural and functional deficiencies. Reconstitution of germ-free animals with a microbiota restores most of these deficiencies, suggesting that gut bacteria provide important and specific tasks to the host's homeostasis.

Metabolic functions consist in the fermentation of non-digestible dietary substrates and endogenous mucus. Gene diversity among the microbial community provides a variety of enzymes and biochemical pathways that are distinct from the host's own constitutive resources. Fermentation of carbohydrates is a major source of energy in the colon for bacterial growth and produces short-chain fatty acids that can be absorbed by the host (Figure 15.2). This results in salvage of dietary energy, and favors the absorption of ions (Ca, Mg, Fe) in the cecum. Metabolic functions also include the production of vitamins (K, B_{12}, biotin, folic acid, panthotenate) and synthesis of aminoacids from ammonia or urea (Metges 2000).

Protective functions of gut microbes include the barrier effect that prevents invasion by pathogens. The resident bacteria represent a crucial line of resistance to the colonization by exogenous microbes or opportunistic bacteria that are present in the gut, but their growth is restricted. The equilibrium between species of resident bacteria provides stability in the microbial population, but use of antibiotics can disrupt the balance (for instance, overgrowth of toxigenic *Clostridium difficile*). The barrier effect is based on the ability of certain bacteria to secrete antimicrobial substances, bacteriocins, which inhibit the growth of pathogens, and also in the competition for ecological niches.

Trophic functions of the gut microbiota include the control of epithelial cell proliferation and differentiation. Epithelial cell turnover is reduced in colonic crypts of germ-free animals as compared to the colonized controls. Cell differentiation is highly influenced by the interaction with resident microorganisms as shown by the expression of a variety of genes in germ-free animals mono-associated with specific bacteria strains (Hooper et al. 2001), and in humans fed with probiotic lactobacilli (van Baarlen et al. 2011). The microbiota suppresses intestinal epithelial cell expression of a circulating lipoprotein-lipase inhibitor, fasting-induced adipose factor (Fiaf), thereby promoting the storage of triglycerides in adipocytes (Backhed et al. 2005).

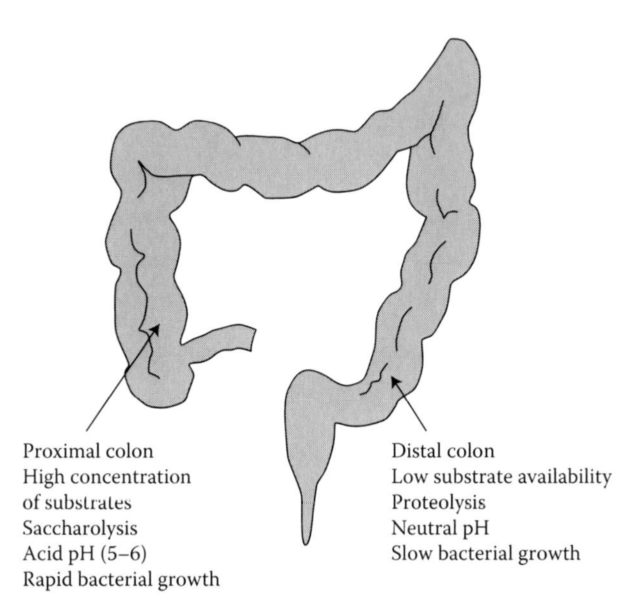

FIGURE 15.2 The human proximal colon is a saccharolytic environment. Fermentation of undigested carbohydrates is intense with high production of short-chain fatty acids, and rapid bacterial growth. By contrast, carbohydrate availability decreases in the distal colon and putrefactive processes of proteins and amino acids are the main energy source for bacteria. (Adapted from Guarner, F. and J. R. Malagelada. 2003. *Lancet* 361:512–9, in Figure 1.)

Gut bacteria play important trophic effects on mucosal immunocompetent cells and are critical for the development of a healthy immune system. Animals bred in a germ-free environment show low densities of lymphoid cells in the gut mucosa; the specialized follicle structures are small and circulating immunoglobulin levels are low. Immediately after exposure to microbes, the number of mucosal lymphocytes expands; germinal centers and immunoglobulin producing cells appear rapidly in follicles and in the lamina propria, and there is a significant increase in the serum immunoglobulin levels (Yamanaka et al. 2003, Bouskra et al. 2008).

During life, multiple and diverse interactions between microbes, epithelium, and gut lymphoid tissues are constantly reshaping local and systemic mechanisms of immunity. Commensal microbes play a major role in the induction of regulatory T cells in the gut lymphoid follicles (Atarashi et al. 2011). Controlled pathways mediated by regulatory T cells are essential homeostatic mechanisms by which the host can tolerate the massive burden of innocuous antigens within the gut or on other body surfaces without resulting in inflammation (Guarner et al. 2006, Round and Mazmanian 2009, MacDonald et al. 2011) (Figure 15.3).

Distant trophic effects include a certain role of the microbiota on the central nervous system. The ability of the gut microbiota to communicate with the brain and thus influence behavior is emerging as an exciting concept (Dinan et al. 2013). Reports suggest that microbial colonization impacts mammalian brain development and subsequent adult behavior (Neufeld et al. 2011). Germ-free mice have increased

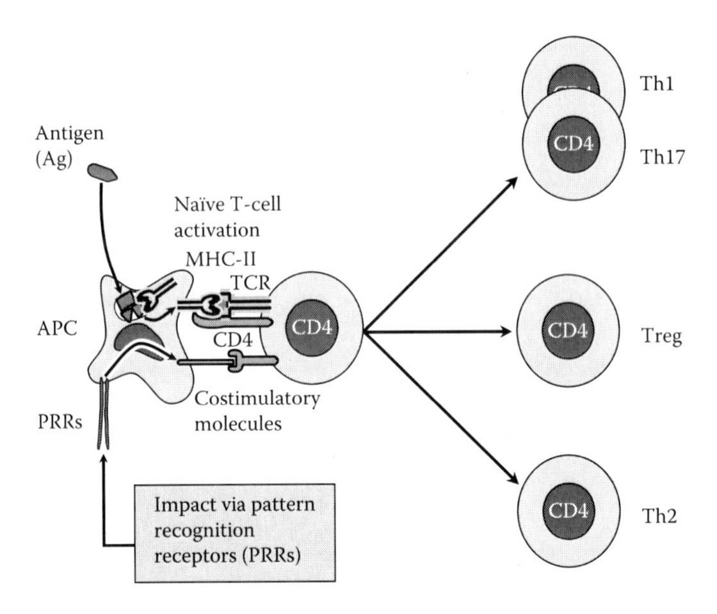

FIGURE 15.3 The specialized lymphoid follicles of the gut mucosa are the major sites for induction and regulation of immune responses. Gut microbes stimulate clonal expansion of lymphocytes, which may differentiate into Th1, Th2, Th17 or Treg cells, with different effector or regulatory capabilities. Innate recognition of microbe associated molecular patterns by antigen-presenting cells (APC) plays a decisive role for the induction of either effector or regulatory pathways.

locomotor activity and reduced anxiety as compared with conventionally colonized mice, and this behavioral phenotype is associated with the altered expression of critical genes in brain regions implicated in motor control and anxiety-like behavior (Diaz Heijtz et al. 2011). When these germ-free mice are reconstituted with a fecal microbiota early in life, they display similar behavior and brain characteristics as conventional mice. Thus, experimental evidence suggests that the enteric microbiota can affect brain development.

15.2.3 Structure of the Human Gut Microbiota

The advent of high-throughput sequencing technologies has lead to a turning point in our understanding of the microbial colonization of the human gut. Analysis of the genetic material in an environment allows the characterization of the microbial communities as a whole and provides the global profile of all the community members and their relative abundance. The new approach has lead to coin the term "metagenomics," which is defined as the study of the genetic material recovered directly from environmental samples by-passing the need to isolate and culture individual community members (Frank and Pace 2008).

The most common approach consists on the extraction of DNA from a biological sample, followed by the amplification and sequencing of 16S ribosomal RNA (rRNA) gene in the sample. The 16S rRNA gene is present in prokaryotes (bacteria and archea) and contains both conserved and variable regions. Thus, similarities and differences in the sequence of nucleotides of the 16S rRNA gene allow taxonomic identification ranging from the domain and phylum level to the species or strain level. Taxonomic identification is based on comparison of 16S rRNA sequences in the sample with reference sequences in the database.

The most powerful molecular approach is not limited to 16S rRNA sequencing but it addresses all the genetic material in the sample. The decreasing cost and increasing speed of DNA sequencing, coupled with the advances in the computational analyses of large datasets, have made it feasible to analyze complex mixtures of entire genomes with a reasonable coverage. The resulting information describes the collective genetic content of the community from which functional and metabolic networks can be inferred. Thus, the full metagenomic approach has the advantage of not only providing the taxonomic characterization of prokaryotic members of the community, but it also tells about non-prokaryotic cells (virus, yeast, protist) and biological functions present in the community.

Molecular studies based either on 16S rRNA gene or full metagenomic sequencing have highlighted that only 7 to 9 of the 55 known divisions or phyla of the domain bacteria are detected in faecal or mucosal samples from the human gut (Eckburg et al. 2005, Arumugam et al. 2011, Human Microbiome Project 2012, Qin et al. 2010) (Figure 15.4). Moreover, such studies also revealed that more than 90% of all the bacterial taxa belong to just two divisions: Bacteroidetes and Firmicutes. The other divisions that have been consistently found in samples from the human distal gut are Proteobacteria, Actinobacteria, Fusobacteria, and Verrucomicrobia. At a species

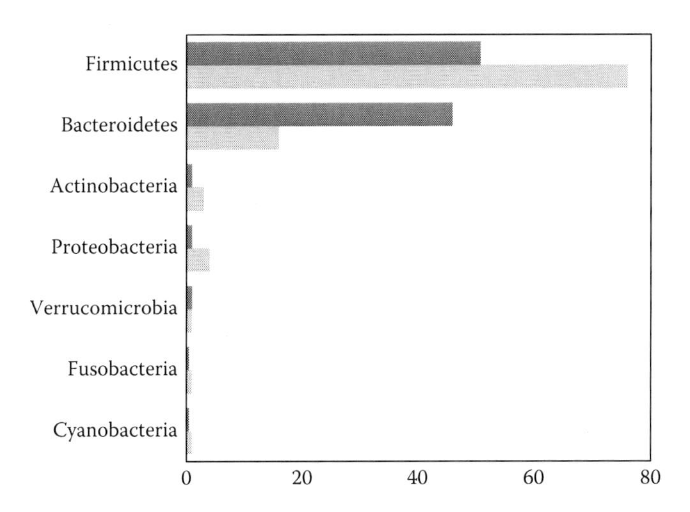

FIGURE 15.4 Composition of the human enteric microbiota as determined by 16S rRNA sequencing of fecal and mucosal samples from the gastrointestinal tract. Only 7 to 9 of the 55 known divisions or phyla of the domain Bacteria are detected. The graph shows number of species or phylotypes (dark columns) of each bacterial division, and total number of strains (light columns) of each division. More than 90% of strains belong to 2 divisions: the Bacteroidetes and the Firmicutes. (Data from the study by Eckburg, P. B. et al., 2005. *Science* no. 308 (5728):1635–8.)

TABLE 15.1
The Human Gut Microbiome

Microbial Genes in the Human Gut	Number of Genes
Number on non-redundant genes in the cohort	
Median gene set per individual	590,384
Common genes (present in at least 50% of individuals)	294,110
Rare genes (present in less than 20% of individuals)	2,375,655

Source: Data from Qin et al. 2010. *Nature* no. 464 (7285):59–65. doi: 10.1038/nature08821.

or strain level, there is a considerable variation in the composition of the faecal microbiota among human individuals. Strain diversity between individuals is highly remarkable so that studies have found that a large proportion of the identified strain-level phylotypes are unique to each person (Eckburg et al. 2005). Each individual harbors his or her own distinctive pattern of bacterial composition. Intra-individual variability is remarkable; and factors, such as diet, drug intake, traveling, or colonic transit time, have an impact on microbial composition in faecal samples over time in a unique host (Caporaso et al. 2011).

Full metagenomic analysis of faecal samples from a cohort of European adult subjects identified a total of 3.3 million non-redundant microbial genes (Qin et al. 2010). This effort provided for the first time a gene catalogue of the human gut microbiome. Each individual carries an average of 600,000 non-redundant microbial genes in the gastrointestinal tract, and around 300,000 microbial genes are common in the sense that they are present in at least 50% of the individuals (Table 15.1). Interestingly, *Bacteroides*, *Faecalibacterium*, and *Bifidobacterium* are the most abundant genera but their relative proportion is highly variable across individuals (Arumugam et al. 2011).

Network analysis of species abundance across different individuals suggested that the human microbiome conforms well-balanced host-microbial symbiotic states driven by groups of co-occurring species and genera (Arumugam et al. 2011). Multidimensional cluster analysis and principal component analysis of fecal samples from American, European, and Japanese individuals revealed that all individual samples formed three robust clusters, in terms of overall similarity, which were designated as "enterotypes." Each of the three enterotypes is identifiable by the variation in the levels of one of the three genera: *Bacteroides* (enterotype 1), *Prevotella* (enterotype 2), and *Ruminococcus* (enterotype 3). The basis for the enterotype clustering is unknown but appears independent of nationality, sex, age, or body mass index. The three enterotypes partition has also been shown in Chinese population (Qin et al. 2012).

15.3 PROBIOTICS AND PREBIOTICS

15.3.1 Concept

The Nobel Prize winner Ilya Metchnikoff, a microbiologist working at the Pasteur Institute in Paris at the beginning of the twentieth century, advocated the theory that aging is caused by toxic bacteria in the gut and that lactic acid could prolong life. Sour milk (yogurt) owes its peculiar flavor and texture to the lactic acid released during the fermentation of lactose by lactic acid bacteria. Until the 1900s, yogurt was common in the diets of the people in the Russian Empire (and especially central Asia and the Caucasus), Turkey and southeastern Europe/Balkans. Based on his theory, Metchnikoff used to drink yogurt every day, and hypothesized that regular consumption of yogurt was responsible for the long lifespans of Bulgarian peasants.

The first reference to the term "probiotic" dates back to 1965 by Lilly and Stillwell (1965), who defined probiotics as "active substances that are essential for a healthy development of life." Some years later, the term was mainly applied to animal-feed supplements containing living micro-organisms, specifically designed to improve animal health. In 2001, a group of experts appointed by FAO and WHO redefined the concept of probiotic as "live micro-organisms which when administered in adequate amounts confer a health benefit on the host," not only amplifying the benefits to human health but also providing guidelines on functional and safety aspects of probiotics (FAO/WHO 2001). According to the guidelines, probiotics must be characterized at three levels: genus, species, and strain; it is essential to highlight the idea that their properties depend on all three and cannot be attributed to other strains, even if they share the same genus and species. Safety of well-characterized bacterial species traditionally used in food products is well established, and probiotics based on these strains are generally recognized as safe (GRAS in the USA and QPS status in Europe). No significant adverse events have been observed despite widespread use of such traditional strains (Salminen et al. 2002). New probiotic strains should undergo a process, a safety assessment, as recommended by the FAO/WHO guidelines.

The term prebiotic refers to "a nondigestible food ingredient that beneficially affects the host by selectively stimulating growth and/or activity of one or a limited number of bacteria in the colon" (Gibson and Roberfroid 1995). A prebiotic should not be hydrolyzed by human intestinal enzymes; it should be selectively fermented by beneficial bacteria, and this selective fermentation should result in a beneficial effect on health or well-being of the host. Most prebiotics described so far are nondigestible carbohydrates that promote the growth of endogenous lactobacilli or bifidobacteria in the large bowel (Table 15.2). Finally, the combination of probiotics and prebiotics is termed "synbiotic," and is an appealing concept to optimize the impact of bacteria on health.

Dysfunction of the microbiota is being incriminated in several diseases or disorders (Table 15.3). Probiotics, prebiotics, and synbiotics can be used to restore homestasis by improving composition and functions of the gut microbial ecosystem and thus providing benefits to the host. This chapter describes some of these benefits under the framework of the main functions gut microbiota in humans.

15.3.2 Metabolic Effects

Probiotics and prebiotics have been used for improving metabolic functions of the gut microbiota like digestion of lactose, reduction of anaerobic degradation of proteins (putrefaction), modulation of colonic gas content, production of short-chain fatty acids, etc.

TABLE 15.2
Products with Established Prebiotic Effect

INULIN-TYPE FRUCTANS	
Linear β (2→1) Fructosyl-Fructose Polymers. Glucose-Fructose$_n$ and/or Fructose-Fructose$_n$	
Short to large size polymers (DP 2-60)	Inulin (especially chicory inulin) (DP_{av} 12)
Short oligomers (DP 2-8)	Fructo-oligosaccharides FOS scFOS (enzymatic synthesis from sucrose) (DP_{av} 3-6) Oligofructose (enzymatic partial hydrolysis of inulin) (DP_{av} 4)
Large size polymers (DP 10-60)	High molecular weight inulin (physical purification) (DP_{av} 25) lcFOS
Mixture (DP 2-8) + (DP 10-60)	Mixture of oligomers and large size polymers
GALACTANS	
Mixture of β (1 → 6); β (1 → 3); β (1 → 4) Galactosyl-Galactose	
Disaccharide Galactosyl-Fructose	Lactulose
Short oligomers Galactose$_n$-Galactose, and/or Galactose$_n$-Glucose (DP2-8)	Galacto-oligosaccharides GOS Trans-galactooligosaccharides TOS (enzymatic transgalactosylsation of lactose)
Mixture of galactans and inulin-type fructans GOS-FOS	Galacto-oligosaccharides and high molecular weight inulin, usually known as GOS-FOS or scGOS-lcFOS

Note: DP, degree of polymerisation; DP_{av}, average degree of polymerization; ITF, inulin-type fructans; FOS, fructo-oligosaccharides; scFOS, short-chain fructo-oligosaccharides; lcFOS, long-chain fructo-oligosaccharides; GOS, galacto-oligosaccharides; scGOS, short-chain galacto-oligosaccharides; TOS, trans-galactooligosaccharides.

15.3.2.1 Lactose Digestion

The disaccharide lactose, mainly found in milk and dairy products, is hydrolyzed to glucose and galactose by lactase (a beta-galactosidase), that is present in the brush border of epithelial cells in the small intestine. However, a sensible percentage of the adult population develops a deficiency of intestinal lactase after weaning. Prevalence of lactose malabsorption in adult populations is high, and varies between 5 to 15% in northern European and American countries and 50 to 100% in African, Asian, and south American countries (de Vrese et al. 2001). These subjects may develop gastrointestinal symptoms such as abdominal bloating, pain, flatulence, and diarrhoea after ingestion of lactose, so that they tend to eliminate milk and dairy products

TABLE 15.3
Microbiota Dysfunction and Potential Impacts on Disease

Disorder	Claimed Microbiota Dysfunction
Infectious diarrhea, antibiotic-associated diarrhea	Altered composition/structure of microbial community
Septic complications: multisystem organ failure, diverticulitis, appendicitis	Deficient barrier function
Necrotizing enterocolitis	Altered composition/structure of microbial community Deficient barrier function
Hepatic encephalopathy	Metabolic dysfunction Deficient barrier function
Functional disorders: constipation, bloating, irritable bowel syndrome	Metabolic dysfunction Defects in trophic functions on motility, immunity
Obesity, type 2 diabetes, metabolic syndrome	Metabolic dysfunction Deficient barrier function Defects in trophic functions on immunity
Atopy, inflammatory bowel diseases, certain autoimmune disorders (?)	Defects in trophic functions on immunity
Colon cancer	Metabolic dysfunction: generation of genotoxic metabolites Defects in trophic functions on epithelial cells
Anxiety (?), autism (?)	Defects in trophic functions on Central Nervous System

from their diet and consequently, their calcium intake may be deficient. The bacteria used as starter culture in yogurt (*Streptococcus thermophilus* and *Lactobacillus delbrueckii* subsp. bulgaricus) can improve lactose digestion and eliminate symptoms in lactase deficient individuals. The benefit is due to the presence of microbial beta-galactosidase in the bacteria that hydrolizes lactose during its transit through the small bowel (Kolars et al. 1984). However, the enzyme is destroyed by gastric secretions if the yogurt is pasteurized or sterilized before consumption (bacterial cell wall protects the enzyme from gastric juice). A large number of human studies in which the consumption of live yogurt cultures was compared with the consumption of heat-killed bacteria demonstrated better lactose digestion and absorption as well as reduction of gastrointestinal symptoms in subjects that consumed yogurt with live cultures (Savaiano et al. 1984, Lerebours et al. 1989, Marteau et al. 1990). The benefit of yogurt bacteria on lactose absorption was also demonstrated in healthy subjects without lactose maldigestion (Rizkalla et al. 2000).

15.3.2.2 Calcium Absorption

Certain prebiotics can improve calcium absorption in adolescents and adults. In controlled human studies, dietary intake of inulin and/or oligofructose at doses from 8 to 15 g/day increased calcium absorption by 18 to 54% (Cashman 2002, Abrams et al. 2007). Inulin is a polysaccharide composed of glucose and a linear chain of fructose moieties linked by specific beta (2-1) bonds. Oligofructose is an inulin-type oligosaccharide that contains only two to ten fructose moieties in the linear chain. Both inulin and oligofructose are poorly digested in humans and its recovery from the distal small intestine is equivalent to that of an unabsorbable polyethylenglycol marker. However, they are completely fermented by the microflora of the colon, particularly by bacteria with a specific fructosidase that hydrolyzes the fructose chain. The products of hydrolysis, fructose, and glucose, are highly efficient substrates for the growth of saccharolytic bacteria, including lactobacilli and bifidobacteria. Oligofructose and inulin have been shown to increase the number of fecal bifidobacteria in healthy humans, and reduce the concentration of bacteroides and clostridia (Gibson et al. 1995). As a result of the fermentation of inulin, the production of short-chain fatty acids within the colonic lumen increases, and a slight acidification of colonic contents is observed. At a lower luminal pH, more calcium is soluble and thus is more readily absorbed by epithelial cells in the cecum and proximal colon. Short-chain fatty acids also enhance calcium absorption.

15.3.2.3 Hepatic Encephalopathy

HE is a serious neuropsychiatric complication of both acute and chronic liver failure. A network of organs is involved in ammonia homeostasis and there is a convincing body of evidence to suggest that hyperammonemia in liver failure results from an altered interorgan trafficking of ammonia. Ammonia produced by the gut and kidney is removed primarily by the liver as urea and glutamine and also by muscle and brain as glutamine. In liver failure, urea and glutamine production is impaired, so that the main organ to offset the remaining ammonia is muscle. These, along with intra- and extrahepatic portosystemic shunts, are the main causes of HE. Minimal HE (MHE) is characterized by subtle neurocognitive deficits without overt clinical manifestations.

The prebiotic lactulose is useful for prevention and treatment of HE in patients with advanced liver disease. A systematic review (Als-Nielsen et al. 2004) suggested that there is insufficient evidence to support or refute the use of non-absorbable disaccharides for hepatic encephalopathy, but the review did not distinguish between the prebiotic lactulose and the non-fermentable disaccharide lactitol. Lactulose is fermented in the colon, decreases proteolytic activity of the microbiota, and thus generation of ammonia (de Preter et al. 2008).

Malaguarnera et al. (2010) tested a mixture of *Bifidobacterium* species and prebiotic fructo-oligosaccharides (FOS) for 12 weeks versus lactulose in patients with MHE, showing similar effects by reducing blood ammonia levels and improving the validated neuropsychological test scores. A meta-analysis assessing efficacy of probiotics, prebiotics, or synbiotics for treating MHE, included nine clinical trials, five of which used lactulose. The remaining four studies used different probiotic species or combinations including FOS. Treatment was associated with significant improvement in MHE (Shukla et al. 2011).

In summary, several probiotics, prebiotics, like lactulose or FOS, and synbiotics are useful and have a safe profile for treating HE or MHE. This effect reflects the ability to decrease microbial proteolytic activity (putrefaction) within the gut by consumption of such probiotics and prebiotics.

15.3.2.4 Irritable Bowel Syndrome

The irritable bowel syndrome (IBS) is a common clinical entity, and, though usually non-severe, results in an impaired quality of life and increases the health-care burden. The pathogenesis of IBS remains undefined and the known risk factors are multifactorial. The increased risk of developing IBS following gastroenteritis, the co-existence of dysbiosis, elevated luminal gas production, and immune activation provide a body of evidence to aim at the enteric microbiota as a therapeutic target. Symptoms of abdominal pain or discomfort, typically associated with defecation or a change in bowel transit, bloating, and flatulence are commonly seen in patients with IBS. Fermentations taking place in the colon generate a variable volume of gas. However, some gut bacteria degrade metabolic substrates without producing gas, and even some other species may consume gas, particularly hydrogen. Hypothetically, administration of appropriate bacteria strains could reduce gas accumulation within the bowel in these patients.

Different meta-analyses conclude that probiotics may have beneficial effects in the management of IBS (McFarland and Dublin 2008, Hoveyda et al. 2009, Moayyedi et al. 2010), and the benefits are strain-specific. In particular, Bifidobacterium lactis DN-173010 seems to improve objectively measured abdominal bloating and gastrointestinal transit, as well as reduced symptomatology (Agrawal et al. 2009). Likewise, another placebo controlled trial with 25 patients concluded that a probiotic mixture (VSL#3) was useful for the relief of abdominal bloating in patients with diarrhoea predominant IBS (Kim et al. 2005). Besides, the same mixture has proven efficacy reducing flatulence (Kim et al. 2003). Probiotics need to be evaluated further but they appear to be useful for the control of the symptoms related with the altered handling or perception of intestinal gas in this group of patients, and they are currently recommended for functional bowel disorders by consensus guidelines (Hungin et al. 2013).

15.3.2.5 Non-Alcoholic Fatty Liver

Non-alcoholic fatty liver disease (NAFLD) comprises a spectrum of conditions that range from steatosis to cirrhosis, at the most serious end of the spectrum. Several studies have demonstrated a strong link between obesity and NAFLD. Experimental evidence suggest that gut-derived products, including bacterial lipopolysaccharide and endotoxin, are involved in the pathogenesis of steatohepatitis, so that it has been shown, increased hepatotoxicity and decreased survival after exposure to LPS in obese mice strains (Yang et al. 1997). Under this hypothesis, some studies evaluated the therapeutic role of probiotics for treating NAFLD. Aller et al. (2011) tested the effect of *Lactobacillus bulgaricus* and *Streptococcus thermophilus* in patients with NAFLD. The study showed an improvement of liver function tests (reduction in plasma levels ALT, AST, and gamma GTP); however, the anthropometric parameters and cardio-metabolic risk factors remained unchanged after treatment. In the other study, Malaguarnera et al. (2012) evaluated the effect of a synbiotic product (*Bifidobacterium longum* with FOS) in patients with non-alcoholic steatohepatitis. A total of 66 patients were recruited and randomly divided into two groups. The synbiotic significantly reduced serum AST levels, insulin resistance (HOMA-IR), serum endotoxin, steatosis, and the NASH activity index. In contrast, negative results were reported by Solga et al. in a (2008) study that assessed liver steatosis by an imaging technique (proton magnetic resonance spectroscopy) and observed an increase of steatosis in three out of four patients treated with the mixture of probiotics VSL#3 for 4 months. However, a larger randomized controlled trial employing a mixture of probiotics (*Lactobacillus plantarum, Lactobacillus deslbrueckii, Lactobacillus acidophilus, Lactobacillus rhamnosus,* and *Bifidobacterium bifidum*) showed significant reduction of liver fat, assessed by magnetic resonance and serum AST level (Wong et al. 2013).

In summary, certain probiotics and prebiotics are an attractive therapeutic option for this clinical condition. Studies have tested single probiotic or multiple species products, and combinations with prebiotics, and current recommendations are limited to the products tested until further studies provide confirmative data and supportive information on mechanisms of action.

15.3.2.6 Metabolic Syndrome and Obesity

Obesity emerges as a major health problem in Western countries due to its associated comorbidities. The increased incidence is probably due to a combination of different causes. A sedentary lifestyle, changing traditional dietary patterns in developed countries or genetic factors are some of the factors that contribute to the onset of obesity. It is known that adipose tissue has the capacity to secrete adipokines (leptin, TNF-alpha, interleukin-6, etc.). These adipokines are related to inflammatory and metabolic processes that contribute to atherosclerosis, dyslipidemia, hypertension, insulin resistance, and type 2 diabetes, NAFLD, and are a possible link between adiposity and cardiovascular complications. Some recent data on the metabolic syndrome suggest that changes in gut microbiome composition may play a role in the disorder. In animal models, fecal microbiota transplantation from obese conventional mice to non-obese germ-free mice resulted in transfer of metabolic syndrome-associated features from the donor to the recipient (Blaut and Klaus 2012). Moreover, Vrieze et al. (2012) in a randomizaed controlled trial, studied in humans the effects of infusing intestinal microbiota from lean donors to recipients with type 2 diabetes and metabolic syndrome. Six weeks after infusion of microbiota from lean donors, insulin sensitivity of recipients improved along with increased levels of butyrate-producing gut microbiota. The mechanisms advocated are the provision of additional energy by the conversion of dietary fiber to SCFA, effects on gut-hormone production, and increased intestinal permeability, causing elevated systemic levels of lipopolysaccharides. The contact with these antigens seems to contribute to low-grade inflammation, a characteristic trait of obesity and the metabolic syndrome. A number of clinical trials are currently evaluating the role of prebiotics and probiotics for prevention and control of obesity associated with metabolic syndrome.

15.3.3 Protective Effects

Probiotics and prebiotics may improve barrier function and help against infections (Figure 15.5).

15.3.3.1 Gastrointestinal Infections

Probiotics are useful for treatment of acute infectious diarrhoea in children, this being the most well-established indication for probiotics. Different strains, including *Lactobacillus reuteri*, *L. rhamnosus strain* GG, *L. acidophilus,* and the yeast

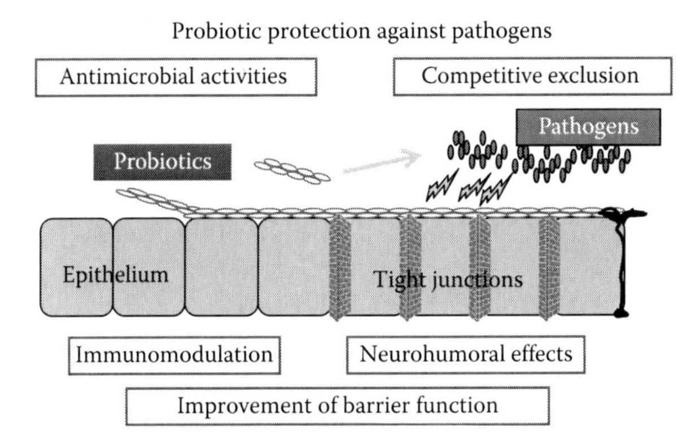

FIGURE 15.5 Probiotics can protect against gastrointestinal infections by different mechanisms of action. Some strains have effects at the intestinal luminal site and produce bacteriocins with antimicrobial activity against pathogens or compete with them for the available substrates and niches. Some strains have effects on the mucosal site by strengthening barrier function (mucus secretion, tight junction improvement) or stimulating immune defense.

Sacharomyces cerevisae (boulardii), have been tested in controlled clinical trials and were proven useful in reducing the severity and duration of diarrhoea. Several meta-analyses of controlled clinical trials have been published, as well as a systematic review from the Cochrane Centre (Allen et al. 2010).

A large number of clinical trials have tested the efficacy of probiotics in the prevention of acute diarrheal conditions, including antibiotic-associated diarrhoea (AAD), nosocomial, and community-acquired infectious enteritis, and traveler's diarrhoea (Sazawal et al. 2006). Prophylactic use of probiotics has proven useful for the prevention of acute diarrhoea in infants admitted into the hospital ward for a chronic disease condition. Probiotics may also be useful in the prevention of community-acquired diarrhoea (Sur et al. 2011).

Several studies have investigated the efficacy of probiotics in the prevention of traveler's diarrhea in adults, and a meta-analysis suggests that probiotics may offer a safe and effective method to prevent traveler's diarrhea (McFarland 2007).

AAD is described as unexplained diarrhea that occurs in association with the use of oral or parenteral antibiotics. Microbiota alteration by antibiotics may change microbial metabolism with the decreased degradation of food residues and osmotic diarrhea as a result. Another consequence of antibiotic therapy leading to diarrhea is the overgrowth of potentially pathogenic organisms such as *Clostridium difficile* (CD). AAD can be caused by multiple organisms other than CD, including *Clostridium perfringens, Staphylococcus aureus,* and *Candida.*

The bacterium CD is an anaerobic pathogen capable of forming spores and secreting enterotoxins. CD is a member of the indigenous gut microbiota, and under normal circumstances, proliferation of this bacterium is suppressed by dominant anaerobes. Antibiotic therapy may perturb the normal balance and impairs the barrier effect of commensals, allowing the overgrowth of CD and access to mucosal niches normally unavailable. The rationale for probiotic administration in order to prevent CD overgrowth includes competition with the pathogen and restoration of the barrier effect.

A meta-analysis (Johnston et al. 2012) showed that probiotic prophylaxis reduces the incidence of diarrhea by CD, with an NNT (number needed to treat) of 26. Different probiotic preparations including *Saccharomyces boulardii*, *Lactobacillus rhamnosus* GG, and others, were tested. Only two of the individual trials reached a statistically significant effect in favor of the probiotic, whereas the meta-analysis of 20 trials showed a clear significant effect of the treatment. This fact is explained by the low number of episodes of diarrhea due to CD in each of the individual trials, so that pooling the data is necessary for a proper evaluation of the effect. Hence, 108 cases of CD infection were observed in the placebo groups versus only 40 cases in probiotic treated arms.

Another randomized, double-blind, placebo-controlled trial (Allen et al. 2013) in which nearly 3000 subjects aged 65 years or older were included, tested a multistrain preparation for 21 days during antibiotic treatment. The mixture failed to prove more effective than placebo for the prevention of CD diarrhea. However, 12 (0.8%) cases were reported in the probiotic group versus 17 (1.2%) in the placebo group (OR: 0.7 [0.34–1.48]; P = 0.35), and a type 2 error may explain the lack of significance.

Prevention of AAD other than CD mediated is a well-established indication for probiotics both in adults and children. To summarize evidence gained during the last 20 years, the meta-analysis (Videlock and Cremonini 2012) of 34 controlled trials indicates that probiotics significantly reduce risk of presenting diarrhea during antibiotic therapy (relative risk is 0.53 with 95% CI 0.44–0.63), with a number needed to treat of 8 (95% CI 7–11). Results were similar when compared between subgroups the probiotic species, population age and sex, and duration of antibiotic and probiotic use. Hence, the use of probiotics has been proven effective in the prevention of antibiotic-associated diarrhea, and is now widely recommended by clinical guidelines (Guarner et al. 2012).

15.3.3.2 Prevention of Systemic Infections

Dysfunction of the gut mucosal barrier may result in the passage through the epithelium of a variable quantity of viable microorganisms that can disseminate throughout the body producing sepsis. Bacterial translocation and its complications have been shown to occur in some pathologic conditions such as post-operative sepsis, severe acute pancreatitis, advanced liver cirrhosis, multisystem organ failure, etc.

Probiotics have been used to prevent sepsis in patients with severe acute pancreatitis. Their efficacy in this setting has been a matter of ongoing debate. In a randomized double-blind trial, patients were treated with either *Lactobacillus plantarum* or placebo. Infected pancreatic necrosis and abscesses occurred at a significantly lower rate in *L. plantarum*-treated patients than in controls (Olah et al. 2002). A large, randomized, double-blind trial, the PROPATRIA study, involved 296 patients in 15 hospitals, and compared the use of a multi-species probiotics preparation (six strains) with a placebo found no difference in infective complications, but mortality was higher in the probiotic group (16 versus 6%), largely due to bowel ischemia (6 versus 0%; Besselink et al. 2008). The authors hypothesized that the combination of severe pancreatitis, organ failure, reduction in mucosal blood flow, and an increased (probiotic) bacterial load could have led to increased local inflammation, with further compromise of mucosal blood supply, resulting in bowel ischemia (Besselink et al. 2009).

A meta-analysis that included seven studies concluded that there is insufficient evidence to support the use of probiotics to prevent infections in acute pancreatitis. The studies included were heterogeneous (Zhang et al. 2010).

A randomized study involving 95 liver transplant patients compared the incidence of infections among three groups of patients submitted to different prophylaxis procedure: selective bowel decontamination with antibiotics, administration of live *L. plantarum* supplemented with fermentable fiber (synbiotic), and administration of heat-killed *L. plantarum* with the fiber supplement. Post-operative infections were recorded in 15 out of 32 patients (48%) in the antibiotics group, 4 out of 31 (13%) in the live *L. plantarum* group, and 11 out of 32 (34%) in the heat-killed *L. plantarum* group, being significant the difference between antibiotics and live *L. plantarum* groups (Bengmark 2003). In a second study by the same group, patients were randomized to receive a synbiotic preparation (including four probiotic strains and four fermentable fibers) or a placebo consisting of the four fibers only. Post-operative infection occurred in only one patient in the treatment group ($n = 33$), in contrast to 16 out of 33 in the placebo group (Rayes et al. 2005). The difference was highly significant. A study of 80 patients undergoing pancreas resection showed significantly fewer post-operative bacterial infections when given Synbiotic 2000 (5 of 40) compared to patients that received fibers only (16 of 40) In addition, the duration of antibiotic therapy was significantly shorter in the latter group (Rayes et al. 2007). In a study of 100 patients undergoing surgery for colorectal cancer who received *L. plantarum*, *L. acidophilus*, and *B. longum*. ($n = 50$) pre- and post-operatively had less post-operative infection complications (14%) compared to the control group (46%; Liu et al. 2011). A meta-analysis, that included nine RCTs, concluded that the use of probiotics or synbiotics reduced post-operative infections after abdominal surgery (for any infection OR: 0.26, 95% CI: 0.12–0.55). These results should be interpreted with caution due to the heterogeneity of the included studies (Pitsouni et al. 2009).

15.3.4 Trophic Effects

Probiotics and prebiotics can be used to modulate immuno-inflammatory responses of the intestinal mucosa. They may potentially influence epithelial growth and proliferation. Finally, additional effects on mood and behavior have been proposed.

15.3.4.1 Necrotizing Enterocolitis

Necrotizing enterocolitis is a severe inflammatory condition of the bowel that may occur in low birth weight neonates due to immaturity and dysfunction of the gut mucosal barrier. Several controlled studies have demonstrated that the use of probiotic mixtures in low-birth-weight infants significantly reduces the incidence and severity of necrotizing enterocolitis and also prevents mortality of immature babies. Meta-analysis of the published trials suggests that probiotics reduce the risk of developing necrotizing enterocolitis by two-thirds and risk of death by one-half (Deshpande et al. 2010). These data are impressive since very few other strategies have proven effective in decreasing the incidence of necrotizing enterocolitis in preterm infants.

15.3.4.2 Inflammatory Bowel Diseases

Clinical and experimental evidence suggests that abnormal activation of the mucosal immune system against the enteric flora is a key event in intestinal inflammatory conditions. Several factors contribute to the pathogenesis of the aberrant immune response toward the autologous flora, including genetic susceptibility, a defect in mucosal barrier function, and a microbial imbalance. In Crohn's disease and ulcerative colitis, patients show an increased mucosal secretion of IgG antibodies against commensal bacteria (Macpherson et al. 1996), whereas the normal physiological response is based on IgA antibodies. Moreover, mucosal T-lymphocytes are hyperreactive against antigens of the common flora (Pirzer et al. 1991). In patients with inflammatory bowel disease the composition of the gut microbiota is characterized by a low diversity of species, but high density of mucosal surface colonization and epithelial invasion in areas with active disease. Also there is a reduction of *F. prausnitzii* (Manichanh et al. 2012). Interactions of gut-commensal microbiota have a central role in promoting homeostatic functions such as immunomodulation, upregulation of cytoprotective genes, prevention and regulation of apoptosis, and maintenance of barrier function (Patel and Lin 2010, Neish et al. 2000). *Bifidobacterium infantis* and *Faecalibacterium prausnitzii* have been shown to induce regulatory T cells and result in the production of the anti-inflammatory interleukin (IL)-10 (O'Mahony et al. 2008, Manichanh et al. 2012). Certain lactobacilli reduce the release of TNFα by inflamed mucosa from Crohn's disease patients (Borruel et al. 2002). Thus, a favorable local microecology could restore the homeostasis of the mucosal immune system and lead to the resolution of the lesions.

Probiotics and prebiotics have been tested in animal models of bowel inflammation. Selected probiotic strains (Madsen et al. 1999, Schultz et al. 2002, McCarthy et al. 2003), including a bacterium genetically engineered to secrete the anti-inflammatory cytokine IL-10 (Steidler et al. 2000), and the prebiotic inulin were proven effective for prevention and treatment of mucosal inflammation. Both probiotics and prebiotics have also been tested in clinical studies.

A Cochrane review that assessed the efficacy of probiotics for maintenance of remission in ulcerative colitis found no difference in probiotics and mesalazine for maintenance of remission in ulcerative colitis. They found a high risk of bias on the studies (Naidoo et al. 2011). A recent meta-analysis showed a benefit for induction of remission of probiotic group compared to placebo (RR: 1.51 [95% CI: 1.10–2.06]), however, there was significant heterogeneity (Shen et al. 2014). Subgroup analysis of type of probiotics showed that only VSL#3 significantly increased the rate of remission/response (RR: 1.74 [95% IC 1.19–2.55]). This study also found probiotics can provide the similar effect as 5-aminosalicylic acid on maintaining remission of UC. Probiotics were not effective for induction or maintenance of remission in Crohn's disease patients. The VSL#3 mixture has been proven highly effective for maintenance of remission of chronic relapsing pouchitis, after induction of remission with antibiotics. In the first study (Gionchetti et al. 2000), a relapse occurred in only 3 out of 20 patients of the VSL#3 group and in all the 20 patients of the placebo group. Of interest, all patients on remission in the probiotic arm had relapses within 4 months after stopping treatment at conclusion of the trial. In the second study, the probiotic mixture was administered in a once-a-day schedule, and similar efficacy was demonstrated (Mimura et al. 2004). Treatment with VSL#3 is also effective in the prevention of the onset of pouchitis after ileal pouch-anal anastomosis (Gionchetti et al. 2003). VSL#3 used at higher doses has been shown to induce remission in patients with acute pouchitis (Gionchetti et al. 2007).

The efficacy of Lactobacillus GG in post-operative recurrence of Crohn's disease has been tested in a randomized, double blind trial. The probiotic showed no effect in the prevention of clinical and endoscopic recurrence as compared with placebo (Prantera et al. 2002). A second clinical trial confirmed the lack of efficacy of this strain in patients with Crohn's disease (Schultz et al. 2004). The same probiotic strain was ineffective as a primary therapy for induction of a clinical or endoscopic response in patients with chronic pouchitis (Kuisma et al. 2003).

The prebiotic inulin has been tested in patients with an ileal pouch-anal anastomosis and mild chronic pouchitis. Compared with placebo, 3 weeks of dietary supplementation with inulin-reduced endoscopic and histological scores (Welters et al. 2002). The effect was associated with an increase in fecal butyrate and a decrease in Bacteroides counts.

In summary, the therapeutical manipulation of the luminal microecology with probiotics and prebiotics for the control and prevention of inflammatory bowel diseases is an attractive concept. Probiotics and prebiotics are safe and well tolerated by IBD patients but clinical trials so far have shown little evidence of efficacy. VSL#3 is effective in preventing pouchitis, which is currently the main indication for probiotics in intestinal inflamationary conditions. There is less evidence of the efficacy of probiotics for inducing and maintaining remission in patients with UC, and no evidence is available to support the use of probiotics in CD.

15.3.4.3 Atopic Diseases

Atopic diseases are due to exaggerated or imbalanced immune responses to environmental and harmless antigens (allergens). Prevalence of allergic diseases in Western societies is increasing at an alarming rate whereas it is much lower in the developing world. It has been suggested that this may be the result of inappropriate microbial stimulus during infancy due to improved hygienic conditions. Some epidemiological and experimental studies have indicated that stimulation of the immune system by certain microbes or microbial products may be effective in the prevention and management of allergic diseases (Matricardi et al. 2003).

The effectiveness of probiotic therapy in the prevention of allergic diseases has been clearly demonstrated in randomized controlled trials (Majamaa and Isolauri 1997, Lodinova-Zadnikova et al. 2003, Lodinova-Zadnikova et al. 2010). A Cochrane review evaluated 12 studies, allergic disease and/or food hypersensitivity outcomes were assessed by 6 studies enrolling 2080 infants, but outcomes for only 1549 infants were reported. Meta-analysis of five studies reporting the outcomes of 1477 infants found a significant reduction in infant eczema (typical RR: 0.82, 95% CI: 0.70–0.95).

There was a significant and substantial heterogeneity between studies (Osborn and Sinn 2007).

A meta-analysis that included 14 studies concluded that probiotic use decreased the incidence of atopic dermatitis (RR: 0.79, [95% CI 0.71–0.88]) and the favorable effect was similar regardless of the time of probiotic use (pregnancy or early life) or the subject(s) receiving probiotics (Pelucchi et al. 2012). Data on a single strain was generally very limited. The only exception was *L. rhamnosus* GG, included among probiotic strains of 6 trials, for which the summary RR was 0.74 (95% CI [0.61–0.90]. Several studies reported a significant reduction in eczema with a combination of probiotics (*B. bifidum*, *B. lactis*, and *Lactococcus lactis* (Niers et al. 2009); *B. bifidum*, *B. lactis*, and *L. acidophilus* (Kim et al. 2010); *L. rhamnosus* LPR and *B. longum* or *L. paracasei* and *B. longum* (Rautava et al. 2012)), compared with placebo. And a recent meta-analysis concluded that probiotics containing mixed bacterial strains may reduce incidence of eczema in infants aged <2 years (Dang et al. 2013).

While the data on prevention are encouraging, a number of studies and meta-analysis did not show a clear benefit of probiotics when used for treatment of atopic eczema (Nermes et al. 2013). Heat-inactivated probiotics have not been clinically effective but recent studies suggest that they can supress a pro-allergic response (Cukrowska et al. 2010).

There are few studies that investigate the effect of probiotics on challenge-confirmed food allergy. In an open, non-randomized trial that included 260 children, 5 different dietary treatment strategies where evaluated according to the rate of acquisition of tolerance in infants with cow's milk allergy. After treatment for 12 months, tolerance to cow's milk protein was significantly higher in the groups receiving extensively hydrolyzed casein formula (EHCF) (43.6%) or EHCF + LGG (78.9%) than in the other groups, implying the ability of LGG to enhance tolerance development (Nermes et al. 2013).

A randomized, double-blind study of infants with challenge-proven cow's milk allergy, administration of L. casei CRL431 and B. lactis Bb12 did not accelerate cow milk tolerance (Hol et al. 2008). Little is known about the efficacy of probiotics in preventing other types of food allergy. Further clinical studies are needed to identify if specific dosing regimens, and specific strains or combinations, are more effective than others. Additionally, more studies are necessary to evaluate if interventions should be tailored to specific subgroups.

15.3.4.4 Colon Cancer

Experimental studies clearly demonstrate a protective effect of prebiotics, such as oligofructose, and probiotics, such as some Lactobacillus and Bifidobacteria strains, or the combination of prebiotics and probiotics, against colon cancer. They can prevent the establishment, growth, and metastasis of transplantable and chemically induced tumours. Several possible mechanisms of protection have been identified (Rafter 2002).

A study on 37 colon cancer patients and 43 polypectomized patients that received a synbiotic food–oligofructose-enriched inulin + *L. rhamnosu* and *B. lactis* or placebo for 12 weeks. Intake of the synbiotic had positive changes in bacterial flora and reduced the colorectal proliferation in the adenoma patients, but these changes were not seen in the cancer patients (Rafter et al. 2007). There are two completed trials assessing the role of probiotics on gut microbiota and colorectal and rectal cancer but results are awaited (Pericleous et al. 2013).

15.3.4.5 Psychobiotics

Increasing evidence has emerged about the influence of the gut microbiota on the brain-gut-axis. A psychobiotic has been defined as a living organism that, when ingested in adequate amounts, produces a health benefit in patients suffering from psychiatric illness. These bacteria are capable of producing and delivering neuroactive substances such as gamma-aminobutyric acid (GABA) and serotonin, which act on the brain-gut axis (Dinan et al. 2013). Lactobacillus rhamnosus had a direct effect on GABA receptors in the central nervous system of a normal, healthy animal. Feeding the strain, reduced stress-induced corticosterone and anxiety- and depression-related behavior (Bravo et al. 2011).

Intestinally, derived strains of lactobacilli and bifidobacteria have the ability to produce GABA from monosodium glutamate (Barrett et al. 2012). Plasma serotonin levels are lower in germ-free mice demonstrating the capacity of the microbiota to influence levels (Collins and Bercik 2009). Probiotics that were shown in vitro and in animal studies to produce neuroactive compounds are currently being tested for psychobiotic potential. While this might become an option in the future, there are no data so far to support the use of probiotics and prebiotics for psychological or psychiatric indications in humans.

REFERENCES

Abrams, S. A., I. J. Griffin, and K. M. Hawthorne. 2007. Young adolescents who respond to an inulin-type fructan substantially increase total absorbed calcium and daily calcium accretion to the skeleton. *J Nutr* no. 137 (11 Suppl):2524S–2526S.

Agrawal, A., L. A. Houghton, J. Morris, B. Reilly, D. Guyonnet, N. Goupil Feuillerat, A. Schlumberger, S. Jakob, and P. J. Whorwell. 2009. Clinical trial: The effects of a fermented milk product containing Bifidobacterium lactis DN-173 010 on abdominal distension and gastrointestinal transit in irritable bowel syndrome with constipation. *Aliment Pharmacol Ther* no. 29 (1):104–14. doi: 10.1111/j.1365-2036.2008.03853.x.

Allen, S. J., E. G. Martinez, G. V. Gregorio, and L. F. Dans. 2010. Probiotics for treating acute infectious diarrhoea. *Cochrane Database Syst Rev* (11):CD003048. doi: 10.1002/14651858.CD003048.pub3.

Allen, S. J., K. Wareham, D. Wang, C. Bradley, H. Hutchings, W. Harris, A. Dhar, H. Brown, A. Foden, M. B. Gravenor, and D. Mack. 2013. Lactobacilli and bifidobacteria in the prevention of antibiotic-associated diarrhoea and Clostridium difficile diarrhoea in older inpatients (PLACIDE): A randomised, double-blind, placebo-controlled, multicentre trial. *Lancet* no. 382 (9900):1249–57. doi: 10.1016/S0140-6736(13)61218-0.

Aller, R., D. A. De Luis, O. Izaola, R. Conde, M. Gonzalez Sagrado, D. Primo, B. De La Fuente, and J. Gonzalez. 2011. Effect of a probiotic on liver aminotransferases in nonalcoholic fatty liver disease patients: A double blind randomized clinical trial. *Eur Rev Med Pharmacol Sci* no. 15 (9):1090–5.

Als-Nielsen, B., L. L. Gluud, and C. Gluud. 2004. Non-absorbable disaccharides for hepatic encephalopathy: Systematic review of randomised trials. *BMJ* no. 328 (7447):1046. doi: 10.1136/bmj.38048.506134.EE.

Arumugam, M., J. Raes, E. Pelletier, D. Le Paslier, T. Yamada, D. R. Mende, G. R. Fernandes, J. Tap, T. Bruls, J. M. Batto et al. 2011. Enterotypes of the human gut microbiome. *Nature* no. 473 (7346):174–80. doi: 10.1038/nature09944.

Atarashi, K., T. Tanoue, T. Shima, A. Imaoka, T. Kuwahara, Y. Momose, G. Cheng, S. Yamasaki, T. Saito, Y. Ohba et al. 2011. Induction of colonic regulatory T cells by indigenous Clostridium species. *Science* no. 331 (6015):337–41. doi: 10.1126/science.1198469.

Backhed, F., R. E. Ley, J. L. Sonnenburg, D. A. Peterson, and J. I. Gordon. 2005. Host-bacterial mutualism in the human intestine. *Science* no. 307 (5717):1915–20. doi: 10.1126/science.1104816.

Barrett, E., R. P. Ross, P. W. O'Toole, G. F. Fitzgerald, and C. Stanton. 2012. gamma-Aminobutyric acid production by culturable bacteria from the human intestine. *J Appl Microbiol* no. 113 (2):411–7. doi: 10.1111/j.1365-2672.2012.05344.x.

Bengmark, S. 2003. Use of some pre-, pro- and synbiotics in critically ill patients. *Best Pract Res Clin Gastroenterol* no. 17 (5):833–48.

Besselink, M. G., H. C. van Santvoort, E. Buskens, M. A. Boermeester, H. van Goor, H. M. Timmerman, V. B. Nieuwenhuijs, T. L. Bollen, B. van Ramshorst, B. J. Witteman et al. and Group Dutch Acute Pancreatitis Study. 2008. Probiotic prophylaxis in predicted severe acute pancreatitis: A randomised, double-blind, placebo-controlled trial. *Lancet* no. 371 (9613):651–9. doi: 10.1016/S0140-6736(08)60207-X.

Besselink, M. G., H. C. van Santvoort, W. Renooij, M. B. de Smet, M. A. Boermeester, K. Fischer, H. M. Timmerman, U. Ahmed Ali, G. A. Cirkel, T. L. Bollen et al. and Group Dutch Acute Pancreatitis Study. 2009. Intestinal barrier dysfunction in a randomized trial of a specific probiotic composition in acute pancreatitis. *Ann Surg* no. 250 (5):712–9. doi: 10.1097/SLA.0b013e3181bce5bd.

Blaut, M. and S. Klaus. 2012. Intestinal microbiota and obesity. *Handb Exp Pharmacol* (209):251–73. doi: 10.1007/978-3-642-24716-3_11.

Borruel, N., M. Carol, F. Casellas, M. Antolin, F. de Lara, E. Espin, J. Naval, F. Guarner, and J. R. Malagelada. 2002. Increased mucosal tumour necrosis factor alpha production in Crohn's disease can be downregulated ex vivo by probiotic bacteria. *Gut* no. 51 (5):659–64.

Bouskra, D., C. Brezillon, M. Berard, C. Werts, R. Varona, I. G. Boneca, and G. Eberl. 2008. Lymphoid tissue genesis induced by commensals through NOD1 regulates intestinal homeostasis. *Nature* no. 456 (7221):507–10. doi: 10.1038/nature07450.

Bravo, J. A., P. Forsythe, M. V. Chew, E. Escaravage, H. M. Savignac, T. G. Dinan, J. Bienenstock, and J. F. Cryan. 2011. Ingestion of Lactobacillus strain regulates emotional behavior and central GABA receptor expression in a mouse via the vagus nerve. *Proc Natl Acad Sci USA* no. 108 (38):16050–5. doi: 10.1073/pnas.1102999108.

Caporaso, J. G., C. L. Lauber, E. K. Costello, D. Berg-Lyons, A. Gonzalez, J. Stombaugh, D. Knights, P. Gajer, J. Ravel, N. Fierer et al. 2011. Moving pictures of the human microbiome. *Genome Biol* no. 12 (5):R50. doi: 10.1186/gb-2011-12-5-r50.

Cashman, K. D. 2002. Calcium intake, calcium bioavailability and bone health. *Br J Nutr* no. 87 (Suppl 2):S169–77. doi: 10.1079/BJNBJN/2002534.

Collins, S. M. and P. Bercik. 2009. The relationship between intestinal microbiota and the central nervous system in normal gastrointestinal function and disease. *Gastroenterology* no. 136 (6):2003–14. doi: 10.1053/j.gastro.2009.01.075.

Cukrowska, B., I. Rosiak, E. Klewicka, I. Motyl, M. Schwarzer, Z. Libudzisz, and H. Kozakova. 2010. Impact of heat-inactivated Lactobacillus casei and Lactobacillus paracasei strains on cytokine responses in whole blood cell cultures of children with atopic dermatitis. *Folia Microbiol (Praha)* no. 55 (3):277–80. doi: 10.1007/s12223-010-0041-6.

Cummings, J. H., J. M. Antoine, F. Azpiroz, R. Bourdet-Sicard, P. Brandtzaeg, P. C. Calder, G. R. Gibson, F. Guarner, E. Isolauri, D. Pannemans et al. 2004. PASSCLAIM—gut health and immunity. *Eur J Nutr* no. 43 (Suppl 2):II118–II173. doi: 10.1007/s00394-004-1205-4.

Dang, D., W. Zhou, Z. J. Lun, X. Mu, D. X. Wang, and H. Wu. 2013. Meta-analysis of probiotics and/or prebiotics for the prevention of eczema. *J Int Med Res* no. 41 (5):1426–36. doi: 10.1177/0300060513493692.

de Preter, V., T. Vanhoutte, G. Huys, J. Swings, P. Rutgeerts, and K. Verbeke. 2008. Baseline microbiota activity and initial bifidobacteria counts influence responses to prebiotic dosing in healthy subjects. *Aliment Pharmacol Ther* no. 27 (6):504–13. doi: 10.1111/j.1365-2036.2007.03588.x.

de Vrese, M., A. Stegelmann, B. Richter, S. Fenselau, C. Laue, and J. Schrezenmeir. 2001. Probiotics—compensation for lactase insufficiency. *Am J Clin Nutr* no. 73 (2 Suppl): 421S–429S.

Deshpande, G., S. Rao, S. Patole, and M. Bulsara. 2010. Updated meta-analysis of probiotics for preventing necrotizing enterocolitis in preterm neonates. *Pediatrics* no. 125 (5):921–30. doi: 10.1542/peds.2009-1301.

Dethlefsen, L., M. McFall-Ngai, and D. A. Relman. 2007. An ecological and evolutionary perspective on human-microbe mutualism and disease. *Nature* no. 449 (7164):811–8. doi: 10.1038/nature06245.

Diaz Heijtz, R., S. Wang, F. Anuar, Y. Qian, B. Bjorkholm, A. Samuelsson, M. L. Hibberd, H. Forssberg, and S. Pettersson. 2011. Normal gut microbiota modulates brain development and behavior. *Proc Natl Acad Sci USA* no. 108 (7):3047–52. doi: 10.1073/pnas.1010529108.

Dinan, T. G., C. Stanton, and J. F. Cryan. 2013. Psychobiotics: A novel class of psychotropic. *Biol Psychiatry* no. 74 (10):720–6. doi: 10.1016/j.biopsych.2013.05.001.

Eckburg, P. B., E. M. Bik, C. N. Bernstein, E. Purdom, L. Dethlefsen, M. Sargent, S. R. Gill, K. E. Nelson, and D. A. Relman. 2005. Diversity of the human intestinal microbial flora. *Science* no. 308 (5728):1635–8. doi: 10.1126/science.1110591.

FAO/WHO. 2001. Report of a Joint FAO/WHO Expert Consultation on Evaluation of Health and Nutritional Properties of Probiotics in Food Including Powder Milk with Live Lactic Acid Bacteria, 1–4 October, at Córdoba, Argentina.

Frank, D. N. and N. R. Pace. 2008. Gastrointestinal microbiology enters the metagenomics era. *Curr Opin Gastroenterol* no. 24 (1):4–10. doi: 10.1097/MOG.0b013e3282f2b0e8.

Gibson, G. R., E. R. Beatty, X. Wang, and J. H. Cummings. 1995. Selective stimulation of bifidobacteria in the human colon by oligofructose and inulin. *Gastroenterology* no. 108 (4):975–82.

Gibson, G. R. and M. B. Roberfroid. 1995. Dietary modulation of the human colonic microbiota: Introducing the concept of prebiotics. *J Nutr* no. 125 (6):1401–12.

Gionchetti, P., F. Rizzello, U. Helwig, A. Venturi, K. M. Lammers, P. Brigidi, B. Vitali, G. Poggioli, M. Miglioli, and M. Campieri. 2003. Prophylaxis of pouchitis onset with probiotic therapy: A double-blind, placebo-controlled trial. *Gastroenterology* no. 124 (5):1202–9.

Gionchetti, P., F. Rizzello, C. Morselli, G. Poggioli, R. Tambasco, C. Calabrese, P. Brigidi, B. Vitali, G. Straforini, and M. Campieri. 2007. High-dose probiotics for the treatment of active pouchitis. *Dis Colon Rectum* no. 50 (12):2075–82; discussion 2082–4. doi: 10.1007/s10350-007-9068-4.

Gionchetti, P., F. Rizzello, A. Venturi, P. Brigidi, D. Matteuzzi, G. Bazzocchi, G. Poggioli, M. Miglioli, and M. Campieri. 2000. Oral bacteriotherapy as maintenance treatment in patients with chronic pouchitis: A double-blind, placebo-controlled trial. *Gastroenterology* no. 119 (2):305–9.

Guarner, F., R. Bourdet-Sicard, P. Brandtzaeg, H. S. Gill, P. McGuirk, W. van Eden, J. Versalovic, J. V. Weinstock, and G. A. Rook. 2006. Mechanisms of disease: The hygiene hypothesis revisited. *Nat Clin Pract Gastroenterol Hepatol* no. 3 (5):275–84. doi: 10.1038/ncpgasthep0471.

Guarner, F., A. G. Khan, J. Garisch, R. Eliakim, A. Gangl, A. Thomson, J. Krabshuis, T. Lemair, P. Kaufmann, J. A. de Paula et al. and Organisation World Gastroenterology. 2012. World Gastroenterology Organisation Global Guidelines: Probiotics and prebiotics October 2011. *J Clin Gastroenterol* no. 46 (6):468–81. doi: 10.1097/MCG.0b013e3182549092.

Guarner, F. and J. R. Malagelada. 2003. Gut flora in health and disease. *Lancet* no. 361 (9356):512–9. doi: 10.1016/S0140-6736(03)12489-0.

Hol, J., E. H. van Leer, B. E. Elink Schuurman, L. F. de Ruiter, J. N. Samsom, W. Hop, H. J. Neijens, J. C. de Jongste, E. E. Nieuwenhuis, Elimination Cow's Milk Allergy Modified by, and group Lactobacilli study. 2008. The acquisition of tolerance toward cow's milk through probiotic supplementation: A randomized, controlled trial. *J Allergy Clin Immunol* no. 121 (6):1448–54. doi: 10.1016/j.jaci.2008.03.018.

Hooper, L. V., T. Midtvedt, and J. I. Gordon. 2002. How host-microbial interactions shape the nutrient environment of the mammalian intestine. *Annu Rev Nutr* no. 22:283–307. doi: 10.1146/annurev.nutr.22.011602.092259.

Hooper, L. V., M. H. Wong, A. Thelin, L. Hansson, P. G. Falk, and J. I. Gordon. 2001. Molecular analysis of commensal host–microbial relationships in the intestine. *Science* no. 291 (5505):881–4. doi: 10.1126/science.291.5505.881.

Hoveyda, N., C. Heneghan, K. R. Mahtani, R. Perera, N. Roberts, and P. Glasziou. 2009. A systematic review and meta-analysis: Probiotics in the treatment of irritable bowel syndrome. *BMC Gastroenterol* no. 9:15. doi: 10.1186/1471-230X-9-15.

Human Microbiome Project, Consortium. 2012. Structure, function and diversity of the healthy human microbiome. *Nature* no. 486 (7402):207–14. doi: 10.1038/nature11234.

Hungin, A. P., C. Mulligan, B. Pot, P. Whorwell, L. Agreus, P. Fracasso, C. Lionis, J. Mendive, J. M. Philippart de Foy, G. Rubin et al. Gastroenterology European Society for Primary Care. 2013. Systematic review: Probiotics in the management of lower gastrointestinal symptoms in clinical practice—an evidence-based international guide. *Aliment Pharmacol Ther* no. 38 (8):864–86. doi: 10.1111/apt.12460.

Johnston, B. C., S. S. Ma, J. Z. Goldenberg, K. Thorlund, P. O. Vandvik, M. Loeb, and G. H. Guyatt. 2012. Probiotics for the prevention of Clostridium difficile-associated diarrhea: A systematic review and meta-analysis. *Ann Intern Med* no. 157 (12):878–88.

Kim, H. J., M. Camilleri, S. McKinzie, M. B. Lempke, D. D. Burton, G. M. Thomforde, and A. R. Zinsmeister. 2003. A randomized controlled trial of a probiotic, VSL#3, on gut transit and symptoms in diarrhoea-predominant irritable bowel syndrome. *Aliment Pharmacol Ther* no. 17 (7):895–904.

Kim, H. J., M. I. Vazquez Roque, M. Camilleri, D. Stephens, D. D. Burton, K. Baxter, G. Thomforde, and A. R. Zinsmeister. 2005. A randomized controlled trial of a probiotic combination VSL#3 and placebo in irritable bowel syndrome with bloating. *Neurogastroenterol Motil* no. 17 (5):687–96. doi: 10.1111/j.1365-2982.2005.00695.x.

Kim, J. Y., J. H. Kwon, S. H. Ahn, S. I. Lee, Y. S. Han, Y. O. Choi, S. Y. Lee, K. M. Ahn, and G. E. Ji. 2010. Effect of probiotic mix (Bifidobacterium bifidum, Bifidobacterium lactis, Lactobacillus acidophilus) in the primary prevention of eczema: A double-blind, randomized, placebo-controlled trial. *Pediatr Allergy Immunol* no. 21 (2 Pt 2):e386–93. doi: 10.1111/j.1399-3038.2009.00958.x.

Kolars, J. C., M. D. Levitt, M. Aouji, and D. A. Savaiano. 1984. Yogurt—an autodigesting source of lactose. *N Engl J Med* no. 310 (1):1–3. doi: 10.1056/NEJM198401053100101.

Kuisma, J., S. Mentula, H. Jarvinen, A. Kahri, M. Saxelin, and M. Farkkila. 2003. Effect of Lactobacillus rhamnosus GG on ileal pouch inflammation and microbial flora. *Aliment Pharmacol Ther* no. 17 (4):509–15.

Lerebours, E., C. N'Djitoyap Ndam, A. Lavoine, M. F. Hellot, J. M. Antoine, and R. Colin. 1989. Yogurt and fermented-then-pasteurized milk: Effects of short-term and long-term ingestion on lactose absorption and mucosal lactase activity in lactase-deficient subjects. *Am J Clin Nutr* no. 49 (5):823–7.

Lilly, D. M. and R. H. Stillwell. 1965. Probiotics: Growth-promoting factors produced by microorganisms. *Science* no. 147 (3659):747–8.

Liu, Z., H. Qin, Z. Yang, Y. Xia, W. Liu, J. Yang, Y. Jiang, H. Zhang, Z. Yang, Y. Wang et al. 2011. Randomised clinical trial: The effects of perioperative probiotic treatment on barrier function and post-operative infectious complications in colorectal cancer surgery—a double-blind study. *Aliment Pharmacol Ther* no. 33 (1):50–63. doi: 10.1111/j.1365-2036.2010.04492.x.

Lodinova-Zadnikova, R., B. Cukrowska, and H. Tlaskalova-Hogenova. 2003. Oral administration of probiotic Escherichia coli after birth reduces frequency of allergies and repeated infections later in life (after 10 and 20 years). *Int Arch Allergy Immunol* no. 131 (3):209–11. doi: 71488.

Lodinova-Zadnikova, R., L. Prokesova, I. Kocourkova, J. Hrdy, and J. Zizka. 2010. Prevention of allergy in infants of allergic mothers by probiotic Escherichia coli. *Int Arch Allergy Immunol* no. 153 (2):201–6. doi: 10.1159/000312638.

MacDonald, T. T., I. Monteleone, M. C. Fantini, and G. Monteleone. 2011. Regulation of homeostasis and inflammation in the intestine. *Gastroenterology* no. 140 (6):1768–75. doi: 10.1053/j.gastro.2011.02.047.

Macpherson, A., U. Y. Khoo, I. Forgacs, J. Philpott-Howard, and I. Bjarnason. 1996. Mucosal antibodies in inflammatory bowel disease are directed against intestinal bacteria. *Gut* no. 38 (3):365–75.

Madsen, K. L., J. S. Doyle, L. D. Jewell, M. M. Tavernini, and R. N. Fedorak. 1999. Lactobacillus species prevents colitis in interleukin 10 gene-deficient mice. *Gastroenterology* no. 116 (5):1107–14.

Majamaa, H. and E. Isolauri. 1997. Probiotics: A novel approach in the management of food allergy. *J Allergy Clin Immunol* no. 99 (2):179–85.

Malaguarnera, M., M. P. Gargante, G. Malaguarnera, M. Salmeri, S. Mastrojeni, L. Rampello, G. Pennisi, G. Li Volti, and F. Galvano. 2010. Bifidobacterium combined with fructo-oligosaccharide versus lactulose in the treatment of patients with hepatic encephalopathy. *Eur J Gastroenterol Hepatol* no. 22 (2):199–206. doi: 10.1097/MEG.0b013e328330a8d3.

Malaguarnera, M., M. Vacante, T. Antic, M. Giordano, G. Chisari, R. Acquaviva, S. Mastrojeni, G. Malaguarnera, A. Mistretta, G. Li Volti et al. 2012. Bifidobacterium longum with fructo-oligosaccharides in patients with non alcoholic steatohepatitis. *Dig Dis Sci* no. 57 (2):545–53. doi: 10.1007/s10620-011-1887-4.

Manichanh, C., N. Borruel, F. Casellas, and F. Guarner. 2012. The gut microbiota in IBD. *Nat Rev Gastroenterol Hepatol* no. 9 (10):599–608. doi: 10.1038/nrgastro.2012.152.

Marteau, P., B. Flourie, P. Pochart, C. Chastang, J. F. Desjeux, and J. C. Rambaud. 1990. Effect of the microbial lactase (EC 3.2.1.23) activity in yoghurt on the intestinal absorption of lactose: An in vivo study in lactase-deficient humans. *Br J Nutr* no. 64 (1):71–9.

Matricardi, P. M., B. Bjorksten, S. Bonini, J. Bousquet, R. Djukanovic, S. Dreborg, J. Gereda, H. J. Malling, T. Popov, E. Raz et al. Eaaci Task Force. 2003. Microbial products in allergy prevention and therapy. *Allergy* no. 58 (6):461–71.

McCarthy, J., L. O'Mahony, L. O'Callaghan, B. Sheil, E. E. Vaughan, N. Fitzsimons, J. Fitzgibbon, G. C. O'Sullivan, B. Kiely, J. K. Collins et al. 2003. Double blind, placebo controlled trial of two probiotic strains in interleukin 10 knockout mice and mechanistic link with cytokine balance. *Gut* no. 52 (7):975–80.

McFarland, L. V. 2007. Meta-analysis of probiotics for the prevention of traveler's diarrhea. *Travel Med Infect Dis* no. 5 (2):97–105. doi: 10.1016/j.tmaid.2005.10.003.

McFarland, L. V. and S. Dublin. 2008. Meta-analysis of probiotics for the treatment of irritable bowel syndrome. *World J Gastroenterol* no. 14 (17):2650–61.

Metges, C. C. 2000. Contribution of microbial amino acids to amino acid homeostasis of the host. *J Nutr* no. 130 (7):1857S–64S.

Mimura, T., F. Rizzello, U. Helwig, G. Poggioli, S. Schreiber, I. C. Talbot, R. J. Nicholls, P. Gionchetti, M. Campieri, and M. A. Kamm. 2004. Once daily high dose probiotic therapy (VSL#3) for maintaining remission in recurrent or refractory pouchitis. *Gut* no. 53 (1):108–14.

Moayyedi, P., A. C. Ford, N. J. Talley, F. Cremonini, A. E. Foxx-Orenstein, L. J. Brandt, and E. M. Quigley. 2010. The efficacy of probiotics in the treatment of irritable bowel syndrome: A systematic review. *Gut* no. 59 (3):325–32. doi: 10.1136/gut.2008.167270.

Moran, N. A. 2006. Symbiosis. *Curr Biol* no. 16 (20):R866–71. doi: 10.1016/j.cub.2006.09.019.

Naidoo, K., M. Gordon, A. O. Fagbemi, A. G. Thomas, and A. K. Akobeng. 2011. Probiotics for maintenance of remission in ulcerative colitis. *Cochrane Database Syst Rev* (12):CD007443. doi: 10.1002/14651858.CD007443.pub2.

Neish, A. S., A. T. Gewirtz, H. Zeng, A. N. Young, M. E. Hobert, V. Karmali, A. S. Rao, and J. L. Madara. 2000. Prokaryotic regulation of epithelial responses by inhibition of IkappaB-alpha ubiquitination. *Science* no. 289 (5484):1560–3.

Nermes, M., S. Salminen, and E. Isolauri. 2013. Is there a role for probiotics in the prevention or treatment of food allergy? *Curr Allergy Asthma Rep* no. 13 (6):622–30. doi: 10.1007/s11882-013-0381-9.

Neufeld, K. M., N. Kang, J. Bienenstock, and J. A. Foster. 2011. Reduced anxiety-like behavior and central neurochemical change in germ-free mice. *Neurogastroenterol Motil* no. 23 (3):255–64, e119. doi: 10.1111/j.1365-2982.2010.01620.x.

Niers, L., R. Martin, G. Rijkers, F. Sengers, H. Timmerman, N. van Uden, H. Smidt, J. Kimpen, and M. Hoekstra. 2009. The effects of selected probiotic strains on the development of eczema (the P and A study). *Allergy* no. 64 (9):1349–58. doi: 10.1111/j.1398-9995.2009.02021.x.

O'Hara, A. M. and F. Shanahan. 2006. The gut flora as a forgotten organ. *EMBO Rep* no. 7 (7):688–93. doi: 10.1038/sj.embor.7400731.

O'Mahony, C., P. Scully, D. O'Mahony, S. Murphy, F. O'Brien, A. Lyons, G. Sherlock, J. MacSharry, B. Kiely, F. Shanahan et al. 2008. Commensal-induced regulatory T cells mediate protection against pathogen-stimulated NF-kappaB activation. *PLoS Pathog* no. 4 (8):e1000112. doi: 10.1371/journal.ppat.1000112.

Olah, A., T. Belagyi, A. Issekutz, M. E. Gamal, and S. Bengmark. 2002. Randomized clinical trial of specific lactobacillus and fibre supplement to early enteral nutrition in patients with acute pancreatitis. *Br J Surg* no. 89 (9):1103–7.

Osborn, D. A. and J. K. Sinn. 2007. Probiotics in infants for prevention of allergic disease and food hypersensitivity. *Cochrane Database Syst Rev* (4):CD006475. doi: 10.1002/14651858.CD006475.pub2.

Patel, R. M. and P. W. Lin. 2010. Developmental biology of gut-probiotic interaction. *Gut Microbes* no. 1 (3):186–95. doi: 10.4161/gmic.1.3.12484.

Pelucchi, C., L. Chatenoud, F. Turati, C. Galeone, L. Moja, J. F. Bach, and C. La Vecchia. 2012. Probiotics supplementation during pregnancy or infancy for the prevention of atopic dermatitis: A meta-analysis. *Epidemiology* no. 23 (3):402–14. doi: 10.1097/EDE.0b013e31824d5da2.

Pericleous, M., D. Mandair, and M. E. Caplin. 2013. Diet and supplements and their impact on colorectal cancer. *J Gastrointest Oncol* no. 4 (4):409–23. doi: 10.3978/j.issn.2078-6891.2013.003.

Pirzer, U., A. Schonhaar, B. Fleischer, E. Hermann, and K. H. Meyer zum Buschenfelde. 1991. Reactivity of infiltrating T lymphocytes with microbial antigens in Crohn's disease. *Lancet* no. 338 (8777):1238–9.

Pitsouni, E., V. Alexiou, V. Saridakis, G. Peppas, and M. E. Falagas. 2009. Does the use of probiotics/synbiotics prevent postoperative infections in patients undergoing abdominal surgery? A meta-analysis of randomized controlled trials. *Eur J Clin Pharmacol* no. 65 (6):561–70. doi: 10.1007/s00228-009-0642-7.

Prantera, C., M. L. Scribano, G. Falasco, A. Andreoli, and C. Luzi. 2002. Ineffectiveness of probiotics in preventing recurrence after curative resection for Crohn's disease: A randomised controlled trial with Lactobacillus GG. *Gut* no. 51 (3):405–9.

Qin, J., R. Li, J. Raes, M. Arumugam, K. S. Burgdorf, C. Manichanh, T. Nielsen, N. Pons, F. Levenez, T. Yamada et al. 2010. A human gut microbial gene catalogue established by metagenomic sequencing. *Nature* no. 464 (7285):59–65. doi: 10.1038/nature08821.

Qin, J., Y. Li, Z. Cai, S. Li, J. Zhu, F. Zhang, S. Liang, W. Zhang, Y. Guan, D. Shen et al. 2012. A metagenome-wide association study of gut microbiota in type 2 diabetes. *Nature* no. 490 (7418):55–60. doi: 10.1038/nature11450.

Rafter, J. 2002. Lactic acid bacteria and cancer: Mechanistic perspective. *Br J Nutr* no. 88 Suppl 1:S89–94. doi: 10.1079/BJN2002633.

Rafter, J., M. Bennett, G. Caderni, Y. Clune, R. Hughes, P. C. Karlsson, A. Klinder, M. O'Riordan, G. C. O'Sullivan, B. Pool-Zobel et al. 2007. Dietary synbiotics reduce cancer risk factors in polypectomized and colon cancer patients. *Am J Clin Nutr* no. 85 (2):488–96.

Rautava, S., E. Kainonen, S. Salminen, and E. Isolauri. 2012. Maternal probiotic supplementation during pregnancy and breast-feeding reduces the risk of eczema in the infant. *J Allergy Clin Immunol* no. 130 (6):1355–60. doi: 10.1016/j.jaci.2012.09.003.

Rayes, N., D. Seehofer, T. Theruvath, M. Mogl, J. M. Langrehr, N. C. Nussler, S. Bengmark, and P. Neuhaus. 2007. Effect of enteral nutrition and synbiotics on bacterial infection rates after pylorus-preserving pancreatoduodenectomy: A randomized, double-blind trial. *Ann Surg* no. 246 (1):36–41. doi: 10.1097/01.sla.0000259442.78947.19.

Rayes, N., D. Seehofer, T. Theruvath, R. A. Schiller, J. M. Langrehr, S. Jonas, S. Bengmark, and P. Neuhaus. 2005. Supply of pre- and probiotics reduces bacterial infection rates after liver transplantation—a randomized, double-blind trial. *Am J Transplant* no. 5 (1):125–30. doi: 10.1111/j.1600-6143.2004.00649.x.

Rizkalla, S. W., J. Luo, M. Kabir, A. Chevalier, N. Pacher, and G. Slama. 2000. Chronic consumption of fresh but not heated yogurt improves breath-hydrogen status and short-chain fatty acid profiles: A controlled study in healthy men with or without lactose maldigestion. *Am J Clin Nutr* no. 72 (6):1474–9.

Round, J. L. and S. K. Mazmanian. 2009. The gut microbiota shapes intestinal immune responses during health and disease. *Nat Rev Immunol* no. 9 (5):313–23. doi: 10.1038/nri2515.

Salminen, M. K., S. Tynkkynen, H. Rautelin, M. Saxelin, M. Vaara, P. Ruutu, S. Sarna, V. Valtonen, and A. Jarvinen. 2002. Lactobacillus bacteremia during a rapid increase in probiotic use of Lactobacillus rhamnosus GG in Finland. *Clin Infect Dis* no. 35 (10):1155–60. doi: 10.1086/342912.

Savaiano, D. A., A. AbouElAnouar, D. E. Smith, and M. D. Levitt. 1984. Lactose malabsorption from yogurt, pasteurized yogurt, sweet acidophilus milk, and cultured milk in lactase-deficient individuals. *Am J Clin Nutr* no. 40 (6):1219–23.

Sazawal, S., G. Hiremath, U. Dhingra, P. Malik, S. Deb, and R. E. Black. 2006. Efficacy of probiotics in prevention of acute diarrhoea: A meta-analysis of masked, randomised, placebo-controlled trials. *Lancet Infect Dis* no. 6 (6):374–82. doi: 10.1016/S1473-3099(06)70495-9.

Schultz, M., A. Timmer, H. H. Herfarth, R. B. Sartor, J. A. Vanderhoof, and H. C. Rath. 2004. Lactobacillus GG in inducing and maintaining remission of Crohn's disease. *BMC Gastroenterol* no. 4:5. doi: 10.1186/1471-230X-4-5.

Schultz, M., C. Veltkamp, L. A. Dieleman, W. B. Grenther, P. B. Wyrick, S. L. Tonkonogy, and R. B. Sartor. 2002. Lactobacillus plantarum 299V in the treatment and prevention of spontaneous colitis in interleukin-10-deficient mice. *Inflamm Bowel Dis* no. 8 (2):71–80.

Shen, J., Z. X. Zuo, and A. P. Mao. 2014. Effect of probiotics on inducing remission and maintaining therapy in ulcerative colitis, Crohn's disease, and pouchitis: Meta-analysis of randomized controlled trials. *Inflamm Bowel Dis* no. 20 (1):21–35. doi: 10.1097/01.MIB.0000437495.30052.be.

Shukla, S., A. Shukla, S. Mehboob, and S. Guha. 2011. Meta-analysis: The effects of gut flora modulation using prebiotics, probiotics and synbiotics on minimal hepatic encephalopathy. *Aliment Pharmacol Ther* no. 33 (6):662–71. doi: 10.1111/j.1365-2036.2010.04574.x.

Solga, S. F., G. Buckley, J. M. Clark, A. Horska, and A. M. Diehl. 2008. The effect of a probiotic on hepatic steatosis. *J Clin Gastroenterol* no. 42 (10):1117–9. doi: 10.1097/MCG.0b013e31816d920c.

Steidler, L., W. Hans, L. Schotte, S. Neirynck, F. Obermeier, W. Falk, W. Fiers, and E. Remaut. 2000. Treatment of murine colitis by Lactococcus lactis secreting interleukin-10. *Science* no. 289 (5483):1352–5.

Sur, D., B. Manna, S. K. Niyogi, T. Ramamurthy, A. Palit, K. Nomoto, T. Takahashi, T. Shima, H. Tsuji, T. Kurakawa et al. 2011. Role of probiotic in preventing acute diarrhoea in children: A community-based, randomized, double-blind placebo-controlled field trial in an urban slum. *Epidemiol Infect* no. 139 (6):919–26. doi: 10.1017/S0950268810001780.

van Baarlen, P., F. Troost, C. van der Meer, G. Hooiveld, M. Boekschoten, R. J. Brummer, and M. Kleerebezem. 2011. Human mucosal in vivo transcriptome responses to three lactobacilli indicate how probiotics may modulate human cellular pathways. *Proc Natl Acad Sci USA* no. 108 Suppl 1:4562–9. doi: 10.1073/pnas.1000079107.

Videlock, E. J. and F. Cremonini. 2012. Meta-analysis: Probiotics in antibiotic-associated diarrhoea. *Aliment Pharmacol Ther* no. 35 (12):1355–69. doi: 10.1111/j.1365-2036.2012.05104.x.

Vrieze, A., E. Van Nood, F. Holleman, J. Salojarvi, R. S. Kootte, J. F. Bartelsman, G. M. Dallinga-Thie, M. T. Ackermans, M. J. Serlie, R. Oozeer et al. 2012. Transfer of intestinal microbiota from lean donors increases insulin sensitivity in individuals with metabolic syndrome. *Gastroenterology* no. 143 (4):913–6 e7. doi: 10.1053/j.gastro.2012.06.031.

Welters, C. F., E. Heineman, F. B. Thunnissen, A. E. van den Bogaard, P. B. Soeters, and C. G. Baeten. 2002. Effect of dietary inulin supplementation on inflammation of pouch mucosa in patients with an ileal pouch-anal anastomosis. *Dis Colon Rectum* no. 45 (5):621–7.

Wong, V. W., G. L. Won, A. M. Chim, W. C. Chu, D. K. Yeung, K. C. Li, and H. L. Chan. 2013. Treatment of nonalcoholic steatohepatitis with probiotics. A proof-of-concept study. *Ann Hepatol* no. 12 (2):256–62.

Wostmann, B. S. 1981. The germfree animal in nutritional studies. *Annu Rev Nutr* no. 1:257–79. doi: 10.1146/annurev.nu.01.070181.001353.

Yamanaka, T., L. Helgeland, I. N. Farstad, H. Fukushima, T. Midtvedt, and P. Brandtzaeg. 2003. Microbial colonization drives lymphocyte accumulation and differentiation in the follicle-associated epithelium of Peyer's patches. *J Immunol* no. 170 (2):816–22.

Yang, S. Q., H. Z. Lin, M. D. Lane, M. Clemens, and A. M. Diehl. 1997. Obesity increases sensitivity to endotoxin liver injury: Implications for the pathogenesis of steatohepatitis. *Proc Natl Acad Sci USA* no. 94 (6):2557–62.

Zhang, M. M., J. Q. Cheng, Y. R. Lu, Z. H. Yi, P. Yang, and X. T. Wu. 2010. Use of pre-, pro- and synbiotics in patients with acute pancreatitis: A meta-analysis. *World J Gastroenterol* no. 16 (31):3970–8.

16 Treatment of the Common Cold with Zinc

Ananda S. Prasad

CONTENTS

16.1 INTRODUCTION

Adults and children in the USA experience two to six episodes of common cold per year [1,2] and the morbidity and loss of working hours due to this are substantial. The complications of the common cold include otitis media, sinusitis, and exacerbations of reactive airway diseases. The clinical syndrome of the common cold is caused by a variety of different viruses [3]. The rhinoviruses are the most frequent.

The effect of zinc lozenges on the duration or severity of common cold symptoms has been examined in at least 14 different studies since 1984 when Eby et al. [4] reported for the first time its efficacy in treatment of this disorder. Later trials gave inconclusive results. Results of trials in which no effect of zinc was demonstrated were criticized as having inadequate sample sizes or using inadequate doses of zinc or improper formulations of zinc that reduced the release of zinc ions from the lozenges. In some studies, a significant effect of zinc lozenges for the treatment of common cold was criticized for inadequate blinding either by the use of poorly matched placebos or because the active preparation was associated with a high incidence of adverse effects [3].

In this chapter, we will summarize our data of two trials of controlled trial of zinc lozenges for the treatment of common cold and propose possible mechanisms of zinc effect on common cold.

16.2 METHODS

16.2.1 First Trial

16.2.1.1 Participants

We recruited 50 volunteers from Detroit Medical Center, Detroit, Michigan, to participate in a randomized, placebo-controlled trial of the efficacy of zinc acetate lozenges in treating the common cold [6]. Two participants in the placebo group dropped out on day 2. We, therefore, had complete data on 48 participants.

Participants were medical students, graduate and undergraduate students, staff, and employees at Wayne State University, who were older than 18 years of age. Participants were informed of the placebo-controlled, double blind nature of the study, and the study protocol was approved by the Human and Animal Investigation Committee of Wayne State University.

Volunteers were recruited if they had had cold symptoms for 24 h or less and had at least 2 of the following 10 symptoms: cough, headache, hoarseness, muscle ache, nasal drainage, nasal congestion, scratchy throat, sore throat, sneezing, and fever. We excluded persons who were pregnant, had a known immunodeficiency disorder, had a chronic illness, had had symptoms of the common cold for more than 24 hours, or had previously used zinc lozenges to treat the common cold.

16.2.1.2 Intervention

Each zinc lozenge consisted of 42.96 mg of zinc acetate dihydrate (USP; Heico Chemicals, Delaware Water Gap, Pennsylvania), 6.0 mg of peppermint oil (National

Formulary; Bell Flavors, North Brook, Illinois), 16.0 mg of silica gel (National Formulary; Siloid 244 FP, Davidson Chemical, Baltimore, Maryland), 4.0 mg of stevia extract powder (90% pure steviodside), 3835.04 mg of directly compressible dextrose (USP; Unidex 2034), and 100 mg of glycerol monostearate (Myvaplex TM 600 P, Eastman Chemical, Kingsport, Tennessee). Each lozenge contained 12.8 mg of zinc. Each placebo lozenge contained 0.25 mg of sucrose octa acetate, 6.0 mg of peppermint oil, 16.0 mg of silica gel, 3877.75 mg of dextrose DC, and 100 mg of glycerol monostearate. The placebo and zinc lozenges were identical in weight (4000 mg), appearance, flavor, and texture.

A research consultant prepared the randomization code and the packages of medication. The packages were identical in appearance except for the randomization numbers. A research assistant, who was blinded to treatment assignments, distributed the study medication. Participants were given 50 lozenges and were asked to dissolve one lozenge in their mouths every 2–3 h while awake for as long as they had cold symptoms. They were instructed not to take other cold preparations during the study period.

16.2.1.3 Outcome Measures

Our primary end point was the average duration of cold symptoms. Secondary end points were plasma levels of zinc and proinflammatory cytokines.

Participants were asked to complete a daily log documenting the severity of symptoms and the medications taken throughout the duration of the cold. Everyday, the participants graded each symptom as 0 for none, 1 for mild, 2 for moderate, and 3 for severe. Total symptom scores were calculated by summing the scores of 10 symptoms for each day. Resolution of cold symptoms was defined as resolution of all symptoms (a total symptom score of 0) or resolution of all but one mild symptom (a total symptom score of 1). The participants were not asked to rate their overall illness in terms of severity.

We obtained plasma samples for assay of zinc and proinflammatory cytokines. Zinc was assayed by using methods established in our laboratory that are based on atomic absorption spectrophotometry [7]. Every precaution was taken to avoid contamination during collection, preparation, and analysis.

We measured levels of three proinflammatory cytokines before and after treatment: soluble interleukin-1 receptor antagonist, soluble tumor necrosis factor (TNF) receptor, and neopterin. We also recruited 17 healthy adult volunteers with no symptoms of cold for a comparison assay of plasma proinflammatory cytokines and zinc. Cytokines were analyzed by using enzyme-linked immunosorbent assay. Quantikine assay kits for soluble TNF receptor and soluble interleukin-1 receptor antagonist were obtained from R and D Systems, Minneapolis, Minnesota, and kits for analysis of neopterin were obtained from American Laboratory Products Company Ltd., Windham, New Hampshire. All cytokine assays were run on the same day.

To assess side effects of the treatment, participants were given a questionnaire to be filled out at the end of the trial. Participants provided "yes" or "no" answers to questions about nausea, vomiting, abdominal pain, diarrhea, constipation, dry mouth, bad taste, and mouth irritation.

Participants returned to the clinic for the final visit within 1 day of resolution of cold symptoms. At this time, they returned unused lozenges. This was done to check adherence and confirm that cold symptoms had resolved.

16.2.1.4 Maintenance of Blinding

Comparability in taste between zinc and placebo was tested in healthy volunteers. Ten participants were given a zinc lozenge and ten received a placebo lozenge. One week later, the participants who received zinc were given placebo and those who received placebo were given zinc. At each visit, the participants filled out a questionnaire in which they were asked to guess whether they received a zinc or placebo lozenge. They had seven choices: certainly placebo, certainly zinc, do not know, possibly placebo, possibly zinc, probably placebo, and probably zinc. Volunteers who selected "certainly," "probably," or "possibly" and were correct about the type of lozenge they received, were considered correct. We therefore categorized participants as "correct," "incorrect," or "do not know."

We assessed the adequacy of blinding among study participants by administering the questionnaire used to assess comparability of taste in healthy volunteers. Participants filled out the questionnaire at the beginning and at the end of the trial.

16.2.1.5 Statistical Analysis

We compared the change in outcomes before and after intervention in the zinc and placebo groups. When changes in both groups were normally distributed, as determined by using the Shapiro–Wilk W test, we used the *t*-test to compare mean changes. When they were not normally distributed, the differences between changes were compared by using the non-parametric Wilcoxon rank-sum test. Multivariate analysis of variance with repeated measures was used to determine the effect of treatment X times on severity scores over the study period. The Fisher exact test was used to determine group differences in side effects. Chisquare analyses were performed to determine group differences in correctly identifying lozenges at baseline and after treatment.

The *t*-test was used to compare plasma zinc and cytokine levels before group assignment with levels in healthy controls. This was done to determine whether participants with colds differed from controls.

All statistical analyses were done by using JMP version 3.2.2 on a Macintosh computer (SAS Institute, Inc., Cary, North Carolina).

16.3 RESULTS

Table 16.1 shows the demographic characteristics of the study participants in the first trial.

16.3.1 Duration and Severity of Cold Symptoms

The average duration of cold symptoms was 4.5 days in zinc recipients and 8.1 days in the placebo group ($P < 0.01$; Table 16.2). The duration of cough (3.1 versus 6.3 days; $P < 0.001$) and nasal discharge (4.1 and 5.8 days; $P = 0.02$) were shorter in zinc

TABLE 16.1
Demographic Characteristics of Study Participants in Trial 1[a]

Variable	Zinc Group (η = 25)	Placebo Group (η = 23)
Mean age 6 SD, *y*	36.4 ± 11.1	37.8 ± 10.9
Sex, *n*		
Male	7	11
Female	18	12
Ethnicity, *n*		
Black	5	11
White	19	12
Middle Eastern Arab	1	0
Smoker, *n*		
No	20	15
Yes	5	8
History of allergy, *n*		
No	23	19
Yes	2	4

Source: Prasad AS et al. 2000. *Annals Int Med* 133:245–52.

[a] Twenty-five volunteers were initially recruited in each group. Two persons in the placebo group dropped out on day 2 and were lost to follow-up. One of the two persons had a sore mouth, and the other developed an ear infection for which care was transferred to a physician outside of Detroit Medical Center.

recipients than in placebo group. Fifty percent of the participants in the zinc group were well in 3.8 days, and 50% of the placebo group were well in 7.7 days.

Repeated-measures analysis of severity scores indicated a treatment X time interaction over the 12 days of the study ($P = 0.002$). At baseline, the average severity score was higher in the zinc group than in the placebo group (10.8 versus 8.9). However, by day 4, the average severity score in the zinc group was half that in the placebo group (2.7 versus 5.4).

16.3.2 Adverse Effects

The zinc and placebo groups did not differ significantly in incidence of nausea (0 versus 1 [0% versus 4%]; $P > 0.2$), vomiting (0 versus 0), abdominal pain (0 versus 2 [0% versus 9%]; $P > 0.2$), diarrhea (2 versus 1 [8% versus 4%]; $P > 0.2$), bad taste (13 versus 6 [52% versus 26%]; $P = 0.08$), or mouth irritation (10 versus 4 [40% versus 17%]; $P = 0.12$). Compared with placebo recipients, zinc recipients reported more mouth dryness (18 versus 6 [72% versus 26%]; $P = 0.003$) and constipation (6 versus 0 [24% versus 0%]; $P = 0.02$).

TABLE 16.2
Duration of Symptoms of the Common Cold in Trial 1

Variable	Mean Duration of Cold Symptoms (95% CI)		P Value
	Zinc Group (η = 25)	Placebo Group (η = 23)	
	d		
Overall symptoms[a]	4.5 6 ± 1.6	8.1 ± 1.8	<0.01
Specific symptoms[b]			
Sore throat	2.0 (1.2 to 2.7)	3.0 (1.8 to 4.3)	>0.2
Nasal discharge	4.1 (3.3 to 4.9)	5.8 (4.3 to 7.3)	0.025
Nasal congestion	3.3 (2.3 to 4.3)	4.7 (3.1 to 6.2)	0.133
Sneezing	2.7 (1.9 to 3.5)	4.4 (3.0 to 5.9)	0.069
Cough	3.1 (2.1 to 4.1)	6.3 (4.9 to 7.7)	0.001
Scratchy throat	2.8 (1.9 to 3.7)	2.8 (1.4 to 4.2)	>0.2
Hoarseness	2.0 (1.0 to 3.0)	1.2 (0.3 to 2.7)	>0.2
Muscle ache	1.4 (0.6 to 2.2)	1.5 (0.3 to 2.7)	>0.2
Fever	0.4 (0.0 to 0.8)	0.2 (–0.1 to 0.5)	>0.2
Headache	2.0 (1.1 to 2.8)	2.4 (1.4 to 3.4)	>0.2

Source: Prasad AS et al. 2000. *Annals Int Med* 133:245–52.

[a] Expressed as the mean ± SD. The difference in overall duration of symptoms between groups was 3.6 days (95% CI, 2.6 to 4.6 days). Because the data on overall duration of symptoms were normally distributed according to the Shapiro–Wilk W test ($P = 0.13$ for both the zinc group and the placebo group; $P = 0.07$ when the groups were combined), a *t*-test was used to analyze the differences between groups.

[b] For each symptom, the Wilcoxon rank-sum test was used to determine differences between groups.

16.3.2.1 Adequacy of Blinding

Out of the 20 participants who received zinc, 5% correctly guessed that they were receiving active therapy. Of 20 participants who received placebo, 10% correctly guessed that they were receiving placebo. Therefore, participants did not correctly guess which type of lozenge they were receiving much better than by chance. In addition, at the beginning of the trial, 48% of zinc recipients and 26% of placebo recipients correctly identified the lozenges ($P > 0.2$). At the end of the study, 56% of zinc recipients and 26% of placebo recipients correctly identified the lozenges ($P = 0.09$). None of these percentages exceeded 50%, indicating that blinding was adequate at the outset and was maintained throughout the study.

16.3.3 Proinflammatory Cytokines

Levels of proinflammatory cytokines in healthy controls and study participants with colds before group assignment are shown in Table 16.3. Only levels of soluble interleukin-1 receptor antagonist and neopterin were increased in participants with the common cold compared with healthy controls. Plasma zinc levels were normal in both groups.

TABLE 16.3
Plasma Levels of Zinc and Proinflammatory Cytokines in Controls and Participants with the Common Cold in Trial 1

	Before Treatment Assignment[a]		After Treatment Assignment[a,b]				Mean Change		
			Zinc Group		Placebo Group				
Variable	Controls[c]	Patients with Cold on Study Group Day 1	Before Treatment	After Treatment	Before Treatment	After Treatment	Zinc Group	Placebo Group	Between-Group Difference in Mean (95% CI)
Plasma zinc level, mmolL/(n)	14.3 (17)	14.6 (47)	14.8 (25)	17.7 (25)	15.1 (22)	14.3 (22)	2.9	20.8	3.7 (2.2 to 5.0)
P value		0.2[d]					<0.001[d]		
Plasma cytokines									
Soluble interleukin-1 receptor antagonist level, pg/mL(n)	279.9 (17)	457.3 (39)	493.6 (22)	340.1 (22)	412.8 (17)	348.8 (17)	−153.5	−64.0	−89.4 (−243.6 to 64.8)
P value		0.022[d]					>0.2[d]		
Soluble TNF receptor level, pg/mL (n)	914.8 (17)	925.0 (37)	900.3 (20)	767.9 (20)	957.6 (17)	853.9 (17)	−132.4	−103.7	−28.7 (−222.7 to 165.3)
P value		>0.2[d]					>0.2[d]		
Neopterin level, pmol/mL (n)	3.6 (17)	6.5 (38)	6.1 (22)	4.9 (22)	7.0 (16)	5.9 (16)	−21.1	−1.1	0 (23.2 to 3.2)
P value		<0.001[d]					0.2[e]		

Source: Prasad AS et al. 2000. *Annals Int Med* 133:245–52.

[a] Although duration of cold and specific symptoms was studied in 25 participants in the zinc group and 23 participants in the placebo group, blood samples were not available from all participants for laboratory analysis. The numbers in parentheses are the number of participants for whom data on zinc and cytokine levels were available.

[b] Only patients with cold on study day 1 were assigned to receive treatment or placebo.

[c] Healthy volunteers who were free of illness or cold.

[d] Use of the Shapiro–Wilk W test revealed that the distribution of mean differences in the zinc and placebo groups in levels of zinc, soluble interleukin-1 receptor antagonist, and soluble TNF receptor were normal. Therefore, these variables were analyzed by using an unpaired *t*-test.

[e] Use of the Shapiro–Wilk W test revealed that the distribution of mean differences in the zinc and placebo groups in levels of neopterin was not normal. Therefore, these variables were analyzed by using the non-parametric Wilcoxon rank-sum test.

The zinc and placebo groups differed significantly only in mean changes in plasma zinc level. The mean change in soluble interleukin-1 receptor antagonist level was greater in the zinc group than in the placebo group (–153.5 versus –64.0 pg/ml), but this difference was not statistically significant ($P > 0.2$). The lack of significant difference in mean changes in cytokine levels between the two groups may have been due to the fact that the blood samples were drawn approximately 3 days later in the placebo group than in the zinc group, after cold symptoms had resolved (the average duration of symptoms was 4.48 days in the zinc group and 8.1 days in the placebo group). The differences in mean changes in cytokine level between the two groups may have been more pronounced if blood for analysis had been drawn in the placebo group on day 5.

Adherence to therapy was determined by lozenge count. The average number of lozenges taken daily was 6.2 in the zinc group and 5.8 in the placebo group ($P = 0.2$).

16.4 THE SECOND TRIAL

16.4.1 Participants

We recruited 50 volunteers from the Detroit Medical Center (Detroit, Michigan) to participate in a randomized, placebo-controlled trial of the efficacy of zinc acetate lozenges in treating the common cold [8]. The group of participants came from similar background as in Trial 1. Participants were informed of the placebo-controlled, double-blind nature of the study, and the study protocol was approved by the Human Investigation Committee of Wayne State University. We recruited healthy volunteers who were free of any illness for various laboratory tests as control subjects. The criteria for recruitment of subjects for this trial were similar to the first trial.

16.4.2 Intervention

The lozenges were cherry oil-flavored Fast Dry zinc acetate lozenges, manufactured by F & F Foods (Chicago, IL). The active lozenges contained 13.3 mg of zinc as zinc acetate in a hard candy that contained 3.8 g of sucrose and corn syrup and that was prepared using the open-pot batch method, with the active ingredient added last. One hundred percent of the zinc was available at physiologic pH 7.4 in positively charged, ionic form. The placebo lozenges were of identical composition, except that they contained 0.25 mg of sucrose octaacetate rather than the active ingredient, zinc. There were no fats, metal chelators, or other zinc ion-binding agents in either the active or placebo lozenges. The placebo and zinc lozenges were identical in weight, appearance, flavor, and texture and were supplied by George Eby. Randomization method and blinding technique were same as in Trial 1.

16.4.3 Outcome Measures

Our primary end point was the average duration of cold symptoms. Secondary end points were plasma levels of (1) zinc; (2) soluble interleukin (IL)–1 receptor antagonist (sIL-1ra) and soluble TNF receptor (sTNF-R) 1; and (3) the plasma adhesion molecules, soluble vascular endothelial cell adhesion molecule (sVCAM)–1 and soluble intercellular adhesion molecule (sICAM)–1.

Participants were asked to complete a daily log documenting the severity of symptoms and the medications taken throughout the duration of the cold as in the first trial.

Plasma samples were collected and assayed for levels of zinc, sIL-1ra, sTNF-R1, sVCAM-1, and sICAM-1. Zinc was assayed by flameless atomic absorption spectrophotometry [7]. Every precaution was taken to avoid contamination during collection, preparation, and analysis. Variables were analyzed using Quantikine ELISA kits for sIL-1ra, sTNF-R1, sVCAM-1, and sICAM-1 (R&D Systems).

To assess adverse effects of the treatment, participants were given a questionnaire to fill out at the end of the trial as in the first trial. Participants returned to the clinic on the fifth day for a blood sampling and again for the final visit within 1 day of resolution of cold symptoms. At this time they returned unused lozenges; lozenges were collected to check adherence and to confirm that cold symptoms had resolved.

16.4.4 Maintenance of Blinding

Comparability in taste between zinc and placebo was tested in the participants at the beginning and at the end of the trial just as in the first trial.

16.4.5 Statistical Analysis

We compared the change in outcomes before and after intervention for the zinc and placebo groups. If the changes were normally distributed in both groups, as determined by the Shapiro-Wilk test, we used the unpaired *t* test to compare mean changes. If the changes were not normally distributed, the differences were examined using the non-parametric Wilcoxon rank-sum test. Multivariate analysis of variance with repeated measures was used to determine the effect of treatment x time on severity scores. Fisher's exact test was used to determine group differences in adverse effects. χ^2 analyses were performed to determine group differences in correctly identifying lozenges at baseline and after treatment. Statistical analyses were completed using JMP IN software (version 5.1.2; SAS Institute) on a MacBook Pro Computer.

16.5 RESULTS

16.5.1 Demographics

Table 16.4 shows the demographic characteristics of the study subjects in the second Trial.

16.5.1.1 Duration and Severity of Cold Symptoms

Table 16.5 shows the duration and severity of cold symptoms in the zinc and placebo groups. The average duration of cold symptoms was 4.0 days in the zinc group and 7.1

TABLE 16.4
Demographic Characteristics of the Second Trial

Variable	Zinc Group ($n = 25$)	Placebo Group ($n = 25$)
Age, mean ± SD (95% CI), years	34.52 ± 14.06 (28.71–40.32)	35.88 ± 13.40 (30.34–41.40)
Sex		
Male	7	9
Female	18	16
Ethnicity		
Black	8	7
White	14	17
Middle Eastern Arab	1	0
Chinese	1	0
Other	1	1
Cigarette Smoker		
No	19	16
Yes	6	9
History of Allergies		
No	19	21
Yes	6	4

Source: Prasad AS et al. 2008. *J of Inf Dis* 197:795–802.
Note: Data are no. of participants, unless otherwise indicated. CI, confidence interval.

days in the placebo group ($P < 0.0001$). The durations of cough, nasal discharge, and muscle ache were significantly shorter in the zinc group than in the placebo group (Table 16.5). In 56% of the zinc-group subjects the cold was completely resolved on day 4, and no subject in the placebo group was free of cold symptoms on day 4.

Repeated-measures analysis of severity scores indicated a significant effect for treatment x time for the zinc group compared with the placebo group over 10 days ($P = .0002$). At baseline, the average severity scores for the zinc and placebo groups were 8.32 and 7.78, respectively; by day 4, these scores were 3.45 and 5.61, respectively.

16.5.1.2 Adequacy of Blinding

In the zinc group at the beginning of the study, only 1 subject identified the lozenges as certainly zinc, and 2 subjects identified them as probably zinc. Thus, 3 (12%) of 25 subjects in this group were correct. At the end of the study, 2 (8%) were correct; 1 subject identified the lozenges as certainly zinc, and another subject identified them as probably zinc.

In the placebo group at the beginning of the study, one subject said that the lozenges were certainly placebo, and another subject identified them as probably placebo. Thus, 2 subjects (8%) in this group were correct. At the end of the study, none of the subjects identified the placebo lozenge correctly.

TABLE 16.5
Duration of Common Cold Symptoms in the Second Trial

	Duration of Cold Symptoms, Mean ± SD (95% CI), Days					
	All Subjects			Blinded Subjects[b]		
Variable	Zinc Group (n = 25)	Placebo Group (n = 25)	P^a	Zinc Group (n = 22)	Placebo Group (n = 23)	P^a
Overall symptoms	4.00 ± 1.04 (3.57–4.42)	7.12 ± 1.26 (6.59–7.64)	<0.0001	3.54 ± 0.96 (3.11–3.97)	7.39 ± 0.98 (6.96–7.81)	<0.0001
Specific symptoms						
Sore throat	1.96 ± 1.83 (1.20–2.71)	3.24 ± 2.93 (2.02–4.45)	0.07	2.00 ± 1.90 (1.15–2.84)	3.35 ± 2.98 (2.05–4.63)	0.07
Nasal discharge	3.00 ± 1.63 (2.32–3.67)	4.56 ± 3.01 (3.31–5.80)	0.02	3.00 ± 1.72 (2.23–3.76)	4.70 ± 3.05 (3.37–6.01)	0.02
Nasal congestion	2.20 ± 2.02 (1.36–3.03)	2.56 ± 2.88 (1.36–3.75)	0.61	2.18 ± 2.06 (1.26–3.09)	2.43 ± 2.97 (1.15–3.71)	0.70
Sneezing	2.64 ± 1.62 (1.96–3.31)	2.60 ± 2.27 (1.66–3.53)	0.94	2.59 ± 1.71 (1.83–3.34)	2.74 ± 2.30 (1.72–3.73)	0.80
Cough	2.16 ± 1.70 (1.45–2.86)	5.08 ± 2.97 (3.85–6.30)	<0.0001	2.14 ± 1.70 (1.38–2.89)	5.35 ± 2.46 (4.07–6.62)	<0.0001
Scratchy throat	1.68 ± 1.54 (1.04–2.31)	1.92 ± 2.30 (0.96–2.87)	0.66	1.73 ± 1.58 (1.02–2.42)	1.91 ± 2.41 (0.87–2.95)	0.76
Hoarseness	1.00 ± 1.44 (0.40–1.59)	2.20 ± 2.90 (1.00–3.39)	0.07	1.00 ± 1.45 (0.35–1.64)	2.17 ± 3.02 (0.86–3.48)	0.10
Muscle ache	0.80 ± 1.22 (0.29–1.30)	2.00 ± 2.25 (1.06–2.93)	0.02	0.82 ± 1.30 (0.24–1.38)	1.70 ± 2.08 (0.70–2.59)	0.09
Fever	0.52 ± 1.35 (0.04–1.05)	1.12 ± 2.00 (0.29–1.94)	0.22	0.55 ± 1.44 (0.09–1.18)	1.13 ± 2.07 (0.23–2.02)	0.27
Headache	1.20 ± 1.32 (0.65–1.74)	1.48 ± 1.71 (0.77–2.18)	0.52	1.23 ± 1.38 (0.61–1.83)	1.30 ± 1.66 (0.58–2.02)	0.86

Source: Prasad AS et al. 2008. *J of Inf Dis* 197:795–802.

Note: CI, confidence interval.

[a] Because the data on duration of symptoms were normally distributed according to the Shapiro-Wilk test, a t test was used to analyze the differences between the groups.

[b] Blinded subjects: we excluded 3 in the zinc group and 2 in the placebo group who correctly identified their lozenges as zinc or placebo at the beginning of the study.

Contingency analysis of correctness by group at the beginning of the study yielded $P = 1.0$, by the χ^2 test (Fisher's exact test). At the end of the study, the same test yielded $P = 0.489$. Thus, there was no significant difference between the two groups.

From these data, we concluded that the blinding of the subjects was adequate. In addition, we analyzed the effect of clinical variables for the 22 completely blinded subjects in the zinc group and the 23 in the placebo group; these data are shown in Table 16.5. For completely blinded subjects, cold symptoms lasted for a mean ± SD of 3.54 ± 0.96 days in the zinc group and 7.39 ± 0.98 days in the placebo group ($P < 0.0001$). The durations of cough and nasal discharge were also significantly shorter in the zinc group (Table 16.5).

16.5.1.3 Adverse Effects

Adverse effects of the zinc and placebo lozenges are compared in Table 16.6. The zinc and placebo groups did not differ significantly in the incidences of any of the adverse effects, including diarrhea, constipation, sweet taste, sour taste, bitter taste, aftertaste, dry mouth, mouth irritation, or bad taste. None of the subjects complained either of abdominal pain or vomiting.

Adherence to therapy was determined by lozenge count. The average number of lozenges taken daily was 6.9 in the zinc group and 6.5 in the placebo group.

Table 16.7 shows the results of treatment on plasma levels of zinc, sIL-1ra, sTNF-R1, sVCAM-1, and sICAM-1. The plasma zinc level increased significantly in the zinc group. The plasma sIL-1ra level decreased significantly in the zinc group after treatment but increased in the placebo group. A comparison of the mean changes (before versus after therapy) in plasma sTNF-R1 and sVCAM-1 levels in the two

TABLE 16.6
Adverse Effects of Zinc and Placebo Lozenges in the Second Trial

	No. (%) of Participants		
Adverse Effect	**Zinc Group ($n = 25$)**	**Placebo Group ($n = 25$)**	**P[a]**
Nausea	3 (12)	1 (4)	0.61
Constipation	2 (8)	1 (4)	0.22
Diarrhea	1 (4)	1 (4)	1.00
Sweet taste	11 (44)	14 (56)	0.57
Sour taste	7 (28)	2 (8)	0.13
Bitter taste	8 (32)	12 (48)	0.38
Aftertaste	20 (80)	18 (72)	0.47
Bad taste	15 (60)	13 (52)	0.67
Dry mouth	13 (52)	17 (68)	0.37
Mouth irritation	1 (4)	2 (8)	1.00

Source: Prasad AS et al. 2008. *J of Inf Dis* 197:795–802.
[a] Fisher's exact test was used to determine group differences.

TABLE 16.7

Plasma Levels of Zinc, Anti-Inflammatory Cytokines, and Adhesion Molecules in the Second Trial

	Control		Before Treatment		After Treatment		Mean Change		
Variable	**Subjects[a]**	**Zinc Group**	**Placebo Group**	**Zinc Group**	**Placebo Group**	**Zinc Group**	**Placebo Group**	**P^b Changes (95% CI)**	**Between-Group Differences in Mean**
Zinc, μg/dL	110 ± 10 (31)	96.0 ± 13.6 (25)	101.2 ± 20.5 (25)	111.2 ± 15.5 (25)	99.5 ± 21.1 (25)	15.2 ± 14.8 (25)	−1.7 ± 12.5 (25)	<0.0001	16.9 (9.0 to 24.7)
sIL-1ra, pg/mL	293 ± 262 (16)	300 ± 299 (23)	327 ± 186 (24)	264 ± 220 (23)	452 ± 397 (24)	−36.3 ± 182.4 (23)	124.7 ± 304 (24)	0.033	−161.1 (−309.1 to −12.2)
sTNF-R1, pg/mL	835 ± 192 (16)	810 ± 300 (24)	883 ± 253 (25)	760 ± 181 (24)	857 ± 297 (25)	−49.3 ± 246 (24)	−25.2 ± 314 (25)	0.76	−24.09 (−186.7 to 138.5)
sVCAM-1, pg/mL	492 ± 224 (25)	441 ± 266 (25)	497 ± 257 (24)	492 ± 224 (25)	490 ± 249 (24)	50.9 ± 252 (25)	−6.3 ± 259 (24)	0.43	57.3 (−89.6 to 204.2)
sICAM-1, pg/mL	248 ± 82.7 (18)	285 ± 162 (25)	227 ± 149 (24)	229 ± 144 (25)	229 ± 114 (24)	−56.1 ± 95.4 (25)	2.2 ± 103.7 (24)	0.04	−58.4 (−115.7 to −1.1)

Source: Prasad AS et al. 2008. *J of Inf Dis* 197:795–802.

Note: Data are mean ± SD values (no. of subjects), except as indicated. CI, confidence interval; sICAM, soluble intercellular adhesion molecule; sIL-1ra, soluble interleukin-1 receptor antagonist; sTNF-R, soluble tumor necrosis factor receptor; sVCAM, soluble vascular endothelial cell adhesion molecule.

[a] The control group included healthy volunteers who were free of any illness or colds.

[b] *P* values are for the difference between pre- and post-treatment values for the indicated group. The Shapiro-Wilk test revealed that the distributions of mean differences in the zinc and placebo groups were normal for all tests. Therefore, the variables were analyzed using an unpaired *t* test.

groups showed no significant differences between groups. Plasma sICAM-1 levels decreased significantly after treatment in the zinc group.

16.6 DISCUSSION

We found that treatment with zinc acetate lozenges was associated with a decrease in the average duration and severity of the common cold in the first trial [6,8]. Five previous trials failed to show a beneficial effect of zinc [9–13], perhaps because inadequate doses or inappropriate formulations of zinc were used, resulting in the lack of bioavailable zinc [5,13]. Hatch and Berthon [14] reported that zinc acetate releases essentially 100% of its zinc as Zn^{++} ions at a physiologic pH, suggesting that zinc acetate lozenges may be the best choice for treatment of common cold.

Except for mouth dryness and constipation, no statistically significant side effects occurred in zinc recipients compared with placebo recipients in the first trial. In the second trial, we observed no side effects. This may be due to the difference in zinc preparations between the two trials. The bad taste, mouth irritation, dry mouth, nausea, and gastric irritation in the zinc group as reported by Mossad et al. [15] and Eby et al. [4] may have been related to the use of different ligands (gluconate-glycine) rather than to zinc itself.

Our test in healthy controls showed that the zinc and placebo lozenges were indistinguishable in taste. Because the participants received only one type of lozenge, it is unlikely that differences in dryness of mouth would give them a basis for deciding whether the lozenge assigned to them contained zinc.

Many of the symptoms observed in the common cold resemble the effects of proinflammatory cytokines [16–18]. Fever, lack of appetite, leukocytosis, hypoferremia, and induction of acute-phase reactant proteins are known effects of interleukin-1β production, released by monocytes and macrophages due to infection. Proinflammatory cytokines have been found in nasal secretions of patients with colds [19,20], and production of cytokines has been detected in human rhinovirus–infected epithelial cells in vitro [19–21]. It has been, therefore, suggested that the symptoms of the common cold are thought to result from an inflammatory “cytokine disease” [19]. We previously showed that interleukin-1β production by mononuclear cells is increased in zinc-deficient subjects and is normalized by zinc supplementation, suggesting that zinc modulates the proinflammatory cytokines released by macrophages and monocytes [22]. In our two studies, we found that symptomatic improvement in the zinc group was associated with increased plasma levels of zinc, suggesting that zinc may have modulated proinflammatory cytokines [6].

Tremacamra, a drug which blocks the receptor, where the Rhino viruses attach at soluble intercellular adhesion molecule 1 (ICAM-1) was recently used to treat experimentally induced rhinovirus infection [23]. Tremacamra was shown to be effective in decreasing the severity of common cold symptoms; however, it was not clear whether the duration of the cold was also decreased [23]. In contrast, we found that the use of zinc was associated with a decrease in both the duration and severity of the common cold. Zinc, therefore may be a less expensive treatment option than tremacamra. In addition, zinc is non-toxic at physiological levels and is non-mutagenic, whereas the toxicity and mutagenicity of tremacamra remains to be ascertained.

In the first trial, zinc-treated participants received approximately 80 mg of elemental zinc per day for 4–5 days, more than five times the recommended daily dietary allowance of 15 mg zinc [6]. Because this high dose was given for a short time, we believe that the effect of zinc was therapeutic and was not related to correction of zinc deficiency. As long as high-dose zinc was administered for a short time (for example, 5 days), it would be unlikely to cause copper deficiency. However, with indiscriminate use of high-dose zinc lozenges for 6–8 weeks, copper deficiency is likely to occur [24]. Thus, zinc therapy for the common cold should be limited to less than a week.

In the second trial also, our results showed that the mean duration and severity of cold symptoms, cough, nasal discharge, and muscle aches were significantly decreased in the zinc group compared with the placebo group [8]. The blinding of therapy was adequate and our analysis of clinical variables in completely blinded subjects showed that the mean durations of cold symptoms, cough, and nasal discharge were significantly decreased in the zinc group compared to the placebo group.

Figure 16.1 summarizes our hypothesis as to how zinc may be acting as an antioxidant and anti-inflammatory agent and how it may decrease ICAM-1 levels. Infection and oxidative stress activate NF-κB, which increases generation and gene

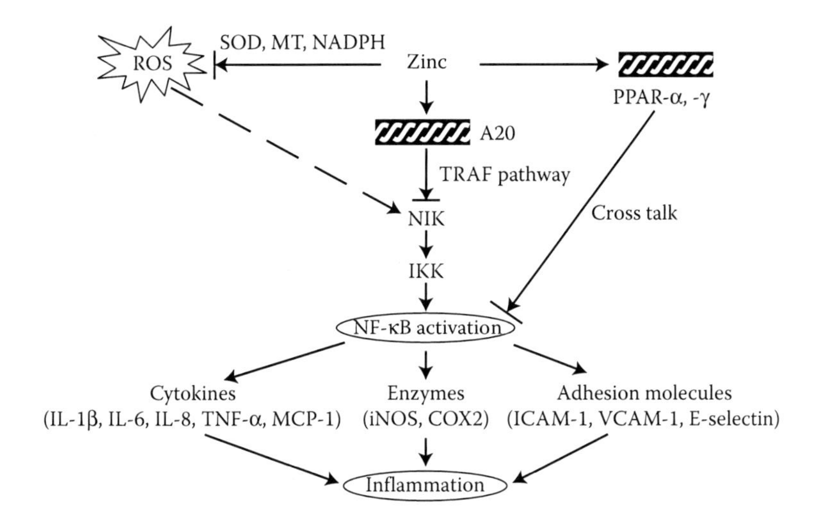

FIGURE 16.1 Action of zinc as an antioxidant by various mechanisms. Zinc is essential for superoxide dismutase (SOD) and is an inhibitor of NADPH oxidase. Zinc also induces metallothionein (MT), which is an excellent scavenger for OH ions. Via A20 induction, zinc inhibits NF-κB activation, and this decreases the gene expression and protein generation of various inflammatory cytokines. Decreased activation of NF-κB by zinc also results in decreased gene expression and generation of intercellular adhesion molecule 1 (ICAM-1) (short solid lines indicate blocked activity, and dashed arrow indicates activation). COX, cyclooxygenase; IKK, IκB kinase; IL, interleukin; iNOS, inducible nitric oxide synthase; MCP, macrophage chemoattractant protein; NIK, NF-κB–inducible kinase; PPAR, peroxisome proliferator–activated receptor; ROS, reactive oxygen species; TNF, tumor necrosis factor; TRAF, TNF receptor–associated factor; VCAM, vascular endothelial cell adhesion molecule. (Adapted from Prasad AS et al. 2008. *J of Inf Dis* 197:795–802.)

expression of inflammatory cytokines (such as TNF-α, IL-1β, and IL-8) and adhesive molecules (such as VCAM-1 and ICAM-1) [25,26]. Zinc decreases oxidative stress and also induces the zinc-dependent transcription factor A20 in monocytes and macrophages, which inhibits NF-κB activation via the TNF-R–associated factor pathway [25]. Zinc decreases oxidative stress by several mechanisms [24,27]. Zinc is an inhibitor of NADPH oxidase, an enzyme that initiates the generation of free radicals; it is essential for SOD and it induces the generation of MT, a low molecular weight protein that removes ˙OH ion effectively (Figure 16.1).

Inflammatory cytokines, generated by activated monocytes and macrophages, are also known to generate greater amounts of reactive oxygen species (ROS) [26]. Zinc supplementation in healthy human subjects aged 20–50 years reduced the concentration of the plasma oxidative stress markers, inhibited the ex vivo induction of TNF-α and IL-1β mRNA in mononuclear cells, and provided protection against TNF-α– induced NF-κB activation in isolated peripheral blood mononuclear cells [25]. We previously provided evidence that, in the human promyelocytic leukemia cell line HL-60, which differentiates to the monocyte and macrophage phenotype in response to phorbol-12-myristate-13-acetate (PMA), zinc increases the expression of A20 and the binding of A20 transactivating factor to DNA, which inhibits NF-κB activation [25,28]. NF-κB is involved in the gene expression of TNF-α and IL-1β in monocytes and macrophages in human and HL-60 cells, and the effect of zinc in inhibiting the gene expression of TNF-α and IL-1β is cell specific [25,28]. In a recent study, we showed that, in elderly persons [55–87 years old], ex vivo generation of TNF-α and plasma oxidative stress markers was significantly lower in the zinc-supplemented group than in the placebo group [27]. Given that increased activation of NF-κB in monocytes and macrophages due to viral infection increases the generation and gene expression of adhesive molecules, such as ICAM-1, our observation that only the zinc group showed a significant decrease in plasma ICAM-1 levels suggests that zinc decreased the generation and gene expression of ICAM-1. Human rhinovirus type 14 "docks" with ICAM-1 on the surface of somatic cells [3,29]. Thus, zinc may in effect act as an antiviral agent by reducing ICAM-1 levels. Another possibility is that zinc ions may form a complex with ICAM-1, preventing the binding of rhinovirus to cells [29].

The ICAM-1 levels at baseline were higher in the zinc group than in the placebo group. Interestingly, the zinc group had more severe cold symptoms than the placebo group at the outset, suggesting that greater severity may have been responsible for higher plasma levels of ICAM-1. More studies are needed to prove this hypothesis.

We propose that the beneficial clinical effects seen in the zinc group were due to the antioxidant and anti-inflammatory effects of zinc. We also suggest that a decrease in plasma ICAM-1 levels due to zinc therapy may have decreased the docking of the cold viruses on the surface of somatic cells.

Cochrane collaboration published their meta-analysis of the effect of zinc on common cold in 2011 [30]. They included 13 therapeutic trials (966 participants) and two preventive trials (394 participants) in their analysis. Therapeutic zinc lozenges was associated with a significant reduction in the duration (standardized mean difference (SMD): 0.97; 95% confidence interval (CIO: −1.56 – 0.38); $P = 0.001$), and severity of common cold (SMD −0.39; 95% CI: −0.77 – 0.02; $P = 0.04$). There was a significant difference between the zinc and control group for the proportion of participants symptomatic after 7 days of treatment (OR: 0.45; 95% CI: 0.2–1.00; $P = 0.05$). The incidence rate ratio (IRR) of developing a cold (IRR: 0.64; 95% CI: 0.47–0.88; $P = 0.006$), school absence ($P = 0.0003$) and prescription of antibiotics ($P = 0.00001$) was lower in the zinc group. Overall adverse events (OR: 1.59; 95% CI: 0.97–2.58; $P = 0.06$), bad taste (OR: 2.64; 95% CI: 1.91–3.64; $P < 0.00001$) and nausea (OR: 2.15; 95% CI: 1.44–3.23; $P = 0.002$) were higher in the zinc group. The Cochrane group concluded that zinc lozenges administered within 24 h of onset of symptoms reduced the duration and severity of the common cold in healthy people [30].

Zinc supplementation for at least 5 months reduced incidence, school absenteeism, and prescription of antibiotics for children with the common cold. People taking zinc lozenges are more likely to experience adverse events such as bad taste and nausea [30].

Another meta-analysis of zinc treatment for common cold was published by Hemilä from Finland in 2011 [31]. Thirteen placebo-controlled trials were examined for the therapeutic effect of zinc lozenges on the duration of common cold. The total number of common cold episodes in these trials was 1407. In five trails when the total zinc used was less than 75 mg/day, there was no effect of zinc on the duration and severity of common cold. In seven of the eight trials which used over 75 mg zinc/day found a statistically significant benefit was observed. In one trial, the benefit was restricted to the symptom severity at the late phase of the colds [31]. The benefits of zinc were restricted to trials when the doses of zinc were greater than 75 mg/day.

The solution chemistry of zinc complexes gives further understanding of the differences between the zinc trials. A direct correlation between daily dosages of all positively charged zinc species at physiologic pH released from lozenges and reductions in duration of common cold has been hypothesized [5]. The analysis of 10 double-blind, placebo controlled zinc trials by solution chemistry methods showed a significant correlation between total daily dosages of positively charged zinc species and a reduction in the mean duration of common colds [5]. Zinc gluconate and zinc acetate have very low chemical stability and mainly release positively charged zinc ions in aqueous solutions at physiologic pH, but stronger complexes do not [4]. Adding a strong zinc binding ligand, such as glycine, citric acid, tartaric acid, mannitol, and sorbitol to a solution containing a zinc complex that is weakly bonded results in the sequestration of zinc to the stronger ligand, reducing or eliminating the benefits of zinc lozenges [5].

A recent publication by Das and Singh [32] confirms that the duration of common cold is significantly decreased by the use of zinc lozenges.

16.7 CONCLUSION

Administration of zinc lozenges was associated with significant reduced duration and severity of common cold symptoms. The therapy with zinc lozenges must be started within 24 h of the onset of symptoms. The daily dosages of elemental zinc should be 75 mg or higher. The solution chemistry of zinc lozenges must be optimal. Zinc acetate and zinc gluconate lozenges are effective, however, if other binders such as glycine, citrate, tartarate, mannitol, or sorbitol are added, the release of zinc ions is not optimal and the therapeutic effect of zinc may be compromised.

The improvement of cold symptoms following zinc therapy is most likely related to the antioxidant and anti-inflammatory properties of zinc. A significant decrease in plasma ICAM-1 levels in zinc group was observed. Human rhinovirus type 14" docks with ICAM-1 on the surface of the somatic cells. Thus zinc may in effect act as an antiviral agent by reducing ICAM-1 levels. Another possibility is that zinc ions may form a complex with ICAM-1, preventing the binding of rhinovirus to cells.

ABBREVIATIONS

COX2	cyclo-oxygenase 2
ICAM-1	soluble intercellar adhesion molecule-1
IκB	Inhibitory protein of NF-κB
IKK	Iκ kinase
IL-1β	Interleukin-1β
IL-8	Interleukin 8
iNOS	inducible nitric oxide synthase
MAPK	mitogen activated protein kinase
MDA	malondehyde
MT	metallothionein
NF-κB	nuclear factor kappa B
NIK	NF-κB inducible kinase
ROS	reactive oxygen species
sICAM-1	soluble intercellular adhesion molecule-1
sIL-1rα	soluble interleukin-1 receptor antagonist
SOD	superoxide dismutase

ACKNOWLEDGMENTS

Funding for our research in part by NIH grant no. 5 R01 A150698-04 and The George and Patsy Eby Foundation, Austin, Texas.

REFERENCES

1. Dingle JH, Badger GF, Jordan WS Jr. 1964. Illness in the home: Study of 25,000 illnesses in a group of Cleveland families. Cleveland, Ohio: Western Reserve University Press.
2. Gwaltney JM Jr, Hendley JO, Simon G, Jordan WS Jr. 1966. Rhinovirus infections in an industrial population. I. The occurrence of illness. *N Engl J Med* 275:1261–8.
3. Turner RB. 2001. The treatment of rhinovirus infections: Progress and potential. *Antiviral Res* 49:1–4.
4. Eby GA, Davis DR, Halcomb WW. 1984. Reduction in duration of common cold by zinc gluconate lozenges in a double-blind study. *Antimicrob Agents Chemother* 25:20–4.
5. Eby GA. 1995. Linearity in dose-response from zinc lozenges in treatment of common colds. *J Pharm Technol* 11:110–22.
6. Prasad AS, Fitzgerald JT, Bao B, Beck FWJ, Chandrasekal PH. 2000. Duration of symptoms and plasma cytokine levels in patients with the common cold treated with zinc acetate. *Annals Int Med* 133:245–52.

7. Prasad AS. 1993. Techniques for measurement of zinc in biological samples. In: *Biochemistry of Zinc*. New York: Plenum, 279–89.
8. Prasad AS, Beck FWJ, Bao B, Snell D, Fitzgerald JT. 2008. Duration and severity of symptoms and levels of plasma interleukin-1 receptor antagonists, soluble tumor necrosis factor receptor, and adhesion molecules in patients with common cold treated with zinc acetate. *J of Inf Dis* 197:795–802.
9. Farr BM, Conner EM, Betts RF, Oleske J, Minnefor A, Gwaltney JM Jr. 1987. Two randomized controlled trials of zinc gluconate lozenge therapy of experimentally induced rhinovirus cold. *Antimicrob Agents Chemother* 31:1183–7.
10. Douglas RM, Miles HB, Moore BW, Ryan P, Pinnock CB. 1987. Failure of effervescent zinc acetate lozenges to alter the course of upper respiratory tract infection of Australian adults. *Antimicrob Agents Chemother* 31:1263–5.
11. Smith DS, Helzner EC, Nuttall CE Jr, Collins M, Rofman BA, Ginsberg D, Goswick CB, Magner A. 1989. Failure of zinc gluconate in treatment of acute upper respiratory tract infections. *Antimicrob Agents Chemother* 33:646–8.
12. Weismann K, Jakobsen JP, Weismann JE, Hammer UM, Nyholm SM, Hansen KE, Lomholt and engineer Schmidt K. 1990. Zinc gluconate lozenges for common cold. A double-blind clinical trial. *Dan Med Bull* 37:279–81.
13. Macknin ML, Piedmonte M, Calendine C, Janosky J, Wald E. 1998. Zinc gluconate lozenges for treating common cold in children. *JAMA* 279:1962–7.
14. Hatch B, Berthon G. 1987. Metal ion-FTS nonapeptide interactions. A quantitative study of zinc (II)-nonapeptide complexes (thymulin) under physiological conditions and assessment of their biological significance. *Inorganica Chimica Acta* 136:165–71.
15. Mossad SB, Macknin ML, Medendorp SV, Mason P. 1996. Zinc gluconate lozenges for treating the common cold. A randomized, double-blind, placebo-controlled study. *Ann Intern Med* 125:81–8.
16. Koch AE, Kunkel SL, Strieter RM. 1995. Cytokines in rheumatoid arthritis. *J Invest Med* 43:28–38.
17. Bui LM, Dressendorfer RH, Keen CL, Summary JJ, Dubick MA. 1994. Zinc status and interleukin-1 b-induced alterations in mineral metabolism in rats. *Proc Soc Exp Biol Med* 206:438–44.
18. Wahl SM, Wong H, McCartney-Francis N. 1989. Role of growth factors in inflammation and repair. *J Cell Biochem* 40:193–9.
19. Pitkaranta A, Hayden FG. 1998. What's new with common colds? Pathogenesis and diagnosis. *Infections in Medicine* 15:50–9.
20. Noah TL, Henderson FW, Wortman IA, Devlin RB, Handy J, Koren HS, Becker S. 1995. Nasal cytokine production in viral acute upper respiratory infections of childhood. *J Infect Dis* 171:584–92.
21. Stockl J, Vetr H, Majic O, Zlabinger G, Kuechler E, Knapp W. 1999. Human major group rhinoviruses downmodulate the accessory function of monocytes by inducing IL-10. *J Clin Invest* 104:957–65.
22. Beck FW, Prasad AS, Kaplan J, Fitzgerald JT, Brewer GJ. 1997. Changes in cytokines production and T cell subpopulations in experimentally induced zinc-deficient humans. *Am J Physiol* 272:E1002–7.
23. Turner RB, Wecker MT, Pohl G, Witek TJ, McNally E, St. George R, Winther B, Hayden FG. 1999. Efficacy of tremacamra, a soluble intercellular adhesion molecule 1, for experimental rhinovirus infection: A randomized clinical trial. *JAMA* 281:1797–804.
24. Prasad AS. 1993. Interactions of zinc with other micronutrients. In: *Biochemistry of Zinc*. New York: Plenum, 259–78.
25. Prasad AS, Bao B, Beck FWJ, Kucuk O, Sarkar FH. 2004. Antioxidant effect of zinc in humans. *Free Radic Biol Med* 37:1182–90.
26. Prasad AS. 2007. Zinc: Mechanisms of host defense. *J Nutr* 137:1345–9.

27. Prasad AS, Beck FWJ, Bao B, Fitzgerald JT, Snell DC, Steinberg JD, Cardozo LJ. 2007. Zinc supplementation decreases incidence of infections in the elderly: Effect of zinc on generation of cytokines and oxidative stress. *Am J Clin Nutr* 85:837–44.
28. Bao B, Prasad AS, Beck FWJ, Godmere M. 2003. Zinc modulates mRNA levels of cytokines. *Am J Physiol Endocrinol Metab* 285:E1095–102.
29. Novick SG, Godfrey JC, Godfrey NH, Wilder HR. 1996. How does zinc modify the common cold? *Med Hypotheses* 46:295–302.
30. Singh M, Das RR. 2011. Zinc for the common cold. The Cochrane Collaboration, Issue 2, published by John Wiley and Sons, Ltd.
31. Hemilä H. 2011. Zinc lozenges may shorten the duration of colds: A systematic review. *The Open Respiratory Med J* 5:51–58.
32. Das RR, Singh M. 2014. Oral zinc for the common cold. *JAMA* 311:1440–41.

Index

C

F

L

M

N

O

P

T

U

V

W

Y

Z

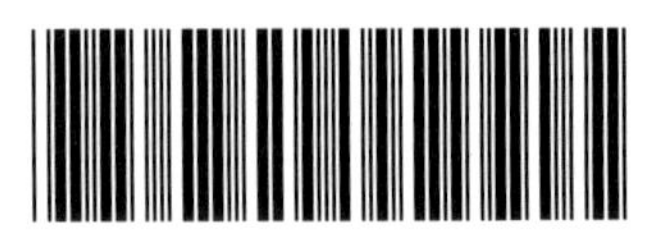